FIRST AID ...

Pediatrics Clerkship

Third Edition

Latha G. Stead, MD, MS, FACEP
Chief, Division of Clinical Research
Professor of Emergency Medicine
University of Florida College of Medicine
Gainesville, Florida
Adjunct Professor of Emergency Medicine
Mayo Clinic, College of Medicine
Rochester, Minnesota

Matthew S. Kaufman, MD
Assistant Professor
Albert Einstein College of Medicine
Department of Hematology
North Shore—Long Island Jewish Medical Center
New Hyde Park, New York

Muhammad Waseem, MD
Associate Professor
Emergency Medicine (Clinical Pediatrics)
Weill Medical College of Cornell University
New York, New York

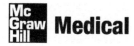 **Medical**

New York / Chicago / San Francisco / Lisbon / London / Madrid / Mexico City
Milan / New Delhi / San Juan / Seoul / Singapore / Sydney / Toronto

First Aid for the® Pediatrics Clerkship, Third Edition

Copyright © 2011 by The McGraw-Hill Companies, Inc. All rights reserved. Printed in the United States of America. Except as permitted under the United States Copyright Act of 1976, no part of this publication may be reproduced or distributed in any form or by any means, or stored in a data base or retrieval system, without the prior written permission of the publisher.

First Aid for the® is a registered trademark of The McGraw-Hill Companies, Inc.

8 9 10 11 12 13 QVS/QVS 20 19 18 17 16

ISBN 978-0-07-166403-5
MHID 0-07-166403-3

This book was set in Electra LH by Rainbow Graphics.
The editors were Catherine A. Johnson and Cindy Yoo.
The production supervisor was Catherine Saggese.
Project management was provided by Rainbow Graphics.
Quad/Graphics was printer and binder.

This book is printed on acid-free paper.

Library of Congress Cataloging-in-Publication Data

Stead, Latha G.
  First aid for the pediatrics clerkship / Latha G. Stead, Matthew S.
Kaufman. -- 3rd ed. / volume editor, Muhammad Waseem.
     p. ; cm.
  Includes index.
  ISBN-13: 978-0-07-166403-5 (pbk. : alk. paper)
  ISBN-10: 0-07-166403-3 (pbk. : alk. paper) 1. Pediatrics–Outlines,
syllabi, etc. 2. Clinical clerkship–Outlines, syllabi, etc. I.
Kaufman, Matthew S. II. Waseem, Muhammad. III. Stead, Latha G. First aid
for the pediatrics clerkship. IV. Title.
  [DNLM: 1. Pediatrics. 2. Clinical Clerkship. 3. First Aid. WS 205
S799f 2010]
  RJ48.3.S74 2010
  618.92'0025--dc22
                                                    2010020734

CONTENTS

CONTRIBUTORS

IRFAN ALI, MD

Fellow, Child Neurology
Department of Child Neurology
Nationwide Children's Hospital
Columbus, Ohio
Neurologic Disease

MUHAMMAD ASLAM, MD

Instructor, Pediatrics
Harvard Medical School
Neonatologist, Children's Hospital Boston
Boston, Massachusetts
Gestation and Birth
Prematurity

FARHEEN BAWAHAB, MD

Research Assistant
National Children's Study
Mount Sinai School of Medicine
New York, New York
Gastrointestinal Disease

NICHOLAS D. CAPUTO, MD, MSc

Resident, Emergency Medicine
Lincoln Medical & Mental Health Center
Bronx, New York
Pediatric Life Support

ALI FARZAD

Medical Student
Class of 2010
St. George's University School of Medicine
Granada, West Indies
Renal, Gynecologic, and Urinary Disease

FARHAT GHAZNAWI

Medical Student
Class of 2010
St. George's University School of Medicine
Granada, West Indies
Renal, Gynecologic, and Urinary Disease

MUSHTAQ A. GODIL, MD

Associate, Pediatric Endocrinology
Department of Pediatrics
Geisinger Medical Center
Danville, Pennsylvania
Endocrine Diseases

IRENE GRINBERG, MD

Resident, Emergency Medicine
Lincoln Medical & Mental Health Center
Bronx, New York
Hematologic Disease

MARC P. KANTER, MD

Chief Resident, Emergency Medicine
Lincoln Medical & Mental Health Center
Bronx, New York
Musculoskeletal Disease

SAQIBA KHAN, MD

Attending Physician, Pediatric Emergency Department
Lincoln Medical & Mental Health Center
Bronx, New York
Special Organs—Eye, Ear, and Nose

VIRAJ S. LAKDAWALA, MD

Chief Resident
Lincoln Medical & Mental Health Center
Bronx, New York
Congenital Malformations and Chromosomal Abnormalities

MAGDA D. MENDEZ, MD

Pediatric Residency Program Director
Lincoln Medical & Mental Health Center
Bronx, New York
Assistant Professor, Clinical Pediatrics
Site Director Pediatric Clerkship
Weill Medical College of Cornell University
New York, New York
Growth & Development
*Health Supervision and Prevention of Illness and Injury in Children
    and Adolescents*

UMARFAROOK J. MIRZA, DO

Resident
Department of Emergency Medicine
Lincoln Medical & Mental Health Center
Bronx, New York
Weill Medical College of Cornell University
New York, New York
Cardiovascular Disease

TAZUDDIN AZMI MOHAMMED, MD

Resident
Department of Pediatrics
Lincoln Medical & Mental Health Center
Bronx, New York
Respiratory Disease

ANDREW J.M. PALIGA, MD, MSc, MHM

Resident
Department of Emergency Medicine
Lincoln Medical & Mental Health Center
Bronx, New York
Weill Medical College of Cornell University
New York, New York
Nutrition

HEIDI M. PINKERT, MD

Attending Physician
Lincoln Medical & Mental Health Center
Bronx, New York
Assistant Professor, Emergency Medicine (Clinical Pediatrics)
Weill Medical College of Cornell University
New York, New York
Dermatologic Disease

ANDALEEB RAJA, MD

Resident, Emergency Medicine
Lincoln Medical & Mental Health Center
Bronx, New York
Psychiatric Disease

SYED K. SHAH, MD

Resident
Department of Pediatrics
Bronx Lebanon Hospital
Bronx, New York
Metabolic Disease

YEKATERINA SITNITSKAYA, MD

Department of Pediatrics
Lincoln Medical & Mental Health Center
Bronx, New York
Assistant Professor
Weill Medical College of Cornell University
New York, New York
Immunologic Disease
Infectious Disease

MUHAMMAD ALI SYED, MD

Resident
Department of Pediatrics
Lincoln Medical & Mental Health Center
Bronx, New York
Respiratory Disease

STUDENT REVIEWERS

LESLIE K. HALE

Medical Student
Class of 2010
University of Rochester School of Medicine and Dentistry
Rochester, New York

STEPHANIE D. HENDERSON

Medical Student
Class of 2011
University of Rochester School of Medicine and Dentistry
Rochester, New York

SAMUEL HORR

Medical Student
Class of 2010
University of Rochester School of Medicine and Dentistry
Rochester, New York

BRIAN JENSSEN

Medical Student
Class of 2010
University of Rochester School of Medicine and Dentistry
Rochester, New York

AJAY E. KURIYAN

Medical Student
Class of 2010
University of Rochester School of Medicine and Dentistry
Rochester, New York

STEPHEN OU

Medical Student
Class of 2010
University of Rochester School of Medicine and Dentistry
Rochester, New York

TARA WEISELBERG

Medical Student
Class of 2010
University of Rochester School of Medicine and Dentistry
Rochester, New York

How to Succeed in the Pediatrics Clerkship

INTRODUCTION

This clinical study aid was designed in the tradition of the First Aid series of books. You will find that rather than simply preparing you for success on the clerkship exam, this resource will also help guide you in the clinical diagnosis and treatment of many of the problems seen by pediatricians. The content of the book is based on the objectives for medical students laid out by the Council on Medical Student Education in Pediatrics (COMSEP). Each of the chapters contains the major topics central to the practice of pediatrics and has been specifically designed for the third-year medical student learning level.

The content of the text is organized in the format similar to other texts in the First Aid series. Topics are listed by bold headings, and the "meat" of the topic provides essential information. The outside margins contain mnemonics, diagrams, summary or warning statements, and tips. Tips are categorized into typical scenarios **Typical Scenario**, exam tips , and ward tips .

The pediatric clerkship is unique among all the medical school rotations. Even if you are sure you do not want to be a pediatrician, it can be a very fun and rewarding experience. There are three key components to the rotation: (1) what to do on the wards, (2) what to do on outpatient, and (3) how to study for the exam.

ON THE WARDS . . .

Be on time. Most ward teams begin rounding around 8 AM. If you are expected to "pre-round," you should give yourself at least 15 minutes per patient that you are following to see the patient, look up any tests, and learn about the events that occurred overnight. Like all working professionals, you will face occasional obstacles to punctuality, but make sure this is occasional. When you first start a rotation, try to show up at least an extra 15 minutes early until you get the routine figured out. There may be "table rounds" followed by walking rounds, but the emphasis is patient-centered.

Find a way to keep your patient information organized and handy. By this rotation, you may have figured out the best way for you to track your patients, a miniature physical, medications, labs, test results, and daily progress. If not, ask around—other medical students or your interns can show you what works for them and may even make a copy for you of the template they use. We suggest index cards, a notebook, or a page-long template for each patient kept on a clipboard.

Dress in a professional manner. Even if the resident wears scrubs and the attending wears stiletto heels, you must dress in a professional, conservative manner. It would be appropriate to ask your resident what would be suitable for you to wear (it may not need to be a full suit and tie or the female equivalent). Wear a short white coat over your clothes unless discouraged.

> **Men** should wear long pants, with cuffs covering the ankle, a long-sleeved, collared shirt, and a tie—no jeans, no sneakers, no short-sleeved shirts.
> **Women** should wear long pants or a knee-length skirt and blouse or dressy sweater—no jeans, sneakers, heels greater than 1½ inches, or open-toed shoes.

Both men and women may wear scrubs during overnight call. Do not make this your uniform.

Act in a pleasant manner. Inpatient rotations can be difficult, stressful, and tiring. Smooth out your experience by being nice to be around. Smile a lot and learn everyone's name. If you do not understand or disagree with a treatment plan or diagnosis, do not "challenge." Instead, say "I'm sorry, I don't quite understand, could you please explain . . ." Be empathetic toward patients.

Be aware of the hierarchy. The way in which this will affect you will vary from hospital to hospital and team to team, but it is always present to some degree. In general, address your questions regarding ward functioning to interns or residents. Address your medical questions to residents, your senior, or the attending. Make an effort to be somewhat informed on your subject prior to asking attendings medical questions.

Address patients and staff in a respectful way. Address your pediatric patients by first name. Address their parents as Sir, Ma'am, or Mr., Mrs., or Miss. Do not address parents as "honey," "sweetie," and the like. Although you may feel these names are friendly, parents will think you have forgotten their name, that you are being inappropriately familiar, or both. Address all physicians as "doctor" unless told otherwise. Nurses, technicians, and other staff are indispensable and can teach you a lot. Please treat them respectfully.

Take responsibility for your patients. Know everything there is to know about your patients—their history, test results, details about their medical problem, and prognosis. Keep your intern or resident informed of new developments that he or she might not be aware of, and ask for any updates of which you might not be aware. Assist the team in developing a plan, and speak to radiology, consultants, and family. Never give bad news to patients or family members without the assistance of your supervising resident or attending.

Respect patients' rights.
  - All patients have the right to have their personal medical information kept private. This means do not discuss the patient's information with family members without that patient's consent, and do not discuss any patient in hallways, elevators, or cafeterias.
  - All patients have the right to refuse treatment. This means they can refuse treatment by a specific individual (e.g., you, the medical student) or of a specific type (e.g., no nasogastric tube). Patients can even refuse lifesaving treatment. The only exceptions to this rule are patients who are deemed to not have the capacity to make decisions or understand situations, in which case a health care proxy should be sought, and patients who are suicidal or homicidal.
  - All patients should be informed of the right to seek advanced directives on admission (particularly DNR/DNI orders). Often, this is done in a booklet by the admissions staff. If your patient is chronically ill or has a life-threatening illness, address the subject of advanced directives. The most effective way to handle this is to address this issue with every patient. This will help to avoid awkward conversations, even with less ill patients, because you can honestly tell them that you ask these questions of all your patients. These issues are particularly imminent with critically ill patients; however, the unexpected can happen with any patient.

Volunteer. Be self-propelled, self-motivated. Volunteer to help with a procedure or a difficult task. Volunteer to give a 20-minute talk on a topic of your choice. Volunteer to take additional patients. Volunteer to stay late. Bring in relevant articles regarding patients and their issues—this shows your enthusiasm, your curiosity, your outside reading, and your interest in evidence-based medicine.

Be a team player. Help other medical students with their tasks; teach them information you have learned. Support your supervising intern or resident whenever possible. Never steal the spotlight, steal a procedure, or make a fellow medical student or resident look bad.

Be prepared. Always have medical tools (stethoscope, reflex hammer, penlight, measuring tape), medical tape, pocket references often electronic these days, patient information, a small toy for distraction/gaze tracking, and stickers for rewards readily available. That way you will have what you need when you need it, and possibly more importantly, you will have what someone else needs when they are looking for it! The key is to have the necessary items with you without looking like you can barely haul around your heavy white coat.

Be honest. If you don't understand, don't know, or didn't do it, make sure you always say that. Never say or document information that is false (a common example: "bowel sounds normal" when you did not listen).

Present patient information in an organized manner. The presentation of a new patient will be much more thorough than the update given at rounds every morning. Vital information that should be included in a presentation differs by age group. Always begin with a succinct chief complaint—always a symptom, not a diagnosis (e.g., "wheezing," not "asthma")—and its duration. The next line should include identifiers (age, sex) and important diagnoses carried (e.g., this is where you could state "known asthmatic" or other important information in a wheezer).

Here is a template for the "bullet" presentation for inpatients the days subsequent to admission:

> This is a [age] year old [gender] with a history of [major/pertinent history such as asthma, prematurity, etc. or otherwise healthy] who presented on [date] with [major symptoms, such as cough, fever, and chills], and was found to have [working diagnosis]. [Tests done] showed [results]. Yesterday/overnight the patient [state important changes, new plan, new tests, new medications]. This morning the patient feels [state the patient's words], and the physical exam is significant for [state major findings]. Plan is [state plan].

Some patients have extensive histories. The whole history should be present in the admission note, but in a ward presentation it is often too much to absorb. In these cases it will be very much appreciated by your team if you can generate a good summary that maintains an accurate picture of the patient. This usually takes some thought, but it is worth it.

How to Present a Chest Radiograph (CXR)

Always take time to look at each of your patients' radiographs; don't just rely on the report. It is good clinical practice and your attending will likely ask you if you did. Plus, it will help you look like a star on rounds if you have seen the film before.

(continued)

- First, confirm that the CXR belongs to your patient and is the most recent one.
- If possible, compare to a previous film.

Then, present in a systematic manner:

1. *Technique*
   Rotation, anteroposterior (AP) or posteroanterior (PA), penetration, inspiratory effort (number of ribs visible in lungfields).

2. *Bony structures*
   Look for rib, clavicle, scapula, and sternum fractures.

3. *Airway*
   Look at the glottal area (steeple sign, thumbprint, foreign body, etc.), as well as for tracheal deviation, pneumothorax, pneumomediastinum.

4. *Pleural space*
   Look for fluid collections, which can represent hemothorax, chylothorax, pleural effusion.

5. *Lung parenchyma*
   Look for infiltrates and consolidations. These can represent pneumonia, pulmonary contusions, hematoma, or aspiration. The location of an infiltrate can provide a clue to the location of a pneumonia:

   - Obscured right (R) costophrenic angle = right lower lobe
   - Obscured left (L) costophrenic angle = left lower lobe
   - Obscured R heart border = right middle lobe
   - Obscured L heart border = left upper lobe

6. *Mediastinum*
   - Look at size of mediastinum—a widened one (> 8 cm) suggests aortic rupture.
   - Look for enlarged cardiac silhouette (> ½ thoracic width at base of heart), which may represent congestive heart failure (CHF), cardiomyopathy, hemopericardium, or pneumopericardium.

7. *Diaphragm*
   - Look for free air under the diaphragm (suggests perforation).
   - Look for stomach, bowel, or NG tube above diaphragm (suggests diaphragmatic rupture).

8. *Tubes and lines*
   - Identify all tubes and lines.
   - An endotracheal tube should be 2 cm above the carina. A common mistake is right mainstem bronchus intubation.
   - A chest tube (including the most proximal hole) should be in the pleural space (not in the lung parenchyma).
   - An NGT should be in the stomach and uncoiled.
   - The tip of a central venous catheter (central line) should be in the superior vena cava (not in the right atrium).
   - The tip of a Swan–Ganz catheter should be in the pulmonary artery.
   - The tip of a transvenous pacemaker should be in the right atrium.

A sample CXR presentation may sound like:

This is the CXR of [child's name]. The film is an AP view with good inspiratory effort. There is an isolated fracture of the 8th rib on the right. There is no tracheal deviation or mediastinal shift. There is no pneumo- or hemothorax. The cardiac silhouette appears to be of normal size. The diaphragm and heart borders on both sides are clear, no infiltrates are noted. There is a central venous catheter present, the tip of which is in the superior vena cava. This shows improvement over the CXR from [number of days ago] as the right lower lobe infiltrate is no longer present.

How to Present an Electrocardiogram (ECG)

See chapter on cardiovascular disease for specific rhythms.

- First, confirm that the ECG belongs to your patient and is most recent one.
- If possible, compare to a previous tracing.

Then, present in a systematic manner:

1. Rate (see Figure 1-1)
   "The rate is [number of] beats per minute."
   - The ECG paper is scored so that one big box is .20 seconds. These big boxes consist of five little boxes, each of which are .04 seconds.
   - A quick way to calculate rate when the rhythm is regular is the mantra: 300, 150, 100, 75, 60, 50 (= 300 / # large boxes), which is measured as the number of large boxes between two QRS complexes. Therefore, a distance of one large box between two adjacent QRS complexes would be a rate of 300, while a distance of five large boxes between two adjacent QRS complexes would be a rate of 60.
   - For irregular rhythms, count the number of complexes that occur in a 6-second interval (30 large boxes) and multiply by 10 to get a rate in bpm.

2. Rhythm
   "The rhythm is [sinus]/[atrial fibrillation]/[atrial flutter]."
   - If p waves are present in all leads, and upright in leads I & AVF, then the rhythm is sinus. Lack of p waves usually suggests an atrial rhythm. A ventricular rhythm (V Fib or V Tach) is an unstable one (could spell imminent death)—and you should be getting ready for advanced cardiac life support (ACLS).

3. Axis (see Figure 1-2 on page 7)
   "The axis is [normal]/[deviated to the right]/[deviated to the left]."
   - If I and aVF are both upright or positive, then the axis is normal.
   - If I is upright and aVF is upside down, then there is left axis deviation (LAD).
   - If I is upside down and aVF is upright, then there is right axis deviation (RAD).
   - If I and aVF are both upside down or negative, then there is extreme RAD.

4. Intervals (see Figure 1-3 on page 7)
   "The [PR]/[QRS] intervals are [normal]/[shortened]/[widened]."
   - Normal PR interval = .12–.20 seconds.
   - Short PR is associated with Wolff-Parkinson-White syndrome (WPW).
   - Long PR interval is associated with heart block of which there are three types:
     - First-degree block: PR interval > .20 seconds (one big box).
     - Second-degree (Wenckebach) block: PR interval lengthens progressively until a QRS is dropped.
     - Second-degree (Mobitz) block: PR interval is constant, but one QRS is dropped at a fixed interval. *(continued)*

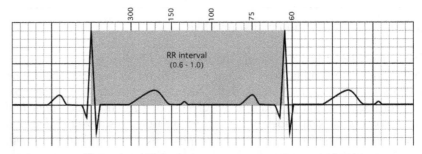

FIGURE 1-1. ECG rate.

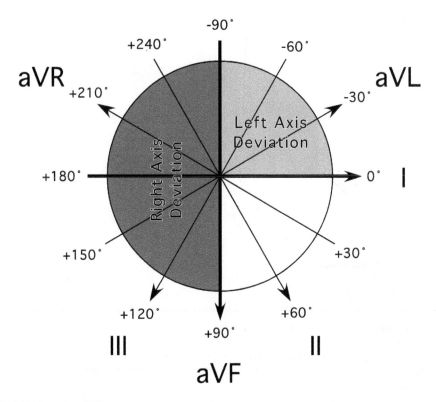

FIGURE 1-2. ECG axes.

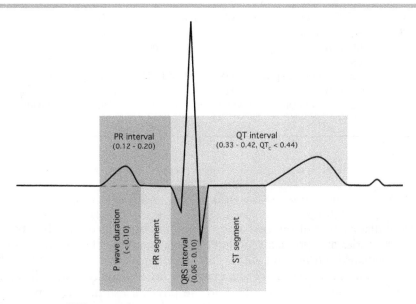

FIGURE 1-3. ECG segments.

- Third-degree block: Complete AV dissociation, prolonged presence is incompatible with life.
- Normal QRS interval ≤ .12 seconds.
- Prolonged QRS is seen when the beat is initiated in the ventricle rather than the sinoatrial node, when there is a bundle branch block, and when the heart is artificially paced with longer QRS intervals. Prolonged QRS is also noted in tricyclic overdose and WPW. *(continued)*

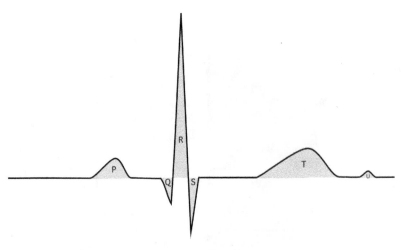

FIGURE 1-4. ECG waves.

5. Wave morphology (see Figure 1-4)
   a. Ventricular hypertrophy
      ■ "There [is/is no] [left/right] [ventricular/atrial] hypertrophy."
   b. Atrial hypertrophy
      ■ Clue is presence of tall p waves.
   c. Ischemic changes
      ■ "There [are/are no] S-T wave [depressions/elevations] or [flattened/in-verted] T waves." Presence of Q wave indicates an old infarct.
   d. Bundle branch block (BBB)
      ■ "There [is/is no] [left/right] bundle branch block."
      ■ Clues:
        ■ Presence of RSR' wave in leads V1–V3 with ST depression and T wave inversion goes with RBBB.
        ■ Presence of notched R wave in leads I, aVL, and V4–V6 goes with LBBB.

ON OUTPATIENT

The ambulatory part of the pediatrics rotation consists of mainly two parts—focused histories and physicals for acute problems and well-child visits. In the general pediatrics clinic, you will see the common ailments of children, but don't overlook the possibilty of less common ones. Usually, you will see the patient first, to take the history and do the physical exam. It is important to strike a balance between obtaining a thorough exam and not upsetting the child so much that the attending won't be able to recheck any pertinent parts of it. For acute cases, present the patient distinctly, including an appropriate differential diagnosis and plan. In this section, be sure to include possible etiologies, such as specific bacteria, as well as a specific treatment (e.g., a particular antibiotic, dose, and course of treatment). For presentation of well-child visits, cover all the bases, but focus on the patients' concerns and your findings. There are specific issues to discuss depending on the age of the child. Past history and development is important, but so is anticipatory guidance–prevention and expectations for what is to come. The goal is to be both efficient and thorough.

Pediatric History and Physical Exam

HISTORY
ID/CC: Age, sex, symptom, duration

HPI:
Symptoms—location, quality, quantity, aggravating and alleviating factors
Time course—onset, duration, frequency, change over time
Rx/Intervention—medications, medical help sought, other actions taken
Exposures, ill contacts, travel

Current Health:
Nutrition—breast milk/formula/food, quantity, frequency, supplements, problems (poor suck/swallow, reflux)
Sleep—quantity, quality, disturbances (snoring, apnea, bedwetting, restlessness), intervention, wakes up refreshed
Elimination—bowel movement frequency/quality, urination frequency, problems, toilet training
Behavior—toward family, friends, discipline
Development—gross motor, fine motor, language, cognition, social/emotional

PMH:
Pregnancy (be sensitive to adoption issues)—gravida/para status, maternal age, duration, exposures (medications, alcohol, tobacco, drugs, infections, radiation); complications (bleeding, gestational diabetes, hypertension, etc.), occurred on contraception?, planned?, emotions regarding pregnancy, problems with past pregnancies
Labor and delivery—length of labor, rupture of membranes, fetal movement, medications, presentation/delivery, mode of delivery, assistance (forceps, vacuum), complications, Apgars, immediate breathe/cry, oxygen requirement/intubation and duration
Neonatal—birth height/weight, abnormalities/injuries, length of hospital stay, complications (respiratory distress, cyanosis, anemia, jaundice, seizures, anomalies, infections), behavior, maternal concerns
Infancy—temperament, feeding, family reactions to infant
Illnesses/hospitalizations/surgeries/accidents/injuries—dates, medications/interventions, impact on child/family—don't forget circumcision
Medications—past (antibiotics, especially), present, reactions
Allergies—include reaction
Immunizations—up to date, reactions
Family history—relatives, ages, health problems, deaths (age/cause), miscarriages/stillbirths/deaths of infants or children
Social history—parents' education and occupation, living arrangements, pets, water (city or well), lead exposure (old house, paint), smoke exposure, religion, finances, family dynamics, risk-taking behaviors, school/daycare, other caregivers

ROS:
General—fever, activity, growth
Head—trauma, size, shape
Eyes—erythema, drainage, acuity, tearing, trauma
Ears—infection, drainage, hearing
Nose—drainage, congestion, sneezing, bleeding, frequent colds
Mouth—eruption/condition of teeth, lesions, infection, odor
Throat—sore, tonsils, recurrent strep pharyngitis
Neck—stiff, lumps, tenderness
Respiratory—cough, wheeze, chest pain, pneumonia, retractions, apnea, stridor
Cardiovascular—murmur, exercise intolerance, diaphoresis, syncope
Gastrointestinal—appetite, constipation, diarrhea, poor suck, swallow, abdominal pain, jaundice, vomiting, change in bowel movements, blood, food intolerances
GU—urine output, stream, urgency, frequency, discharge, blood, fussy during menstruation, sexually active
Endocrine—polyuria/polydipsia/polyphagia, puberty, thyroid, growth/stature
Musculoskeletal—pain, swelling, redness, warmth, movement, trauma
Neurologic—headache, dizziness, convulsions, visual changes, loss of consciousness, gait, coordination, handedness
Skin—bruises, rash, itching, hair loss, color (cyanosis)
Lymph—swelling, redness, tender glands

(continued)

PHYSICAL EXAM

General—smiling, playful, cooperative, irritable, lethargic, tired, hydration status
Vitals—temperature, heart rate, respiratory rate, blood pressure
Growth—weight, height, head circumference and percentiles, BMI if applicable
Skin—inspect, palpate, birthmarks, rash, jaundice, cyanosis
Hair—whorl, lanugo, Tanner stage
Head—anterior fontanelle, sutures
Eyes—redness, swelling, discharge, red reflex, strabismus, scleral icterus
Ears—tympanic membranes (DO LAST!)
Nose—patent nares, flaring nostrils
Mouth—teeth, palate, thrush
Throat—oropharynx (red, moist, injection, exudate)
Neck—range of motion, meningeal signs
Lymph—cervical, axillary, inguinal
Cardiovascular—heart rate, murmur, rub, pulses (central/peripheral; bilateral upper and lower extremities including femoral), perfusion/color
Respiratory—rate, retractions, grunting, crackles, wheezes
Abdomen—bowel sounds, distention, tenderness, hepatosplenomegaly, masses, umbilicus, rectal
Back—scoliosis, dimples
Musculoskeletal—joints—erythema, warmth, swelling tenderness, range of motion
Neurologic—gait, symmetric extremity movement, strength/tone/bulk, reflexes (age-appropriate and deep tendon reflexes), mentation, coordination
Genitalia—circumcision, testes, labia, hymen, Tanner staging
Note: The COMSEP website (http://comsep.org) has a video clip demonstrating the pediatric physical exam. It can be found under "curriculum" then "curriculum support resources."

YOUR ROTATION GRADE

Usually, the clerkship grade is broken down into three or four components:

- *Inpatient evaluation:* This includes evaluation of your ward time by residents and attendings and is based on your performance on the ward. Usually, this makes up about half your grade, and can be largely subjective.
- *Ambulatory evaluation:* This includes your performance in clinic, including clinic notes and any procedures performed in the outpatient setting.
- *National Board of Medical Examiners (NBME) examination:* This portion of the grade is anywhere from 20% to 50%, so performance on this multiple-choice test is vital to achieving honors in the clerkship.
- *Objective Structured Clinical Examination (OSCE):* Some schools now include an OSCE as part of their clerkship evaluation. This is basically an exam that involves standardized patients and allows assessment of a student's bedside manner and physical examination skills. This may comprise up to one fourth of a student's grade.

HOW TO STUDY

Make a list of core material to learn. This list should reflect common symptoms, illnesses, and areas in which you have particular interest or in which you feel particularly weak. Do not try to learn every possible topic.

Symptoms
- Fever
- Failure to thrive
- Sore throat
- Wheezing
- Vomiting
- Diarrhea
- Abdominal pain
- Jaundice
- Fluid and electrolyte imbalance
- Seizures

The knowledge you need on the wards is the day-to-day management know-how (though just about anything is game for pimping!). The knowledge you want by the end-of-rotation examination is the epidemiology, risk factors, pathophysiology, diagnosis, and treatment of major diseases seen in pediatrics.

As you see patients, note their major symptoms and diagnosis for review. Your reading on the symptom-based topics above should be done with a specific patient in mind. For example, if a patient comes in with diarrhea, read about common infectious causes of gastroenteritis and the differences between and complications of them, noninfectious causes, and dehydration in the review book that night.

Select your study material. We recommend:
- This review book, *First Aid for the Pediatrics Clerkship*
- A major pediatric textbook—*Nelson's Textbook of Pediatrics* (also available on MD Consult) and its very good counterpart, *Nelson's Essentials*
- *The Harriet Lane Handbook*—the bible of pediatrics: medicine, medications, and lab values as they apply to children

Prepare a talk on a topic. You may be asked to give a small talk once or twice during your rotation. If not, you should volunteer! Feel free to choose a topic that is on your list; however, realize that the people who hear the lecture may consider this dull. The ideal topic is slightly uncommon but not rare, for example, Kawasaki disease. To prepare a talk on a topic, read about it in a major textbook and a review article not more than 2 years old. Then search online or in the library for recent developments or changes in treatment.

Procedures. You may have the opportunity to perform a couple of procedures on your pediatrics rotation. Be sure to volunteer to do them whenever you can, and at least actively observe if participation is not allowed. These may include:
- Lumbar puncture
- Intravenous line placement
- Nasogastric tube placement
- Venipuncture (blood draw)
- Pulling central (and other) lines
- Foley (urinary) catheter placement
- Ankle–brachial index (ABI) measurement
- Transillumination of scrotum
- Intraosseous line placement
- Transcranial doppler study

If you have read about your core illnesses and core symptoms, you will know a great deal about pediatrics. It is difficult but vital to balance reading about your specific patients and covering all of the core topics of pediatrics. To study for the clerkship exam, we recommend:

2–3 weeks before exam: Read this entire review book, taking notes.
10 days before exam: Read the notes you took during the rotation on your core content list, and the corresponding review book sections.
5 days before exam: Read the entire review book, concentrating on lists and mnemonics.
2 days before exam: Exercise, eat well, skim the book, and go to bed early.
1 day before exam: Exercise, eat well, review your notes and the mnemonics, and go to bed on time. Do not have any caffeine after 2 P.M.

Other helpful studying strategies include:

Study with friends. Group studying can be very helpful. Other people may point out areas that you have not studied enough and may help you focus on the goal. If you tend to get distracted by other people in the room, limit this to less than half of your study time.

Study in a bright room. Find the room in your house or in your library that has the best, brightest light. This will help prevent you from falling asleep. If you don't have a bright light, get a halogen desk lamp or a light that simulates sunlight (not a tanning lamp).

Eat light, balanced meals. Make sure your meals are balanced, with lean protein, fruits and vegetables, and fiber. A high-sugar, high-carbohydrate meal will give you an initial burst of energy for 1 to 2 hours, but then you'll drop.

Take practice exams. The point of practice exams is not so much the content that is contained in the questions, but the training of sitting still for 3 hours and trying to pick the best answer for each and every question.

Tips for answering questions. All questions are intended to have one best answer. When answering questions, follow these guidelines:

Read the answers first. For all questions longer than two sentences, reading the answers first can help you sift through the question for the key information.
Look for the words "EXCEPT, MOST, LEAST, NOT, BEST, WORST, TRUE, FALSE, CORRECT, INCORRECT, ALWAYS, and NEVER." If you find one of these words, circle or underline it for later comparison with the answer.

Finally, remember—children are not just small adults. They present with a whole new set of medical and social issues. More than ever, you are treating families, not just individual patients.

The following "cards" contain information that is often helpful during the pediatrics rotation. We advise that you make a copy of these cards, cut them out, and carry them in your coat pocket when you are on the wards.

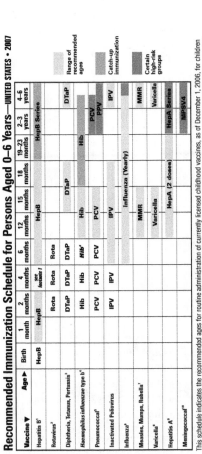

Recommended Immunization Schedule for Persons Aged 0–6 Years—UNITED STATES • 2007

This schedule indicates the recommended ages for routine administration of currently licensed childhood vaccines, as of December 1, 2006, for children aged 0–6 years. Additional information is available at http://www.cdc.gov/nip/recs/child-schedule.htm. Any dose not administered at the recommended age should be administered at any subsequent visit, when indicated and feasible. Additional vaccines may be licensed and recommended during the year. Licensed combination vaccines may be used whenever any components of the combination are indicated and other components of the vaccine are not contraindicated and if approved by the Food and Drug Administration for that dose of the series. Providers should consult the respective Advisory Committee on Immunization Practices statement for detailed recommendations. Clinically significant adverse events that follow immunization should be reported to the Vaccine Adverse Event Reporting System (VAERS). Guidance about how to obtain and complete a VAERS form is available at http://www.vaers.hhs.gov or by telephone, 800-822-7967. **FOOTNOTES ON REVERSE SIDE**

© 2011 by The McGraw-Hill Companies. From Stead et al, *First Aid for the Pediatrics Clerkship: Third Edition.*

© 2011 by The McGraw-Hill Companies. From Stead et al, *First Aid for the Pediatrics Clerkship: Third Edition.*

FOOTNOTES
1. **Hepatitis B vaccine (HepB).** *(Minimum age: birth)*
   At birth:
   - Administer monovalent HepB to all newborns before hospital discharge.
   - If mother is hepatitis surface antigen (HBsAg)-positive, administer HepB and 0.5 mL of hepatitis B immune globulin (HBIG) within 12 hours of birth.
   - If mother's HBsAg status is unknown, administer HepB within 12 hours of birth. Determine the HBsAg status as soon as possible and if HBsAg-positive, administer HBIG (no later than age 1 week).
   - If mother is HBsAg-negative, the birth dose can only be delayed with physician's order and mother's negative HBsAg laboratory report documented in the infant's medical record.
   After the birth dose:
   - The HepB series should be completed with either monovalent HepB or a combination vaccine containing HepB. The second dose should be administered at age 1–2 months. The final dose should be administered at age ≥ 24 weeks. Infants born to HBsAg-positive mothers should be tested for HBsAg and antibody to HBsAg after completion of ≥ 3 doses of a licensed HepB series, at age 9–18 months (generally at the next well-child visit).
   4-month dose:
   - It is permissible to administer 4 doses of HepB when combination vaccines are administered after the birth dose. If monovalent HepB is used for doses after the birth dose, a dose at age 4 months is not needed.
2. **Rotavirus vaccine (Rota).** *(Minimum age: 6 weeks)*
   - Administer the first dose at age 6–12 weeks. Do not start the series later than age 12 weeks.
   - Administer the final dose in the series by age 32 weeks. Do not administer a dose later than age 32 weeks.
   - Data on safety and efficacy outside of these age ranges are insufficient.
3. **Diphtheria and tetanus toxoids and acellular pertussis vaccine (DTaP).** *(Minimum age: 6 weeks)*
   - The fourth dose of DTaP may be administered as early as age 12 months, provided 6 months have elapsed since the third dose.
4. **Haemophilus influenzae type b conjugate vaccine (Hib).** *(Minimum age: 6 weeks)*
   - TriHiBit (DTaP/Hib) combination products should not be used for primary immunization but can be used as boosters following any Hib vaccine in children aged ≥ 12 months.
   - If PRP-OMP (PedvaxHIB or ComVax [Merck]) is administered at ages 2 and 4 months, a dose at age 6 months is not required.
5. **Pneumococcal vaccine.** *(Minimum age: 6 weeks for pneumococcal conjugate vaccine [PCV]; 2 years for pneumococcal polysaccharide vaccine [PPV])*
   - Administer PCV at ages 24–59 months in certain high-risk groups. Administer PPV to children aged ≥ 2 years in certain high-risk groups. See MMWR 2000;49(No. RR-9):1–35.
6. **Influenza vaccine.** *(Minimum age: 6 months for trivalent inactivated influenza vaccine [TIV]; 5 years for live, attenuated influenza vaccine [LAIV])*
   - All children aged 6–59 months and close contacts of all children aged 0–59 months are recommended to receive influenza vaccine.
   - Influenza vaccine is recommended annually for children aged ≥ 59 months with certain risk factors, health-care workers, and other persons (including household members) in close contact with persons in groups at high risk. See MMWR 2006;55(No. RR-10):1–41.
   - For healthy persons aged 5–49 years, LAIV may be used as an alternative to TIV.
   - Children receiving TIV should receive 0.25 mL if aged 6–35 months or 0.5 mL if aged ≥ 3 years.
   - Children aged < 9 years who are receiving influenza vaccine for the first time should receive 2 doses (separated by ≥ 4 weeks for TIV and ≥ 6 weeks for LAIV).
7. **Measles, mumps, and rubella vaccine (MMR).** *(Minimum age: 12 months)*
   - Administer the second dose of MMR at age 4–6 years. MMR may be administered before age 4–6 years, provided ≥ 4 weeks have elapsed since the first dose and both doses are administered at age ≥ 12 months.
8. **Varicella vaccine.** *(Minimum age: 12 months)*
   - Administer the second dose of varicella vaccine at age 4–6 years. Varicella vaccine may be administered before age 4–6 years, provided that ≥ 3 months have elapsed since the first dose and both doses are administered at age ≥ 12 months. If second dose was administered ≥ 28 days following the first dose, the second dose does not need to be repeated.
9. **Hepatitis A vaccine (HepA).** *(Minimum age: 12 months)*
   - HepA is recommended for all children aged 1 year (i.e., aged 12–23 months). The 2 doses in the series should be administered at least 6 months apart.
   - Children not fully vaccinated by age 2 years can be vaccinated at subsequent visits.
   - HepA is recommended for certain other groups of children, including in areas where vaccination programs target older children. See MMWR 2006;55(No. RR-7):1–23.
10. **Meningococcal polysaccharide vaccine (MPSV4).** *(Minimum age: 2 years)*
   - Administer MPSV4 to children aged 2–10 years with terminal complement deficiencies or anatomic or functional asplenia and certain other high-risk groups. See MMWR 2005;54(No. RR-7):1–21.
   CS108190

Legend:
- Range of recommended ages
- Catch-up immunization
- Certain high-risk groups

13

Recommended Immunization Schedule for Persons Aged 7–18 Years—UNITED STATES • 2007

Vaccine ▼	Age ▶	7–10 years	11–12 YEARS	13–14 years	15 years	16–18 years
Tetanus, Diphtheria, Pertussis[1]		see footnote 1	Tdap	Tdap		
Human Papillomavirus[2]		see footnote 2	HPV (3 doses)	HPV Series		
Meningococcal[3]		MPSV4	MCV4		MCV4	MCV4
Pneumococcal[4]			PPV			
Influenza[5]			Influenza (Yearly)			
Hepatitis A[6]			HepA Series			
Hepatitis B[7]			HepB Series			
Inactivated Poliovirus[8]			IPV Series			
Measles, Mumps, Rubella[9]			MMR Series			
Varicella[10]			Varicella Series			

Range of recommended ages

Catch-up immunization

Certain high-risk groups

This schedule indicates the recommended ages for routine administration of currently licensed childhood vaccines, as of December 1, 2006, for children aged 7–18 years. Additional information is available at **http://www.cdc.gov/nip/recs/child-schedule.htm**. Any dose not administered at the recommended age should be administered at any subsequent visit, when indicated and feasible. Additional vaccines may be licensed and recommended during the year. Licensed combination vaccines may be used whenever any components of the combination are indicated and other components of the vaccine are not contraindicated and if approved by the Food and Drug Administration for that dose of the series. Providers should consult the respective Advisory Committee on Immunization Practices statement for detailed recommendations. Clinically significant adverse events that follow immunization should be reported to the Vaccine Adverse Event Reporting System (VAERS). Guidance about how to obtain and complete a VAERS form is available at **http://www.vaers.hhs.gov** or by telephone, **800-822-7967. FOOTNOTES ON REVERSE SIDE**

© 2011 by The McGraw-Hill Companies. From Stead et al, *First Aid for the Pediatrics Clerkship: Third Edition.*

© 2011 by The McGraw-Hill Companies. From Stead et al, *First Aid for the Pediatrics Clerkship: Third Edition.*

FOOTNOTES
1. **Tetanus and diphtheria toxoids and acellular pertussis vaccine (Tdap).** *(Minimum age: 10 years for BOOSTRIX® and 11years for ADACEL™)*
   - Administer at age 11–12 years for those who have completed the recommended childhood DTP/DTaP vaccination series and have not received a tetanus and diphtheria toxoids vaccine (Td) booster dose.
   - Adolescents aged 13–18 years who missed the 11–12 year Td/Tdap booster dose should also receive a single dose of Tdap if they have completed the recommended childhood DTP/DTaP vaccination series.
2. **Human papillomavirus vaccine (HPV).** *(Minimum age: 9 years)*
   - Administer the first dose of the HPV vaccine series to females at age 11–12 years.
   - Administer the second dose 2 months after the first dose and the third dose 6 months after the first dose.
   - Administer the HPV vaccine series to females at age 13–18 years if not previously vaccinated.
3. **Meningococcal vaccine.** *(Minimum age: 11 years for meningococcal conjugate vaccine [MCV4]; 2 years for meningococcal polysaccharide vaccine [MPSV4])*
   - Administer MCV4 at age 11–12 years and to previously unvaccinated adolescents at high school entry (at approximately age 15 years).
   - Administer MCV4 to previously unvaccinated college freshmen living in dormitories; MPSV4 is an acceptable alternative.
   - Vaccination against invasive meningococcal disease is recommended for children and adolescents aged ≥ 2 years with terminal complement deficiencies or anatomic or functional asplenia and certain other high-risk groups. See *MMWR* 2005;54(No. RR-7);1–21. Use MPSV4 for children aged 2–10 years and MCV4 or MPSV4 for older children.
4. **Pneumococcal polysaccharide vaccine (PPV).** *(Minimum age: 2 years)*
   - Administer for certain high-risk groups. See *MMWR* 1997;46(No. RR-8);1–24, and *MMWR* 2000;49(No. RR-9);1–35.
5. **Influenza vaccine.** *(Minimum age: 6 months for trivalent inactivated influenza vaccine [TIV]; 5 years for live, attenuated influenza vaccine [LAIV])*
   - Influenza vaccine is recommended annually for persons with certain risk factors, health-care workers, and other persons (including house-hold members) in close contact with persons in groups at high risk. See *MMWR* 2006;55(No. RR-10);1–41.
   - For healthy persons aged 5–49 years, LAIV may be used as an alternative to TIV.
   - Children aged < 9 years who are receiving influenza vaccine for the first time should receive 2 doses (separated by ≥ 4 weeks for TIV and ≥ 6 weeks for LAIV).
6. **Hepatitis A vaccine (HepA).** *(Minimum age: 12 months)*
   - HepA is recommended for certain other groups of children, including in areas where vaccination programs target older children. See *MMWR* 2006;55(No. RR-7):1–23.
   - The 2 doses in the series should be administered at least 6 months apart.
7. **Hepatitis B vaccine (HepB).** *(Minimum age: birth)*
   - Administer the 3-dose series to those who were not previously vaccinated.
   - A 2-dose series of Recombivax HB® is licensed for children aged 11–15 years.
8. **Inactivated poliovirus vaccine (IPV).** *(Minimum age: 6 weeks)*
   - For children who received an all-IPV or all-oral poliovirus (OPV) series, a fourth dose is not necessary if the third dose was administered at age ≥ 4 years.
   - If both OPV and IPV were administered as part of a series, a total of 4 doses should be administered, regardless of the child's current age.
9. **Measles, mumps, and rubella vaccine (MMR).** *(Minimum age: 12 months)*
   - If not previously vaccinated, administer 2 doses of MMR during any visit, with ≥ 4 weeks between the doses.
10. **Varicella vaccine.** *(Minimum age: 12 months)*
    - Administer 2 doses of varicella vaccine to persons without evidence of immunity.
    - Administer 2 doses of varicella vaccine to persons aged < 13 years at least 3 months apart. Do not repeat the second dose, if administered ≥ 28 days after the first dose.
    - Administer 2 doses of varicella vaccine to persons aged ≥ 13 years at least 4 weeks apart.

CS108190

SECTION II

High-Yield Facts

Gestation and Birth

Gestational/Embryologic Landmarks

See Table 2-1.

Germ Layers

See Table 2-2.

Heart

- ▪ **Week 3:** Paired heart tubes begin to work.
- ▪ **Week 4:**
  - ▪ Primordial atrium is divided into left and right by septa primum and secundum.
  - ▪ Septum primum forms the valve of the foramen ovale, which closes about 3 months after birth.
  - ▪ Failure of the foramen ovale to close results in an **atrial septal defect (ASD).**
- ▪ **Week 7:**
  - ▪ The single ventricle is divided into left and right; prior to that the interventricular foramen communicates between left and right sides.
  - ▪ Failure of the interventricular foramen to close results in a **ventricular septal defect (VSD).**

The main source of energy for a growing fetus is carbohydrates.

Bicuspid aortic valve and VSD are the most common congenital heart defects.

TABLE 2-1. Gestational/Embryologic Landmarks

Week 1	Fertilization, usually in fallopian tube ampulla Implantation begins
Week 2	Implantation complete Endoderm and ectoderm form (bilaminar embryo)
Week 3	Mesoderm formed (trilaminar embryo)
Week 5	Subdivisions of forebrain, midbrain, and hindbrain are formed
Week 7	Heart formed
Week 8	Primary organogenesis complete Placentation occurs
Week 9	Permanent kidneys begin functioning
Week 10	Midgut returns from umbilical cord, where it was developing, to abdominal cavity, while undergoing counterclockwise rotation
Week 24	Primitive alveoli are formed and surfactant production begins
Week 26	Testicles descend

HIGH-YIELD FACTS

GESTATION AND BIRTH

TABLE 2-2. Summary of Germ Layer Derivatives

ECTODERM	NEURAL CREST CELLS (ECTODERM)	MESODERM	ENDODERM
CNS, peripheral nervous system (PNS)	Spinal nerves; cranial nerves V, VII, IX, X; sensory neurons	Connective tissue, cartilage, bone	Epithelial lining of gastrointestinal tract, respiratory tract, and middle ear, including eustachian tube
Sensory epithelia of eye, ear, nose	Autonomic ganglia	Striated and smooth muscle	
Epidermis, hair, nails	Adrenal medulla	Blood and lymphatic systems	Tonsil parenchyma
Mammary glands, pituitary gland, subcutaneous glands	Meninges	Ovaries, testes, genital ducts	Thymus
	Pigment cells, glial cells of peripheral nerves	Serous membranes lining body cavities	Parathyroid and thyroid glands
Tooth enamel		Spleen, adrenal cortex	Liver, pancreas

Upper portion of fetal body is perfused much better than lower because of the way fetal circulation functions.

Circulation

- See Figure 2-1.
- Well-oxygenated blood returns from placenta through umbilical vein, where half of it enters the inferior vena cava through the ductus venosus (continuation of the umbilical vein beyond the branching of the left

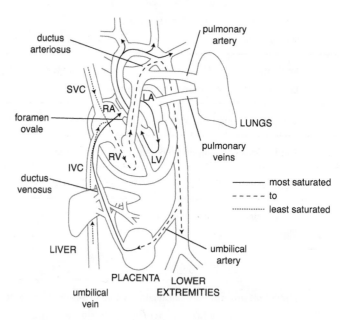

TO BRAIN, HEART
UPPER EXTREMITIES

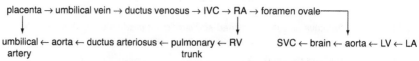

placenta → umbilical vein → ductus venosus → IVC → RA → foramen ovale

umbilical ← aorta ← ductus arteriosus ← pulmonary ← RV   SVC ← brain ← aorta ← LV ← LA
artery   trunk

FIGURE 2-1. Fetal circulation.

and right portal veins), and the rest enters the hepatic circulation (preferentially through the left portal vein).

- Despite the fact that the umbilical venous blood joins the inferior vena cava prior to entering the right atrium, the streams do not mix substantially. Blood from the artery to vein is preferentially shunted through the foramen ovale to the left atrium, while blood from the lower inferior vena cava, right hepatic circulation, and superior vena cava enters the right ventricle.
- The major portion of blood exiting the right ventricle is then shunted to the aorta through the ductus arteriosus because the lungs are collapsed and pulmonary artery pressures are high.
- Sixty-five percent of blood in the descending aorta returns to the umbilical arteries for reoxygenation at the placenta; the remainder supplies the inferior part of the body.
- After birth, pulmonary artery pressure drops because the lungs expand, reducing flow across the ductus arteriosus and stimulating its closure (usually within first few days of life). (See Figure 2-2.)
- Pressure in the left atrium becomes higher than that in the right atrium after birth due to the ↑ pulmonary return, which stimulates closure of the foramen ovale (usually complete by third month of life).

Closure of the ductus arteriosus can be prevented by prostaglandin E₁ and facilitated by indomethacin (via inhibition of prostaglandin synthesis).

Failure of kidneys to develop can → **oligohydramnios** (↓ fluid in the amniotic cavity).

Hemoglobin

Fetal erythropoiesis occurs in the yolk sac (3–8 weeks), liver (6–8 weeks), spleen (9–28 weeks), and then bone marrow (28 weeks onward).

Failure of kidneys to migrate can → ectopic kidneys.

Genitourinary Tract

- Metanephri (permanent kidneys) start functioning at 9 weeks; urine is excreted into amniotic cavity.
- Initially, kidneys lie in the pelvis; by 8 weeks they migrate into their adult position.
- Morphologic sexual characteristics do not develop until 7 weeks' gestation.
- In males, testis-determining factor induces primary sex cords to develop as male gonads, with testosterone production by 8 weeks.
- Testicles develop intra-abdominally and then descend through inguinal canals into the scrotum by 26 weeks.
- Ovaries are identified by 10 weeks; primary sex cords develop into female gonads with primordial follicles developing prenatally.

A horseshoe kidney gets caught on the inferior mesenteric artery (IMA) during ascent.

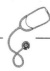

Failure of testicle(s) to descend, cryptorchidism, may need to be corrected surgically to prevent progressive dysplasia and may affect fertility.

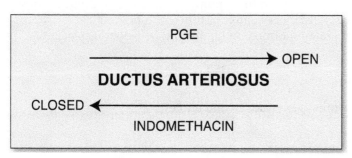

FIGURE 2-2. Mechanism of ductus arteriosus patency/closure.

Gastrointestinal Tract

- By 10 weeks, the midgut returns from the umbilical cord, where it was developing, to the abdominal cavity, while undergoing counterclockwise rotation.
- Insufficient rotation of the midgut, called **malrotation,** can present in neonatal period as intestinal obstruction.
- Incomplete separation of foregut and primitive airway can → **tracheoesophageal fistula (TEF).**
- Failure of the intestine to return to the abdominal cavity with intestinal contents remaining at the base of the umbilical cord causes **gastroschisis,** a full-thickness abdominal wall defect with extruded intestine.

Lungs

By 24 weeks, primitive alveoli are formed and surfactant production is begun.

Central Nervous System (CNS)

- During week 3, the neural tube is formed on the ectodermal surface.
- Neural tube openings (rostral and caudal) are closed by 25–27 days.
- By week 5, subdivisions of forebrain, midbrain, and hindbrain are formed.
- Failure of caudal neural tube to close completely can result in **spina bifida** (unfused vertebral arch with or without unfused dura mater and spinal cord), commonly seen in the lumbar area. Failure of the rostral neural tube to close can result in anencephaly.

PLACENTA

Development

- Fetal portion of placenta is formed from chorionic sac.
- Maternal portion is derived from endometrium.

Transport

- Nutrients, electrolytes, water, and gases are diffused or transported across the placenta.
- Most drugs pass through placenta and can be detected in fetal plasma (eg, warfarin, morphine, propylthiouracil, and drugs of abuse).
- A few substances cannot pass because of their size or charge (eg, heparin); protein hormones (eg, insulin) do not cross placenta.

Metabolism

Placenta synthesizes glycogen and cholesterol.

Infants born prior to 30 weeks are given exogenous surfactant to prevent respiratory distress syndrome (RDS). Mom is given steroids.

Lecithin-to-sphingomyelin ratio in the amniotic fluid greater than 3 indicates fetal lung maturity.

Folic acid supplements during pregnancy reduce incidence of neural tube defects.

Maternal α-fetoprotein (AFP) is *high in:*
- Multiple gestations (most common)
- Fetal neural tube defects
- Gastroschisis

Endocrine Function

Placenta produces β-human chorionic gonadotropin (β-hCG), human chorionic adrenocorticotropic hormone (ACTH), human placental lactogen, and human chorionic somatomammotropin.

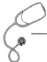
Infections

Infants who have experienced an intrauterine infection have a higher-than-average incidence of being small for gestational age, hepatosplenomegaly, congenital defects, microcephaly, and intracranial calcifications.

TOXOPLASMOSIS

- Maternal infection is due to ingestion of oocysts from feces of infected cats and is asymptomatic.
- Clinical features in infants include microcephaly, hydrocephalus, intracranial calcifications, chorioretinitis, and seizures.

RUBELLA

- Congenital rubella syndrome is rare due to the effectiveness of the rubella vaccine.
- Maternal infection early in pregnancy can result in congenital rubella syndrome, which includes meningoencephalitis, microcephaly, cataracts, sensorineural hearing loss, and congenital heart disease (patent ductus arteriosus and pulmonary artery stenosis).

CYTOMEGALOVIRUS (CMV)

- Common—occurs in 1% of newborns.
- Newborn disease is associated with primary maternal infection with a 50% chance of infection.
- In those affected, only 5% have neurologic deficits.
- Infection occurs in 1% of pregnancies with recurrent or reactivated infection.
- CMV transmitted intrapartum, through infected blood or through breast milk, is not associated with neurologic deficits.
- Clinical features include intrauterine growth retardation (IUGR), low birth weight, petechiae and purpura, jaundice and hepatosplenomegaly, microcephaly, chorioretinitis, and intracranial calcifications.
- Late manifestations like learning and hearing deficits can occur in 10% of clinically inapparent infections.

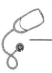

Toxins and Teratogens

ALCOHOL

- Most common teratogen.
- The amount of alcohol consumed correlates with the severity of spectrum of effects in the neonate, ranging from mild reduction in cerebral function to classic fetal alcohol syndrome (see Figure 2-3).

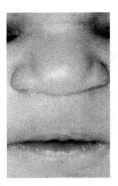

FIGURE 2-3. Fetal alcohol syndrome.

Notice the depressed nasal bridge, flat philtrum, long upper lip, and thin vermillion border. (Reproduced, with permission, from Stoler JM, Holmes LB. Underrecognition of prenatal alcohol effects in infants of known alcohol abusing women. *Journal of Pediatrics* 135(4):430–436, 1999.)

- Clinical manifestations include microcephaly and mental retardation, IUGR, facial dysmorphism (midfacial hypoplasia, micrognathia, shortened nasal philtrum, short palpebral fissures, and a thin vermillion border), renal and cardiac defects, and hypospadias.

COCAINE

 Term, 5-lb., 2-day-old infant has irritability, nasal stuffiness, and coarse tremors. He feeds poorly and has diarrhea. *Think: Cocaine or heroin withdrawal.*

Cocaine readily crosses the placental barrier, placing the fetus at risk. Symptoms of cocaine withdrawal include tremors, high-pitched cry, irritability, excess suck, apnea, and tachycardia, which can become evident within the first 72 hours of life. Opiates also cross the placenta. Tremor and irritability are the common symptoms of opiate withdrawal. Vague autonomic symptoms such as yawning and sneezing are often present.

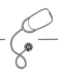

Cocaine use is associated with placental abruption.

- Causes maternal hypertension and constriction of placental circulation → ↓ uterine blood flow and fetal hypoxia.
- Associated with a higher risk of spontaneous abortion, placental abruption, fetal distress, meconium staining, preterm birth, IUGR, and low Apgar scores at birth.
- Associated with intracranial hemorrhage and necrotizing enterocolitis; cardiac, skull, and genitourinary malformations; and ↑ incidence of sudden infant death syndrome (SIDS).
- Cocaine withdrawal in an infant causes irritability, ↑ tremulousness, and poor feeding, as well as ↑ incidence of learning difficulties and attention and concentration deficits later on.

NARCOTICS

Heroin and methadone are associated with IUGR, SIDS, and infant narcotic withdrawal syndrome.

TOBACCO

Smoking is associated with ↓ birth weight.

PHENYTOIN

Phenytoin is associated with **fetal hydantoin syndrome,** which includes IUGR, mental retardation, dysmorphic facies, and hypoplasia of nails and distal phalanges.

TETRACYCLINE

Tetracycline causes tooth discoloration and inhibits bone formation.

ISOTRETINOIN (ACCUTANE)

Accutane is associated with hydrocephalus, microtia, micrognathia, and aortic arch abnormalities.

WARFARIN

- Warfarin causes abnormal cartilage development, mental retardation, deafness, and blindness.
- Warfarin is no longer used in pregnant women due to the advent of low-molecular-weight heparin, which has fewer side effects and is well tolerated.

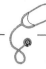

Infants of narcotic-abusing mothers should never be given naloxone in the delivery room because it may precipitate seizures.

MATERNAL CONDITIONS

Diabetes

- Associated with macrosomia (weight > 4 kg), which can → birth-related injury.
- Fetal complications are related to degree of control of maternal diabetes.
- Other fetal/neonatal complications include metabolic disorders (hypoglycemia, hypocalcemia, and hypomagnesemia), perinatal asphyxia, respiratory distress syndrome, hyperbilirubinemia, polycythemia and hyperviscosity, and congenital malformations including cardiac, renal, gastrointestinal, neurologic, and skeletal defects.

Others

- Hypertension and renal and cardiac disease are associated with small-for-gestational-age babies and prematurity.
- Maternal lupus is related to first-degree atrioventricular (AV) block in affected infants.

Elevation of maternal glucose causes elevated fetal glucose, → fetal hyperinsulinism, which can → hypoglycemia in the newborn.

Vascular disease of placenta, caused by maternal illness (such as diabetes or lupus) can → insufficient supply of nutrients to fetus and IUGR.

25

Delivery Room Care

- Once the head is delivered, the nose and mouth are suctioned.
- Once the whole body is delivered, the newborn is held at the level of the table and the umbilical cord is clamped.
- Newborn is then placed under radiant warmer and is dried with warm towels.
- Mouth and nose are gently suctioned.
- Gentle rubbing of the back or flicking of the soles of the feet, if needed to stimulate breathing.
- When the umbilical cord is clamped and cut, absent blood flow within the umbilical vein → the closure of the ductus venosus.

Apgar Scoring

- Practical method of assessing newborn infants immediately after birth to help identify those requiring resuscitation on a scale of 0–10. It is not a substitute for assessing the ABCs in neonatal resuscitation.
- Assessment at 1 and 5 minutes; further assessments at 10 and 15 minutes may indicate success of resuscitation (see Table 2-3). Resuscitation efforts should not be delayed or interrupted to assign an Apgar score.
- A poor Apgar score alone cannot be used to diagnose asphyxia or predict the development of cerebral palsy.

Prophylaxis

- Gonococcal and chlamydial eye infection prophylaxis is with erythromycin or tetracycline ointment.
- Vitamin K is given intramuscularly (IM) to prevent hemorrhagic disease of the newborn.

Cord Blood/Stem Cells

- Blood gas study should be sent if fetal distress is present.
- Can be used to test for infant's blood type.
- Rich in stem cells, which are pleuripotential cells that have potential use in malignancies and gene therapy.

TABLE 2-3. Apgar Scoring

	Activity (Muscle Tone)	Pulse	Grimace (Reflex Irritability)	Appearance (Skin Color)	Respiration
0	Absent	Absent	No response	Blue-gray, pale all over	Absent
1	Arms and legs flexed	Below 100 bpm	Grimace	Normal, except for extremities	Slow, irregular
2	Active movement	Above 100 bpm	Sneeze, cough, pull away	Normal all over	Good crying

Total out of 10: 7–10 normal newborn; 4–7 may require some resuscitative measures; ≤ 3 require immediate resuscitation.

General Appearance

Plethora (high hematocrit secondary to chronic fetal hypoxia), jaundice, sepsis and TORCH infections, cyanosis (with congenital heart and lung disease), pallor (anemia, shock, patent ductus arteriosus).

Skin

- Erythema toxicum is a pustular rash distributed over the trunk, face, and extremities, which resolves over a week.
- Mongolian spots are bluish spots present over the buttocks and back that are seen in infants of African, Asian, and Native American descent that tend to fade over a year.
- Capillary hemangiomas ("stork bites") are pink spots over the eyelids, forehead, and back of the neck that tend to fade with time.
- See Dermatologic Disease chapter.

Head

- Anterior fontanelle closes at 9–12 months.
- Large fontanelle is seen in hypothyroidism, osteogenesis imperfecta, and some chromosomal abnormalities.
- Absent anterior fontanel is associated with craniosynostosis.

Face

- Mouth—look for cleft lip/palate and macroglossia (large tongue is seen with hypothyroidism, Down's, and Beckwith-Wiedemann syndrome).
- Coarse facial features are associated with mucopolysaccharidoses.
- Look for dysmorphic features, including micrognathia, bossing of the forehead, hypertelorism (widely spaced eyes), and low-set ears (Down syndrome) (see Congenital Malformations and Chromosomal Abnormalities chapter).

Eyes

- Check for red reflex with ophthalmoscope. An absent red reflex in one or both eyes signifies blockage of the passageway between the cornea and retina such as associated with cataracts or eye tumor (retinoblastoma).
- Look for cataracts, Brushfield spots (salt-and-pepper speckling of the iris seen in Down syndrome), leukocoria (white pupil) with retinoblastoma (rare), and subconjunctival hemorrhage, which can occur after a traumatic delivery.
- See Special Organs—Eye, Ear, Nose chapter.

Neck

- Inspect for thyroid enlargement and palpate along the sternocleidomastoid for hematoma.
- Check for any fistula or tracts, which are associated with branchial closure malformations.

Prenatal infections that most commonly cause birth defects:

TORCH

Toxoplasmosis
Other (hepatitis B, syphilis, varicella-zoster virus)
Rubella
Cytomegalovirus
Herpes simplex virus/ human immunodeficiency virus (HSV/HIV)
See Figure 2-4.

A bulging fontanelle is seen with ↑ intracranial pressure, hydrocephalus, and meningitis.

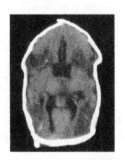

FIGURE 2-4. Head CT consistent with TORCH infection—marked ventricular dilation, extensive encephalomalacia involving both cerebral hemispheres, absent corpus callosum, periventricular calcifications, skull deformity with overriding sutures.

Chest

- Symmetry/equality of breath sounds.
- Retractions and grunting may signify respiratory distress (nasal flaring, intercostal retractions, use of accessory muscles).
- Breasts may be enlarged from the effects of maternal estrogens.

Cardiovascular

- Heart rate rhythm, quality of heart sounds, and the presence of a murmur. Murmur in a newborn infant can be due to open ductus arteriosus, but persistent murmur is always pathologic and needs evaluation.
- Check pulses and compare brachial with femoral pulse to get an estimate of vascular volume and also to rule out aortic arch obstruction (aortic stenosis, coarctation of aorta), where the femoral pulses will be weak or absent.

Abdomen

- Palpate for masses.
- Examine umbilicus for omphalocele and gastroschisis.
- Inspect the umbilical cord for single umbilical artery (normally two); if present, may indicate congenital anomalies.

Extremities

- Check both clavicles for any step off especially in the midclavicular area, where most clavicles fractures occur.
- Primitive reflexes (see Growth and Development chapter).
- Examine for congenital hip dysplasia.

Back

Look for dimples or tufts of hair that may indicate spina bifida.

Genitalia

- Girls may have vaginal bleeding and swollen labia secondary to withdrawal of maternal estrogens.
- In boys, palpate for the presence of testicles in scrotum and look for hypo- or epispadias (urethral opening proximal to normal position either on the dorsal or ventral surface).

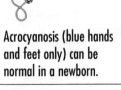

Acrocyanosis (blue hands and feet only) can be normal in a newborn.

Papilledema does not occur in infants with open cranial sutures.

SMALL OR LARGE FOR GESTATIONAL AGE

Small for Gestational Age (SGA)

- Birth weight less than the tenth percentile for gestational age.
- There are two broad categories, early and late onset.
- Early onset:
  - Insult that begins before 28 weeks' gestational age.

- Head circumference and height are proportionally small-sized (**symmetric**).
- Seen in infants born to mothers with severe vascular disease with hypertension, renal diseases, congenital anomalies, infections, and chromosomal abnormalities.
- Late onset or **asymmetric** IUGR.
    - Occurs with an insult after 28 weeks' gestational age.
    - Sparing of the head circumference.
    - Can occur with multiple gestation and preeclampsia.

Large for Gestational Age (LGA)

- Birth weight greater than the 90th percentile for gestational age.
- Those at risk are infants of diabetic mothers, postmature infants, and those with Beckwith-Wiedemann syndrome.
- Most LGA infants have large parents and are constitutionally large.
- Macrosomic infants are those with a birth weight > 4 kg.

BIRTH TRAUMA

Clavicular Fracture

- Most common bone fracture during delivery.
- Complete fracture symptoms involve ↓ or absent movement, gross deformity of clavicle, tenderness on palpation, and localized crepitus.
- Greenstick (partial) fractures have no symptoms and the diagnosis is made at 7–10 days because of callus formation.
- Management is often conservative (pin arm inside sleeve to shirt to ↓ movement).

Caput Succedaneum

- Area of edema over the presenting portion of the scalp during a vertex delivery.
- Associated with bruising and petechiae.
- Can cross suture lines.

Cephalohematoma

- Caused by bleeding that occurs below the periosteum of the overlying bone (usually the parietal).
- Associated with skull fractures in 5–10%, most often linear.
- Contained within the periosteum: does not cross suture lines.
- Subgaleal bleed:
    - Usually associated with delivery trauma or a bleeding disorder.
    - Always between the aponeurosis and periosteum layers, with bleeding into the loose areolar tissue.
    - Crosses suture lines and feels very boggy with localization to the dependent area.
    - Risk factor for significant indirect hyperbilirubinemia in the infant.

Absent breath sounds may signify a tension pneumothorax or atelectasis; bowel sounds in the thorax may indicate congenital diaphragmatic hernia.

Diminished femoral pulses are seen in coarctation of the aorta.

The most common cause of an abdominal mass in a newborn is an enlarged kidney.

Layers of the skull can be remebered by this mnemonic:
SCALP
Skin
Cutaneous tissue
Aponeurosis
Loose areolar tissue
Periosteum

Circumcision should be avoided in boys with hypo- or epispadias, as foreskin can be used to repair these defects later on.

All macrosomic infants should be examined for signs of birth trauma and checked for hypoglycemia.

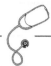

Complete clavicular fractures will → absence of Moro reflex.

Caput succedaneum is external to the periosteum and crosses the midline of the skull and suture lines versus a cephalohematoma, which is below the periosteum and does not cross suture lines.

Brachial plexus injuries can occur during birth when traction is used with shoulder dystocia.

Skull Fracture/Epidural Hematoma

- Skull fractures are uncommon; most are linear and associated with cephalohematoma. Depressed fractures are often visible and may require surgery.
- Epidural hematomas are rare and may require prompt surgical evacuation.

Molding

- Temporary asymmetry of the skull from the overlapping of bones that occurs following prolonged labor and vaginal deliveries.
- Normal head shape is regained within a week.

Klumpke Palsy

- Involves the lower arm and affects the seventh and eighth cervical and first thoracic nerve roots. The hand is paralyzed and has an absent grasp reflex, causing a "claw hand" deformity.
- It is rare to have an isolated Klumpke palsy.
- Is often accompanied by Horner syndrome.

Erb Palsy

- Erb-Duchenne involves the upper arm and is the most common type.
- Involves the fifth and sixth cervical roots, and the arm is adducted and internally rotated, but the grasp reflex is intact (see Figure 2-5).

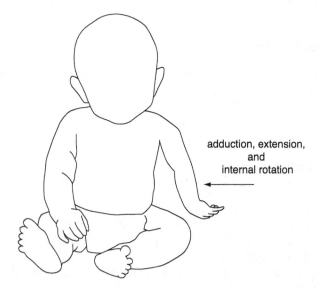

adduction, extension, and internal rotation

FIGURE 2-5. Erb palsy

Risk Factors

- Rupture of amniotic membranes for 18 hours or more.
- Chorioamnionitis.
- Intrapartum maternal fever.
- Maternal group B *Streptococcus* (GBS) colonization.
- Prematurity.
- Maternal UTI with gram-negative organisms is emerging as the common cause due to perinatal GBS prophylaxis.

Degree of functional return in birth brachial plexus injuries depends on the severity of the nerve injury (stretch, rupture, avulsion).

Group B *Streptococcus* (GBS)

- Major cause of severe systemic infection in neonates.
- Vertical transmission most important route of transmission.
- Two patterns of disease:
  - Early-onset disease (< 1 week of age):
    - Presents shortly after birth (usually < 12 hours) as sepsis, pneumonia, or meningitis.
    - Infants < 24 hours of age may not have fever.
    - Can be associated with persistent pulmonary hypertension of the newborn (PPHN).
  - Late-onset disease (1 week–3 months): Occurs after the first week of life and most often manifests as bacteremia without a source. The most common focal infection is meningitis (35%) and presents with bulging fontanelle, lethargy, irritability, vomiting, and seizures.
- Diagnosis is confirmed by GBS isolation from sterile body fluid (blood, cerebrospinal fluid).
- Empiric therapy with ampicillin and gentamicin should be started only if infant is symptomatic (ie, apnea, low temperature, feeding intolerance).
- If infant is asymptomatic, monitoring for 48 hours is sufficient since infant will typically show signs of infection within a 48-hour period.
- Intrapartum therapy with penicillin G does not prevent late onset disease but protects against early onset disease.

Twenty percent of pregnant women are colonized with GBS. It is recommended that all pregnant women be screened (vaginal, rectal swabs) at 35–37 weeks of gestation, and be given intrapartum antibiotics if positive.

Escherichia coli

- Principal cause of gram-negative sepsis and meningitis in newborn.
- Commonly colonize genitourinary (GU) and gastrointestinal (GI) tracts.
- Risk factors include maternal urinary tract infection (UTI) during last month of pregnancy in addition to previously mentioned risk factors.
- Clinical manifestations include sepsis, meningitis, UTI, pneumonia.
- Diagnosis is confirmed by *E coli* isolation from normally sterile body fluids.
- Treatment should be based on antibiotic sensitivity data, but a third-generation cephalosporin should be used as an empiric agent.
- *E coli* infection in the infant is common in infants with galactosemia.

Listeria monocytogenes

- Important cause of neonatal sepsis.
- Colonizes GU tract.
- Clinical manifestations include sepsis and meningitis.
- Diagnosis is confirmed by *L monocytogenes* isolation from sterile body fluid.
- Treatment is with penicillin or ampicillin.

Herpes Simplex

Cesarean section is performed for women with primary genital herpes and vaginal lesions in late gestation.

- Prevalence rate for adults with genital herpes is about 20%.
- Risk of neonatal disease is much higher with primary maternal infection (44%), and only 3% for a recurrent one.
- Ninety percent of neonatal infection is acquired through infected secretions during birth.
- There are three distinct patterns of disease:
  - Cutaneous disease:
    - Involves skin, mouth, and eyes.
    - Vesicular eruptions appear around 7–10 days of life, usually on presenting part.
    - If not recognized promptly, can progress to disseminated disease.
  - Encephalitic disease:
    - Occurs at second to third week of life.
    - Clinical signs include lethargy, irritability, poor suck, seizures.
    - Cutaneous lesions may be absent.
  - Disseminated disease:
    - Sepsis-like clinical picture (apnea, irritability, hypotonia, hypotension).
    - Cutaneous lesions may be absent.

DIAGNOSIS

- HSV can be isolated in cell culture from skin lesions or nasopharyngeal swabs.
- Polymerase chain reaction (PCR) is a sensitive tool for HSV detection.

TREATMENT

- Acyclovir is very effective in treatment of HSV infection.
- Course of treatment is often prolonged (21 days) for encephalitic and disseminated forms.

Chlamydia

A 3-week-old infant presents with paroxysmal cough and tachypnea, but no fever; bilateral diffuse crackles, hyperinflation, and patchy infiltrates on x-ray; he had conjunctivitis at 10 days of age. *Think: Chlamydia trachomatis.*

The incubation period of chlamydial conjunctivitis is between 5 and 14 days; usually manifests later than gonococcal conjunctivitis (occurs 2–5 days after birth). It is commonly acquired from the birth canal during delivery. It is the most common infectious cause of conjunctivitis in the neonates. Generally, gonococcal conjunctivitis usually has a more rapid and progressive course than *Chlamydia.*

- Acquired during passage through the birth canal of an infected mother.
- Causes conjunctivitis (few days to several days) and pneumonia (between 3 and 19 weeks).
- Characteristic "staccato" cough may not be evident in newborn infants, and may present with frequent apneic episodes.

DIAGNOSIS

Culture.

TREATMENT

Erythromycin orally for 14 days.

Erythromycin use has been associated with development of pyloric stenosis.

Syphilis

- Results from transplacental transfer of *Treponema pallidum*.
- Common features include intermittent fever, osteitis and osteochondritis, hepatosplenomegaly, lymphadenopathy, persistent rhinitis ("snuffles"), and a maculopapular rash involving the palms and the soles.
- Late manifestations include a saddle nose deformity, saber shins, frontal bossing, Hutchison teeth and mulberry molars, sensorineural, and Clutton's joints (painless joint effusions).

DIAGNOSIS

- Rapid plasma reagin (RPR) titers and the flourescent treponemal antibody-absorption test (FTA-ABS).
- Treponemes can also be seen on darkfield microscopy of nasal discharge.

TREATMENT

Penicillin G.

HIV

- Up to 25% of pediatric human immunodeficiency virus (HIV) infection results from maternal-fetal vertical transmission.
- Transmission from infected breast milk can occur; however, exclusively breast-fed infants have lower transmission rates.
- Clinical features in the infant include persistent thrush, lymphadenopathy and hepatosplenomegaly, severe diarrhea, failure to thrive, and recurrent infections.
- Strategies to reduce transmission:
  - Maternal treatment with ZDV during pregnancy.
  - Consider elective C-section at 38 weeks when feasible.
  - Mothers who are HIV positive should be advised not to breast-feed due to risk of transmission.

Maternal treatment with zidovudine (ZDV) in the second trimester reduces the rate of transmission by > 70%.

DIAGNOSIS

Detection of p24 antigen in peripheral blood, PCR to detect viral nucleic acid in peripheral blood, and enzyme-linked immunosorbent assay (ELISA) for the detection of antibodies.

TREATMENT

Nutritional support, *Pneumocystis jiroveci* prophylaxis, antiviral therapy, and anti-infective agents for specific infections.

SELECTED PROBLEMS IN FULL-TERM INFANTS

Developmental Dysplasia of the Hip (DDH)

- Occurs in ~1 in 800 births.
- More common in white females with breech presentation, and is more likely to be unilateral and involve the left hip.
- Signs include asymmetry of the skin folds in the groin and shortening of the affected leg.
- Evaluation maneuvers:
  - Ortolani—abduction of the hips by using gentle inward and upward pressure over the greater trochanter.
  - Barlow—adduct the hips by using the thumb to apply outward and backward pressure; "clunking" of reduction and dislocation are elicited in patients with hip dislocation.
- Diagnosis is confirmed by ultrasound. Current American Academy of Pediatrics (AAP) guidelines ask for ultrasound only in female infants with breech presentation and a hip click.
- Can be treated with a special brace (Pavlik harness) or sometimes casting. See Musculoskeletal Disease/Orthopedics chapter.

Meconium Ileus/Aspiration

A full-term male infant was born after a prolonged second stage of labor and thick meconium at delivery. He was depressed at birth, requiring intubation and suction of the meconium from below the vocal cords. His condition improved quickly, and he was vigorous at 3 minutes of life. Apgar score was 3 and 7 at 1 and 5 minutes of life, respectively. He was doing well in the well-baby nursery until at 3 hours of life, when he was noted to have dusky episode and was transferred to the special care nursery where his O_2 saturation was noted to be 82% breathing room air. He was placed in oxyhood oxygen climbing up to 100% with borderline O_2 saturation in the mid-80s. He was intubated and started on mechanical ventilation. His chest x-ray is shown in the figure. What is the likely diagnosis and management of this infant?

The infant described has characteristic meconium aspiration syndrome as seen by nodular appearance of both lung fields on the chest x-ray. He is developing persistent pulmonary hypertension of the newborn (PPHN), management of which includes aggressive ventilation, inhaled nitric oxide, and close monitoring of the gas exchange. An echocardiogram is useful to provide details on the elevated pulmonary pressures as well as to rule out any cardiac defects. Infants are at risk of hypotension and shunting of pulmonary flow via the ductus arteriosus into the systemic circulation resulting in differential O_2 saturation in the upper and lower extremities and require pressor support (dopamine, dobutamine, epinephrine) to elevate systemic blood pressure to the level above pulmonary pressure to prevent hypotension and shunting.

> Delivery room management of a meconium-stained infant consists of nasopharyngeal suctioning before the delivery of the thorax. Infants with respiratory depression require intubation and tracheal suctioning.

- Meconium is the first intestinal discharge of a newborn infant and is composed of epithelial cells, fetal hair, mucus, and bile.
- Intrauterine stress may cause passage of meconium into the amniotic fluid, which can cause airway obstruction and a severe inflammatory response, → severe respiratory distress known as meconium aspiration syndrome.
- Meconium ileus occurs when meconium becomes obstructed in the terminal ileum; presentation is with failure to pass stool, abdominal distention, and vomiting.
- Infants with meconium ileus should be tested for cystic fibrosis.

Meconium ileus is the most common presentation of cystic fibrosis in the neonatal period.

Hypoxic/Ischemic Encephalopathy

- Hypoxic ischemic encephalopathy is an important cause of permanent damage to the cells of the CNS that occurs secondary to hypoxia (↓ oxygen delivery) and ischemia (↓ blood flow).
- Can be caused by maternal conditions (hypertension), placental insufficiency, severe neonatal blood loss, and overwhelming infection.
- Neurologic manifestations include hypotonia, coma, and seizures.
- It can result in death, cerebral palsy (CP), and mental retardation.
- Newer modalities of treatment include selective head cooling or whole body cooling, which are used at several tertiary care neonatal intensive care units (NICUs) in the United States.

Ninety percent of full-term infants pass their first stool within the first 24 hours of life.

Congenital Diaphragmatic Hernia (CDH)

- Associated with chromosomal abnormalities, low birth weight, and IUGR.
- Can be diagnosed on prenatal ultrasound (between 16 and 24 weeks).
- Signs and symptoms include respiratory distress immediately on delivery, tachypnea, poor breath sounds over affected side of chest (most commonly **left**), and scaphoid abdomen.
- Prenatally diagnosed diaphragmatic hernia in a neonate warrants an ex-utero intrapartum treatment (EXIT) procedure, where neonatologists and surgeons are present at delivery and infant is intubated and central extracorporeal membrane oxygenation (ECMO) catheters placed at the delivery of the head and neck.
- Respiratory distress is a cardinal sign in neonates with CDH.

Only 10% of patients with cerebral palsy have birth events associated with asphyxia; the cause of the majority of cases of CP remains unknown.

Jaundice

- Common causes of hyperbilirubinemia include ABO incompatibility, breast milk jaundice (see Nutrition chapter), Rh iso-immunization, and infection.
- **Conjugated hyperbilirubinemia (direct):**
  - When an infant's direct (conjugated) bilirubin is > 3 mg/dL or more than 20% of the total bilirubin.
  - Most common causes are idiopathic neonatal hepatitis (diagnosis of exclusion) and biliary atresia.
- **Unconjugated hyperbilirubinemia (indirect):**
  - When an infant's indirect (unconjugated) serum bilirubin level is > 10 mg/dL in term infants. Nomograms developed by AAP are used

High indirect serum bilirubin levels in the first 24 hours of life are never physiologic.

In neonates there is a cephalopedal progression of jaundice; approximate levels for involvement:

- Head and neck: 4–8 mg/dL
- Upper trunk: 5–12 mg/dL
- Lower trunk and thighs: 8–16 mg/dL
- Arms and lower legs: 11–18 mg/dL
- Palms and soles: > 15 mg/dL

Early diagnosis of hypothyroidism and treatment with thyroid hormone prior to 3 months of age can greatly improve intellectual outcome.

to plot bilirubin levels and to categorize infants into low or high risk group and need for treatment.

- Most common cause of neonatal jaundice, seen in up to 50% of neonates.
- Secondary to ↑ bilirubin load, defective uptake and conjugation, and impaired excretion into bile.
- Physiologic hyperbilirubinemia is seen after the first 24 hours of life, peaks at 3 days, and resolves over 2 weeks.
- **Kernicterus:**
  - Bilirubin neurotoxicity secondary to persistently elevated bilirubin levels, which exceed albumin-binding capacity of the blood resulting in deposition of bilirubin in the basal ganglia.
  - This can result in subtle neurologic deficits, hearing loss, profound encephalopathy, and death.
- Treatment is initiated to prevent kernicterus.
  - Phototherapy with blue-green light converts bilirubin in skin to non-toxic isomers that are excreted without conjugation.
  - Elevated bilirubin levels (12–20 mg/dL) are usually treated with phototherapy.
  - Exchange transfusion should be considered at higher levels (20–25 mg/dL).

Neonatal Screening

- Available for various genetic, metabolic, hematologic, and endocrine disorders.
- All states have screening programs, although specific tests required vary.
- Tests performed on heel puncture include those for hypothyroidism, galactosemia, adrenal hyperplasia, cystic fibrosis, phenylketonuria, and other organic acid and aminoacidopathies.

Auditory Screening

- Hearing impairment can affect speech and language development and occurs in 5 in 1000 births.
- All infants should be screened with otoacoustic emission hearing testing.

Prematurity

DEFINITIONS

- Premature infant: Live-born newborn delivered prior to 37 weeks from the first day of last menstrual period.
- Low birth weigh (LBW): < 2500 g.
- **Very low birth weight (VLBW): 1500 g.**
- **Extremely low birth weight (ELBW): < 1000 g.**
- Extremely low gestational age neonate (ELGAN): < 750 g and/or gestational age 26 weeks.

ETIOLOGY

- Most premature births have no identifiable causes.
- Identifiable contributors include maternal, fetal, and obstetric:
  - Maternal:
    - Low socioeconomic status.
    - Preeclampsia.
    - Infections (urinary tract infections, group B streptococcus, etc).
    - Chronic medical illness (hypertension, renal disease, diabetes, cyanotic heart disease, etc).
    - Drug use.
  - Fetal:
    - Multiple gestation.
    - Fetal distress (from hypoxia, etc).
    - Congenital anomalies.
  - Obstetric:
    - Incompetent cervix.
    - Polyhydramnios.
    - Chorioamnionitis.
    - Premature rupture of membranes.
    - Placenta previa and abruptio placenta.

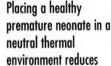

Placing a healthy premature neonate in a neutral thermal environment reduces calories burned.

COMMON PROBLEMS IN PREMATURE NEWBORNS

Respiratory Distress Syndrome (RDS; Hyaline Membrane Disease of the Newborn)

ETIOLOGY/PATHOPHYSIOLOGY

- Occurs secondary to insufficiency of lung surfactant due to immaturity of surfactant producing type 2 alveolar cells.
- Alveoli are small, inflate with difficulty, and do not remain gas-filled between inspirations.
- Rib cage is weak and compliant.
- High surface tension and propensity for alveolar collapse.
- Alveolar collapse results in progressive atelectasis, intrapulmonary shunting, hypoxemia, and cyanosis.

EPIDEMIOLOGY

- Usually seen in infants < 32 weeks' gestational age, but has been seen in full-term infants, especially when the mother has maternal diabetes.
- The incidence of RDS is inversely proportional to gestational age.

SIGNS AND SYMPTOMS

- Seen within the first 4 hours of life.
- Tachypnea.
- Grunting.
- Cyanosis.

DIAGNOSIS

Chest x-ray with fine, diffuse reticulogranular or "ground glass" pattern and air bronchograms (see Figure 3-1).

TREATMENT

- Aggressive respiratory support, including oxygen, continuous positive airway pressure (CPAP), intubation, and mechanical ventilation.
- To ↓ barotrauma, novel methods of ventilation are sometimes used—high-frequency oscillation, jet ventilation, and liquid ventilation.
- Exogenous surfactant replacement (instillation via endotracheal tube) has dramatically reduced mortality in infants with RDS.

Bronchopulmonary Dysplasia (BPD)

DEFINITION

- Chronic lung disease that develops in preterm neonates treated with oxygen and positive-pressure ventilation.
- Need for supplemental oxygen beyond 28 days of life.
- Characterized by squamous metaplasia and hypertrophy of small airways.

Production of surfactant can be accelerated by maternal steroid (betamethasone) administration; best if given 24–48 hours prior to delivery.

Most of these neonates also receive antibiotics because clinically and radiographically RDS and congenital pneumonia are indistinguishable.

Antenatal steroids have shown to reduce the incidence of RDS.

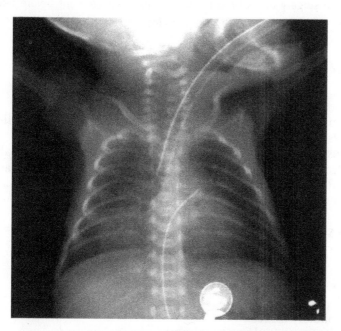

FIGURE 3-1. Chest x-ray demonstrating "ground glass" infiltrates consistent with respiratory distress syndrome (with a more focal area of infiltrate or atelectasis in the medial right lung base).

Etiology

- Multifactorial.
- Lung immaturity.
- Prolonged mechanical ventilation.
- Barotrauma (from mechanical ventilation).
- Oxygen toxicity to the lungs.

Diagnosis

Chest x-ray with hyperaeration and atelectasis.

Treatment

- Supplemental oxygen as needed.
- Oral steroids.
- Bronchodilators.

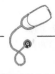

Necrotizing Enterocolitis (NEC)

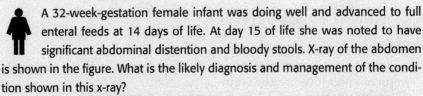

A 32-week-gestation female infant was doing well and advanced to full enteral feeds at 14 days of life. At day 15 of life she was noted to have significant abdominal distention and bloody stools. X-ray of the abdomen is shown in the figure. What is the likely diagnosis and management of the condition shown in this x-ray?

X-ray of this infant is consistent with necrotizing enterocolitis with evident pneumatosis (free air within the bowel wall) in the descending colon area. Management includes serial x-rays to detect perforation of the bowel wall, which requires immediate surgery to seal the bowel. Medical management before perforation includes NPO, IV fluids, and IV antibiotics for a period of 14 days.

The most common gastrointestinal emergency in the premature infants.

Etiology

- Seen primarily in premature infants, but can occur in full-term neonates (5–25%).
- Caused by bowel ischemia and bacterial invasion of intestinal wall.
- More common in premature infants treated with indomethacin for patent ductus arteriosus. Indomethacin may cause splanchnic vasoconstriction.

Signs and Symptoms

- Intolerance of oral feeding (vomiting, bilious aspirates, and large volume residue in stomach).
- Abdominal distention.
- Temperature instability.
- Respiratory distress.
- Acidosis, sepsis, shock.

Diagnosis

- Distended loops of bowel.
- Abdominal x-ray with "pneumatosis intestinalis"—air bubbles within the bowel wall (see Figure 3-2).

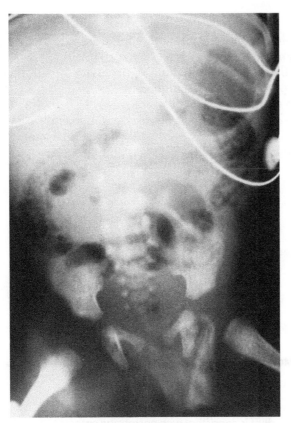

FIGURE 3-2. Necrotizing enterocolitis.

Distended loops of bowel and pneumatosis intestinalis.

An absolute indication for operative intervention in NEC is pneumoperitoneum.

Most common complication is stricture.

- Air in portal vein.
- Free air under diaphragm (in case of perforation).
- Occult blood in stool.

TREATMENT

- Discontinue feeds.
- Nasogastric decompression.
- Intravenous fluids.
- Antibiotics.
- Surgery (bowel necrosis, intestinal perforation, pneumoperitoneum, failure of medical treatment).

Retinopathy of Prematurity (ROP)

Disease that affects immature vasculature in the eyes of premature infants.

ETIOLOGY

- Caused by proliferation of immature retinal vessels due to excessive use of oxygen.
- Can → retinal detachment and blindness in severe cases.
- Multifactorial; the number one cause has been noted to be hyperoxia.
- Characterized by neovascularization of retina and vascular congestion that can → retinal detachment and ↓ visual acuity in severe cases.

Currently, severe retinopathy of prematurity is rare due to judicious use of oxygen.

All infants < 1500 g birth weight or younger than 32 weeks' gestational age at birth are at risk of developing ROP.

DIAGNOSIS

- All very-low-birth-weight infants should be screened for ROP with an ophthalmoscopic exam.
- An ophthalmology evaluation is necessary in all premature infants < 1500 g, < 32 weeks' gestation.
- First eye exam:
  - At 27–28 weeks (for 23–24 weeks' gestational age).
  - At 4th or 5th week (> 25–28 weeks' gestational age).
  - Before discharge (> 29 weeks' gestational age).

TREATMENT

Laser surgery may be needed in severe cases.

Intraventricular Hemorrhage (IVH)

DEFINITION

- Rupture of germinal matrix blood vessels due to hypoxic or hypotensive injury.
- Most IVHs occur within 72 hours after birth.

PREDISPOSING FACTORS

- Prematurity.
- RDS.
- Hypo- or hypervolemia.
- Shock.
- Bleeding disorders.

SIGNS AND SYMPTOMS

- Most are asymptomatic.
- Apnea.
- Hypertension or hypotension.
- Changes in muscle tone.
- Lethargy.
- Poor suck.
- Seizure.
- Bulging fontanelle.

DIAGNOSIS

Cranial ultrasound (through anterior fontanelle).

TREATMENT

- Directed toward correction of underlying conditions (RDS, shock, etc).
- In cases of associated hydrocephalus, placement of ventriculoperitoneal shunt may be required.
- Prognosis is dependent on the grade of IVH:
  - Grades I and II: Good outcome.
  - Grade III: Significant cognitive impairment.
  - Grade IV: Major neurologic problems.

All premature, very-low-birth-weight infants should have a cranial ultrasound in the first week of life to look for intraventricular hemorrhage.

- Disorders related to prematurity and low birth weight (BW) are the leading cause of neonatal death.
- Only 20% of neonates with BW of 500–600 g survive.
- Survival of infant with BW of 1250–1500 g is ~ 90%.
- There is no worldwide, universal gestational age that defines viability.
- In the United States, chance of normal survival is 50% after 24 weeks.

SPECIAL NEEDS OF EX-PREEMIES

- Heat loss: ↑ susceptibility to heat loss (high body surface area-to-body weight ratio, ↓ brown fat stores, nonkeratinized skin, and ↓ glycogen supply). Minimize heat loss by:
  - Warmed blankets or cellophane wrap.
  - Plastic film over the baby immediately after drying.
- Hypoglycemia.
- Fluid and electrolyte imbalance.
- Hyperbilirubinemia.
- Due to their bronchopulmonary dysplasia, ex-preemies can experience recurrent wheezing episodes and severe course of respiratory infections, especially respiratory syncytial virus (RSV).
- Due to ↑ work of breathing and "catch-up" growth, ex-preemies should receive high-calorie diet to allow for this additional caloric expenditure.
- Routine vaccination should be given based on postnatal (not gestational) age.
- Early identification and intervention is needed for infants with developmental problems.

Ex-preemies can receive RSV prophylaxis with RSV monoclonal antibodies during RSV season (IM injections once a month).

Premature infants have proportionally more fluid in the extracellular fluid compartment than the intracellular compartment and are at risk for fluid and electrolyte imbalance.

Optimal parenteral nutrition can be achieved by total parenteral nutrition (TPN)—specialized solution consisting of amino acids, dextrose, minerals, and electrolytes.

Breast milk is the best choice for enteral feeding for premature infants.

HIGH-YIELD FACTS

PREMATURITY

Growth and Development

- Understanding normal growth patterns of childhood is important because it is an indication of the overall health of a child.
- Growth is influenced by both genetics and environment.

Growth Charts

- Height, weight, and head circumference are plotted on growth curves to compare the patient to the population.
- Growth charts compare individual children with the 5th, 10th, 25th, 50th, 75th, 90th, and 95th percentiles.
- Serial plotting of a patient's growth allows the clinician to observe patterns of growth over time.
- Body mass index (BMI) is plotted on growth curves for males and females from 2 to 20 years of age. BMI above 85% classifies as overweight and above 95% as obese.
- Potential limitations of particular growth charts include possible development from small population sizes, ethnic differences, and whether they represent growth potential versus proper care and feeding.
- Specialized charts exist for children who are premature (Babson), have Down syndrome, myelomeningocele, Prader-Willi syndrome, cerebral palsy, or Williams syndrome.

Early Growth Trends

- A term infant regains birth weight by 2 weeks.
- During the first 3 months, a child is expected to gain 20 to 30 g/day or close to 1 kg/month.
- A child doubles birth weight by the fifth month of life and triples by his or her first birthday.
- Growth chart recording should be adjusted for gestational age until the infant is 2 years old.
- Children with genetic short stature may have normal length and weight at birth but their growth percentiles decline within the first 2–3 years.
- Appetite normally ↓ in the second year of life coincident with the slowing of the growth rate.

Intrauterine Factors

- Insulin-like growth factor (IGF) is important for fetal growth.
- Growth hormone and IGF are both important for postnatal growth.
- Thyroid hormone is important for central nervous system (CNS) development, but not important for fetal growth.
- Fetal weight gain is greatest during the third trimester.
- Teratogens, TORCH infections (toxoplasmosis, other [hepatitis B, syphilis, varicella-zoster virus], rubella, cytomegalovirus, herpes simplex virus/human immunodeficiency virus), and chromosomal abnormalities (trisomy 21, Turner syndrome) can impair fetal growth.

Having only one point on a growth chart is like having no point; the trend over time is what is important.

In the normal child, the greatest growth occurs in the first year of life.

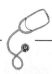

Carefully plotting on a growth chart is the most accurate method by which to follow a child's physical growth.

Teeth

- By age 2½, children should have all of their primary teeth including their second molars.
- Central incisors are first to erupt, between 5 and 8 months.
- Second molars are last to erupt, between 20 and 30 months.
- Secondary (permanent) teeth begin to erupt by age 6–7 years.
- Early or late tooth eruption may be within normal limits, though it can be an indicator of a nutritional, genetic, or metabolic problem.
- Delayed eruption:
  - Endocrine disorders (hypothyroidism).
  - Genetic abnormalities (Down syndrome).

SPECIFIC GROWTH PROBLEMS

Microcephaly

DEFINITION

Head circumference > 3 standard deviations below the mean for age and sex.

ETIOLOGY

- Genetic (familial, isolated).
- Syndromic:
  - Chromosomal: Trisomy 21, 13, 18.
  - Contiguous gene deletion: Cri-du-chat syndrome, Williams syndrome.
  - Single-gene defects: Cornelia de Lange syndrome, Smith-Lemli-Opitz syndrome.
- Prenatal insults (radiation, alcohol, hydantoin, TORCH infections, maternal phenylketonuria [PKU] and maternal diabetes, ↓ placental blood flow).
- Perinatal hypoxic-ischemic encephalopathy.
- Structural malformation (eg, lissencephaly),

Measure parents' and siblings' head circumference to check for familial cause of microcephaly.

IMPACT

A small brain predisposes to cognitive/motor delay, mental retardation, and seizures.

Weight is affected first in FTT, followed by height and head circumference.

Macrocephaly

DEFINITION

Head circumference > 3 standard deviations above the mean.

ETIOLOGY

- Familial in 50% of cases.
- Hydrocephalus.
- Other causes: Large brain (megalencephaly), cranioskeletal dysplasia, Sotos syndrome.

Psychosocial reasons account for most cases of FTT in the United States.

Signs of FTT:
SMALL KID
Subcutaneous fat loss
Muscle atrophy
Alopecia
Lagging behind norms
Lethargy
Kwashiorkor/marasmus
Infection
Dermatitis

Failure to Thrive (FTT)

DEFINITION

FTT is defined as a weight below the third percentile or a fall off the growth chart by two percentiles.

ETIOLOGY

- Organic causes include disease of any organ system.
- Nonorganic causes include abuse, neglect, and improper feeding (see Table 4-1).

SIGNS AND SYMPTOMS

- Expected age norms for height and weight not met.
- Hair loss.
- Loss of muscle mass.
- Subcutaneous fat loss.
- Dermatitis.
- Lethargy.
- Recurrent infection.
- Kwashiorkor—protein malnutrition.
- Marasmus—inadequate nutrition.

DIAGNOSIS

- Detailed history:
  - Gestation, labor, and delivery.
  - Neonatal problems (feeding or otherwise).
  - Breast-feeding mother's diet and medications.
  - Types and amounts of food, who prepares and how the formula or food is prepared, who feeds.
  - Vomiting, diarrhea, infection.
  - Sick parents or siblings.
  - Major family life events/chronic stressors.
  - Travel outside the United States.
  - Any injuries to child.
- Observation of parent-child interactions, especially at feedings, is critical for diagnosis.
- Lack of weight gain after adequate caloric feedings is characteristic of nonorganic failure to thrive.
- Screening tests for common causes include complete blood count (CBC), electrolytes, blood urea nitrogen (BUN), creatinine, and albumin and thyroid-stimulating hormone (TSH).

Organic versus nonorganic FTT is best distinguished by a detailed history and physical exam.

TREATMENT

- If a nonorganic cause is suspected or the child is severely malnourished, hospitalization may be required.
- If organic, treat the cause.

PROGNOSIS

FTT during the first year of life has a poor outcome due to the rapid growth of the brain during the first 6 months.

TABLE 4-1. Etiology of FTT

Gastrointestinal

Nutritional
- Kwashiorkor
- Marasmus
- Zinc/iron deficiency

Feeding Disorder
- Oral-motor apraxia
- Cleft palate
- Dentition disorder

Vomiting
- Gastrointestinal reflux
- Structural anomalies
- Pyloric stenosis
- Central nervous system (CNS) lesions
- Hirschsprung disease

Diarrhea
- Chronic toddler diarrhea
- Milk protein allergy/intolerance
- Infectious
  - Bacterial
  - Parasitic
- Malabsorption
  - Cystic fibrosis
  - Celiac disease
  - Inflammatory bowel disease

Pulmonary
- Tonsillar hypertrophy
- Cystic fibrosis
- Bronchopulmonary dysplasia
- Asthma
- Structural abnormalities
- Obstructive sleep apnea

Renal
- Chronic pyelonephritis
- Renal tubular acidosis
- Fanconi syndrome
- Chronic renal insufficiency
- Urinary tract infection
- Diabetes insipidus

Endocrine
- Hypothyroidism
- Rickets
- Vitamin D deficiency
- Vitamin D resistance
- Hypophosphatemia
- Growth hormone resistance/deficiency
- Adrenal insufficiency/excess
- Parathyroid disorders
- Diabetes mellitus

CNS
- Pituitary insufficiency
- Diencephalic syndrome
- Cerebral palsy
- Cerebral hemorrhages
- Degenerative disorders

Congenital
- Inborn errors of metabolism
- Trisomy 13, 18, 21
- Russell-Silver syndrome
- Prader-Willi syndrome
- Cornelia de Lange syndrome
- Perinatal infection
- Fetal alcohol syndrome

Other
- Prematurity
- Oncologic disease/treatment
- Immunodeficiency
- Collagen vascular disease
- Lead poisoning

Nonorganic Causes
- Child neglect/abuse
- Poverty
- Lack of true caregivers
- Mental illness within the family
- Marital discord/spousal abuse in the home

Hepatic
- Chronic hepatitis
- Glycogen storage disease

Infectious
- Tuberculosis
- HIV

Cardiac
- Congenital heart malformations

A child smiles spontaneously, babbles, sits without support, reaches, and feeds herself a cookie but has no pincer grasp. What is her approximate age? *Think: 8–9 months* (immature pincer grasp at 10 months). Fine pincer grasp of an object between the thumb and forefinger generally develops at 12 months of age.

- Attainment of developmental milestones is an indicator of a child's overall neurologic function.
- Maturation of intellectual, social, and motor function should occur in a predictable manner.
- It is essential that the physician recognize normal patterns in order to identify deviations.

Developmental Milestones

- Each new motor, language, and social skill should be acquired during an expected age range in a child's life.
- Each new skill is built on an earlier skill, and skills are rarely skipped (see Table 4-2).

TABLE 4-2. **Developmental Milestones**

AGE	MOTOR	LANGUAGE	SOCIAL	OTHER
1 month	Reacts to pain	Responds to noise	Regards human face Establishes eye contact	
2 months	Eyes follow object to midline **Head up prone**	Vocalizes Coos by 3 months	Social **smile** Recognizes parent	
4 months	Eyes follow object past midline **Rolls over**	**Laughs and squeals**	**Regards hand**	

6 months	**Sits well unsupported**
	Transfers objects hand to
	  hand (switches hands)
	Rolls prone to supine
		Babbles	Recognizes strangers	6abbles (babbles)
				Six strangers *switch*
				  sitting at *six months*

9 months	**Pincer grasp, immature (10
	  months)**
	Crawls
	Cruises (walks holding
	  furniture)
		Mama/dada,
		  nonspecific
		Bye-bye
			Starts to explore
			Stranger anxiety
				Can crawl, therefore can
				  explore
				It takes 9 months to be a
				  "mama"
				Pinches furniture to walk

TABLE 4-2. **Developmental Milestones** *(continued)*

12 months	**Walks with one hand held** Throws object	Mama/dada specific and knows **1–3 words** **Follows one-step command with gesture**		Walking away from mom causes anxiety Knows 1 word at 1 year
2 years	**Walks up and down stairs** Copies a line **Runs** **Kicks ball**	**2–3-word phrases** One half of speech is understood by strangers Refers to self by name **Pronouns**	Parallel play	Puts 2 words together at 2 At age 2, ⅔ (½) of speech understood by strangers
3 years	**Copies a circle** **Pedals a tricycle** Can build a bridge of 3 cubes Repeats 3 numbers	Speaks in sentences Three fourths of speech is understood by strangers Recognizes 3 colors	Group play **Plays simple games** Knows gender Knows first and last name	*Tri*cycle, 3 cubes, 3 numbers, 3 colors, 3 kids make a group At age 3, ¾ of speech understood by strangers
6 years	Draws a person with 6 parts Ties shoes	Identifies left and right		At 6 years: *skips, shoes, person with 6 parts*
4 years	Identifies body parts Copies a cross Copies a square (4.5 years) **Hops on one foot**	Speech is completely understood by strangers Uses past tense **Tells a story**	Plays with kids, social interaction	Song "head, shoulder, knees, and toes," 4 parts reminds you that at age 4 body parts can identify
4 years	**Throws overhand**			At age 4, ⅘ of speech is understood by strangers When using past tense, speaks of things that happened be*fore* If a 2-year-old can copy one line, a 4-year-old can copy two lines to draw a cross and a square, which has 4 sides
5 years	Copies a triangle Catches a ball Skips with alternating feet Partially dresses self	Writes name Counts 10 objects		

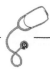

For age adjustment between birth and 2 years, subtract the number of weeks of prematurity from the chronological age. For an 18-month-old baby who is an ex-preemie at 30 weeks, the difference from full term at 40 weeks is 10 weeks, so the corrected age is 18 months minus 10 weeks = 15½ months.

Neurologic Development

- Myelination of the nervous system begins midgestation and continues until 2 years of age.
- Myelination occurs in an orderly fashion, from head to toe (cephalo-caudal).
- Brain at birth weighs approximately 10% of the newborn's body weight (adult brain, 2% of body weight).
- Primitive reflexes are present after birth and diminish by 6 months (see Table 4-3).

Age Adjustment for Preterm Infants

- Preterm infants may differ from full-term infants with regard to development.
- Age correction should be done until the child is 24 months old for children born more than 2 weeks early.
- Use the corrected age when assessing developmental progress and growth.

TABLE 4-3. Primitive Reflexes

REFLEX	TIMING	ELICIT	RESPONSE
Moro	Birth to 5–6 months	While supine, allow head to suddenly fall back approximately 3 cm	Symmetric extension and adduction, then flexion, of limbs
Startle	Birth to 5–6 months	Startle	Arms and legs flex immediately
Galant	Birth to 2–6 months	While prone, stroke the paravertebral region of the back	Pelvis will move in the direction of the stimulated side
Sucking	Becomes voluntary at 3 months	Stimulate lips	Sucks
Babinski	Birth to 4 months	Stroke from toes to heel	Fanning of toes
Tonic neck	Birth to 6–7 months	While supine, rotate head laterally	Extension of limbs on chin side, and flexion of limbs on opposite side (fencing posture)
Rooting	Less prominent after 1 month	Stroke finger from mouth to earlobe	Head turns toward stimulus and mouth opens
Palmar/plantar grasp	Birth to 2–3 months	Stimulation of palm or plantar surface of foot	Palmar grasp/plantar flexion
Parachute	Appears at 9 months remains throughout life	Horizontal suspension and quick thrusting movement toward surface	Extension of extremities

An 18-month-old infant brought in for temper tantrums has normal gross and fine motor skills but lacks language development and is cooperative and alert on exam. *Think: Hearing loss.*

Screening for hearing in the newborn nursery before discharge has resulted in earlier detection of hearing loss. Hearing impairment impacts language development. Inattention may be the initial presentation. It can also affect behavior and academic achievement.

DEFINITION

- Performance significantly below average in a given skill area.
- Global developmental delay: Significant delay in two or more areas of development (gross or fine motor, speech and language, cognition, social and personal, and activities of daily living).
- Early detection of delay is important because brain development is most malleable in the early years of life.

ETIOLOGY

- Cerebral palsy.
- Mental retardation.
- Learning disabilities.
- Hearing and vision deficits.
- Autism.
- Neglect.
- Attention deficit/hyperactivity disorder (ADHD).
- Lack of exposure.

DIAGNOSIS

- The Denver Development Assessment Test (Denver II) is a screening tool intended to be performed at well-child visits to identify children with developmental delay.
  - For children up to the age of 6 years.
  - Evaluates personal-social, fine motor, gross motor, and language skills.
- Clinical Adaptive Test (CAT)/Clinical Linguistic Auditory and Milestone Scale (CLAMS) rates problem solving, visual motor ability, and language development from birth to 36 months of age.
- Early intervention is important because the younger children are treated, the better the outcome.

- Present in 3–10% of children.
- To make a diagnosis of learning disability, the child must have a normal IQ.

Developmental Evaluation

12 months: No babbling and no gesture

16 months: No single word

24 months: No two-word phrase

At age 1 year, a child uses one word and follows a one-step command.

At age 2 years, a child uses two- to three-word phrases and follows two-step commands, and others can understand half of the child's language.

At age 3 years, a child uses three-word sentences, and others can understand three fourths of the child's language.

At age 4 years, a child should be 40 lbs. and 40 inches tall, and be able to draw a four-sided figure.

- Include difficulties with reading (dyslexia), arithmetic (dyscalculia), and writing (dysgraphia).
  - Dyslexia is one of the most common learning disabilities.
  - Failure to acquire reading skills in the usual time course.
  - These children have excellent spoken language.
  - Presents with different degrees of severity.

SLEEP PATTERNS

- Infants sleep 18 hours per day, with 50% rapid eye movement (REM) sleep, compared to an adult with 20% REM sleep.
- By age 4 months, nighttime sleep becomes consolidated.
- Two sleep stages are REM (irregular pulse and time when dreaming occurs) and non-REM (deep sleep).
- Parasomnias (sleep disorders) begin near age 3 years.
- Nightmares occur during REM sleep—the child awakens in distress about a dream.
- Night terrors occur in non-REM sleep—the child appears awake and frightened but is not responsive, and then is amnestic about the event the next morning.
- Somnambulism (sleepwalking) occurs in non-REM sleep; most common in ages 4–8 years.
- Somniloquy (talking) is very common throughout life, sometimes accompanying night terrors and sleepwalking.

Nutrition

Term infants, due to loss of extracellular water and suboptimal caloric intake, may lose up to 10% of their birth weight in the first few days of life but regain their birth weight by the end of the second week.

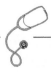

Don't put baby to sleep with a bottle; it can ↑ dental caries.

Breast milk predominant protein is whey (whey-to-casein ratio: 70:30).

Immunoglobulin A (IgA) accounts for 80% of the protein in colostrum.

Whole cow's milk is not recommended before 1 year of age, because an infant's gastrointestinal (GI) tract is not developed enough to digest (poor absorption), predisposing to allergy, → GI blood loss and iron deficiency.

Newborn Feeding Tips

- For term newborns, caloric requirement is 100–120 kcal/kg/day (as compared to 1-year-old, 75 kcal/kg/day).
- Newborns grow at a rate of about 30 g/day.
- Newborns usually begin feeding within the first 6 hours of life.
- Newborns should be breast- or formula-fed every 3–4 hours thereafter.
- *Supply = demand*—the more often the baby breast-feeds, the more milk will be produced.
- After a period of 4–6 months of exclusive breast-feeding the mother should begin to introduce solid foods into the child's diet.
- If the child has stopped losing weight by 5–7 days and begins to gain weight by 12–14 days, then feeding is adequate.
- Hunger is not the only reason infants cry. They don't need to be fed every time they cry.
- Human milk is ideal for a term infant in first year of life.
- Whole cow's milk is not suitable for infants because the higher intake of sodium, potassium, and protein ↑ renal solute load.
- Cow's milk can be introduced after the first birthday.
- Optimal protein requirement of term infant is 2.2 g/kg body weight per day.

Colostrum

- The first milk produced after birth.
- Usually a deep lemon color.
- Helps to clear bilirubin from the gut, produced from the high red blood cell turnover during blood volume contraction in the first weeks of life, which helps prevent jaundice.
- High in protein, minerals, immunologic factors, and antimicrobial peptides such as lactoferrin and lactoperoxidase; low in carbohydrates and fat.

Benefits of Breast-Feeding

- Infant:
  - ↓ incidence of infection (ie, otitis media, pneumonia, meningitis, bacteremia, diarrhea, urinary tract infection [UTI], botulism, necrotizing enterocolitis).
  - **Higher levels of immunologic factors**—immunoglobulins, complement, interferon, lactoferrin, lysozyme.
  - ↓ **exposure to enteropathogens.**
  - Other postulated benefits include higher IQ, better vision, ↓ risk of sudden infant death syndrome (SIDS), less fussy eaters.
  - ↓ incidence of chronic disease (type 1 diabetes, lymphoma, Crohn disease/ulcerative colitis [UC], allergies).
- Maternal:
  - ↑ maternal oxytocin levels.
  - ↓ postpartum bleeding.
  - More rapid involution of uterus.
  - Less menstrual blood loss.

- Delayed ovulation.
- Improved bone mineralization.
- ↓ risk of ovarian and breast cancer.
- Psychological benefits: ↑ maternal-child bonding.
- Other: Saves money for family and society, no risk of mixing errors, correct temperature, convenient, no preparation.

Common Problems with Breast-Feeding

- Soreness of nipples: Not due to prolonged feeding—due to improper positioning and poor removal.
- Engorgement: Unpleasant/painful swelling of the breasts when feeding cycle is ↓ suddenly (relieved by ↑ feeding on affected breast).
- Maternal fatigue, stress, and anxiety. Affects hormones needed for lactation.
- Fear of inadequate milk production, → formula milk supplementation.
- As the infant begins to feed less often, less milk is naturally produced. This often causes mother to misconceive that she is not producing enough milk to nourish the baby. Because of this, mother will frequently begin supplementing her milk with bottle milk, beginning a cycle of longer intervals between feeding, which causes less and less milk to actually be produced.
- Jaundice (see Table 5-1 and Gestation and Birth chapter).
- Possible vitamin deficiencies—A, D, K, B$_{12}$, thiamine, riboflavin.
- Infants who are exclusively breast-fed should receive vitamin drops after age 4 months.

Contraindications to Breast-Feeding

- Breast cancer.
- Cancer chemotherapy.
- Some medications (such as antimetabolites, chloramphenicol methimazole, tetracycline).
- Street drugs.
- Herpetic breast lesions.

TABLE 5-1. Breast-Feeding versus Breast Milk Jaundice

BREAST-FEEDING JAUNDICE	BREAST MILK JAUNDICE
Also called "not enough milk jaundice"—usually due to ↓ or poor milk intake.	Syndrome of prolonged unconjugated hyperbilirubinemia that is thought to be due to an inhibitor to bilirubin conjugation in the breast milk of some mothers.
Occurs *during* first week of life.	Begins *after* first week of life; peaks usually after second to third week.
Reduced enteral intake, → infrequent and scanty bowel movements and ↑ enterohepatic circulation of bilirubin.	Transient unless severe unconjugated hyperbilirubinemia.
	No treatment necessary.

Cow's milk predominant protein is casein (78%).

Breast-fed infant requires the following supplements:
- Vitamin K 1 mg IM at birth
- Vitamin D 400 IU/day
- Fluoride (after 6 months)
- Iron from 4 to 12 months

Tell the breast-feeding mother: If the baby doesn't let go, break the suction by inserting finger into corner of mouth; don't pull.

Breast-Feeding jaundice occurs in the First week. Breast Milk jaundice occurs Many weeks later.

Oral contraceptive is not a contraindication for breast-feeding.

Not every woman will feel "milk letdown" despite proper breast-feeding.

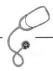

The common cold and flu are not contraindications to breast-feeding.

Most common cause of FTT is inadequate caloric intake.

Mastitis: Tender erythematous swelling of portion of breast usually associated with fever. Most common organism is *Staphylococcus*, transmitted from oropharynx of asymptomatic infant. Infant should continue to feed on affected breast.

Undernutrition has the greatest effect on brain development from 1 to 3 months of age.

- Untreated, active tuberculosis.
- Cytomegalovirus (CMV) infection.
- Human immunodeficiency virus (HIV) infection.
- In developing countries where food is scarce and HIV is endemic, the World Health Organization recommends breast-feeding by HIV-infected moms because the benefits outweigh the risks.
- Galactosemia: Infants with galactosemia should not ingest lactose-containing milk.

Signs of Insufficient Feeding of Infant

- Fewer than six wet diapers per day after age 1 week (before that, count one wet diaper per age in days for first week of life).
- Continual hunger, crying.
- Continually sleepy, lethargic baby.
- Fewer than seven feeds per day.
- Long intervals between feedings.
- Sleeping through the night without feeding.
- Loss of > 10% of weight.
- ↑ jaundice.

Reasons for Failure to Grow and Gain Weight

An 18-month-old African immigrant male is brought in by his parents for a health evaluation. The family members are refugees. As you examine the child, you find that he is in the bottom 2% in both height and weight and is thin looking. The parents deny any childhood illnesses and state that the child has never been severely ill. Blood tests including complete blood count, chemistry, and liver function tests are within normal limits, and albumin is 2.3. What is the diagnosis? Failure to thrive (FTT). It is a condition when physical growth of a child is below the 3rd or 5th percentile. Nonorganic or psychosocial FTT is more common. The laboratory evaluation is usually normal and should be obtained judiciously. Obtaining a detailed history is the most important part of evaluation, which helps to determine whether the cause is organic or nonorganic.

- Improper formula preparation.
- Use of skim and 2% milk before age 2.
- Prolonged used of diluted formula.
- Prolonged used of BRAT (bananas, rice, applesauce, toast) diet after illness.
- Excessive juice or water.
- Inappropriate feeding schedule.

Formula

- Types (see Table 5-2).
- Inappropriate formulas (see Table 5-3).
- Hydrolysate formula:
  - Formula with peptides: Nutramigen, Progestimil, Alimentum.
  - Formulas with free amino acids: Neocate, Elecare.

TABLE 5-2. Formulas

FORMULA	INDICATIONS	FORMULATIONS
Cow's milk based (Examples: Enfamil, Similac)	Premature	Lactose-free
	Transitional	Low electrolyte
		Low iron
		Whey hydrosylate
Soy protein based (Examples: Isomil, Prosobee)	Galactosemia	Carbohydrate free
	Lactose intolerance	Fiber-containing
		Sucrose free Lower whey-to-casein ratio
Protein hydrosylate	Malabsorption	
	Food allergies	
Amino acid based	Food allergies	
	Short gut	
High medium-chain triglyceride oil	Chylous ascites Chylothorax	
Metabolic		Lofenelac
		Phenex-1—phenylketonuria (PKU)
		Propimex-1—propionic acidemia

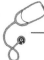

Anemia in infant receiving goat milk = megaloblastic anemia.

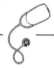

Feed at earliest sign of hunger; stop at earliest sign of satiety.

Predominant fat in preterm infant formula is medium-chain triglycerides.

Formula for an infant who is allergic to both cow milk and soy protein: Hydrolysate formula.

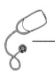

Do not give an infant under 6 months of age water or juice (water fills them up; juice contains empty calories, and excess sugar can cause diarrhea).

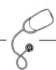

Do not use 2% milk before 2 years of age or skim milk before 5 years.

Solid Foods

- Solid food should be introduced between 4 and 6 months; introducing solids before this time does not contribute to a healthier child, nor does it help the infant to sleep better.
- New foods should be introduced individually and about a week apart; this is done to identify any allergies and intolerance the child may have. There are many suggested orders in which to introduce new food. A common one is vegetable first, green to orange, and then fruits, to introduce foods from most bland to sweetest.

Readiness for Solid Foods

- Hand-to-mouth coordination.
- ↓ tongue protrusion reflex.
- Sits with support.

HIGH-YIELD FACTS

NUTRITION

Typical formulas contain 20 kcal/ounce.

Avoid foods that are choking risks, including small fruits, raw vegetables, nuts, candy, and gum.

TABLE 5-3. Inappropriate Formulas

Cow's milk	↓ iron, essential fatty acids, vitamin E
	↑ sodium, potassium, chloride, and protein
Goat's milk	Allergen potential
	Very high potential renal solute load High protein
	Low in folate and iron
	Questionable pasteurization
Rice milk	Very low in protein and fat
	Low in electrolytes and almost all vitamins and minerals
Commercial soy milk (not soy formula)	Soy induces L-thyroxine depletion through fecal waste, creating an ↑ requirement for iodine, potentially → goiter

- Improved head control.
- Drooling.
- Opens mouth to spoon.

Caloric Requirements

Estimated average requirement: Basal metabolic rate × physical activity level (see Table 5-4).

TABLE 5-4. Daily Caloric Requirements

AGE	MALES (KCAL)	FEMALES (KCAL)
0–3 months	545	515
4–6 months	690	645
7–9 months	825	765
10–12 months	920	865
1–3 years	1230	1165
4–6 years	1715	1545
7–10 years	1970	1740
11–14 years	2220	1845
15–18 years	2755	2110

Physiologic Compartments

TOTAL BODY WATER (TBW)

TBW makes up 50–75% of the total body mass depending on age, sex, and fat content.

DISTRIBUTION

- Intracellular fluid accounts for two thirds of TBW and 50% of total body mass.
- Extracellular fluid accounts for one third of TBW and 25% of total body mass.

EXTRACELLULAR FLUID (ECF)

ECF is composed of plasma (intravascular volume) and interstitial fluid (ISF).

DEHYDRATION

- Definition: Body fluid depletion (see Table 5-5).
- Causes can be divided into two categories:
  - ↓ intake.
  - ↑ loss (e.g., vomiting, diarrhea).
- → hypovolemia, gradually affecting each organ system.

TABLE 5-5. Signs and Symptoms of Dehydration

	MILD	**MODERATE**	**SEVERE**
% Body weight loss	3–5%	6–9%	> 10%
General	Consolable	Irritable	Lethargic/obtunded
Heart rate	Regular	↑	More ↑
Blood pressure	Normal	Normal/low	Low
Tears	Normal	Reduced	None
Urine	Normal	Reduced	Oliguric/anuric
Skin turgor	Normal	Tenting	None
Anterior fontanel	Flat	Soft	Sunken
Capillary refill	< 2 sec	2–3 sec	> 3 sec
Mucous membranes	Moist	Dry	Parched/cracked

Neonates have a greater percentage of TBW per weight than do adults (about 70–75%).

You know a patient is dehydrated when he or she is **PARCHED:**
Pee, **P**ressure (blood)
Anterior fontanel
Refill, capillary
Crying
Heart rate
Elasticity of skin
Dryness of mucous membranes

Percentage of dehydration can be estimated using (pre-illness weight – illness weight / pre-illness weight) × 100%.

HIGH-YIELD FACTS

NUTRITION

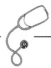

For convenience, use the Holliday-Segar method to determine maintenance intravenous (IVF) requirements:
- Give 100 mL/kg of water for the first 10 kg.
- For a child over 10 kg but under 20 kg, give 1000 mL + 50 mL/kg for each kilogram over 10 kg.

1 kg = 2.2 pounds

Calculations for fluid therapy are just estimates—you must monitor the success of fluid replacement by measuring ins and outs, body weight, and clinical picture (see Table 5-6).

4-2-1 IVF RULE: To determine rate in milliliters per hour, use 4 (for first 10 kg) × 10 kg + 2 (for second 10 kg) × 10 kg + 1 (for remainder) × remaining kg = 65 mL/hr.

Fluid Therapy

GOALS

Rapidly expand the ECF volume and restore tissue perfusion, replenish fluid and electrolyte deficits, meet the patient's nutritional needs, and replace ongoing losses.

METHODS

- Fluid requirements can be determined from caloric expenditure.
- For each 100 kcal metabolized in 24 hours, the average patient will require 100 mL of water, 2 to 4 mEq Na^+, and 2 to 3 mEq K^+.
- This method overestimates fluid requirements in neonates under 3 kg.
- For a child over 20 kg, give 1500 mL + 20 mL/kg for each kilogram over 20 kg.

MAINTENANCE

- Replacement of *normal* body fluid loss.
- Causes of normal fluid loss include:
  - Insensible fluid loss (ie, lungs and skin).
  - Urinary loss.
- Water requirements (mL/100 calories metabolized/day): Insensible— skin, 30; lungs, 15; stool, 5; urine, 50.

DEFICIT

- Replacement of *abnormal* fluid and electrolyte loss (ie, from vomiting, diarrhea, etc).
- Example: For a 25-kg patient, 100 (for first 10 kg) × 10 + 50 (for second 10 kg) × 10 + 20 (for remainder) × 10 = 1600 mL/day or 65 mL/hr when divided by 24 hours.

Deficit Therapy

HYPONATREMIA

In hypotonic (hyponatremic) dehydration, serum $Na^+ < 130$ mEq/L.

EPIDEMIOLOGY

- Most common electrolyte abnormality.
- More common in infants fed on tap water.

TABLE 5-6. Calculating Maintenance Fluids per Day

BODY WEIGHT (KG)	MILLILITERS PER DAY	MILLILITERS PER HOUR
0–10	100/kg	4/kg
11–20	1000 + 50/kg over 10	40 + 2/kg over 10
>20	1500 + 20/kg over 20	60 + 1/kg over 20

ETIOLOGY

- Hypervolemic hyponatremia—fluid retention:
  - Congestive heart failure (CHF).
  - Cirrhosis.
  - Nephrotic syndrome.
  - Acute or chronic renal failure.
- Hypovolemic hyponatremia—↑ sodium loss:
  - Due to renal loss:
    - Diuretic excess, osmotic diuresis, salt-wasting diuresis.
    - Adrenal insufficiency, pseudohypoaldosteronism.
    - Proximal renal tubular acidosis.
    - Metabolic alkalosis.
  - Due to extra-renal loss:
    - Gastrointestinal (GI)—vomiting, diarrhea, tubes, fistula.
    - Sweat.
    - Third-spacing—pancreatitis, burns, muscle trauma, peritonitis, effusions, ascites.
- Euvolemic hyponatremia:
  - Syndrome of inappropriate antidiuretic hormone secretion (SIADH):
    - Hospitalized children are at ↑ risk for nonphysiologic secretion of ADH.
    - Tumors.
    - Chest disorders.
    - Central nervous system (CNS) disorders—infection, trauma, shunt failure.
    - Drugs—vincristine, vinblastine, diuretics, carbamazepine, amitriptyline, morphine, isoproterenol, nicotine, adenine arabinoside, colchicine, barbiturates.
  - Glucocorticoid deficiency.
  - Hypothyroidism.
  - Water intoxication due to intravenous (IV) therapy, tap water enema, or psychogenic (excess water drinking).
  - Polydipsia.

SIGNS AND SYMPTOMS

- Symptoms may occur at serum concentrations of ≤ 125 mEq/L.
- Cerebral edema—more pronounced in acute.
- Early: Anorexia, nausea, headache.
- Mental status changes.
- Later: Beware of brain herniation—posturing, autonomic dysfunction, respiratory depression, seizures, and coma.
- Central pontine myelinolysis can occur if hyponatremia is corrected too quickly.

DIAGNOSIS

- Volume status.
- Acute versus chronic.
- Serum and urine osmolality and sodium concentration, blood urea nitrogen (BUN), creatinine, other labs (glucose, aldosterone, thyroid-stimulating hormone [TSH], etc).

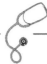

Hyponatremia can be factitious in the presence of high plasma lipids or proteins; consider the presence of another osmotically active solute in the ECF such as glucose or mannitol when hypotonicity is absent.

SIADH:
- Euvolemia
- Low urine output
- High urinary sodium loss
- Treat with fluid restriction

The rise in serum Na+ in the correction of chronic hyponatremia should not exceed 2 mEq/L/hr or cerebral pontine myelinosis may occur secondary to fluid shifts from the intracellular fluid.

The fluid deficit plus maintenance calculations generally approximate 5% dextrose with 0.45% saline; 6 mL/kg of 3% NaCl will raise the serum Na+ by 5 mEq/L.

Look for a low urine specific gravity (< 1.010) in diabetes insipidus. These patients appear euvolemic because most of the free water loss is from intracellular and interstitial spaces, not intravascular.

A hypervolemic hypernatremic condition can be caused by the administration of improperly mixed formula, or this may present as a primary hyperaldosteronism. Always demonstrate the proper mixing of formula to parents who use powdered preparations.

If the serum Na⁺ falls rapidly, cerebral edema, seizures, and cerebral injury may occur secondary to fluid shifts from the ECF into the CNS.

TREATMENT

- Na^+ deficit: (Na⁺ desired – Na⁺ observed) × body weight (kg) × 0.6.
- One half of the deficit is given in the first 8 hours of therapy, and the rest is given over the next 16 hours.
- Deficit and maintenance fluids are given together.
- If serum Na^+ is < 120 mEq/L and CNS symptoms are present, a 3% NaCl solution may be given IV over 1 hour to raise the serum Na^+ over 120 mEq/L.

HYPERNATREMIA

In hypertonic (hypernatremic) dehydration, serum Na^+ > 150 mEq/L.

ETIOLOGY

- ↓ water or ↑ sodium intake.
- ↓ sodium or ↑ water output.
- Diabetes insipidus (either nephrogenic or central) can cause hypernatremic dehydration secondary to urinary free water losses.
- Hypovolemic hypernatremia:
  - Extrarenal or renal fluid losses.
  - Adipsic hypernatremia is secondary to ↓ thirst—behavioral or damage to the hypothalamic thirst centers.
- Hypervolemic hypernatremia:
  - Hypertonic saline infusion.
  - Sodium bicarbonate administration.
  - Accidental salt ingestion.
  - Mineralocorticoid excess (Cushing syndrome).
- Euvolemic hypernatremia:
  - Extrarenal losses—↑ insensible loss.
  - Renal free water losses—central diabetes insipidus (DI), nephrogenic DI.

SIGNS AND SYMPTOMS

- Anorexia, nausea, irritability.
- Mental status changes.
- Muscle twitching, ataxia.

TREATMENT

- The treatment of elevated serum Na^+ must be done gradually at a rate of ↓ around 10–15 mEq/L/day.
- Usually, a 5% dextrose with 0.2% saline solution is used to replace the calculated fluid deficit over 48 hours after initial restoration of adequate tissue perfusion using isotonic solution.
- If the serum Na^+ deficit is not correcting, the free water deficit may be given as 4 mL/kg of free water for each milliequivalent of serum Na^+ over 145, given as 5% dextrose water over 48 hours.
- Too rapid correction of hypernatremia can result in cerebral edema.

HYPOKALEMIA

Can be considered at K^+ < 3.5 mEq/L, but is extreme when K^+ < 2.5 mEq/L.

HIGH-YIELD FACTS

NUTRITION

ETIOLOGY

Excess renin, excess mineralocorticoid, Cushing syndrome, renal tubular acidosis (RTA), Fanconi syndrome, Bartter syndrome, villous adenoma of the colon, diuretic use/abuse, GI losses, skin losses, diabetic ketoacidosis (DKA).

SIGNS AND SYMPTOMS

↓ peristalsis or ileus, hyporeflexia, paralysis, rhabdomyolysis, and arrhythmias including premature ventricular contractions (PVCs), atrial nodal or ventricular tachycardia, and ventricular fibrillation.

DIAGNOSIS

- Serum value.
- Electrocardiogram (ECG) may demonstrate flattened T waves, shortened PR interval, and U waves.

TREATMENT

- Consider cardiac monitor.
- **If potassium is dangerously low (< 2.5 mEq/L) and patient is symptomatic, IV potassium must be given.**
- Do not exceed the rate of 0.5 mEq/kg/hr.
- Oral potassium may be given to replenish stores over a longer period of time. Common forms of potassium include the chloride, phosphate, citrate, and gluconate salts.

Hypokalemia can precipitate digitalis toxicity.

For every 0.1-unit reduction in serum pH, there is an ↑ in serum K^+ of about 0.2–0.4 mEq/L.

HYPERKALEMIA

- Mild to moderate: K^+ = 6.0–7.0.
- Severe: K^+ > 7.0.

ETIOLOGY

Renal failure, hypoaldosteronism, aldosterone insensitivity, K^+-sparing diuretics, cell breakdown, metabolic acidosis, transfusion with aged blood.

SIGNS AND SYMPTOMS

Muscle weakness, paresthesias, tetany, ascending paralysis, and arrhythmias including sinus bradycardia, sinus arrest, atrioventricular block, nodal or idioventricular rhythms, and ventricular tachycardia and fibrillation.

DIAGNOSIS

- Serum value.
- ECG may demonstrate peaked T waves and wide QRS.

TREATMENT

- If hyperkalemia is severe or symptomatic, first priority is to stabilize the cardiac membrane. Administer calcium chloride or gluconate (10%) solution under close cardiac monitoring.
- Sodium bicarbonate, albuterol nebulizer, or glucose plus insulin can be given to shift K^+ to the intracellular compartment.
- Kayexalate resin can be given to bind K^+ in the gut (works the slowest).
- Furosemide can be given to enhance urinary K^+ excretion.
- In extreme cases, hemo- or peritoneal dialysis may be necessary.

Fluoride

- Supplement after age 6 months if the water is not fluorinated sufficiently (particularly well water).
- If < 3.3 ppm, supplement with 0.25 mg per day.
- Supplementation is recommended for the exclusively breast-fed infants.
- Deficiency: Dental caries.
- Excess: Fluorosis—mottling, staining, or hypoplasia of the enamel.
- Children under 2 years should not use fluoridated toothpaste, and then only a small pea-sized amount up to age 6 years.

Because of the ↑ risk for fluorosis, don't give fluoride supplements before age 6 months!

Most bottled water is not fluorinated.

Vitamin D

- Vitamin D is critical for skeletal development and cellular function because of its effect on calcium homeostasis (by promoting intestinal calcium absorption).
- Breast milk typically contains about 25 IU/L of vitamin D, which is insufficient for rickets prevention.
- Deficiency can occur if breast-feeding infant's mother has insufficient intake, infant's sun exposure is inadequate, or the infant is fed on whole cow's milk.
- Supplementation is with 400 IU/day.
- Deficiency: Impaired mineralization of bone tissue (osteomalacia) and of growth plates (rickets).
- Vitamin D deficiency can → hypocalcemia.

Iron

A 4-year-old female was brought in by EMS with a complaint from the mother that the child had a sudden onset of diarrhea and vomiting. The mother reports blood in the vomitus. On examination, the child is very irritable. She is breathing very rapidly, and her heart rate is 167 beats/min, with a blood pressure of 96/57 mm Hg. The mother states that she is a healthy child with no recent illnesses and is up to date on all her vaccinations. There has been no recent travel, and the child's 3-year-old brother is not ill. There has been no change in the child's diet. The mother states that she is very conscientious of the diets in the house, as she is trying to get pregnant again and is taking prenatal vitamins. What is the diagnosis? Iron overdose

Iron poisoning is one of the most fatal in children. Iron preparations are readily available due to their widely prescribed use in prenatal care. It is particularly attractive to young children because these brightly colored tablets appear similar to candy. In addition, often some iron preparations are coated with sucrose to make them palatable. Iron poisoning should be considered in a child with acute onset of vomiting and hypoperfusion. Serum iron levels should be obtained and are helpful in predicting the clinical course of the patient.

- Newborn iron stores are sufficient for 6 months in a term infant.
- Therefore, breast-fed infants need iron supplementation 1 mg/kg/day (ie, iron-fortified cereals and baby foods), beginning at 4 to 6 months.
- Preterm breast-fed infants should receive 2 mg/kg/day starting at 2 months of age.
- Deficiency: Anemia (hypochromic microcytic) and growth failure.
- Only iron-fortified formula should be used for weaning or for supplementing breast milk in children younger than 12 months.

Dark-skinned children are more likely to have inadequate sun exposure.

Vitamin K

- Human breast milk is deficient in vitamin K.
- Infant has a limited body store of vitamin K.
- Therefore, it is necessary to administer a 1-mg vitamin K IM injection at birth. Recommended for every newborn, not just breast-fed.
- Deficiency: Thought to contribute to hemorrhagic disease of the newborn.
- Vitamin K is necessary for the synthesis of clotting factors II, VII, IX, and X.
- Fat soluble: Requires bile salts for absorption.

Breast milk has less iron than cow's milk, but the iron in breast milk is more bioavailable.

Zinc

- Deficiency-associated intestinal malabsorption, nutritional intake limited to breast milk.
- Deficiency used to be associated with total parenteral nutrition (TPN); now formulas have zinc in them.
- Deficiency manifests as acrodermatitis, alopecia, and growth failure.

Vitamin A

A 14-month-old infant presents with anorexia, pruritus, and failure to gain weight; he has a bulging anterior fontanel and tender swelling over both tibias. The mother buys all food at a natural foods store. *Think: Hypervitaminosis A.*

Central nervous system, liver, bone, and skin and mucous membranes are the common sites. Acute vitamin A toxicity is not common. Initial presentation is primarily neurologic. Symptoms include irritability, tiredness, and somnolence. A bulging fontanel due to increased intracranial pressure may be present in infants. Pain and tenderness, particularly in the long bones, is often present.

- Hypervitaminosis A.
- Congenital absence of enzymes needed to convert provitamin A carotenoids to vitamin A.
- Acute:
    - Pseudotumor cerebri: Bulging fontanel, drowsiness, cranial nerve palsies.
    - Nausea, vomiting.

- Chronic:
  - Poor weight gain.
  - Irritability.
  - Tender swelling of bones—hyperostosis of long bones, craniotabes; ↓ mineralization of skull.
  - Pruritus, fissures, desquamation.

Other Supplements

- If mother is a strict vegetarian, supplement thiamine and vitamin B_{12}.
- Thiamine deficiency causes beriberi (weakness, irritability, nausea, vomiting, pruritus, tremor, possible congestive heart failure).
- Human milk will have adequate vitamin C only if mother's intake is sufficient.
- Commercial formula is often modified from cow's milk and fortified with vitamins and minerals so that no additional supplements are needed for the full-term infant.

> Vitamin A deficiency is the number 1 worldwide most common cause of blindness in young children.

OBESITY

A 16-year-old female presents to her primary care physician for a routine health visit. Upon questioning she states that she is very concerned about becoming overweight and that she goes to the gym often but wants nutritional advice. On examination, she is very thin and emaciated with very little subcutaneous fat, and you notice a thin layer of hair on her arms. She states that she is not sexually active and her last menstrual period was 4 months ago. What is the diagnosis? Anorexia nervosa

DEFINITION

- Overweight is defined as a body mass index (BMI)-for-age ≥ 95th percentile on the Centers for Disease Control and Prevention (CDC) growth charts.
- BMI is calculated by dividing weight (in kilograms) by height (in meters squared).
- Adults:
  - Normal BMI: 18.5–24.9 kg/m².
  - Overweight: 25.0–29.9 kg/m².
  - Obesity: 30.0–39.9 kg/m².
  - Extreme obesity: > 40 kg/m².
  - Obesity: BMI of ≥ 30.
- Children: "At risk for overweight": BMI 90th–95th percentile for age and sex.

RISK FACTORS

- Excessive intake of high-energy foods ("empty" calories).
- Inadequate exercise in relation to age and activity, sedentary lifestyle.
- Low metabolic rate relative to body composition and mass.
- Genetics: Strong relationship between BMI of children and their biologic parents:

- If one parent is obese, risk of obesity as an adult is 40%.
- If two parents are obese, risk of obesity as an adult is 80%.
  - Certain genetic disorders (Alström syndrome, Carpenter syndrome, Cushing syndrome, Fröhlich syndrome, hyperinsulinism, Laurence-Moon-Bardet-Biedl syndrome, muscular dystrophy, myelodysplasia, Prader-Willi syndrome, pseudohypoparathyroidism, Turner syndrome).

EPIDEMIOLOGY

Most often presents at ages 1 year, 4–5 years, and adolescence.

COMPLICATIONS

- Negative social attitudes: Embarrassment, harassment.
- Respiratory: Sleep apnea.
- Orthopedic: Slipped capital femoral epiphysis (SCFE).
- Metabolic: Type 2 diabetes mellitus.
- Cardiovascular: Hypertension, hyperlipidemia.

PREVENTION

- Early awareness and starting good eating and exercise habits early may hinder the development of overeating and obesity.
- Parent education is paramount in providing guidance in appropriate nutrition and feeding habits to promote healthy lifestyles for children.
- Certain cultures are more predisposed to overfeed children when children are upset.
- Newborns need all the nourishment they can get. They need to be fed on a continuous schedule and on demand.
- Within the first year, offer food only when the child is hungry.
- Have predictable eating schedules and offer child-sized portions using child-sized plates.
- Avoid using food as reward or punishment.

DIAGNOSIS

BMI is the most useful index for screening for obesity. It correlates well with subcutaneous fat, total body fat, blood pressure, blood lipid levels, and lipoprotein concentrations in adolescents.

TREATMENT

- Adherence to well-organized program that involves both a balanced diet and exercise.
- Behavioral modification.
- Involvement of family in therapy.
- Surgery and pharmacotherapy are relatively contraindicated in children.
- Very-low-calorie diets are detrimental to growth and development—all nutritional needs should be met.
- Avoid rapid ↓ in weight.
- Goal of effective weight reduction is not so much to lose pounds but to maintain weight through growth spurt.
- If BMI is > 97th percentile for age and sex, weight reduction may be recommended even prior to pubertal growth spurt.

There is a direct relationship between degree of obesity and severity of medical complications.

Obesity makes **SHADE:**
SCFE
Hypertension
Apnea (sleep)
Diabetes
Embarrassment

HIGH-YIELD FACTS

NUTRITION

Health Supervision and Prevention of Illness and Injury in Children and Adolescents

- The leading cause of death in children **under 1 year of age** is grouped under the term *perinatal conditions*, which include:
  - Congenital malformation, deformations, and chromosomal abnormalities (number one cause).
  - Low birth weight.
  - Sudden infant death syndrome (SIDS).
  - Respiratory distress syndrome.
  - Complications of pregnancy.
  - Perinatal infections.
  - Intrauterine or birth hypoxia.
- From **1 year to 24 years of age,** the leading cause of death is injury (unintentional injuries).

PREVENTION

Prevention is of primary importance in caring for the pediatric patient and is promoted through:

- Parental guidance (anticipatory guidance and counseling).
- Screening tests.
- Immunization.

PARENTAL GUIDANCE

Age-appropriate anticipatory guidance is provided to parents at various well-child visits.

1 Week–1 Month

 A 1-month-old infant is brought to the ED with poor feeding, weak suck, drooling, constipation, and ↓ spontaneous movements. He is exclusively breast-fed, and his mother has been giving him home remedy for "colic". Physical exam is positive for hypotonia. *Think: Botulism* and its relationship with some home remedies prepared with honey. Treatment is with human botulism immune globulin (BIG-IV).

- Place infant to sleep on back to prevent sudden infant death syndrome (SIDS).
- Use a car seat.
- Know signs of an illness.
- Maintain a smoke-free environment (associated with SIDS and ear infections).
- Maintain water temperature at < 120°F (48.8°C).
- Do not give honey to a child under 1 year of age (risk for botulism).
- Discuss normal crying behavior and give some suggestions for how to calm the infant.

Be informed of social services and financial assistance available to parents and patients.

2 Months–1 Year

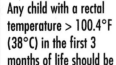

Any child with a rectal temperature > 100.4°F (38°C) in the first 3 months of life should be seen immediately.

- Childproof home to keep children safe from poisons, household cleaners, medications, buckets and tubs filled with water, plastic bags, electrical outlet covers, hot liquids, matches, small and sharp objects, guns, and knives.
- The American Academy of Pediatrics (AAP) does not recommend syrup of ipecac anymore. Explain proper use of syrup of ipecac for poisonings, and give telephone number to local poison control hotline.
- No solid food until 4–6 months.
- Avoid baby walkers.
- Do not put baby to bed with bottle, as it can cause dental caries.
- Breast-feed or give iron-fortified formula, but no whole milk until after 1 year of age.
- Avoid choking hazards such as coins, peanuts, popcorn, carrot sticks, hard candy, whole grapes, and hot dogs.
- May start using cup at 6–9 months.

Falls and drowning are major risks of injury and death in toddlers.

1–5 Years

Most infants drown in their own bathtub.

- Use toddler car seat (ages 1–4) and booster seat (ages 4–8) if proper weight and height.
- Brush teeth, see dentist.
- Wean from bottle (start by 9 months of age with the introduction of cup).
- Make sure home is childproof again.
- Restrict child's access to stairs.
- Allow child to eat with hands or utensils.
- Use sunscreen.
- Wear properly fitting bicycle helmet.
- Provide close supervision, especially near dogs, driveways, streets, and lawnmowers.
- Make appointment with dentist by 1 year of age.
- Ensure that child is supervised when near water; build fence around swimming pool with latched gate.
- Screen for amblyopia, strabismus, and visual acuity in all children younger than 5 years.
  - Strabismus: Cover test or Hirschberg light reflex test in children < 3 years.
  - Visual acuity: > 3 years and screen every 1–2 years throughout childhood.

Temperature of the water heater should be kept below 120°F (49°C) to prevent accidental scalding injuries.

6–10 Years

- Reinforce personal hygiene.
- Teach stranger safety.
- Provide healthy meals and snacks.
- Keep matches and guns out of children's reach.
- Use seat belt always, and booster seat until 4 feet 9 inches in height.

11–21 Years

- Continue to support a healthy diet and exercise.
- Wear appropriate protective sports gear.

- Counsel on safe sex and avoiding alcohol and drugs.
- Promote a healthy social life, balanced diet, and at least 30 minutes of exercise every day.
- Ask about mood or eating disorders (see below).

Blood Pressure

- Routine monitoring of blood pressure should begin at age 3 years.
- Most common cause of high blood pressure reading in children is inappropriate cuff size.

Metabolic Screening

In the first month of life, the neonate should receive screening for various metabolic disorders including hypothyroidism, phenylketonuria (PKU), sickle cell disease, and adrenal cortex abnormalities.

Metabolic screening may vary from state to state in the United States.

Lead Screening

- Exposure is ↑ by:
  - Living in or visiting a house built before 1960 with peeling or chipped paint.
  - Plumbing with lead pipes or lead solder joints.
  - Living near a major highway where soil may be contaminated with lead.
  - Contact with someone who works with lead.
  - Living near an industrial site that may release lead into the environment.
  - Taking home remedies that may contain lead.
  - Having friends/relatives who have had lead poisoning.
- Screen for lead levels at age 12 months.

Hematocrit

- Screen for anemia at 9–12 months of age where certification is needed for WIC (Women, Infants, and Children) or if the appropriate risk factors are present.
- Second test 6 months later in high-risk communities for iron deficiency.
- Anemia: Hemoglobin levels < 11 g/dL.

Hyperlipidemia

- Screen for hyperlipidemia in children older than 2 years with appropriate risk factors:
  - Family history of coronary or peripheral vascular disease before the age of 55 years in parents or grandparents.
  - Parent with a total serum cholesterol level > 240 mg/dL.
  - Obesity.
  - Hypertension.
  - Diabetes mellitus.

- Screening may also be considered in children with inactivity; also in adolescents who smoke.
- Risk factors for anemia include low socioeconomic status, birth weight under 1500 g, whole milk received before 6 months of age, low-iron formula given, low intake of iron-rich foods.

Vision and Hearing

- A hearing screen is recommended shortly after birth.
- Vision screening may begin at age 3 years, sooner if concerns.
- Suspect hearing loss earlier if child's speech is not developing appropriately.
- A child's cooperation is essential to obtaining an accurate result (~3 years).

CAR SEATS

Newborns should not leave the hospital without a car seat.

- Car seats should be used for travel in automobiles for children from birth until the child reaches at least 40 pounds.
- Children under 20 pounds should be in an infant car seat, which belongs in the back seat and is rear-facing.
- Children from 20 pounds to 40 pounds belong in a car seat that is in the back seat but may be forward facing.
- Never place a car seat in front of an air bag (front passenger-side and side-impact air bags). The safest place for the infant is the middle portion of the rear seat.
- Make sure parents understand the proper use of car seats.
- Booster seats should be used until the child is 4 feet 9 inches tall (generally ages 4–8).

VACCINES

- See page 13.
- Site of injection:
  - Infants: Anterolateral thigh.
  - Children: Deltoid.

Hepatitis B

A 25-year-old female who is hepatitis B surface antigen positive is about to deliver a baby and she asks what is the best way to prevent the baby from having hepatitis B. *Think: Prevention.*

Babies born to women who are hepatitis B surface antigen positive receive hepatitis B immunoglobulin and hepatitis B vaccine shortly after birth, and 1–2 months after completing three doses of hepatitis B vaccine, they should be tested for hepatitis B surface antigen as well as the antibody.

- First given intramuscularly (IM) at birth or within first 2 months of life.
- Second dose given 1 month after first dose.

- Third dose given 4 months after first dose and 2 months after second dose, but not before 6 months of age.
- Must give at birth along with hepatitis B immune globulin (HBIG) if baby is exposed transplacentally or if maternal status is unknown.
- Infants born to HBsAg-positive mothers should be tested for HBsAg and antibody to HBsAg 1–2 months after completion of at least three doses of the HepB vaccine, at age 9–18 months.

CONTENT

Adsorbed recombinant hepatitis B surface antigen proteins.

SIDE EFFECTS

- Pain at injection site.
- Fever > 99.9°F (37.7°C) in 1–6%.

CONTRAINDICATIONS

Anaphylactic reaction to vaccine, yeast, or another vaccine constituent.

Diphtheria, Tetanus, and Acellular Pertussis (DTaP)

- Minimum age: 6 weeks.
- Given IM at 2, 4, and 6 months of age, then another between 12 and 18 months of age.
- The fourth dose may be administered as early as age 12 months; **must** allow 6 months between third and fourth doses.
- Administer the final dose at age 4–6 years.

CONTENT

- DTaP is diphtheria and tetanus toxoids with acellular pertussis.
- DTP contains a whole-cell pertussis.

SIDE EFFECTS

- Erythema, pain, and swelling at injection site.
- Fever > 100.9°F (38.3°C) in 3–5%.
- Anaphylaxis in 1/50,000.

CONTRAINDICATIONS

- Anaphylactic reaction to vaccine or another vaccine constituent.
- Encephalopathy not attributable to another cause within 7 days of a prior dose of pertussis vaccine.

Haemophilus influenzae Type B (Hib)

- Minimum age: 6 weeks.
- Given IM at 2, 4, and 6 months of age, then again between 12 and 15 months of age.

CONTENT

Consists of a capsular polysaccharide antigen conjugated to a carrier.

Fever is not a contraindication to receiving immunization. Moderate/severe illness is a contraindication. This holds true for all vaccines.

DTaP is preferred for children under 7 years of age. Td or Tdap is given after 7 years of age.

DTP has greater risks of side effects than DTaP.

DTaP is not a substitute for DTP if a contraindication to pertussis exists.

SIDE EFFECTS

Erythema, pain, and swelling at injection site in 25%.

CONTRAINDICATIONS

Anaphylactic reaction to vaccine or vaccine constituent.

Measles, Mumps, and Rubella

A 12-month-old boy is due for his vaccines in the middle of October. His mother mentions that he developed a skin rash as well as some respiratory problems 1 month prior after she fed him eggs for the first time. He is due for MMR, varicella, and influenza vaccines. *Think: Egg allergy* and the vaccines that are contraindicated: Influenza vaccine, yellow fever vaccine. MMR can be given safely to children with egg allergy.

MMR is a live virus vaccine.

- Minimum age: 12 months.
- First dose given subcutaneously (SC) at 12–15 months of age, and second dose at 4–6 years of age.
- Second dose may be given at any time after 4 weeks from first dose if necessary.
- Must be at least 12 months old to ensure a sufficient response.

CONTENT

Composed of live attenuated viruses.

SIDE EFFECTS

- Fever > 102.9°F (39.4°C) 7–12 days after immunization in 10%.
- Transient rash in 5%.
- Febrile seizures and encephalopathy with MMR vaccine are rare. Transient thrombocytopenia may occur 2–3 weeks after vaccine in 1/40,000.

CONTRAINDICATIONS

- Anaphylactic reaction to prior vaccine.
- Anaphylactic reaction to neomycin or gelatin.
- Immunocompromised states.
- Pregnant women.
- Recent intravenous immune globulin (IVIg) administration requires delaying vaccinations by 12 months.

Inactivated Poliovirus Vaccine (IPV)

- Minimum age: 6 weeks.
- Given SC at 2 and 4 months, then again between 6 and 18 months, then a fourth between 4 and 6 years of age.
- The final dose should be administered on or after the fourth birthday and at least 6 months following the previous dose.
- If four doses are administered prior to age 4 years, a fifth dose should be administered at age 4–6 years.
- OPV is given orally.

CONTENT

- IPV contains inactivated poliovirus types 1, 2, and 3.
- Live oral poliovirus vaccine (OPV) contains live attenuated poliovirus types 1, 2, and 3.

SIDE EFFECTS

- Vaccine-associated paralytic polio (VAPP) with OPV in 1/760,000.
- With prior IPV, risk is reduced by 75–90%.

CONTRAINDICATIONS

- Anaphylaxis to vaccine or vaccine constituent.
- Anaphylaxis to streptomycin, polymixin B, or neomycin.

An all-IPV schedule is recommended in the United States to prevent VAPP (vaccine-associated paralytic polio). Under certain circumstances, OPV may be used.

Varicella

- Minimum age: 12 months.
- Given SC between 12 and 18 months of age; second dose between 4 and 6 years (may be administered before age 4, provided at least 3 months have elapsed since the first dose).
- Susceptible persons > 13 years of age must receive two doses at least 4 weeks apart.

OPV is contraindicated in immunodeficiency disorders or when household contacts are immunocompromised.

CONTENT

Cell-free live attenuated varicella virus.

Varicella vaccine contains live virus.

SIDE EFFECTS

- Erythema and swelling in 20–35%.
- Fever in 10%.
- Varicelliform rash in 1–4%.

CONTRAINDICATIONS

- Anaphylactic reaction to vaccine, neomycin, or gelatin.
- Patients with altered immunity, including corticosteroid use for > 14 days.
- Patients on salicylate therapy.
- Pregnant women.
- Recent blood product or IG administration (defer at least 5 months).

Influenza Vaccine (Seasonal)

- Minimum age: 6 months (trivalent inactivated influenza vaccine [TIV]); 2 years (live attenuated influenza vaccine) [LAIV]).
- Given IM to children > 6 months of age yearly beginning in autumn, usually between October and mid-November (two doses 1 month apart for the first time).
- All children should receive this vaccine, especially high-risk children.
- Caution! LAIV should not be given to children aged 2–4 years who have had wheezing in the past 12 months.

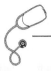

It is especially important to vaccinate for influenza those with asthma, chronic lung disease, cardiac defects, immunosuppressive disorders, sickle cell anemia, chronic renal disease, and chronic metabolic disease.

CONTENT

- Contains three virus strains, usually two type A and one type B, and can be an inactivated whole-virus vaccine or a "split" vaccine containing disrupted virus particles.
- Children < 9 years of age should receive the "split" vaccine only.
- Children without prior exposure to influenza vaccine should receive two vaccines 1 month apart in order to obtain a good response.

SIDE EFFECTS

- Pain, swelling, and erythema at injection site.
- Fever may occur, especially in children < 24 months of age.
- In children > 13 years of age, fever may occur in up to 10%.

CONTRAINDICATIONS

Children with anaphylactic reactions to chicken or egg protein.

Influenza vaccine does not cause the disease. The vaccine has been associated with an ↑ risk of Guillain-Barré syndrome (GBS) in older adults, but no such cases have been reported in children.

H1N1 Vaccine

- Two doses separated by 4 weeks in children under 10 years of age.
- Two preparations:
  - Inactivated vaccine (killed virus).
  - Nasal spray vaccine (live attenuated) approved for children > 2 years old.
- The following patients should receive priority:
  1. Pregnant women.
  2. Caregivers for infants aged < 6 months.
  3. Health care providers.
  4. Children aged 6 months–4 years.
  5. Children and adolescents aged 5–18 years with medical conditions.

CONTRAINDICATIONS

1. Children younger than 6 months of age.
2. Severe allergy to chicken eggs.
3. Severe reaction to an influenza vaccination.
4. People who developed GBS within 6 weeks of getting an influenza vaccine previously.

Chemoprophylaxis against influenza is recommended as an alternative means of protection in those who cannot be vaccinated.

Pneumococcus (Conjugate Vaccine)

- Minimum age: 6 weeks for pneumococcal conjugate vaccine (PCV), 2 years for pneumococcal polysaccharide vaccine (PPSV).
- Babies receive three doses (shots) 2 months apart starting at 2 months, and a fourth dose when they are 12–15 months old.
- Also given to high-risk children ≥ 2 years of age.
- PCV is recommended for all children aged younger than 5 years. Administer one dose of PCV to all healthy children aged 24–59 months who are not completely immunized for their age.
- Administer PPSV ≥ 2 months after last dose of PCV to children aged 2 years or older with certain underlying medical conditions, including a cochlear implant.

The pneumococcal vaccine helps to protect against meningitis, bacteremia, pneumonia, and otitis media caused by serotypes of *Streptococcus pneumoniae*.

- The older PPV-23 vaccine (not indicated under age 2) contains the purified capsular polysaccharide antigens of 23 pneumococcal serotypes. The PPV-23 is usually reserved for high-risk children.
- The newer PCV-7 is the conjugate vaccine described above.

SIDE EFFECTS

- Erythema and pain at injection site.
- Anaphylaxis reported rarely.
- Fever and myalgia are uncommon.

CONTRAINDICATIONS

Usually deferred during pregnancy.

Hepatitis A Vaccine

- Minimum age: 12 months.
- Administer to all children aged 1 year (12–23 months).
- Administer two doses at least 6 months apart.
- Recommended for older children who live in areas where vaccination programs target older children, who are at ↑ risk for infection, or for whom immunity against hepatitis A is desired.

Meningococcal Vaccine

- Minimum age: 2 years for meningococcal conjugate vaccine (MCV4) and meningococcal polysaccharide vaccine (MPSV4).
- Administer MCV4 to children aged 2–10 years with:
  - Persistent complement component deficiency.
  - Anatomic or functional asplenia.

Rotavirus Vaccine

- Minimum age: 6 weeks.
- Administer the first dose at age 6–14 weeks (maximum age: 14 weeks 6 days). Vaccination should not be initiated for infants aged 15 weeks 0 days or older.
- The maximum age for the final dose in the series is 8 months 0 days.
- If Rotarix rotavirus vaccine is administered at ages 2 and 4 months, a dose at 6 months is not indicated.

> Live attenuated vaccines include:
> - MMR
> - VZV
> - Nasal influenza vaccine
> - OPV
> - Smallpox
> - Typhoid
>
> These should be avoided in the immunocompromised.

Respiratory Syncytial Virus (RSV)

- Palivizumab (synagis) is a monoclonal antibody used for prophylaxis against infections with RSV.
- Given IM once a month at the beginning of RSV season, usually beginning in October and ending in March.
- Children < 2 years of age with chronic lung disease who have required medical therapy 6 months before the anticipated RSV season should receive the vaccine.
- Children born at 32 weeks' gestation or earlier with other risk factors for lung disease should receive the vaccine.

CONTENT

RSV immune globulin intravenous (RSV-IGIV) consists of RSV-neutralizing antibodies collected from donors selected for high serum titers.

Tuberculosis (TB)

The Mantoux test contains five tuberculin units of purified protein derivative (PPD).

SCREENING

- Asymptomatic children at high risk for tuberculosis should be screened with a PPD test annually.
- The test is placed intradermally in:
  - Children having contact with persons with confirmed or suspected disease.
  - Children with radiographic or clinical findings of TB.
  - Children from medically underserved populations (eg, low income, homeless, injection drug users).
  - Children with travel history to endemic countries.
  - Children with HIV.
  - Children with clinical conditions that make them high risk.
- Interpretation: See Table 6.1.

TABLE 6-1. Guidelines for Determining a Positive Tuberculin Skin Test Reaction

INDURATION > 5 MM	INDURATION > 10 MM	INDURATION > 15 MM
HIV-positive persons	Recent arrivals (< 5 years) from high-prevalence countries	Persons with no risk factors for TB
Recent contacts of TB case	Injection drug users	
Fibrotic changes on chest radiograph consistent with old TB	Residents and employees[a] of high-risk congregate settings: prisons and jails, nursing homes and other health care facilities, residental facilities for AIDS patients, and homeless shelters	
Patients with organ transplants and other immunosuppressed patients (receiving the equivalent of > 15 mg/d prednisone for > 1 month)	Mycobacteriology laboratory personnel	
Children < 5 years of age are considered to have a positive PPD if the measurement is > 5 mm and < 10 mm	Persons with clinical conditions that make them high risk: silicosis, diabetes mellitus, chronic renal failure, some hematologic disorders (eg, leukemias and lymphomas), other specific malignancies (eg, carcinoma of the head or neck and lung), weight loss of > 10% of ideal body weight, gastrectomy, jejunoileal bypass	
	Children < 4 years of age or infants, children, and adolescents exposed to adults in high-risk categories	

[a] For persons who are otherwise at low risk and are tested at entry into employment, a reaction of > 15 mm induration is considered positive.

(Reproduced, with permission, from the American Thoracic Society. Diagnostic standards and classification of tuberculosis in adults and children. *Am J Respir Crit Care Med* 2000;161: 1376. Copyright © 2000 American Thoracic Society.)

- The QuantiFERON®-TB Gold test (QFT-G) is a newer alternative for detection of TB, approved by the U.S. Food and Drug Administration (FDA) in 2005.
  - Advantages:
    - Requires a single patient visit to draw a blood sample.
    - Results can be available within 24 hours.
    - Does not boost responses measured by subsequent test, which can happen with tuberculin skin tests (TSTs).
    - Is not subject to reader bias that can occur with TSTs.
    - Is not affected by prior BCG (bacille Calmette-Guerin) vaccination.
  - Disadvantages:
    - Blood samples must be processed within 12 hours after collection while white blood cells are still viable.
    - Limited data in children < 17 years of age, among persons recently exposed to *Mycobacterium tuberculosis*, and in immunocompromised persons.
    - Errors in collecting or transporting blood specimens or in running and interpreting the assay can ↓ the accuracy of QFT-G.
    - Limited data on the use of QFT-G to determine who is at risk for developing TB disease.

MEDICATIONS

Only 25% of Food and Drug Administration (FDA)-approved drugs have been approved for pediatric use.

Differences Between Children and Adults

ABSORPTION

- Infants have thinner skin; therefore, topical substances can more likely cause systemic toxicity.
- Children do not have the stomach acidity of adults until age 2, and gastric emptying time is slower and less predictable, → ↑ absorption of some medications.

DISTRIBUTION

- Less predictable in children.
- Total body water ↓ from 90% in infants to 60% in adults.
- Fat stores are similar to adults in term infants, but much less in preterm infants.
- Newborns have smaller protein concentration, therefore less binding of substances in the blood.
- Infants have an immature blood–brain barrier.

METABOLISM

Infants metabolize some drugs more slowly or rapidly than adults and may create a different proportion of active metabolites.

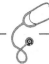

Controls with *Candida*, measles, or diphtheria can be placed along with the PPD to test for anergy, although opinion may vary in practice.

ELIMINATION

Kidney function ↑ with age, so younger children may clear drugs less efficiently.

DOSAGE

Pediatric medications are generally dosed by milligrams per kilogram (mg/kg).

POISONING

EPIDEMIOLOGY

More often accidental in younger children and suicide gestures or attempts in older children/adolescents.

SIGNS AND SYMPTOMS

See Table 6-2.

PREVENTION

- Childproof home, including cabinets and containers.
- Store toxic substances in their original containers and out of children's reach.
- Supervise children appropriately.
- Have poison control center number easily accessible.

MANAGEMENT

- Frequently, ingested substances are nontoxic, but if symptoms arise or there is any question, a poison control center should be contacted.
- History:
  - Precise name of product (generic, brand, chemical—bring container or extra substance/pills).
  - Estimate amount of exposure, time of exposure.
  - Progression of symptoms.
  - Other medical conditions (eg, pregnancy, seizure disorder).
- Gastric decontamination: Emesis (induced by syrup of ipecac) and gastric lavage remove only one third of stomach contents and are not generally recommended, though the combination of the latter with activated charcoal may be most effective.
- Activated charcoal is effective for absorbing many drugs and chemicals, though it does not bind heavy metals, iron, lithium alcohols, hydrocarbons, cyanide. It may be used in conjunction with cathartics such as sorbitol or magnesium sulfate.
- Dilution of stomach contents with milk has limited value except in the case of ingestion of caustic materials.
- Skin decontamination: Remove clothing, use gloves, flood area with water for 15 minutes, use other mild material such as petroleum or alcohol to remove substances not removed by water.
- Ocular decontamination: Rinse eyes with water, saline, or lactated Ringer's for > 15 minutes; consider emergency ophthalmologic exam.

TABLE 6-2. "Toxidromes," Symptoms, and Some Causes

ANTICHOLINERGIC	CHOLINERGIC	EXTRAPYRAMIDAL	HYPER-METABOLIC	OPIATES	WITHDRAWAL	SYMPATHO-MIMETIC
Hyposecretion, thirst, urinary retention	Hypersecretion Muscle fasciculation, weakness	Tremor, rigidity	Fever Tachycardia	CNS depression	Abdominal cramps, diarrhea	Hyperthermia, hypertension, tachypnea
Flushed skin, dilated pupils			Hyperpnea Restlessness Convulsions	Dilated pupils Hypothermia Hypotension	Lacrimation, sweating	Dilated pupils
Tachycardia, respiratory insufficiency	Bronchospasm, arrhythmias		Metabolic acidosis		Tachycardia, restlessness	Psychosis, convulsions
Delirium, hallucinations	Convulsions, coma				Hallucinations	
Belladonna	Organo-phosphates (insecticides)	Haloperidol	Salicylates	Lomotil	Cessation of:	Amphetamines
Some mushrooms	Metoclopramide			Propoxyphene Heroin	Alcohol Benzodiazepines	Cocaine Theophylline
Antihistamines	Some mushrooms			Methadone		Caffeine
Tricyclic antidepressants				Codeine	Barbiturates	
	Black widow spider bites			Morphine Demerol	Opiates	
	Tobacco					

- Respiratory decontamination: Move to fresh air; bronchodilators may be effective, inhaled dilute sodium bicarbonate may help acid or chlorine inhalation.
- Antidotes: See Table 6-3.
- Treat seizures, respiratory distress/depression, hemodynamics, and electrolyte disturbances as they arise.

TABLE 6-3. Drug Toxicities

DRUG	SIGNS AND SYMPTOMS	TREATMENT/ANTIDOTE
Sulfonamides	Kernicterus in infants	
Chloramphenicol	Gray baby syndrome—vomiting, ashen color, cardiovascular collapse	
Quinolones	May cause cartilage defects in children	
Tetracycline	Gray enamel of permanent teeth, affects bone growth (avoid in children < 9 years old)	Not necessary unless massive ingestion
Salicylate	Reye syndrome—hepatic injury, hypoglycemia, vomiting—in children with viral illnesses Hypermetabolic	
Acetaminophen	Generalized malaise, nausea, vomiting Latent period Jaundice and bleeding (direct hepatocellular necrosis) Metabolic acidosis, renal and myocardial damage, coma	*N*-acetylcysteine (Mucomyst)
Tricyclic antidepressants	Anticholinergic Widened QRS, flattened T waves	Intubation and activated charcoal if altered sensorium Sodium bicarbonate IV
Prednisone	Growth retardation Cataracts	
Organophosphates	Cholinergic	Atropine Pralidoxime
Heavy metals (eg, arsenic, mercury, lead, chromium, copper, gold, nickel, zinc)		Dimercaprol Dimercaptosuccinic acid (succimer, DMSA), EDTA
Iron	Abdominal pain, vomiting	Deferoxamine
Methanol, ethylene glycol	Intoxication	Ethanol
	Blindness (methanol)	Fomepizole
Benzodiazepines	Sedation	Flumazenil (recommended only in cases of iatrogenic overdose)

TABLE 6-3. Drug Toxicities *(continued)*

Opiates	Respiratory depression	Naloxone
	Pinpoint pupils	
Anticholinergics	"Mad as a hatter;	
	Dry as a bone;	
	Blind as a bat;	
	Red as a beet;	
	Hot as Hades"	

ADOLESCENCE

- Adolescence comprises the ages between 10 and 21 years.
- The most common health problems seen in this age group include unintended pregnancies, sexually transmitted diseases (STDs), mental health disorders, physical injuries, and substance abuse.

PREVENTION

- Be on the lookout for adolescents at high risk for health problems, including physical, mental, and emotional health.
- Screen for depression. Suicide is the third leading cause of death in adolescents. Depression in the adolescent can manifest as irritability, anger, new drug use, and drop-off in school performance.
- Look for:
  - Decline in school performance, excessive school absences, cutting class.
  - Frequent psychosomatic complaints.
  - Changes in sleeping or eating habits.
  - Difficulty in concentrating.
  - Signs of depression, stress, or anxiety.
  - Conflict with parents.
  - Social withdrawal.
  - Sexual acting-out.
  - Conflicts with the law.
  - Suicidal thoughts, preoccupation with death.
  - Substance abuse.

SCREENING

- Routine health care should involve audiometry and vision screening, blood pressure checks, exams for scoliosis.
- Breast and pelvic exams in females may also be necessary, and self-exams should be emphasized.
- Likewise, examination for scrotal masses is necessary in males with emphasis on self-examination.
- STDs (**gonorrhea and chlamydia**), including HIV should be considered in those adolescents with high-risk behaviors. Counsel sexually active adolescents on contraception and protection against STDs.

The leading causes of death for adolescents are accidents, homicide, and suicide.

One percent of adolescents have made at least one suicide gesture.

HIGH-YIELD FACTS

HEALTH SUPERVISION

- Screen with Pap smears within 3 years of the onset of sexual activity or at 21 years of age.
- Adolescents who are engaged in one risk-taking activity such as smoking cigarettes are at greater risk for experimenting with drugs and alcohol.

PHYSICAL EXAM

Sexual maturity should be assessed at each visit.

Pregnancy

EPIDEMIOLOGY

- Over 750,000 teenage girls become pregnant in the United States each year (see Table 6-4).
- One fifth of all sexually active girls become pregnant each year.

Contraception

EPIDEMIOLOGY

- According to a 2004 Centers for Disease Control and Prevention (CDC) report, 62% of high school seniors report having ever had intercourse.
- Ninety-eight percent of sexually active teens report using at least one form of birth control.
- Thirty-three percent of ninth graders report having had sex.
- Most common contraceptions methods are condoms (94%) and oral contraceptives (61%).

RISK FACTORS

Factors associated with early sexual activity include poor academic performance, lower expectations for education, poor perception of life options, low school grades, and involvement in other high-risk behaviors such as substance abuse.

FORMS OF CONTRACEPTION

- Abstinence, condoms (male and female), diaphragm, cervical cap, spermicides, or some combination of these.

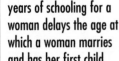

An ↑ in the number of years of schooling for a woman delays the age at which a woman marries and has her first child.

TABLE 6-4. 2002 Teenage Statistics

	PREGNACY RATE (%)	BIRTH RATE (%)	ABORTION RATE (%)
Overall	7.54	4.30	21.7
Blacks	13.4	6.66	49.4
Hispanics	13.2	8.34	28.5

(Data from Guttemacher Institute, 2006.)

- Hormonal methods include oral contraceptive pills and injectable or implantable hormones, and hormone patches.
- Intrauterine devices are not recommended for adolescents because of the ↑ risk of sexually transmitted infections.

COMBINATION ORAL CONTRACEPTIVES

Usually consist of either 50, 35, 30, or 20 μg of an estrogenic substance such as mestranol or ethinyl estradiol plus a progestin.

SIDE EFFECTS

- Short-term effects may include nausea and weight gain.
- Other possible effects include thrombophlebitis, hepatic adenomas, myocardial infarction, and carbohydrate intolerance.

POTENTIAL BENEFITS

Long-range benefits may include ↓ risks of benign breast disease and ovarian disease.

Adolescents who smoke may ↑ their risk for side effects from oral contraceptives.

HIV/AIDS

See the Infectious Disease chapter.

EPIDEMIOLOGY

- HIV/AIDS is the sixth leading cause of death among adolescents aged 15–24 years.
- One half of all new infections in the United States occur in people younger than 25 years of age.

SCREENING

Screening should include adolescents with risk factors such as previous STD, unprotected sex, practicing insertive or receptive anal sex, trading sex for money or drugs, homelessness, intravenous drug or crack cocaine use, being the victim of sexual abuse.

CHILD ABUSE

DEFINITION

Child maltreatment encompasses a spectrum of abusive actions, and lack of action, that result in morbidity or death. Forms of child abuse include:

- Physical abuse
- Sexual abuse
- Neglect

If the story doesn't make sense, suspect abuse.

RISK FACTORS

- Parental risk factors:
  - Low socioeconomic status.
  - Mother's age (young).
  - History of being abused as a child.
  - Alcoholism, substance abuse, psychosis.
  - Social isolation.

Mongolian spots can be confused with bruises.

A baby should never be shaken for any reason.

The most common reason for shaking a baby is inconsolable crying.

Sometimes abusive parents "punish" their children for enuresis or resistance to toilet training by forcibly immersing their buttocks in hot water.

Skeletal injuries suspicious of abuse: "**S**ome **P**arents **A**re **M**aliciously **M**ean" (or Parents Should Manage Anger)

CNS injuries suspicious of abuse: "**M**others, **R**efuse **S**haking!" (**M**etaphyseal fractures, **R**etinal hemorrhages, **S**ubdural hematoma)

- Child risk factors:
    - Children with special needs, handicapped children (chronic illness, congenital malformation, mental retardation).
    - Prematurity.
    - Age < 3 years.
    - Nonbiologic relationship to the caretaker.
    - "Difficult" children.
- Family and environmental factors:
    - Unemployment.
    - Intimate partner violence.
    - Poverty.

Physical Abuse

Suspect if:

- Injury is unexplained or unexplainable.
- Injury is inconsistent with mechanism suggested by history.
- History changes each time it is told.
- There are repeated "accidents."
- There is a delay in seeking care.

SKIN MANIFESTATIONS

Bruises
- Most common manifestation of physical abuse
- Suspicious if:
    - Seen on nonambulatory infants.
    - Have geometric pattern (belt buckles, looped-cord marks).

Burns
- Suspicious if:
    - Involve both hands or feet in stocking-glove distribution or buttocks with sharp demarcation line (forced immersion in hot water).
    - Cigarette burns—if nonaccidental, usually full-thickness, sharply circumscribed.
    - "Branding" injuries (inflicted by hot iron, radiator cover, etc).

SKELETAL INJURIES

Suspicious if:

- Spiral fractures of lower extremities in nonambulatory children (see Figure 6-1A and B).
- Posterior rib fractures (usually caused by squeezing the chest).
- Fractures of different **A**ges.
- Metaphyseal "chip" fractures (usually caused by wrenching).
- Multiple fractures.
- Scapular and clavicle fractures.

CENTRAL NERVOUS SYSTEM (CNS) INJURIES

- Most common cause of death in child abuse: "Shaken baby syndrome."
- Occurs due to violent shakes and slamming against mattress or wall while an infant is held by the trunk or upper extremities.

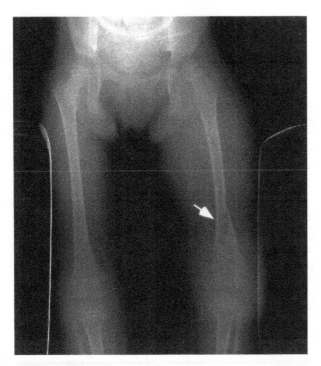
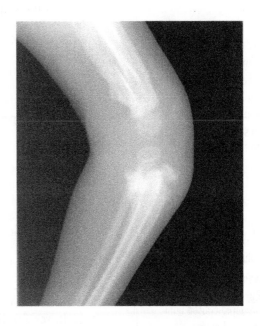

FIGURE 6-1.

A. Spiral fracture (arrow) of the femur in a nonambulatory child, consistent with nonaccidental trauma. B. Same child 2 months later. Note the exuberant callus formation at all the fracture sites in the femur and proximal tibia and fibula.

- Findings include:
  - **R**etinal hemorrhages.
  - **S**ubdural hematoma (from rupturing of bridging veins between dura mater and brain cortex).
- Symptoms include:
  - Lethargy or irritability
  - Vomiting
  - Seizures
  - Bulging fontanelle

Abdominal Injuries

- Second most common cause of death in child abuse.
- Usually no external marks. Most commonly, liver or spleen is ruptured.
- Symptoms include vomiting, abdominal pain or distention, shock.

Sexual Abuse

- Includes genital, anal, oral contact; fondling; and involvement in pornography.
- Most common perpetrators—fathers, stepfathers, mother's boyfriend(s) (adults known to child).
- Suspect if:
  - Genital trauma.
  - STDs in small children.
  - Sexualized behavior toward adults or children.

Epiphyseal-metaphyseal injury is virtually diagnostic of physical abuse in an infant, since an infant cannot generate enough force to fracture a bone at the epiphysis.

Shaken baby syndrome can mimic meningitis or sepsis.

Children too young to talk about what has happened to them (generally younger than 2) should have a complete skeletal survey if you suspect abuse.

A child who presents with multiple fractures at multiple sites and in various stages of healing should be considered abused until proven otherwise.

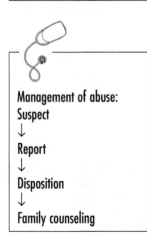

Management of abuse:
Suspect
↓
Report
↓
Disposition
↓
Family counseling

- Unexplained decline in school performance.
- Runaway.
- Chronic somatic complaints (abdominal pain, headaches).
- Symptoms include:
  - May be totally absent.
  - Tears/bleeding in female or male genitalia.
  - Anal tears or hymenal tears (not very reliable symptoms).

Evaluation of Suspected Abuse

PHYSICAL ABUSE

- Bleeding disorders must be ruled out in case of multiple bruises.
- X-ray skeletal survey (skull, chest, long bones) in children < 2 years of age (to look for old/new fractures).
- Computed tomographic (CT) scans of the head/abdomen as indicated.
- Ophthalmology consult.

SEXUAL ABUSE

- Sexual abuse includes *any* sexual activity (nonconsensual and consensual) between an adult and a child.
- Cultures for STDs, test for presence of sperm, if indicated (usually within 72 hours of assault).

MANAGEMENT

- If abuse is suspected, it must be reported to child protective services (CPS) (after medical stabilization, if needed).
- All siblings need to be evaluated for abuse, too (up to 20% of them might have signs of abuse).
- Disposition of the child (ie, whether to discharge the patient back to parents or to a CPS worker if medically cleared) has to be decided by CPS in conjunction with treating physician.
- Family must receive intensive intervention by social services and, if needed, legal authorities.
- *Remember:* If sent back to abusive family without intervention, up to 5% of children can be killed and up to 25% seriously reinjured.

Neglect

DEFINITION

- Neglect is the most common form of reported abuse.
- Neglect to meet nutritional, medical, and/or developmental needs of a child can present as:
  - Failure to thrive.
  - Poor hygiene (severe diaper rash, unwashed clothing, uncut nails).
  - Developmental/speech delay.
  - Delayed immunizations.
  - Not giving treatment for chronic conditions.

MANAGEMENT

If nonorganic (ie, due to insufficient feeding) failure to thrive is suspected:

- Patient should be hospitalized and given unlimited feedings for 1 week; 2 oz/24 hours of weight gain is expected.
  - All suspected cases of neglect must be reported to CPS.

Munchausen Syndrome by Proxy

DEFINITION

- Parent/caregiver either simulates illness, exaggerates actual illness, or induces illness in a child.
- Psychiatrically disturbed parent(s) gain satisfaction from attention and empathy from hospital personnel or their own family because of problems created.

EPIDEMIOLOGY

- Affected children are usually < 6 years old.
- Parent (usually mother) has some medical knowledge.

SIGNS AND SYMPTOMS

- Vomiting (induced by ipecac).
- Chronic diarrhea (from laxatives).
- Recurrent abscesses or sepsis (usually polymicrobial, from injecting contaminated fluids).
- Apnea (from choking the child).
- Fever (from heating thermometers).
- Bloody vomiting or diarrhea (from adding blood to urine or stool specimens).

Baron von Munchausen was an 18th-century nobleman who became famous because of his incredible stories, which included travel to the moon and flying atop a cannonball over Constantinople, as well as visiting an island made of cheese. His name became a synonym for gross confabulations.

DIAGNOSIS

Diagnosis is difficult, but is initiated by removing child from parent via hospitilization. Usually, child without access to parent will have all/most symptoms resolved; testing will also usually be normal.

MANAGEMENT

- Admission to the hospital for observation, possibly using hidden video cameras.
- All cases of suspected Munchausen syndrome by proxy must be reported to CPS.

Sudden Infant Death Syndrome (SIDS)

DEFINITION

- Sudden death of an infant (< 1 year old) that remains unexplained after thorough case investigation, autopsy, and review of the clinical history.
- SIDS is one of the leading causes of death of infants.

ETIOLOGY

Apnea hypothesis.

DIAGNOSIS

Difficult to differentiate from intentional harm.

PREVENTION

- There has been a vast ↓ in the number of cases since the trend of having infants sleep on their backs (supine).
- The number one preventive measure to date is parental education, though the use of cardiorespiratory monitoring in the home is being debated.
- Limiting passive smoke exposure.

Infants unable to roll over should be placed on the back while sleeping.

Congenital Malformations and Chromosomal Anomalies

It is important for all pediatricians in all fields to recognize signs and symptoms of congenital disorders, including dysmorphologic features. It is also important to involve genetics in the patient's care, for appropriate screening and treatment of conditions associated with genetic syndromes, genetic testing, if available and appropriate, and counseling regarding siblings and possible future offspring of the patient. Finally, physicians strive for a unifying diagnosis, and usually one is sufficient, but patients can have more than one thing going on, *and* children with genetic disorders can also get the diseases children without genetic conditions get!

ENVIRONMENTAL FACTORS

 A 3-week-old infant is brought for seizure. On physical examination, the patient has microcephaly. Cerebral calcifications are seen on brain CT scan. What does the infant likely have? **Congenital Cytomegalovirus infection**

Teratogens:

- Cause 10% of all birth defects.
- Include maternal metabolic disorders (diabetes mellitus), maternal/intrauterine infections (TORCHeS [toxoplasmosis, others, rubella, cytomegalovirus, herpes simplex, syphilis]), drugs, radiation, mechanical forces.
- Common teratogenic drugs include ethanol, warfarin, isoretinoin, lithium, valproic acid, fluoroquinolones, tetracyclines, and phenytoin.

GENETIC FACTORS

Include single gene, parental imprinting, molecular cytogenetics.

- Single gene:
  - Autosomal (dominant/recessive).
  - X-linked (dominant/recessive).
- Parental imprinting: Genetic defect is dependent on which parent passes the abnormal gene.
- Molecular cytogenetics:
  - Unstable repeat sequences
  - Uniparental disomy
  - Translocation

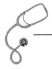

Trisomies:
- Age 13, Puberty: **Patau**
- Age 18, can vote— "Elect": **Edwards syndrome**
- Age 21, can Drink: **Down**

Trisomy 21 (Down Syndrome)

A female infant has slanted palpebral fissures, epicanthal folds, and some delayed development. *Think: Down syndrome.*

This is a classic description of an infant with Down syndrome. The diagnostic clinical features include flat facial profile, oblique palpebral fissures and epicanthic folds are usually evident at birth. It is also a leading cause of severe mental retardation in children. It is the most common chromosomal disorders.

A 33-week-gestation male infant born to a 40-year-old mother was noted to have facial dysmorphism with depressed nasal bridge, wide-spaced eyes, low hairline, and low-set ears. He was also noted to have a single palmar crease in both hands. At 2 hours of life he was noted to have bilious emesis, and an abdominal x-ray was obtained, as shown in the figure. What is the diagnosis and management of this infant?

The infant described was born to a mother with advanced maternal age (> 35 years) and features consistent with trisomy 21 (Down syndrome). X-ray is notable for the classic double-bubble sign, which is pathognomonic for duodenal atresia. Management includes surgical repair of the duodenal atresia and also to confirm the diagnosis of trisomy 21 by chromosome analysis.

- Extra copy of the genetic material on chromosome 21.
- Most common malformation syndrome.
- Most common chromosome disorder.
- Most common genetic cause of moderate mental retardation.

ETIOLOGY

- Ninety-five percent complete trisomy (meiotic nondisjunction of homologous chromosomes).
- Four percent Robertsonian translocation (to chromosome 14).
- One percent mosaicism.

EPIDEMIOLOGY

One in 600 births.

RISK FACTORS

Advanced maternal age.

Patients with Down syndrome develop Alzheimer's dementia early, around age 35.

SIGNS AND SYMPTOMS

Think of duodenal atresia in a newborn with Down syndrome presenting with bilious vomiting.

- More than 100 different physical signs can be present.
- Varying degrees of mental retardation (most with IQs between 35 and 70).
- Generalized hypotonia (of central nervous system [CNS] origin; most meet major motor milestones at 2× normal age).
- Balding scalp hair pattern.
- Upslanted eyes with epicanthal folds (see Figure 7-1).
- Flat nasal bridge.
- Prominent tongue.
- Extra neck skin folds (sometimes visible on prenatal ultrasound).
- Transverse palmar (simian) creases.
- Small ears.
- Short stature.
- Joint laxity.
- Hypoplastic nipples.
- Brushfield spots on irises.
- Subendocardial cushion defect (atrial/ventricular septal defect [ASD/ VSD], atrioventricular [AV] canal).
- Duodenal atresia, Hirschsprung's disease, imperforate anus.
- Hypothyroidsim.
- Amyloid plaques and neurofibrillary tangles in brain—early onset dementia.
- ↑ risk of leukemia (acute lymphocytic leukemia [ALL], acute myelogenous leukemia [AML], acute megakaryocytic leukemia).
- ↑ risk of neonatal leukemoid reactions.
- Atlantoaxial instability becomes an issue later in life.
- Most males with Down syndrome are sterile but some females have been able to reproduce.

Look for "double-bubble sign" in a plain abdominal radiograph.

DIAGNOSIS

- Prenatal diagnosis can be made via amniocentesis or chorionic villus sampling.
- Maternal serum α-fetoprotein (AFP) is ↓.

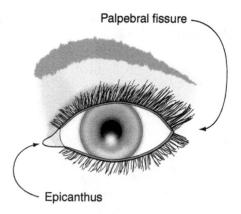

FIGURE 7-1. Location of epicanthus and palpebral fissure.

In Down syndrome, there are epicanthal folds and upwardly slanted palpebral fissures.

- Low maternal serum unconjugated estriol level.
- Elevated maternal beta-human chorionic gonadotropin (β-hCG).

TREATMENT

- Early childhood intervention to maximize social and intellectual capacity.
- Life skills training.
- Surgery for correction of cardiac and duodenal defects.
- At risk for atlantoaxial dislocation and cervical cord compression.
- ↑ risk for leukemia and respiratory tract infections.
- Yearly screening for thyroid disease.

Trisomy 18 (Edwards Syndrome)

ETIOLOGY

- Most common type is complete trisomy.
- Small percentage are due to mosaicism.

EPIDEMIOLOGY

One in 6000 live births; second most common trisomy.

SIGNS AND SYMPTOMS

- Prominent occiput.
- Low-set ears.
- Small mouth.
- Short sternum.
- Thumb and radius agenesis/hypoplasia.
- Camptodactyly (little finger fixed in flexion).
- Redundancy of cardiac valve leaflets.
- Hypertonia.
- Seizures.
- Rocker-bottom feet.

TREATMENT

- Supportive.
- Fifty percent die within first week of life. Most common cause of death is apnea.
- Five to ten percent survive beyond the first year.
- Those who survive are severely mentally retarded.

Trisomy 13 (Patau Syndrome)

Higher frequencies in stillbirths and spontaneous abortions.

ETIOLOGY

- Seventy-five percent complete trisomy.
- Twenty-three percent Robertsonian translocation (to chromosome 14).
- Four percent mosaicism.

EPIDEMIOLOGY

One in 10,000 live births.

SIGNS AND SYMPTOMS

- Holoprosencephaly (failure of telencephalon to divide into two hemi-spheres, resulting in large central ventricle; brain assumes configuration of a fluid-filled ball).
- Microphthalmia and other eye defects (coloboma, cyclops).
- Midline facial defects.
- Polydactyly.
- Scalp cutis aplasia.
- Cystic kidneys.
- VSD.

TREATMENT

- Supportive.
- Eighty percent die within first month; 5% survive past 6 months.

SEX CHROMOSOME ANOMALIES

Turner Syndrome

A newborn infant has lymphedema of the hands and feet, extra skin folds at a short neck, widely spaced nipples, and ↓ femoral pulses. *Think: Gonadal dysgenesis (45,X) Turner syndrome,* and do a chromosomal analysis to confirm the diagnosis.

Many infants with Turner syndrome are recognized at birth due to the presence of edema of the hands and feet and loose skin folds at the nape of the neck. Coarctation of aorta may be present in up to 20%.

Turner syndrome is the most common cause of primary amenorrhea.

ETIOLOGY

45,XO—missing one X chromosome.

EPIDEMIOLOGY

One in 2000–5000 live female births.

RISK FACTORS

Not related to advanced maternal age.

SIGNS AND SYMPTOMS

- Short stature.
- Webbed neck.
- Lymphedema of hands and feet.
- Coarctation of the aorta + biscuspid aortic valve.
- Small mandible.
- Narrow maxilla and high arched palate.
- Epicanthal folds.
- Impaired hearing (sensorineural).
- Delay in motor skill development with normal intelligence.

- Ovarian dysgenesis.
- Phenotypically female.
- Association with spontaneous abortion.

TREATMENT

- Replacement for secondary sex characteristic development.
- Monitor for autoimmune hypothyroidism.
- Refer to an endocrinologist for induction of puberty at an appropriate age.
- Resection of any intra-abdominal gonads to prevent malignancy.

Noonan Syndrome

- Phenotypically similar to Turner syndrome but can affect both sexes.
- Girls with Noonan syndrome have normal XX chromosomes.
- Autosomal dominant.
- Pulmonary stenosis.
- Mental retardation often present.

Klinefelter Syndrome

ETIOLOGY

- Presence of an extra X chromosome in males.
- 47,XXY most common.
- Most common cause of hypogonadism and infertility in males.

EPIDEMIOLOGY

One in 500 males.

RISK FACTORS

Advanced maternal age.

SIGNS AND SYMPTOMS

- Hypogonadism.
- Small testes but puberty occurs at the normal age.
- Most patients are phenotypically normal until puberty.
- Azoospermia (absence of sperm).
- Tall stature (eunuchoid).
- Female hair distribution, gynecomastia.
- Learning disabilities.
- Delay of motor skill development
- Presence of inactivated X chromosome (Barr body).

TREATMENT

- Administration of testosterone during puberty to improve secondary sex characteristics.
- Interventions for developmental delays/learning disabilities.

Imprinting—different phenotype, same genotype.

Angelman Syndrome

ETIOLOGY

- Sixty percent due to **maternal** deletion 15q11–13 (see Prader-Willi syndrome).
- Forty percent have two normal paternal copies of chromosome 15.

EPIDEMIOLOGY

One in 20,000.

SIGNS AND SYMPTOMS

- Happy, laughing disposition—previously known as the "happy puppet" or "marionette joyeuse" syndrome because of this and stereotyped flapping of hands.
- Often, strikingly attractive children with lighter pigmentation than other family members (often blond-haired, blue-eyed).
- Mental retardation (severe).
- Microcephaly.
- Ataxia.
- Hypotonia (ataxia and hypotonia create the characteristic "puppet"-like gait).
- Epilepsy (80%) with characteristic electroencephalographic (EEG) findings.
- Complete absence of speech.
- Unusual facies characterized by a large mandible and open-mouthed expression revealing tongue.
- Inappropriate laughter.

The same chromosomal deletion causes Angelman syndrome and Prader-Willi syndrome. The only difference is that in Angelman syndrome the missing genetic material is maternal, and in Prader-Willi, paternal.

TREATMENT

- Supportive.
- Seizures are often refractory to anticonvulsant therapy.
- Normal life span.

Prader-Willi Syndrome

ETIOLOGY

- Genetic.
- Seventy-five percent **paternal** deletion 15q11–13 (see Angelman syndrome).
- Twenty-five percent maternal disomy.
- Hyperphagia/lack of satiety, ↓ caloric requirement secondary to hypotonia/↓ movement, and obsessions/compulsions that focus on food all contribute to the vicious cycle → obesity in these patients.
- Obesity.
- Small hands and feet.
- Hypogonadism.

EPIDEMIOLOGY

One in 15,000–20,000.

SIGNS AND SYMPTOMS

- Hypotonia and poor feeding (in infancy) progressing to hyperphagia and obesity by childhood.
- Precocious puberty.
- Micropenis.
- Mild mental retardation.
- Sleep disturbances.
- Lighter pigmentation than other family members.
- Significant behavioral problems (stubborn, manipulative, aggressive).
- Fluent speech.
- Obsessive/compulsive traits.

TREATMENT

- Strict diet and behavioral interventions to prevent obesity.
- Growth hormone to promote stature, and other timely hormone supplementation to promote secondary sex characteristics.
- Patients develop complications from obesity that limit their life span.
- Early prevention of obesity is the key to quality and quantity of life in these patients.

MOLECULAR CYTOGENETIC DISORDERS

22q11 Syndrome

- Caused by deletion of a small piece of chromosome 22.
- Seen in DiGeorge syndrome, velocardiofacial syndrome.
- Occurs in 1 in 4000 births.
- Most common features include congenital heart defects (85%), palatal abnormalities, thymic aplasia, immune deficiency (defective T-cell function), hypocalcemia (parathyroid involvement), characteristic facial features.
- Cardiac features include tetralogy of Fallot, interrupted aortic arch.
- Detected by fluorescence in situ hybridization (FISH).

Fragile X Syndrome

ETIOLOGY

Due to ↑ number of repeated nucleotide sequences (CGG).

EPIDEMIOLOGY

- One in 2000 births
- Male-to-female ratio: 2:1.

RISK FACTORS

Family history.

Fragile X is the most common form of heritable mental retardation.

- Mental retardation.
- Macroorchidism in boys.
- Protruding ears, macrocephaly, triangular, elongated facies, flat malar bones.
- Shyness, autistic behavior, avoidance of eye contact.

AUTOSOMAL-DOMINANT CONDITIONS

- People in every generation are affected.
- Examples include adult polycystic kidney disease, familial hypercholesterolemia, Marfan syndrome, neurofibromatosis type 1 (von Recklinghausen disease), von Hippel–Lindau, Huntington disease, familial adenomatous polyposis, and hereditary spherocytosis.
- Marfan syndrome:
  - Connective tissue disorder affecting fibrillin.
  - Chromosome 15.
  - Tall stature, long limbs.
  - Cardiovascular—aortic root dilatation, mitral valve prolapse, aortic regurgitation.
  - Ophthalmologic—lens subluxation.
  - Sudden death usually due to aortic dissection.

AUTOSOMAL-RECESSIVE CONDITIONS

- Skips generations (often a grandparent has had a similar condition).
- Examples include cystic fibrosis and many enzyme deficiencies/metabolic disorders.
- History of early deaths from unknown disorders or multiple miscarriages.
- Consanguinity really ↑ the odds—you must ask if the parents are blood relatives.

X-LINKED RECESSIVE CONDITIONS

- Usually only males are affected; females are unaffected or only partially affected (due to lyonization) carriers of the trait.
- Examples include Duchenne and Becker muscular dystrophies, hemophilia A and B, Fabry disease, glucose-6-phosphate dehydrogenase (G6PD) deficiency, Hunter syndrome, ocular albinism, red–green color blindness, and Alport syndrome.

The X chromosome lyonizes randomly early in embryogenesis when there are relatively few cells. Since all daughter cells lyonize the same X, the odds that a significantly disproportionate inactivation of the "good" X will occur in carrier females, while small, are not infinitesimal. When this occurs, the carrier is affected, and the mechanism is termed *unfortunate lyonization.*

Polydactyly

DEFINITION

- Presence of more than five fingers or toes, which may be rudimentary to fully developed.
- Incidence: 2 per 1000 live births.

ETIOLOGY

- May occur as an isolated defect (whether genetic, toxic, or mechanical) or in conjunction with syndromes such as:
  - Ellis–van Creveld syndrome: With congenital heart disease.
  - Bardet-Biedl syndrome: With obesity, pigmentary retinopathy, mental retardation, hypogonadism, and renal failure.
  - Meckel-Gruber syndrome: Triad of occipital encephalocele, large polycystic kidneys, and postaxial polydactyly. Associated abnormalities include oral clefting, genital anomalies, CNS malformations, fibrosis of the liver, and pulmonary hypoplasia.

DIAGNOSIS

Observation, x-ray, fetal sonogram.

TREATMENT

Surgery, usually at 1 year of age.

Syndactyly

Definition

Webbing or fusing of two or more fingers or toes. May be bony and/or cutaneous. Often looked for between the second and third toes.

PATHOPHYSIOLOGY

Failure of cell apoptosis between digits during development.

TREATMENT

Surgery.

Craniosynostosis

DEFINITION

- Premature closing of one or more cranial sutures due to abnormalities of skull development.
- Can be primary skull/bone defect or a result of failure of brain growth.
- Syndromic craniosynostosis in 20%.
- Most common: Apert syndrome and Crouzon syndrome.

ETIOLOGY

May occur alone or in conjunction with syndromes such as:
- Apert syndrome
- Chotzen syndrome
- Pfeiffer syndrome
- Carpenter syndrome
- Crouzon syndrome

SIGNS AND SYMPTOMS

Early closure of fontanels and sutures.

COMPLICATIONS

- Hydrocephalus.
- ↑ intracranial pressure (ICP).
- Developmental delay.

TREATMENT

- Craniotomy to prevent intracranial and ophthalmologic complications.
- Multidisciplinary approach—genetics, psychology, pediatrics, surgery, neurology.
- Genetic counseling.
- Long-term follow-up.

Amniotic Bands

DEFINITION

- Fibrous strands of membrane stretching across chorionic cavity.
- Form of disruption.

EPIDEMIOLOGY

Not associated with problems in future pregnancies.

ETIOLOGY

- Spontaneous.
- Associated with abdominal trauma.
- May be associated with chorionic villus sampling (CVS).

PATHOPHYSIOLOGY

Caused by early amnion rupture and leakage of chorionic fluid.

SIGNS AND SYMPTOMS

- May be innocent and not cause any harm to the fetus.
- Can → limb or other body part constriction or amputation (amniotic band syndrome).
- May be associated with oligohydramnios and ↓ fetal movement.

DIAGNOSIS

Ultrasound.

TREATMENT

Most bands disappear on their own, not appearing on follow-up ultrasound.

Cleft Palate/Lip

DEFINITION

- Spectrum of defects of the upper lip, philtrum, and hard and soft palates.
- Cleft lip, cleft palate, or both.
- Unilateral or bilateral.

EPIDEMIOLOGY

- Fourth most common birth defect.
- Incidence of orofacial clefting is 1 in 700 live birth.
- Occur more often in infants of Asian, Latino, or Native American descent.
- More common in males.

ETIOLOGY

- Teratogens—ethanol, anticonvulsants, steroids, chemotherapy, maternal vitamin A excess.
- Gestational factors—maternal diabetes, amniotic bands.
- Chromosomal abnormalities.
- Idiopathic (majority).

PATHOPHYSIOLOGY

- Clefting of lip and anterior (primary) palate due to defect in fusing of both maxillary processes with the frontonasal process during weeks 5 and 6.
- Clefting of posterior (secondary) palate due to defect in fusion of palatal shelves during weeks 7 and 8.

SIGNS AND SYMPTOMS

Can affect feeding, speech, illness (colds and ear infections), teething, hearing, and emotional coping.

DIAGNOSIS

Physical exam of lips, palate, and oropharynx.

TREATMENT

- Infants with cleft palate may require assistance with feeding.
- Surgical repair of lip within first months of life, palate around 1 year of life; potential for final repairs and scar revisions in adolescence.
- Cleft team can include plastic and oral surgeons; geneticist; ear, nose, and throat (ENT) specialist; dentist; speech pathologist; audiologist; social worker or psychologist; and nurse coordinator.
- Genetic counseling.

Omphalocele

DEFINITION

Herniation of abdominal contents (usually only intestine, though can include liver and/or spleen) through umbilical root, which is covered only by peritoneum.

In a normal pregnancy, there is approximately 600 mL of amniotic fluid surrounding the baby at 40 weeks' gestation.

Amniotic fluid volume ↓ as gestational age advances beyond 32 or 34 weeks' gestation.

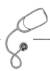

Isolated third-trimester oligohydramnios is not necessarily associated with poor perinatal outcome.

Oligohydramnios becomes most evident after 20 weeks of gestation.

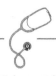

Pulmonary hypoplasia is the most serious complication of oligohydramnios.

EPIDEMIOLOGY

- May be associated with other congenital defects, including chromosomal anomalies, heart defects, and diaphragmatic hernia.
- Association: Beckwith-Wiedemann syndrome (omphalocele, macrosomia, hypoglycemia), trisomies 13 and 18.

DIAGNOSIS

Some may be detected on prenatal ultrasounds.

TREATMENT

- Until any other, more serious conditions have been taken care of, the extruded contents are covered.
- Serial reductions of intestines back into abdomen until skin closure is possible.

Oligohydramnios

DEFINITION

- Abnormally small amount of amniotic fluid (amniotic fluid index [AFI] < 5.0 cm or single pocket of fluid < 2 cm).
- Volume < 500 mL = oligohydramnios.
- Complicates 1–5% of pregnancies.

ETIOLOGY

- Premature rupture of membranes (PROM).
- Intrauterine growth retardation (IUGR).
- Postdates pregnancy.
- Renal anomalies (eg, bilateral renal agenesis, multicystic dysplastic kidneys, posterior urethral valves).
- Other congenital anomalies (eg, aneuploidy).
- Placental abruption.
- Twin-twin transfusion.
- Iatrogenic—nonsteroidal prostaglandin synthetase inhibitors, first-trimester chorionic villus sampling, second-trimester amniocentesis; amniotic fluid level may return to normal.
- Idiopathic.

PATHOPHYSIOLOGY

Amniotic fluid is regulated by fetal urine, as well as fetal oral secretions and respiratory secretions. Any process disrupting this exchange of fluid can → pathological amniotic fluid levels.

COMPLICATIONS

- Fetal demise.
- Pulmonary hypoplasia.
- Facial deformities.
- Skeletal deformities (eg, compressed thorax, twisted feet).

Potter Syndrome

- Potter syndrome specifically refers to bilateral renal agenesis, though other renal anomalies → oligohydramnios have also used the eponym.
- Potter syndrome includes pulmonary hypoplasia, skeletal anomalies, and characteristic facies (sloping forehead; flattened nose; recessed chin; and low-set, floppy ears).
- It is incompatible with neonatal life.
- Death occurs due to pulmonary hypoplasia.

DIAGNOSIS

- Amniotic fluid index (AFI)—sum of the maximum vertical pocket of amniotic fluid in each quadrant of the uterus.
- Best to use average of three readings.

TREATMENT

- Depends on etiology.
- First goal is to remove the inciting cause or correct the underlying problem (eg, discontinue prostaglandin inhibitor, place a shunt).
- Measures to prepare fetus for possible premature birth (corticosteroids and antibiotics for PROM).
- Antepartum testing to determine appropriate time for delivery in IUGR.

Hypospadias

DEFINITION

Improper location of urethral meatus, not at tip of penis, but on underside of penis, even as far back as the scrotum.

ETIOLOGY

Hereditary—if father has, there is a 20% chance that child will.

SIGNS AND SYMPTOMS

- Curvature of penis downward; foreskin "hooding."
- Potentially may have to sit down to urinate.

DIAGNOSIS

Clinical, though radiologic studies may be necessary if other congenital defects possibly present.

TREATMENT

- Surgical correction to extend urethra to end of penis before 18 months of age and chordae repair if sexual function will be affected by bent erect penis.
- May require more than one operation.
- Beware of postoperative bleeding, infections, stenosis, and fistulae.

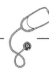

Patients with second-trimester oligohydramnios have a higher prevalence of congenital anomalies and a lower fetal survival rate than those women with oligohydramnios in the third trimester.

Suspect bilateral renal agenesis if maternal ultrasonography shows **oligohydramnios,** nonvisualization of the bladder, and absent kidney.

Infants with hypospadias should not be circumcised at birth, as the foreskin may be useful in the repair.

HIGH-YIELD FACTS

CONGENITAL MALFORMATIONS

Metabolic Disease

DEFINITION

Inherited biochemical disorders.

PATHOPHYSIOLOGY

Mutations affecting proteins involved in the many metabolic pathways of the body. Typically result in deficiency of enzyme production or build-up of toxic metabolites, or both.

EPIDEMIOLOGY

Disorders involving deficiencies of enzymes are often autosomal recessive (please see noted exceptions in this chapter).

SIGNS AND SYMPTOMS

- Often normal at birth, but can show signs early, including metabolic acidosis, poor feeding, vomiting, lethargy, and convulsion.
- Mental retardation, organomegaly, unusual body odor, episodic decompensation.

DIAGNOSIS

- **Newborn metabolic screening:**
  - Standard in United States: Allows for early detection and treatment and can potentially prevent serious consequences.
  - Panel of test varies state by state but phenylketonuria (PKU), hypothyroidism, galactosemia, and hemoglobinopathies are nearly universal.
  - Tandem mass spectrometry is the usual method used for screening.
  - The following conditions are screened in most states:
    - Galactosemia.
    - Hypothyroidism.
    - Hemoglobinopathy.
    - Tyrosinemia.
    - Biotinidase deficiency.
    - Congenital adrenal deficiency.
    - Maple syrup urine disease.
    - Homocystinuria.
    - Cystic fibrosis.
    - Medium-chain acyl-CoA dehydrogenase deficiency (MCAD).
    - Urea cycle defects.
    - HIV is screened in some states.
  - Classification:
    - Amino acid and urea cycle disorders:
      - Homocystinuria.
      - Maple syrup urine disease.
      - Phenylketonuria.
      - Tyrosinemia.
      - **Urea cycle** (arginase deficiency, argininosuccinic academia, citrullinemia, ornithine transport defect).
    - Fatty acid oxidation disorders:
      - Carnitine transport defect.
      - Citrullinemia.
      - Glutaric acidemia type 2.
      - Medium-chain acyl-CoA dehydrogenase deficiency.

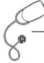

Medium-chain acyl-CoA dehydrogenase deficiency is the most common fatty acid oxidation disorder and may be associated with intermittent severe metabolic crises or sudden death.

TABLE 8-1. **Newborn Screening of Amino Acid Disorders**

DISORDER	SCREENING TEST	AGE OF TREATMENT	CONFIRMATORY TEST
Phenylketonuria (PKU)	Mass spectrometry	First weeks of life	Plasma phenylalanine and mutation testing
Tyrosinemia	Mass spectrometry	First weeks of life	Plasma amino acid profile and urine succinylacetone
Maple syrup urine disease (MSUD)	Mass spectrometry	First weeks of life	Plasma amino acid profile and allo-isoleucine

- Organic acid disorders:
  - 3-hydroxy-3-methyglutaryl-CoA lyase deficiency
  - Glutaric acidemia type I
  - Isovaleric acidemia
  - Methylmalonic acidemia
  - Propionic acidemia
- Many can be detected in the neonatal period or infancy, and some are included in newborn screening (see Table 8-1).

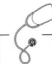

Most fatty acid oxidation disorders present with hypoglycemia.

TREATMENT

- Treatment varies but is often supportive/symptomatic.
- Frequently includes dietary modifications.
- Increasing availability of enzyme or gene-related treatment options.

DEFECTS OF AMINO ACID METABOLISM

See Table 8-2.

TABLE 8-2. **Disorders of Amino Acid Metabolism**

DISEASE	ACCUMULATION	DEFICIENCY	DISTINCTIVE FEATURE	
Phenylketonuria (PKU)	Phenylalanine and metabolites	Usually phenylalanine hydroxylase	Fair hair and skin, blue eyes, mousy odor	AR
Homocystinemia/ Homocystinuria	Homocystine, methionine	Usually cystathionine synthase	Ectopia lentis	AR
Maple syrup urine disease (MSUD)	Branched-chain amino acids: leucine, isoleucine, valine	Branched-chain ketoacid dehydrogenase	Odor of maple syrup in urine, sweat, cerumen	AR
Hartnup disease	Deficiency of neutral amino acids: tryptophan	Sodium-dependent amino acid transport system in renal tubules and intestines	Most are asymptomatic	AR

Phenylketonuria (PKU)

DEFINITION

Inherited disorder of amino acid metabolism in which phenylalanine cannot be converted to tyrosine.

ETIOLOGY

Deficiency of phenylalanine hydroxylase (or its cofactor tetrahydrobiopterin—2% of cases).

PATHOPHYSIOLOGY

- Accumulation of phenylalanine and its phenylketone metabolites disrupt normal metabolism and cause brain damage.
- Tyrosine becomes essential amino acid.

EPIDEMIOLOGY

- Autosomal recessive.
- One in 10,000–20,000 live births.
- Routinely screened for in the United States.

SIGNS AND SYMPTOMS

- Normal at birth.
- Severe mental retardation with IQ of 30 may develop at the end of 1 year (progressive and irreversible).
- Hypopigmentation due to low tyrosine (fair hair and skin, blue eyes).
- Eczema, mousy/musty body odor, hypertonia.

DIAGNOSIS

- Screened in all newborns.
- Serum tested 72 hours after initiation of first protein feed (test may be negative prior to 72 hours).
- If not screened neonatally, diagnosis usually made at 4–6 months of age.
- Prenatal and carrier testing possible.

TREATMENT

- Limit dietary phenylalanine (eg, in artificial sweeteners) and ↑ tyrosine; if started within first 10 days of life, infants can have normal intelligence.
- Strict dietary restriction during pregnancy.

Homocystinemia/Homocystinuria

DEFINITION

Inherited disorder of amino acid metabolism in which homocysteine is present in greater than trace amounts in the urine.

ETIOLOGY

Most commonly a deficiency of cystathionine β-synthase, but can also be a defect of methylcobalamin formation or deficiency of methyltetrahydrofolate reductase.

Phenylketones: phenylacetate, -lactate, and -pyruvate, in urine.

Aspartame contains phenylalanine.

↓ pigmentation in PKU is secondary to the inhibition of tyrosinase by phenylalanine.

Lethargy, anorexia, anemia, rashes, and diarrhea are signs of tyrosine deficiency.

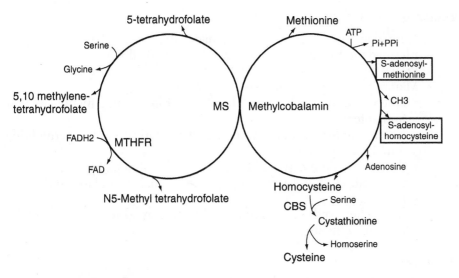

FIGURE 8-1. Homocysteine pathway.

PATHOPHYSIOLOGY

Homocysteine is not remethylated to methionine (see Figure 8-1).

EPIDEMIOLOGY

Autosomal recessive (1 in 200,000 live births).

SIGNS AND SYMPTOMS

- Depends on particular enzyme deficiency.
- Most commonly normal at birth, with failure to thrive and developmental delay subsequently occurring.
- Shares several skeletal and ocular features with Marfan syndrome.
- Later, ectopia lentis, marfanoid body habitus, progressive mental retardation, vaso-occlusive disease, osteoporosis, or fair skin with malar flush can occur.

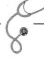

Ectopia lentis is subluxation of the lens, signaled by iridodonesis (quivering of iris) and myopia.

Late complications:
- Astigmatism
- Optic atrophy
- Glaucoma
- Cataracts
- Retinal detachment

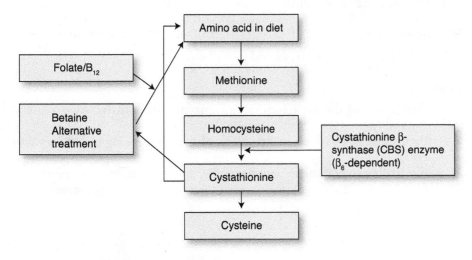

FIGURE 8-2. Methionine metabolism.

DIAGNOSIS

- Normal at birth; diagnosis usually made after 3 years of age.
- Elevated methionine and homocysteine in body fluids.
- Prenatal diagnosis possible.
- Marfan phenotype—differential diagnosis:
  - Homocystinuria: Marfanoid habitus, ectopia lentis, mental retardation, osteoporosis.
  - Ehlers-Danlos syndrome types 1 and 3: Marked joint hypermobility, mitral valve prolapse.
  - Stickler syndrome (hereditary arthro-ophthalmopathy): Tall stature, retrognathia, mitral valve prolapse, midfacial hypoplasia, retinal detachment.
  - Klinefelter syndrome: Marfanoid habitus, small testes and genitalia, learning difficulty.

Branched-chain amino acids are: leucine, isoleucine, valine.

TREATMENT

- Pyridoxine responsive form: 50% are this form and easily missed in the neonatal period. High-dose vitamin B_6.
- Pyridoxine unresponsive form: Restriction of methionine intake and supplementation of cysteine. (May require concurrent folic acid to show response.) Betaine can also play a role in this group.
- Other types may require vitamin B_{12} or methionine supplementation.

In MSUD, plasma leucine levels are usually higher than those of the other accumulating branched amino acids.

Maple Syrup Urine Disease (MSUD) or Branched-Chain Ketoaciduria

DEFINITION

Inherited disorder of branched-chain amino acid metabolism in which elevated quantities of leucine, isoleucine, valine, and corresponding oxoacids accumulate in the body fluids.

ETIOLOGY

Deficiency of branched-chain ketoacid dehydrogenase.

PATHOPHYSIOLOGY

Defect in the decarboxylation of leucine, isoleucine, and valine by a branched-chain ketoacid dehydrogenase.

Correcting the serum glucose level in MSUD does not improve the clinical state.

EPIDEMIOLOGY

One in 250,000 live births in general population.

SIGNS AND SYMPTOMS

- Deficiency of different subunits of enzyme account for wide clinical variability.
- Poor feeding, vomiting in first week of life, proceeding to lethargy and coma.
- Alternating hypertonicity and flaccidity, convulsions, hypoglycemia.
- Odor of maple syrup in urine, sweat, cerumen (burnt sugar smell).

Suspect MSUD:
- Intermittent symptoms (feeding difficulties and apnea) related to protein ingestion
- Sweet-smelling cerumen

DIAGNOSIS

- Elevated plasma and urine levels if leucine, isoleucine, valine, and allo-isoleucine; ↓ plasma alanine.
- Urine precipitant test.
- Neuroimaging in the acute state shows cerebral edema.

TREATMENT

- Chronically, low branched-chain amino acid diet.
- Frequent serum level monitoring.
- Acutely, intravenous administration of amino acids other than branched chain.
- Hemodialysis or peritoneal dialysis can save the patient's life in acidotic crisis, but liver transplantation can definitely treat MSUD.

Hartnup Disease

DEFINITION

Inherited defect in transport of neutral amino acids by intestinal mucosa and renal tubules.

ETIOLOGY

Deficient activity of a sodium-dependent transport system.

PATHOPHYSIOLOGY

Deficiency of tryptophan results in the clinical manifestations.

EPIDEMIOLOGY

Autosomal recessive.

SIGNS AND SYMPTOMS

- Usually asymptomatic.
- Rarely, cutaneous photosensitivity, episodic psychiatric changes.
- Marginal nutrition results in clinical manifestations in predisposed individuals.

DIAGNOSIS

- Aminoaciduria (neutral: alanine, serine, threonine, valine, leucine, isoleucine, phenylalanine, tyrosine, tryptophan, histidine).
- Normal plasma amino acid levels.

TREATMENT

Nicotinic acid/nicotinamide and a high-protein diet in symptomatic patients.

Urinary proline, hydroxyproline, and arginine remain normal in Hartnup disease (unlike in other causes of generalized aminoaciduria, such as Fanconi syndrome).

DEFECTS OF LIPID METABOLISM—LYSOSOMAL STORAGE DISEASES

Lipidoses

See Table 8-3.

Gaucher disease is the most common lysosomal storage disease (1 in 75,000). Splenomegaly is the most common presenting sign.

TABLE 8-3. Lysosomal Storage Diseases—Lipidoses

DISEASE	DEFICIENCY/ACCUMULATION	FEATURE	INHERITANCE
GM1 gangliosidoses	▪ Deficiency of β-galactosidase ▪ Accumulation of GM1 ganglioside	▪ Infantile, juvenile, adult forms (multiple forms) ▪ 50% cherry red spot on macula but clear cornea ▪ Hepatosplenomegaly ▪ Rashes, edema, psychomotor retardation ▪ Coarse facial features, skeletal abnormalities ▪ Blind and deaf by 1 year, death by 3–4 years of age ▪ WBC with inclusions	Autosomal recessive
GM2 gangliosidoses	*Tay-Sachs disease:* ▪ Deficiency of α subunit hexosaminidase A ▪ Results in accumulation of GM2 ganglioside in brain *Sandhoff disease:* ▪ Accumulation of GM2 ganglioside in brain and peripheral organs ▪ Defect of β subunit hexoseaminidases A and B	▪ Infantile and juvenile forms (multiple forms) ▪ Diagnosis at 5–6 months, death by 3–5 years of age ▪ Cherry red spot on macula but clear cornea ▪ Hyperacusis (exaggerated startle response) ▪ Froglike position ▪ No organomegaly in Tay-Sachs ▪ Hepatosplenomegaly in Sandhoff disease ▪ Normal WBC	Autosomal recessive Ashkenazi Jews (Tay-Sachs)
Niemann-Pick disease (six subtypes)	▪ Deficiency of sphingomyelinase ▪ Accumulation of sphingomyelin and cholesterol in reticuloendothelial and parenchymal cells	▪ 50% cherry red spot on macula in type A and normal in B and C types All types with clear cornea ▪ Hepatosplenomegaly, neonatal jaundice ▪ Diagnosis by 4 months, death by 3 years of age (infantile onset) ▪ Varying neurologic signs/deterioration (depending on subtype) ▪ Foam cells in bone marrow aspirates	Autosomal recessive Ashkenazi Jews
Gaucher disease (three types)	▪ Deficiency of β-glucosidase ▪ Accumulation of glucocerebroside in reticuloendothelial system	▪ Type I is most common (Ashkenazi Jews) ▪ Affects bone, liver, spleen, bone marrow, and brain (types II and III) ▪ Pancytopenia ▪ Bone fractures, pain, avascular necrosis ▪ Gaucher cells in bone marrow —"crinkled paper" cytoplasm ▪ Infantile form—rapid neurologic deterioration ▪ Adult form—more common, normal life span ▪ Treated with enzyme replacement	Autosomal recessive

TABLE 8-3. Lysosomal Storage Diseases—Lipidoses *(continued)*

Fabry disease	▪ Deficiency of ceramide trihexosidase or α-galactosidase A ▪ Accumulation of glycosphingolipids in vascular endothelium, nerves, and organs ▪ Clinical onset in childhood and adolescence	▪ Angiokeratomas (dark red punctate macules that do not blanch, occur in clusters, some become papules, distribution is bilateral and symmetric, navel and buttocks most common) and teleangiectasias ▪ First sign is severe neuropathic limb pain ▪ Asymmetric corneal deposits (cornea cloudy on slit lamp examination) ▪ Progressive kidney failure (biopsy shows lipid) and hepatomegaly ▪ Cardiac involvement with disease progression	X-linked recessive
Krabbe disease (globoid cell leukodystrophy)	▪ Deficiency of galactosyl-ceramide β-galactosidase or galactocerebrosidase ▪ Accumulation of ceramide galactose within lysosomes of brain white matter	▪ Progressive central nervous system degeneration; symptoms present within first 6 months of life ▪ Optic atrophy, spasticity, early death but clear cornea ▪ Globoid cells in areas of demyelination (distended, multinucleated bodies found in basal ganglia, pontine nuclei, and cerebellar white matter) ▪ Treatment: Hematopoietic stem cell transplant for infants prior to onset of neurologic symptoms	Autosomal recessive
Farber disease	▪ Deficiency of ceramidase ▪ Accumulation of ceramide in peripheral organs, joints, and lymph nodes	▪ Normal at birth; clinical onset at 4 months of age and diagnosis at 1 year ▪ Nodules (granulomas containing ceramide) on joints, vocal cords (hoarseness, respiratory complications) ▪ Severe mental and motor retardation Clear cornea with cherry red spot in 12% of cases	Autosomal recessive

DEFINITION/ETIOLOGY/PATHOPHYSIOLOGY

Inherited deficiencies of lysosomal hydrolases cause lysosomal accumulation of sphingolipids in brain and viscera.

Fabry disease is X-linked recessive.

EPIDEMIOLOGY

Most are autosomal recessive.

SIGNS AND SYMPTOMS

Depends on site of abnormal accumulations:

- Nervous system: Neurodegeneration, ocular findings.
- Viscera: Organomegaly, skeletal abnormalities, pulmonary infiltration.

Ganglisidoses (eg, GM1 and Tay-Sachs) have cherry red spot on macula in 50% of cases, as does Niemann-Pick.

Hepatosplenomegaly occurs in the GM1 gangliosidoses and Sandhoff disease, but not in Tay-Sachs disease.

Hunter syndrome is X-linked recessive.

DIAGNOSIS

Measurement of specific enzymatic activity in leukocytes or cultured fibroblasts.

TREATMENT

- Usually no specific treatment.
- Supportive/symptomatic therapy.
- Gaucher disease: Recombinant enzyme.
- Krabbe disease: Hematopoietic stem cell transplant.

Mucopolysaccharidoses

DEFINITION/ETIOLOGY/PATHOPHYSIOLOGY

Inherited deficiencies of lysosomal enzymes needed for the degradation of glycosaminoglycans (GAGs) resulting in widespread lysosomal storage of dermatan and heparan sulfates and severe clinical abnormalities. Keratan sulfates accumulate in other mucopolysaccharidoses not mentioned. See Table 8-4.

EPIDEMIOLOGY

Most are autosomal recessive.

SIGNS AND SYMPTOMS

- Normal at birth, diagnosis at 1+ years.
- "Gargoyle" cells containing lysosomes engorged with mucopolysaccharide.

TABLE 8-4. Lysosomal Storage Diseases—Mucopolysaccharidoses

SYNDROME	DEFICIENCY	DISTINCTIVE FEATURES	INHERITANCE
Hurler syndrome (MPS I)	α-L-iduronidase	▪ Severe, progressive; clinical onset at 1 year of age and death by 10 years of age ▪ Mental retardation, heart disease, corneal clouding, organomegaly, coarse facies ▪ Dysostosis multiplex, obstructive airway disease ▪ Enlarged tongue, hearing loss, limited language	Autosomal recessive
Scheie syndrome (milder form of Hurler's)	α-L-iduronidase	▪ Normal intelligence and relatively normal life span ▪ Corneal clouding, stiff joints, aortic regurgitation	Autosomal recessive
Hunter syndrome (MPS I)	Iduronate 2-sulfatase	▪ Mild to severe; clinical onset 1–2 year of age and death before 15 years in severe form ▪ Dysostosis multiplex, mental retardation, organomegaly, coarse facies ▪ Clear cornea but associated with retinitis and papilledema in severe cases	X-linked recessive

MPS, mucopolysaccharidosis.

- Excessive urinary excretion of GAGs.
- Progressive mental and physical deterioration.
- Coarse features.
- Corneal clouding.
- Stiff joints (abnormal hyalinization of collagen).
- Organomegaly.
- Skeletal abnormalities.

DIAGNOSIS

- Detection of enzyme deficiency in leukocytes or cultured fibroblasts.
- Roentgenographic changes consistent with dystosis multiplex.
- Urinary excretion of dermatan and heparan sulfates.

TREATMENT

Supportive therapy. Hurler's can be treated with bone marrow transplant.

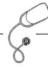

Dysostosis Multiplex
- Large dolichocephalic skull
- Thickened calvarium
- Ovoid vertebral bodies
- Flared iliac bones
- Shallow acetabulae
- Irregular widening of long bones

DEFECTS OF CARBOHYDRATE METABOLISM–GLYCOGEN STORAGE DISEASES

See Table 8-5.

von Gierke Disease

 A 3-month-old, breast-fed infant has failure to thrive, severe hepatomegaly, thin extremities, fasting hypoglycemia, lipemia, and metabolic acidosis. *Think: von Gierke disease.*

von Gierke is an inherited disorder that affect glycogen metabolism. It is due to the deficiency of glucose-6-phosphatase, which results in accumulation of glucose-6-phosphate, which in turns causes ↑ glycolysis and lactic acidosis. It is characterized by growth retardation, hypoglycemia, hepatomegaly, hyperlipidemia, hyperuricemia, lactic acidemia, and seizure. In neonatal period, hypoglycemia and lactic acidosis are the common presentation. Hepatomegaly becomes evident by 3–4 months of age.

TABLE 8-5. Glycogen Storage Diseases

DISEASE	GLYCOGEN ACCUMULATION	DEFICIENCY	TYPE
von Gierke disease	Liver, kidney, and intestine	Glucose-6-phosphatase	I
McArdle disease	Skeletal muscle	Skeletal muscle glycogen phosphorylase	V
Pompe disease	Cardiac and skeletal muscle	α-1,4-glucosidase (acid maltase)	II

DEFINITION

Inherited disorder of glycogen metabolism characterized by deposition of glycogen in the **liver, kidney,** and **intestine.**

ETIOLOGY

Deficiency of glucose-6-phosphatase.

PATHOPHYSIOLOGY

Glycogen-to-glucose metabolism stops at glucose-6-phosphate.

EPIDEMIOLOGY

Autosomal recessive.

SIGNS AND SYMPTOMS

- Fasting hypoglycemia (due to impaired gluconeogenesis, glycogenolysis, and recycling of glucose through the glucose-6-phosphate to glucose system).
- Massive hepatomegaly.
- Elevated serum levels of lactate, uric acid, cholesterol, triglycerides.
- Renal complications (Fanconi syndrome, nephrocalcinosis, focal segmental glomerulosclerosis).
- Slow growth, diarrhea, bleeding disorders, hypotonia, and gout.

DIAGNOSIS

- Normal at birth; diagnosis usually at 5 months.
- Administration of epinephrine, glucagons, galactose, fructose, or glycerol does not provoke normal hyperglycemic response (may precipitate acidosis).
- DNA tests form common mutations.
- In cases where mutation testing is not easily done, enzyme measurements can confirm the diagnosis.
- Liver biopsy demonstrates accumulation of glycogen in cells.

TREATMENT

- Avoid fasting.
- Supportive therapy aimed at maintaining normal glucose levels.
- Nocturnal intragastric, frequent, high-carbohydrate meals, are the main stay of treatment up to 1–2 years age.
- After 2 years of age, snacks or nocturnal intragastric feedings of uncooked cornstarch may be sufficient.
- High-protein diet is not effective.
- Granulocyte colony–stimulating factors to combat neutropenia and inflammation.
- Allopurinol to lower urate levels, bicarbonate or potassium citrate for lactic acidosis.
- Liver transplant for refractory disease.

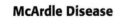
McArdle disease affects the Muscles.

McArdle Disease

DEFINITION

Inherited disorder of glycogen metabolism characterized by deposition of glycogen in skeletal muscle.

Deficiency of muscle glycogen phosphorylase (myophosphorylase).

EPIDEMIOLOGY

Autosomal recessive.

SIGNS AND SYMPTOMS

- Involves only skeletal muscles (accumulations of glycogen predominant in subsarcolemmal location).
- Temporary weakness and cramping of skeletal muscles during or after exercise.
- No rise in blood lactate during exercise.
- Characteristic "second wind" with initiation of fatty acid metabolism.

DIAGNOSIS

- Asymptomatic during infancy. Presents in adolescence/early childhood.
- Muscle biopsy and assay show deficiency of enzyme.
- Myoglobinuria, serum creatine kinase always elevated (elevated CK at rest).

TREATMENT

- Dietary modification (high fat and protein); sucrose prior to aerobic exercise; proper "warm-up" period.
- Prognosis is good with sedentary lifestyle.

Pompe Disease

DEFINITION

Inherited disorder of glycogen metabolism characterized by deposition of glycogen in cardiac and skeletal muscle.

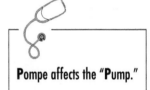

Pompe affects the "Pump."

ETIOLOGY

Deficiency of acid α-1,4-glucosidase (acid maltase).

PATHOPHYSIOLOGY

- Generalized glycogenesis because the defect is in all cells.
- Results in inability to convert mannose to glucose.

EPIDEMIOLOGY

Autosomal recessive.

SIGNS AND SYMPTOMS

- Rapid, progressive cardiomyopathy with massive cardiomegaly, macroglossia, hypotonia, hepatomegaly; death by 1–2 years.
- Juvenile form milder, slowly progressive myopathy, little to no cardiac abnormality. Death usually secondary to respiratory failure.

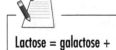

Lactose = galactose + glucose.

DIAGNOSIS

- Electrocardiogram (ECG): May show shortened PR interval.
- Electromyogram (EMG).

TREATMENT

Enzyme replacement with recombinant α-glucosidase delays disease progression.

Galactosemia

> A 2-week-old neonate has jaundice, hepatomegaly, and positive urinary-reducing substance. Odor of urine is normal. *Think: Galactosemia.*
>
> Since galactosemia is included in the newborn screening, it is diagnosed before the symptoms develop. Jaundice, hepatomegaly, vomiting, lethargy, and feeding difficulties are the common initial presentation. Presence of a reducing substance in urine in infants with galactosemia who are ingesting lactose establishes the diagnosis.

DEFINITION

Inborn errors of carbohydrate metabolism that result in elevated galactose and metabolite levels in blood and urine.

ETIOLOGY

Three types:

- Classic: Absence of galactose-1-phosphate uridyltransferase (inability to process lactose/galactose).
- Others: Galactokinase, uridine diphosphate galactose-4-epimerase.

PATHOPHYSIOLOGY

- Ingestion of galactose → ↑ concentrations in the blood and urine.
- Toxic substances, including galactitol, cause organ damage.

EPIDEMIOLOGY

- Autosomal recessive.
- One in 60,000.

SIGNS AND SYMPTOMS

- Cataracts, hepatosplenomegaly, mental retardation, sepsis (*E coli*).
- Triad: **Liver failure** (jaundice and coagulation disorder), **renal tubular dysfunction** (glucosuria, aminoaciduria, and acidosis), and **cataract.**

DIAGNOSIS

- Should be considered in newborn, infant, or child if jaundice, hepatomegaly, vomiting, hypoglycemia, convulsions, lethargy, irritability, feeding difficulties, poor weight gain, diarrhea, aminoaciduria, cataracts, vitreous hemorrhage, hepatic cirrhosis, ascites, splenomegaly, or mental retardation are noted.
- Presence of reducing substance in urine after ingestion of human or cow's milk is suggestive.
- Routinely screened for in the United States (Table 8-6).

When diagnosis of galactosemia is not made at birth, damage to the liver and brain become irreversible.

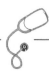

Neonates with galactosemia are at ↑ risk for *Escherichia coli* sepsis.

Elimination of galactose from diet in galactosemia does not ensure reversal of cataract formation.

TABLE 8-6. Screening for Galactosemia and Urea Cycle Defect

DISORDER	SCREENING	AGE OF TREATMENT	CONFIRMATORY TEST
Galactosemia	GALT enzyme measurement	First few days of life	GALT enzyme measurement, DNA mutations, galactose-1-P measurement
Urea cycle	Mass spectrometry	First few days of life	Plasma amino acid profile, DNA mutations

TREATMENT

- Exclude galactose and lactose from diet (example: dairy and breast milk).
- Soy-based formula.

Fructosuria

DEFINITION

Inborn errors of carbohydrate metabolism that result in elevated fructose and metabolite levels in blood and urine.

ETIOLOGY

Deficiency of fructokinase.

PATHOPHYSIOLOGY

- Enzyme is normally found in the liver, kidney, and intestine.
- Ingested fructose is not metabolized.

EPIDEMIOLOGY

Autosomal recessive.

SIGNS AND SYMPTOMS

- Asymptomatic until fructose introduced into diet
- Fructosemia and fructosuria.

DIAGNOSIS

Presence of urinary-reducing substrate without clinical symptoms.

TREATMENT

None indicated.

There is almost no renal threshold for fructose.

Do not confuse fructosuria with heriditary fructose intolerance (aldolase B deficiency), which presents with failure to thrive, hypoglycemia, lactic acidosis, vomiting, and seizures. Typically discovered during infancy at time of weaning with the introduction of fructose or sucrose into diet. Also autosomal recessive.

Lesch-Nyhan Syndrome

DEFINITION

- An X-linked-recessive disorder of purine metabolism resulting in deposition of purines in tissues and subsequent clinical abnormalities.
- Up to 1% of patients with gout may have Lesch-Nyhan syndrome.

ETIOLOGY

Deficiency of **hypoxanthine–guanine phosphoribosyl transferase (HGPRT)**.

Self-injurious behavior in Lesch-Nyhan syndrome can include banging head against wall and biting/mutilating one's fingers.

SIGNS AND SYMPTOMS

- Delayed motor development.
- Extrapyramidal sign resulting in choreoathetosis at approximately 1 year of age.
- Spastic cerebral palsy, self-injurious behavior.
- Hyperuricemia, uricosuria, urinary tract calculi, nephropathy, tophi, gouty arthritis.

DIAGNOSIS

- Normal at birth; diagnosis usually made at 3 months when delayed motor development becomes apparent.
- Uric acid crystalluria may first be noted as orange crystals in the diaper during the first weeks of life.
- Serum uric acid levels.
- Gout generally does not develop until puberty.

Think Lesch-Nyhan syndrome in the presence of self-mutilation and characteristic choreoathetosis; mental retardation.

TREATMENT

- No specific treatment; supportive therapy.
- Allopurinol to reduce serum uric acid levels.
- Prevention of self-injury.
- Death (due to infection or renal failure) in the second or third decade.

See Table 8-7.

- Complex heterozygosity: Different mutations in each gene allele—each individually "silent," but when combined produce clinical or biochemical manifestations.
- Consanguinity (children of first-degree relatives): ↑ risk for inherited disorders, as many are autosomal recessive.
- Sudden infant death syndrome (SIDS) or apparent life-threatening event (ALTE) may be the initial presentation of an inborn error of metabolism.
- Unexplained developmental delay may indicate an underlying metabolic disease.

HIGH-YIELD FACTS

METABOLIC DISEASE

TABLE 8-7. Familial Hyperlipidemias

Disorder	Lipids	Clinical Manifestations	Treatment	Deficiency
Hypercholesterolemia (type II hyperlipoproteinemia)	▪ Large elevations in serum cholesterol (> 500 mg/dL) ▪ Heterozygous form is common: ~1:500 ▪ Homozygous form is very rare: ~1:1,000,000	▪ Tendinous xanthomata ▪ Early atherosclerotic cardiovascular disease (late childhood/early adulthood myocardial infarction)	▪ Statins and cholestyramine for heterozygous form ▪ Liver transplant for rare homozygous form	Genetic defect in low-density lipoprotein (LDL) receptor
Hyperchylomicronemia (type I hyperlipoproteinemia)	▪ Accumulation of chylomicrons ▪ Low/normal LDL ▪ Serum grossly milky	▪ Eruptive xanthomata ▪ Periodic severe abdominal pain (pancreatitis) starting in infancy (colic) ▪ No atherosclerotic disease	▪ Very-low-fat diet may resolve xanthomatosis and reduce the risk of painful (and sometimes fatal) crises	Autosomal recessive (rarer than type II) Deficiency of lipoprotein lipase or cofactor apolipoprotein C-II
Dysbetalipoproteinemia (Type III)	▪ Absent chylomicrons ▪ Abnormal very-low-density lipoprotein (VLDL) and LDL ▪ Moderately severe elevations of cholesterol and triglyceride (TG) levels ▪ Cholesterol-to-TG ratio may equal 1	▪ Planar xanthomata ▪ Premature peripheral vascular disease and coronary artery disease	▪ Planar xanthomata ▪ Weight loss, diet, exercise ▪ Adults with persistent elevations treated with fibric acid derivatives	Abnormal apolipoprotein E
Endogenous hypertriglyceridemia	▪ ↑ VLDL	▪ Obesity, glucose intolerance ▪ Insulin resistance ▪ Hyperinsulinemia ▪ Hyperuricemia	▪ Weight control ▪ Dietary modification	Overproduction or reduced clearance of VLDL

HIGH-YIELD FACTS

METABOLIC DISEASE

HIGH-YIELD FACTS

METABOLIC DISEASE

Immunologic Disease

Transplacental antibodies protect neonates against chickenpox, measles, mumps, and rubella, but **not** chlamydia, gonorrhea, or group B *Streptococcus*.

- First immunoglobulin to appear in the bloodstream after the initial exposure to an antigen (primary antibody response): **IgM**
- Secretory antibody response: **IgA**
- Major antibody to protein antigens: **IgG**

- **Primary lymphoid organs**—development of lymphocytes: Bone marrow, fetal liver, and spleen. Thymus: maturation of T cells.
- **Secondary lymphoid tissue**—sites of antigen recognition: Lymph nodes, spleen, mucosal-associated lymphoid tissues (MALT), and gut-associated lymphoid tissues (GALT).
- Maternal serum antibodies (immunoglobulin G [IgG]) transferred across the placenta protect the infant from birth until approximately 6 months of age, and totally disappear by 12–18 months of age.
- Maternal antibodies (IgA) are transferred to the child's intestinal tract through breast milk.
- A child's IgG antibodies begin developing between 6 months and 1 year of age.
- Children under the age of 2 years develop strong immune response to polysaccharide antigens in a vaccine (*Haemophilus influenzae*, pneumococcal) if they are conjugated to a protein carrier.

HYPERSENSITIVITY REACTIONS

See Table 9-1 for types of hypersensitivity reactions.

- **Urticaria (hives):** Pale or reddened irregular, elevated itchy patches of skin.
- **Angioedema:** Giant wheals caused by localized dilatation and ↑ permeability of the capillaries in the deep dermis.
- **Vesicle:** A collection of fluid underneath epidermis = blister < 5 mm in diameter
- **Bulla:** Blister > 5 mm in diameter with thin walls.

Anaphylaxis

DEFINITION

A severe and potentially life-threatening systemic allergic IgE-mediated reaction caused by release of mediators from tissue mast cells and blood basophils.

TABLE 9-1. Types of Hypersensitivity Reactions

HYPERSENSITIVITY	ANTIBODY	EFFECT	EXAMPLES
Type I	IgE	Mast cells release mediators	Hay fever Anaphylaxis
Type II	IgM, IgG	Cytotoxic: Cell lysis	Goodpasture syndrome
Type III	IgM, IgG	AG-AB complex triggers complement	Serum sickness
Type IV	None	T cells infiltrate	Poison ivy dermatitis, PPD posivity

ETIOLOGY

- Foods: Milk, egg, peanuts, shellfish.
- Drugs: β-lactam antibiotics, sulfa.
- Vaccine, immune globulin, blood products.
- Latex (gloves, Foley catheters, and endotracheal tubes).
- Insect stings.

SIGNS AND SYMPTOMS

- Abrupt onset and rapid progression within 5–30 minutes.
- Generalized pruritus, **urticaria, tearing,** angioedema.
- Flushing, dizziness.
- Vomiting, abdominal cramps.
- Respiratory symptoms: Upper airway obstruction (laryngeal angioedema), bronchospasm.
- Hypotension, shock.

DIAGNOSIS

- History of exposure.
- Clinical presentation.
- **Serum tryptase** (at 1, 4, and 8 hours).
- See Figure 9-1 for National Institute of Allergy and Immunologic Disease/Food Allergy and Anaphylaxis Network diagnostic criteria.

TREATMENT

- Airway, breathing, circulation (ABC).
- Epinephrine (1:1000–0.01 mL/kg subcutaneously). Minimum dose: 0.1 mL. Maximum dose: 0.3. mL.
- Diphenhydramine 1–2 mg/kg IV, IM, or PO q4–6h.
- Cimetidine 5–10 mg/kg IV q6h (refractory cases).
- Admit if upper airway obstruction, significant bronchospasm, blood pressure instability.

Urticaria (Hives)

DEFINITION

Allergic (IgE-mediated), or nonallergic (nonimmunological: physical, chemical)–mediated skin lesions.

ETIOLOGY

- Infections:
  - Viruses (influenza, enterovirus, infectious mononucleosis, hepatitis).
  - Bacteria (group A β-hemolytic streptococci).
- Medications (penicillin, cephalosporin, phenytoin, barbiturate, aspirin).
- Foods.
- Insect stings.
- Autoimmune diseases.
- Malignancies.

SIGNS AND SYMPTOMS

- Raised pale and pink pruritic areas of annular or serpiginous pattern.
- Rash is often **migratory, waxing and waning.**

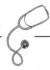

Anaphylactoid Reaction

- Clinically similar to anaphylaxis
- **Not IgE mediated**
- Does **not** require previous exposure

Risk factors for severe anaphylactic reaction:

- Asthma
- β blockade
- Adrenal insufficiency

Prophylaxis:

- Avoid
- ID bracelet
- Self-injectable epinephrine (Epi-pen).

Viral infections are the most common causes of urticaria in children.

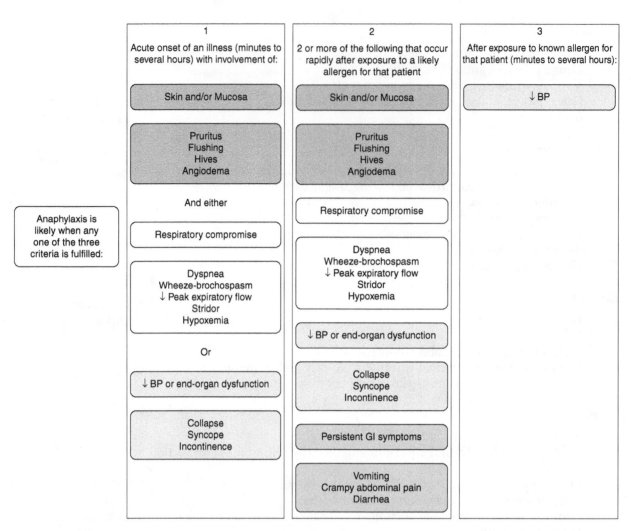

Anaphylaxis is likely when any one of the three criteria is fulfilled:

1
Acute onset of an illness (minutes to several hours) with involvement of:

Skin and/or Mucosa

Pruritus
Flushing
Hives
Angiodema

And either

Respiratory compromise

Dyspnea
Wheeze-brochospasm
↓ Peak expiratory flow
Stridor
Hypoxemia

Or

↓ BP or end-organ dysfunction

Collapse
Syncope
Incontinence

2
2 or more of the following that occur rapidly after exposure to a likely allergen for that patient

Skin and/or Mucosa

Pruritus
Flushing
Hives
Angiodema

Respiratory compromise

Dyspnea
Wheeze-brochospasm
↓ Peak expiratory flow
Stridor
Hypoxemia

↓ BP or end-organ dysfunction

Collapse
Syncope
Incontinence

Persistent GI symptoms

Vomiting
Crampy abdominal pain
Diarrhea

3
After exposure to known allergen for that patient (minutes to several hours):

↓ BP

FIGURE 9-1. Visual representation of National Institute of Allergy and Immunologic Disease/Food Allergy and Anaphylaxis Network diagnostic criteria.

(Reproduced, with permission, from Manivannan V, Decker WW, Stead LG, et al. *Intl J Emerg Med*, 2009.)

DIAGNOSIS

Clinical; no tests needed.

TREATMENT

- Avoiding the precipitating cause.
- Epinephrine (1:1000 at 0.01 mg/kg) if urticaria is severe.
- Diphenhydramine.

Serum Sickness

 For the past 2 weeks, a 6-year-old boy has had puffy eyelids on awakening and swelling of the feet and abdomen in the afternoon. He complains of joint aches and on-and-off fever. His history includes a sting by a yellow jacket. Physical examination is significant for generalized lymphadenopathy. Urinalysis shows protein 3+ and ESR is 35. *Think: Serum sickness.*

DEFINITION

Type III hypersensitivity reaction; does not require prior sensitization.

PATHOPHYSIOLOGY

Antigen-antibody complexes form deposits in blood vessels, particularly in joints and glomeruli of the nephrons, where they activate the classical complement pathway, resulting in vasculitis.

ETIOLOGY

- Antigout medications: Allopurinol, gold salts.
- Antimicrobials: **Cefaclor,** penicillin, griseofulvin, sulfonamides.
- Antiarrhythmics: Quinidine, procainamide.
- Antihypertensives: Captopril, hydralazine.
- Thyroid medications: Thiouracil, iodides.
- Other medications: Barbiturates, phenytoin.
- Serum/blood products, venoms.

SIGNS AND SYMPTOMS

- Onset 1–3 weeks after initial exposure to an offending agent.
- Fever, arthralgia, lymphadenopathy, and rash (serpiginous and urticarial or polymorphous).
- Frequent facial edema.
- **Rare** arthritis, cardiovascular and renal involvement.
- Symptoms persist 7–10 days and resolve spontaneously.

DIAGNOSIS

- Clinical.
- Low levels of C3, C4 (complement components), and CH50.

TREATMENT

Withdrawal of the offending agent.

Drug Reaction

DEFINITION

- Abnormal immunologically mediated hypersensitivity responses.
- Relatively rare.

Most common causes of drug reactions: penicillin, sulfonamide.

Drug Reactions

- Most are afebrile.
- Eruption may worsen before improving after discontinuation of the drug.

The most common site for the manifestation of drug reactions is the skin.

ETIOLOGY

Potentially any drug can cause drug reaction.

PATHOPHYSIOLOGY

- Type I (IgE mediated): Penicillin, cephalosporin.
- Type II (cytotoxic antibody mediated): Penicillin—hemolytic anemia; quinidine—thrombocytopenia.
- Type III (immune complex mediated): Penicillin, sulfonamides, cephalosporin.
- Type IV (cell mediated): Contact dermatitis—Neosporin.

CLINICAL CRITERIA

- Reactions do not resemble pharmacologic action of the drug.
- Similar to those that may occur with other allergens.
- Timing: 7–10 days.
- Reproduced by minute doses.
- Discontinuation may result in resolution.

SIGNS AND SYMPTOMS

- Mild rash to anaphylaxis.
- **Fixed drug eruptions:** Recur at the same site after each administration of causative drug (sulfonamides are the most common).

DIAGNOSIS

- Eosinophilia is a clue but is not diagnostic.
- Skin test is available for penicillin. It is indicated for the patients with a history of penicillin-associated anaphylaxis, urticaria, or serum sickness.
- Radioallergosorbent test (RAST).

DISPOSITION

- Discontinue likely offending agent.
- Admit if:
  - Stevens-Johnson syndrome.
  - Toxic epidermal necrolysis.
  - Severe drug reaction.
  - Respiratory distress.

Penicillin Allergy

TYPES

Wide variety of allergic reactions:

- Type I: Anaphylaxis.
- Type II: Hemolytic anemia.
- Type III: Serum sickness.

AMPICILLIN/AMOXICILLIN RASH

- Not urticaria, seen with infectious mononucleosis.
- Hyperuricemia.

Food Allergy/Sensitivity

PATHOPHYSIOLOGY

- Most of the true **hypersensitivities to food** products are **IgE mediated.** IgE binds to mast cells, resulting in the release of histamine and other mediators. Most common triggers are peanuts, shellfish, and eggs.
- Early presentation in life. Only ~5% of children under the age of 4 years have food hypersensitivity. It is seen even less frequently in older children.
- Most **adverse reactions** to food **do not** have an immunologic basis.
- Nonimmunologic food intolerances are common, like enzyme deficiencies (lactase deficiency, vomiting, diarrhea).

Most common food
allergies:
- Peanut
- Shellfish
- Eggs

SIGNS AND SYMPTOMS

- **IgE-mediated hypersensitivity** reactions start **within minutes** of the responsible food intake, and often are associated with urticaria, edema, and anaphylaxis (see below).
- **Allergic enterocolitis of infancy** with vomiting and diarrhea (becomes bloody) represents hypersensitivity to cow's milk proteins, but is **not** IgE mediated. It → failure to thrive. Half of infants reacting to the cow's milk protein also react to soy protein. Note early presentation in the first month of life.
- **Gluten-sensitive enteropathy** is also a non-IgE-mediated food hypersensitivity (celiac disease), and also → failure to thrive. Gradual onset of symptoms in the **second half of infancy,** when the child starts to eat grains (cereal) containing gluten protein.

TREATMENT

Avoidance of offending agent.

Stevens-Johnson Syndrome (SJS; Erythema Multiforme Major)

DEFINITION

Extreme variant of erythema multiforme (EM) with systemic toxicity and involvement of the mucous membranes.

ETIOLOGY

- Drugs: Sulfonamides and anticonvulsants.
- *Mycoplasma pneumoniae,* herpes simplex virus.

Mild EM does not progress to SJS.

SIGNS AND SYMPTOMS

- Prodromal phase (1–14 days): Fever, headache, malaise.
- Mucosal involvement:
  - Exudative conjunctivitis.
  - Oral erosions on the palate and gingivae.
  - Urethritis, vaginitis.
- Skin involvement: Target lesions—annular, with pink halo surrounding a pale halo and erythematous center. May have central blistering. Palms and soles are involved.
- **Nikolsky's sign:** Separation of normal epidermis at the basal layer caused by sliding finger pressure ("rubbed off" line).
- See Dermatologic Disease chapter.

The oral cavity is almost always involved in erythema mulitforme major.

DIAGNOSIS

- **Clinical criteria:** Cutaneous lesion plus at least two mucosal surfaces involved.
- Skin biopsy is not indicated (would show perivascular mononuclear cell infiltrate).

TREATMENT

- Hospitalization for supportive care.
- Intravenous (IV) hydration.
- Topical steroids and anesthetics as needed.

IMMUNODEFICIENCIES

- Primary (congenital) immune deficiencies (Table 9-2) present at different ages, depending on category of disorder.
- When evaluating a child with recurrent infections, pay attention to the following:
  - **Age of onset:** T-cell deficiency presents in the first 3–4 months of life, whereas B-cell disorders present after 6 months of age, when maternal antibodies disappear.

TABLE 9-2.   Combined and Primary T-Cell Immune Deficiencies

DISORDER	DEFECT	LYMPHOCYTES	IMMUNE GLOBULINS	CLINICAL	INFECTIONS	TREATMENT
SCID group (ADA = one third)	Variable enzyme deficiencies	Low/no T, some/no B	Low/no titers	0–3 months FTT, thrush, ALC < 500	PCP, sepsis, severe VZV	BMT, ADA replacement
DiGeorge	Point mutation Midline defects No thymus	Low/no T	Low/no titers	Low Ca, truncus arteriosus	Same	Thymus transplant (ALC < 100)
Wiskott-Aldrich	X-linked, defective cytoskeleton of the cells	Normal #	High IgA, IgE Low IgM, titers	Eczema, TCP	OIs (PCP), severe HSV and VZV	BMT
Ataxia-telangiectasia	AR, defect in DNA repair	Progressive loss of T4	Low IgA, IgM, and titers	Wobbly gait, red sclerae, lymphomas	OIs, sinopulmonary	Antibioics
Chronic mucocutaneus candidiadis	T cells don't respond to candidal antigens	Normal #	Normal	Endocrinopathy (thyroid)	Persistent thrush, thickened nails	Systemic antifungal

ADA, adenosine deaminase; ALC, absolute lymphocyte count; AR, autosomal recessive; BMT, bone marrow transplantation; FTT, failure to thrive; HSV, herpes simplex virus; OI, opportunistic infection; PCP, *Pneumocystis jiroveci* pneumonia; SCID, severe combined immunodeficiency; TCP, thrombocytopenia; VZV, varicella-zoster virus.

- **X-linked inheritance:** Similar case in a male relative (Bruton's, Wiskott-Aldrich, chronic granulomatous disease [CGD]).
- **Clinical features:**
    - Failure to thrive (FTT): Severe combined immunodeficiency (SCID).
    - Hypertelorism, hypocalcemia, truncus arteriosus: DiGeorge syndrome.
    - Absence of tonsils and lymphatic nodes: Bruton agammaglobulinemia.
    - Coarse features, eczema, lax joints, scoliosis: Job syndrome.
- **Workup:** Thymus shadow on chest x-ray, antibody titers (response to vaccination), absolute lymphocyte count (ALC).
- **Sites of infection:**
    - Phagocytes (CGD): Sinopulmonary and soft tissues.
    - Immunoglobulin deficiencies: Sinopulmonary and gastrointestinal (*Giardia*).
    - T cells: Disseminated (mycobacteria, varicella-zoster virus).
- **Types of microorganisms:** Intracellular infections in T-cell disorders (viruses, mycobacteria, *Pneumocystis*); *Neisseria* infections in late complement deficiency.

Severe Combined Immunodeficiency (SCID)

A 4-month-old female just diagnosed with failure to thrive (FTT) presents with respiratory distress. On physical examination, she has a temperature of 101°F (38.3°C), RR 70 breaths/min, and oxygen saturation 91% (on room air). Oral thrush and bilateral rhonchi were present. There is no lymphadenopathy. Her white blood cell count is 16.2, 83% neutrophils, 11% monocytes. Chest x-ray shows diffuse bilateral interstitial infiltrates. *Think: PCP.*

Infection with opportunistic organisms such as PCP is common in infants with SCID. Absence of lymph nodes in an infant with FTT in the first few months of life is suggestive of SCID. Oral thrush, extensive diaper rash, and failure to thrive are the prominent features.

Onset of SCID at 3 months of age:
- No palpable lymph nodes
- Opportunistic infections
- Failure to thrive

DEFINITION
Abnormalities of both humoral and cellular immunity.

ETIOLOGY
- A group of genetic abnormalities that result in severe T-cell depletion (or dysfunction) and B-cell dysfunction (eg, enzyme deficiencies → defect in stem cell maturation).
- **Adenosine deaminase (ADA) deficiency:** One third of all SCID cases.

SIGNS AND SYMPTOMS

- Presents within first 3 months with diarrhea, pneumonia, otitis, sepsis, FTT, and skin rashes.
- Frequency and severity of infections.
- Persistent infection with **opportunistic organisms** (*Candida*, mycobacteria, herpes viruses, CMV, PCP).
- Absent lymphatic nodes, hypoplastic thymus.

DIAGNOSIS

- Lymphopenia: ALC (absolute lymphocyte count) < 500.
- ↓ serum IgG, IgA, and IgM.
- Low or no T and B cells.

Measures to be taken in SCID:
- Protective isolation
- Irradiation of all blood products

TREATMENT

- Aggressive antimicrobial treatment of even mild infections.
- Recombinant ADA is available for replacement therapy.
- Bone marrow transplantation (BMT).

PROGNOSIS

Death within first 2 years if untreated.

Letterer-Siwe Disease

An 18-month-old female presents with two "bumps on the head." Physical examination shows weight below 3rd percentile; two palpable masses on the scalp; and scaly, greasy patches of rash over the scalp, eyebrows, neck, and in the ear canals; generalized lymphadenopathy; and hepatosplenomegaly. WBC: 5.6, Hb 8.4, platelet count 76. Lateral skull radiograph shows two well-defined lytic lesions. *Think: Letterer-Siwe disease.*

Letter-Siwe disease is the most severe form of Langerhans' cell histiocytosis. Patients with this disease typically present with a scaly seborrhea and eczematous rash that involves the scalp, ear canals, abdomen, and intertriginous areas of the neck and face. Typical age of presentation is under 2 years. There is a potential for pancytopenia because of hematopoietic involvement.

DEFINITION

- The most severe form of Langerhans' cell histiocytosis (LCH).
- Manifestation of complex immune dysregulation.

Letterer-Siwe disease:
- Lytic lesions
- Lymphadenopathy
- Eczema

SIGNS AND SYMPTOMS

- Skeleton involved (80%): Skull, vertebrae (eosinophilic granuloma, lytic lesions).
- Skin (50%): Seborrheic or eczematoid dermatitis in a child of < 2 years of age
- Lymphadenopathy (33%).
- Hepatosplenomegaly (20%).

- Anorexia, FTT
- Exophthalmos.
- Pituitary dysfunction: Growth retardation, diabetes insipidus.
- Systemic manifestations: Fever, weight loss, irritability, FTT.
- Bone marrow suppression: Anemia, thrombocytopenia, neutropenia.

LAB

- Complete blood count (CBC).
- Liver function tests (LFTs).
- Coagulation profile.
- Chest x-ray.
- Skeletal survey.
- Urine osmolality.
- Tissue biopsy (skin or bone lesions).

TREATMENT

- Treatment directed at arresting the progression of lesion (low-dose local radiation).
- Systemic multiagent chemotherapy.
- Spontaneous remission.

DiGeorge Syndrome

> A 2-month-old infant with congenital heart disease and cleft palate is hospitalized with cough and tachypnea. He has a history of a seizure episode. Chest x-ray shows diffuse infiltrates and no thymic shadow. Serum calcium is 6.5 mg/dL. *Think: DiGeorge syndrome.*
>
> DiGeorge syndrome is a T-cell deficiency that results from failure of development of the third and fourth pharyngeal pouches, which are responsible for the development of thymus and parathyroid glands. These result in lack of T-cell-mediated immunity, tetany, and congenital defects of the heart and great vessels. It is important to recognize this diagnosis because without treatment it is fatal.

PATHOPHYSIOLOGY

- Deletion in chromosome 22, resulting in a defect of development of the third and fourth pharyngeal pouches.
- Phenotypical translation into midline defects of the heart, head, parathyroids, and thymus.

SIGNS AND SYMPTOMS

- Dysmorphic features: Hypertelorism, cleft palate.
- Congenital heart disease: **Truncus arteriosus, interrupted aortic arch.**
- Hypoparathyroidism presents as hypocalcemic seizures ("**tetany**").
- Recurrent infections: depending on T-lymphocyte counts. Opportunistic infections (OIs) in severe cases.

CATCH 22
Cardiac abnormality
(tetralogy of Fallot)
Abnormal facies
Thymic aplasia
Cleft palate
Hypocalcemia
(22 abmormality on the 22 chromosome)

DIAGNOSIS

- Calcium level and parathyroid hormone.
- T-cell count (variable).
- Chest x-ray: No thymic shadow.
- Echocardiogram.
- **Fluorescent in situ hybridization (FISH)** test detects the 22q11.2 deletion.

TREATMENT

- Thymic transplant if ALC < 100.
- BMT is not an option because of high risk for graft-versus-host disease (GVHD).
- Use **irradiated blood products** only.

Ataxia-Telangiectasia (AT)

DEFINITION

Autosomal-recessive disorder of DNA repair that presents as telangiectasias, ataxia, and variable extent of T-cell deficiency, with progressive loss of T helpers. Both humoral and cellular immunodeficiency.

SIGNS AND SYMPTOMS

- Usually presents during first 6 years, wheelchair confinement by 10–12 years.
- **Earliest sign: Telangiectasias on the sclerae** (misdiagnosed as "pink eye").
- Progressive cerebellar ataxia.
- Chronic sinusitis, bronchiectases.
- OIs.
- ↑ risk of malignancy (lymphomas, leukemia).

LAB

- Absence of antibodies after vaccination.
- Low IgA and IgM.
- T4 lymphocytes decline over time.
- ↑ serum α-fetoprotein.

TREATMENT

- Supportive therapy.
- Improve pulmonary function.
- Prophylaxis of OIs.

Chronic Mucocutaneous Candidiasis (CMC)

DEFINITION

- T-cell dysfunction: Inability to recognize candidal antigens.
- A heterogeneous group of disorders characterized by recurrent or persistent superficial candidal infections of the skin, nails, and mucous membranes.

Ataxia-telangiectasia:
- Injected sclera
- Ataxia
- Lymphoma

SIGNS AND SYMPTOMS

- Refractory thrush may extend to the esophagus.
- Refractory severe diaper rash.
- Angular cheilitis.
- Nails thickened, significant edema and erythema of the surrounding periungual tissue.
- Often associated with endocrinopathy: Hypo/hyperthyroidism, polyendocrinopathy.

TREATMENT

- Systemic antifungals
- Skin care

Wiskott-Aldrich Syndrome

A 10-month-old boy presents with oral thrush despite 10 days of treatment with nystatin. He had 4 episodes of otitis media. Physical examination shows oral thrush and multiple patches of eczema. Both tympanic membranes are dull. CBC shows the following: WBC 7.6, Hb 11.3, platelet count 97. His uncle died in infancy of infection. *Think: Wiskott-Aldrich syndrome.*

Wiskott-Aldrich syndrome is an X-linked recessive syndrome characterized by the triad of eczema, thrombocytopenia, and immunodeficiency. The initial manifestation usually is petechiae or bleeding in the first few months of life. Classic presentation is thrombocytopenia, eczema, and recurrent otitis media.

Wiskott-Aldrich syndrome:
- Eczema
- Thrmobocytopenia
- ↑ IgA/IgE

DEFINITION

X-linked-recessive disorder of cell cytoskeleton, presenting as eczema, thrombocytopenia (TCP), and ↑ susceptibility to infection.

SIGNS AND SYMPTOMS

- Atopic dermatitis/eczema.
- Thrombocytopenic purpura.
- Recurrent infections in infancy: Pneumococcal (otitis, pneumonia), persistent thrush.
- OIs: *Pneumocystis jiroveci* pneumonia (PCP).

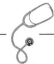

Oral candidiasis at > 6 months of age should arouse suspicion for the presence of an immunodeficiency.

LAB

- ↓ IgM.
- ↑ IgA and IgE.
- Absence of antibodies after vaccination.

Common Variable Immunodeficiency (CVID)

DEFINITION

- A group of disorders of T- and B-cell interaction and cytokine production, resulting in impaired IgM to IgG switch and in the absence of protective antibody titers (see Table 9-3).
- Often (one fourth) familial.
- Involves the formation of autoantibodies.

TABLE 9-3. B-Cell Disorders and Immunoglobulin Deficiencies

DISORDER	DEFECT	LYMPHOCYTES	IMMUNO-GLOBULINS	CLINICAL	INFECTIONS	TREATMENT
Bruton's agamma-globulinemia	X-linked arrest of B-cell maturation	No B Normal T	Low/no titers	No tonsils, no palpable lymph nodes	Pneumococcal Rotaviral *Giardia*	IVIG
Selective IgA deficiency	No switch to IgA	Normal #	Normal IgM, IgG, and titers	Allergies, arthritis, IBD	Mostly respiratory	IVIG is counterindicated
CVID (a group of disorders)	Abnormal T- and B-cell interactions One fourth familial	Normal #	Normal IgM Low IgA, IgG, and titers	Lymphadenopathy, autoimmune lymphomas	Pneumococcal, *Giardia*, sinusitis	IVIG if IgG < 400

CVID, common variable immunodeficiency; IBD, inflammatory bowel disease; IVIG, intravenous immune globulin.

SIGNS AND SYMPTOMS

- Two peak ages of onset: Children aged 1–5 years and 16–20 years old.
- Lymphadenopathy, splenomegaly.
- Association with autoimmune diseases: Inflammatory bowel disease (IBD), sprue-like syndrome, arthritis.
- Lymphoid interstitial pneumonitis, granulomas on various organs.
- ↑ risk of malignancies: Non-Hodgkin lymphoma, gastric carcinoma.
- Sinopulmonary infections: Pneumococcal, *Mycoplasma*.
- Gastrointestinal (GI) infections: *Giardia*.

Bruton's Congenital Agammaglobulinemia

DEFINITION

- X-linked tyrosine kinase deficiency resulting in the arrest of B-cell maturation. Gene defect in Xq22.
- Severe hypogammaglobulinemia.

SIGNS AND SYMPTOMS

- No tonsils.
- No palpable lymphatic nodes.
- Recurrent/chronic sinopulmonary (pneumococcal), GI (*Giardia*) infections.
- ↑ susceptibility to enteroviral meningoencephalitis.

DIAGNOSIS

Very low or absent mature B lymphocytes and all classes of immunoglobulins. No production of protective antibodies (negative titers).

Bruton's agammaglobulinemia:
- Male
- No palpable lymph nodes
- No tonsil
- Respiratory and gastrointestinal infections

Infants with Bruton's agammaglobulinemia remain well for the first 6 months due to the presence of maternal IgG antibodies.

Selective IgA Deficiency

DEFINITION

Deficiency of IgA-predominant immunoglobulin on mucosal surfaces.

EPIDEMIOLOGY

Most common of the primary antibody deficiencies.

SIGNS AND SYMPTOMS

- Mostly respiratory tract infections.
- Allergies.
- Autoimmune diseases: IBD, arthritis.

DIAGNOSIS

- IgA < 5 mg/dL.
- Normal levels of other immunoglobulins and normal response to vaccination.
- Normal cell-mediated immunity.

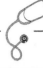

Selective IgA deficiency can → fatal anaphylaxis with blood (IVIG) infusion. **IVIG is contraindicated.**

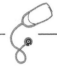

IgA is the major immunoglobulin within the upper airway.

Chédiak-Higashi Syndrome

DEFINITION

Autosomal-recessive syndrome caused by mutations of the lysosomal trafficking regulator gene, resulting in abnormal chemotaxis and fusion of intracellular granules.

SIGNS AND SYMPTOMS

- Recurrent skin infections and pneumonias (*Staphylococcus aureus*).
- Partial oculocutaneous albinism.
- Progressive peripheral neuropathy.

DIAGNOSIS

- Giant gray granules in the cytoplasm of nucleated cells.
- Leukopenia, neutropenia.
- Chemotaxis test.

TREATMENT

- Ascorbic acid has no effect.
- Antibiotics for acute infections.
- BMT (does not prevent or cure peripheral neuropathy).

Thymic hypo- or aplasia → a deficiency of functional T cells.

Chronic Granulomatous Disease (CGD)

A 10-month-old male presents with a temperature of 101.6°F (38.7°C) and a 3 × 4-cm abscess of the left buttock. His WBC count is 19.9, 77% neutrophils. At the age of 5 months he had staphylococcal cervical lymphadenitis that required drainage. His uncle also had recurrent abscesses. *Think: CGD.*

Recurrent infections in the first year of life are usually the first symptom. Granulomatous lesions in the lungs, skin, and liver are common.

PATHOPHYSIOLOGY

- Most common inherited disorder of phagocytosis, X-linked or autosomal recessive.
- Oxidase deficiency in neutrophils and macrophages = defect in generation of oxygen metabolites.
- Chemotaxis and phagocytosis intact.
- Inability to kill **catalase-positive** microorganisms: *S aureus*.

SIGNS AND SYMPTOMS

- Presents in the first years of life.
- Recurrent deep soft tissue abscesses and lymphadenitis.
- Severe staphylococcal and *Burkholderia cepacia* pneumonia and lung abscess, pneumatoceles.
- Osteomyelitis.
- Hepatosplenomegaly (granulomas).

DIAGNOSIS

- Nitroblue tetrazolium test.
- **Leukocytosis.**
- Hypergammaglobulinemia.

TREATMENT

- Aggressive antimicrobial treatment of infection.
- Surgical excision of abscesses.

Job Syndrome (Hyper-IgE)

Job syndrome:
- Eczema
- Eosinophilia
- Lax joints
- Staph infections

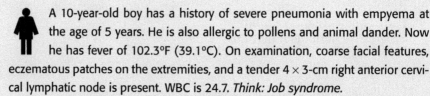

A 10-year-old boy has a history of severe pneumonia with empyema at the age of 5 years. He is also allergic to pollens and animal dander. Now he has fever of 102.3°F (39.1°C). On examination, coarse facial features, eczematous patches on the extremities, and a tender 4 × 3-cm right anterior cervical lymphatic node is present. WBC is 24.7. *Think: Job syndrome.*

Job syndrome is hyperimmunoglobulinemia E with impaired chemotaxis. IgE level should be obtained. *Characteristic findings include* eczema, recurrent "cold," staphylococcal skin abscesses, sinusitis, and otitis media.

DEFINITION

- Neutrophil chemotactic defect.
- Autosomal dominant.

SIGNS AND SYMPTOMS

- Recurrent staphylococcal infections.
- Eczema.
- Coarse facial features, lax joints.

DIAGNOSIS

- IgE > 10,000 IU/mL.
- Eosinophilia.

TABLE 9-4.   Phagocytic and Chemotactic Disorder

DISORDER	INHERITANCE	DEFECT	CLINICAL	INFECTIONS	DIAGNOSIS
Chronic granulomatous disease	X-linked	Pyruvate deficiency in PMNs and macrophages	Gingivitis, seborrheic dermatitis, retinitis pigmentosa	Deep soft tissue abscesses, lymphadenitis, *Staphylococcus, Aspergillus*	Neutrophil oxidation test NBT = old Leukocytosis
Chédiak-Higashi	Autosomal recessive	Abnormal chemotaxis and fusion of intracellular granules	Partial albinism, progressive neuropathy, HSM	Skin and lung *Staphylococcus*	Chemotaxis test, leukopenia
Job (hyper-IgE) syndrome	Autosomal dominant	Connective tissue and chemotaxis disorder	Coarse features, eczema, lax joints	Skin and lung, *Staphylococcus, Aspergillus*	IgE > 10,000, eosinophilia

HSM, hepatosplenomegaly; NBT, nitroblue tetrazolium; PMN, polymorphonuclear neutrophil.

TREATMENT

- Penicillinase-resistant antibiotics.
- BMT.

Complement Deficiency

A 16-year-old female presents with a second episode of meningococcal meningitis. Her CH50 is 78%. *Think: C5–C9 deficiency.*

Patients with complement deficiency are uniquely susceptible to meningococcal infection. Defects in terminal complement are associated with recurrent infections with *Neisseria*.

COMPLEMENT

Complex system of nine serum proteins (C1–C9).

FUNCTIONS OF COMPLEMENT

- Opsonization.
- Bacteria cell lysis.
- Facilitating chemotaxis.

ASSOCIATED DISEASES

- C1q deficiency: Systemic lupus erythematosus (SLE).
- C1 esterase inhibitor (C1 INH) deficiency: Hereditary angioedema.
- C2 deficiency: Pneumococcal infections.
- C5–C9 terminal complement deficiency: Neisserial infection.

Meningococcal vaccination is the best way to protect a patient with complement deficiency.

Hypocomplementemia occurs in patients with lupus nephritis and poststreptococcal glomerulonephritis, but not in Henoch-Schönlein purpura or minimal change disease.

TABLE 9-5. Complement Deficiencies

DEFICIENCY	MECHANISM	INFECTIONS	CH50
C2 (most common)	↓ opsonins	Pyogenic in one fifth	< 10%
Properdin (X-linked)	↓ opsonins	Pyogenic	Normal (AH50 low)
C5–C9	↓ membrane attack	Recurrent *Neisseria meningitidis*	> 50%

DIAGNOSIS

CH50 screening test.

Asplenia

A 7-year-old African-American girl who just immigrated from Togo presents with fever of 104°F (40°C). Physical examination did not reveal any source of fever. There is no palpable spleen. Her WBC count is 28.2, Hct 27.1, and there are Howell-Jolly bodies in RBCs. Blood culture grew *Streptococcus pneumoniae*. Think: *Sickle cell disease.*

Patients with asplenia are at increased risk for the development of sepsis, most commonly due to *S pneumoniae*. Patients with sickle cell disease develop functional asplenia. Howell-Jolly bodies indicate hyposplenism.

Asplenia:
- Howell-Jolly bodies
- Encapsulated organism

DEFINITION

Absence of the functional spleen.

ETIOLOGY

- Associated with some congenital syndromes.
- Functional asplenia may be secondary to **sickle cell disease** (SCD) or other hemoglobinopathies.
- Hyposplenia may be secondary to SLE, rheumatoid arthritis (RA), IBD, GVHD, nephrotic syndrome, or prematurity.
- Splenectomy due to trauma, Hodgkin's lymphoma, and hereditary spherocytosis.

DIAGNOSIS

- ↓ IgM antibodies, alternate complement pathway, and tuftsin.
- ↑ requirement for opsonic antibodies.
- **Howell-Jolly bodies** in erythrocytes.

COMPLICATIONS

Sepsis with encapsulated organisms:

- 0–6 months: Gram-negative enteric (*Klebsiella*, *Escherichia coli*).
- > 6 months of age: *S pneumoniae*, *Haemophilus influenzae* type B. Malaria and babesiosis are more severe.

TREATMENT

- Penicillin prophylaxis.
- Pneumococcal immunization, also *H influenzae* and meningococcal (vaccinations against encapsulated organisms).

Graft-versus-Host Disease (GVHD)

DEFINITION

- Donor lymphocytes detect host as foreign.
- Complication of BMT.

ETIOLOGY

Engraftment by immunocompetent donor lymphocytes in an immunologically compromised host.

PATHOPHYSIOLOGY

Donor T-cell activation by antibodies against host major histocompatibility complex antigens.

SIGNS AND SYMPTOMS

- Acute: < 100 days:
  - Erythroderma.
  - Cholestatic hepatitis—abnormal LFTs.
  - Enteritis—diarrhea and cramps.
  - ↑ susceptibility to infections.
- Chronic: > 100 days:
  - Either:
    - Generalized skin involvement, **or**
    - Localized skin involvement and/or hepatic dysfunction **and** liver histologic evidence of chronic aggressive hepatitis, bridging necrosis, or cirrhosis
  - Or:
    - Involvement of the eye ("keratoconjunctivitis sicca" = dry eye).
    - Involvement of minor salivary glands or oral mucosa (dryness).
    - Involvement of any other target organ.

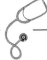

Requirements for the diagnosis of graft-versus-host disease:
- Graft must contain immunocompetent cells.
- Host must be immunocompromised.
- Histocompatibility differences must exist.

TREATMENT

- High-dose glucocorticoids.
- Immunosuppressive therapy.

Infectious Disease

DEFINITION

Fever **without obvious focus** of infection (except otitis media) in a well-appearing child, and positive blood culture for a bacterial pathogen.

ETIOLOGY

Group B strep is the most common cause of neonatal septicemia

Neonates
- Group B streptococci
- *Escherichia coli*
- *Listeria monocytogenes*
- *Staphylococcus aureus*
- Coagulase-negative *Staphylococcus* (preterm infants, catheter-related)
- *Candida albicans* (preterm infants, catheter-related)

Children
- *Streptococcus pneumoniae* (most common)
- *Neisseria meningitidis*
- *Salmonella typhimurium*
- *S aureus*
- Group A streptococci

SIGNS AND SYMPTOMS

- Fever
- Leukocytosis

PREDISPOSING FACTORS

- Loss of external defenses (burns, ulceration, catheter).
- Inadequate immune function.
- Impaired reticuloendothelial function.
- Overwhelming inoculum.

TABLE 10-1. Age-Based Management of Possible Occult Bacteremia in a Low-Risk Infant—Full Term, Previously Healthy, with Negative Laboratory Screen (Normal WBC Count and Urinalysis)

AGE	MANAGEMENT
< 60 days	▪ All considered for hospitalization and parenteral antibiotics. ▪ Ampicillin and gentamicin for newborns. ▪ Ampicillin + cefotaxime for second month of life.
61–90 days	▪ Manage as outpatient if good follow-up, with or without one dose of ceftriaxone. ▪ Unreliable follow-up: CSF exam prior to ampicillin + cefotaxime.
3–36 months	▪ If fever > 102.2°F (39°C): Get WBC; cultures of blood, urine. ▪ Ceftriaxone is optional if nonseptic appearance; follow-up extremely important.

CSF, cerebrospinal fluid; WBC, white blood cell count.

Diagnostic Workup

- Blood and urine cultures.
- Complete blood count (CBC): Normal WBC count is > 5000 and < 15,000 cells/cmL.
- Lumbar puncture if < 60 days old.

Treatment

- Treat to prevent progression to septicemia.
- See Table 10-1 for age-based criteria.

A 3-month-old female is brought to the ED with fever, vomiting × 1, ↓ activity, and poor breast-feeding of 1 day's duration. Previous history is unremarkable. Physical examination shows the following: "ill appearing," temperature of 101.1°F (38.4°C), HR 196 beats/min, and no identifiable focus of infection. *Think: Sepsis.*

Young infants are at ↑ risk for infection. Initial presentation may be nonspecific signs and symptoms, and young infants lack focal signs of infection.

Definition

- A systemic inflammatory response to infection that includes hemodynamic and metabolic derangements.
- Hypoperfusion abnormalities include lactic acidosis, oliguria, an alteration of mental status, and an ↑ alveolar-arterial oxygen gradient.

Diagnostic Criteria

Manifested by ≥ 2 conditions:

- Hyper- or hypothermia (≥ 101.2°F [38.4°C] or < 96.8°F [36°C]).
- Tachycardia (heart rate: infant > 160 bpm, child > 150 bpm).
- Tachypnea (respiratory rate: infant > 60, child > 50).
- WBC count > 15,000 or < 5000 cells/L and bandemia.

Etiology

Same as for occult bacteremia above.

Signs and Symptoms

- Remember, a sick-looking, listless, infant who is not eating in the first 3 months of life with a rectal temperature < 98°F (36.7°C) is **hypothermic** and thus septic.
- Vomiting is usual symptom in **any infant** with fever.

Diagnosis

- Same as for occult bacteremia.
- Ten percent will have negative cultures.

RISK FACTORS

- Younger at greater risk.
- Prematurity.
- Immunodeficiency.
- Catheters.
- Contact with known N *meningitidis* or *Haemophilus influenzae* infection.

Septic Shock

DEFINITION

Shock associated with systemic inflammatory response syndrome (SIRS) is defined as "hypotension persisting despite adequate fluid resuscitation, along with the presence of hypoperfusion abnormalities or organ dysfunction." Septic shock is defined as shock plus clinical evidence of infection.

DIAGNOSTIC CRITERIA

Clinical evidence of infection **plus** meets the criteria for SIRS, **plus** one of the following:

- Hypoperfusion requiring > 40 mL/kg isotonic fluid (crystalloid or colloid) and/or inotropic support.
- Hypotension.
- More than one manifestation of organ hypoperfusion.

TREATMENT

- IV broad-spectrum antibiotics.
- Manage shock with supportive therapy to maintain blood pressure, perfusion, and oxygenation.

Meningococcemia (Figure 10-1)

Meningococcemia
- Fever
- Purpura
- Rapid progression

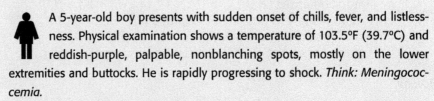

A 5-year-old boy presents with sudden onset of chills, fever, and listlessness. Physical examination shows a temperature of 103.5°F (39.7°C) and reddish-purple, palpable, nonblanching spots, mostly on the lower extremities and buttocks. He is rapidly progressing to shock. *Think: Meningococcemia.*

Typical presentation is sudden onset of fever, vomiting, headache, and lethargy. Most patients have petechiae on presentation. The infection can progress rapidly to profound shock and DIC.

- Presents nonspecifically but progresses rapidly (within hours).
- Most progress to septic shock due to endotoxin.
- First petechiae, then purpura, and finally eschar (one of the rashes seen on palms and soles).
- Typical rash distribution: Buttocks and lower extremities.
- Adrenal hemorrhage (Waterhouse-Friedrichsen syndrome) and insufficiency common.
- Establish diagnosis by culture of blood, cerebrospinal fluid (CSF), and skin lesions.

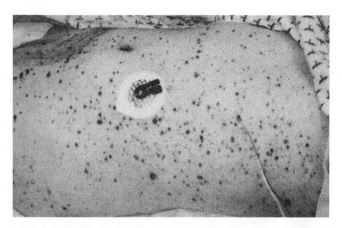

FIGURE 10-1. **Meningococcemia.**

(Reproduced, with permission, from Knoop KJ, Stack LB, Storrow AB, et al. *Atlas of Emergency Medicine*, 3rd ed. New York: McGraw-Hill, 2010: 423. Photo contributor: Richard Strait, MD.)

TREATMENT

- IV ceftriaxone or cefotaxime is treatment of choice until sensitivities are available.
- See Septic Shock.

HUMAN IMMUNODEFICIENCY VIRUS (HIV) IN THE CHILD

ETIOLOGY

- Infants: Vertical transmission from mothers either perinatally or through breast milk (preventable with antiretroviral prophylaxis).
- Adolescents: Sexual transmission or IV drug use.

DIAGNOSIS

- HIV screening is part of prenatal care.
- In non-breast-feeding infants < 18 months of age and born to HIV-infected mothers, *definitive* exclusion of HIV-1 is based on:
  - At least two negative **HIV-1 DNA or RNA virologic tests,** both of which were obtained at ≥ 1 month of age and one of which was obtained at ≥ 4 months of age **or**
  - Two negative HIV-1 **antibody test** results from separate specimens obtained at ≥ 6 months of age **and**
  - No other laboratory or clinical evidence of HIV-1 infection, and no AIDS-defining condition for which there is no other underlying condition of immunosuppression.
- In adolescents of > 13 years of age, rapid oral swab enzyme immunoassay (EIA) is an alternative method. If it is positive, confirmatory enzyme-linked immunosorbent assay (ELISA) and Western blot are required.
- Suspect HIV infection in a child with failure to thrive, oral thrush after 3 months of age, generalized nontender lymphadenopathy, hepatosplenomegaly, and thrombocytopenia.

Perinatal HIV
- Lymphadenopathy
- Hepatosplenomegaly
- Oral thrush
- Failure to thrive

Common presentation:
Infants: PCP
Children: ITP

■ Consider acute HIV syndrome in a sexually active adolescent with mononucleosis-like illness with fever, lymphadenopathy, and hepatosplenomegaly.
■ See Table 10-2 for clinical classifications.

TABLE 10-2. **1993 Centers for Disease Control and Prevention Clinical Classification of HIV Infection in Children < 13 years**

CLINICAL CATEGORY	DIAGNOSTIC CRITERIA
Not symptomatic	If two positive results on separate occasions
Mildly symptomatic	Two or more of following conditions: ■ Lymphadenopathy ■ Hepatomegaly ■ Splenomegaly ■ Dermatitis ■ Parotitis ■ Recurrent or persistent upper respiratory infections, sinusitis, or otitis media
Moderately symptomatic	■ Anemia, neutropenia, or thrombocytopenia persisting for 30 days ■ Bacterial meningitis, pneumonia, or sepsis ■ Candidiasis persisting > 2 months in child > 6 months ■ Cardiomyopathy ■ Cytomegalovirus infection ■ Hepatitis ■ Herpes zoster: two episodes in more than one dermatome ■ Disseminated varicella ■ Herpes simplex virus bronchitis, pneumonitis, or esophagitis ■ Nephropathy ■ Persistent fever (> 1 month) ■ Toxoplasmosis
Severely symptomatic	■ Serious bacterial infection (two in 2 years' time) ■ Disseminated coccidioidomycosis ■ Extrapulmonary cryptococcosis ■ Encephalopathy: more than one finding for > 2 months with no illness to explain ■ Disseminated histoplasmosis ■ Kaposi sarcoma ■ Primary lymphoma in brain ■ Tuberculosis ■ Other mycobacterium infection ■ *Pneumocystis jiroveci* pneumonia ■ Polymorphonuclear leukocytes ■ Wasting syndrome

TREATMENT

- Three classes:
  - Nucleoside reverse transcriptase inhibitors (NRTIs).
  - Non-nucleoside reverse transcriptase inhibitors (NNRTIs).
  - Protease inhibitors.
- HIV rapidly becomes resistant; therefore, multidrug therapy is necessary.

Toxoplasmosis

ETIOLOGY

- *Toxoplasma gondii* (intracellular protozoan).
- Cats excrete cysts in feces.

SIGNS AND SYMPTOMS

- Mononucleosis syndrome including fever, lymphadenopathy, and hepatosplenomegaly.
- Disseminated infection with T cell deficiency.

DIAGNOSIS

Serologic antibody tests, biopsy, visualization of parasites in CSF.

TREATMENT

Pyrimethamine and sulfadiazine used concurrently (both inhibit folic acid synthesis, so replace folic acid).

Cryptococcosis

DEFINITION

- Fungal infection.
- Primary infection in lungs.
- Disseminates to brain, meninges, skin, eyes, and skeletal system in immune compromised.

SIGNS AND SYMPTOMS

- Subacute or chronic meningitis is the most common presentation in AIDS.
- Typically presents with fever, headache, and malaise.
- Postinfectious sequelae commonly including hydrocephalus.
- Change in visual acuity.
- Deafness.
- Cranial nerve palsies.
- Seizures.
- Ataxia.

DIAGNOSIS

- Definitive diagnosis requires isolation of the organism from body fluid or tissue specimens: sputum, bronchopulmonary lavage, or CSF.

- **Niger seed (birdseed)** can ↑ detection in sputum and urine.
- The latex agglutination test and EIA for detection of **cryptococcal capsular polysaccharide antigen in serum or CSF** specimens are excellent rapid diagnostic tests.
- Microscopy: Encapsulated yeast seen as white halos when CSF is mixed with India ink.
- Can be grown in culture (takes up to 3 weeks).
- May also see cryptococcomas on head CT.

TREATMENT

- Treat with combination therapy using amphotericin B and flucytosine.
- Relapse rate is very high. This is a reason for subsequent maintenance therapy with oral fluconazole.

Pneumocystis jiroveci Pneumonia

Formerly *P carinii*, now classified as a fungus.

EPIDEMIOLOGY

- Peak incidence 3–6 months of age.
- Highest mortality rate in infants.

SIGNS AND SYMPTOMS

- Acute onset of fever, tachypnea, dyspnea, dry cough, and **progressive hypoxemia**.
- Chest x-ray—diffuse bilateral interstitial infiltrates or alveolar disease, may have characteristic "ground glass" appearance.

DIAGNOSIS

Diagnosis by **methenamine silver staining of bronchoalveolar fluid lavage (BAL)** to identify cyst walls or Giemsa staining to identify nuclei of trophozoites. LDH > 500.

TREATMENT

- First-line treatment with prednisone is trimethoprim-sulfamethoxazole (TMP-SMX) (TMP: 15–20 mg/kg/24 hr; SMX: 75–100 mg/kg/24 hr) q6h for 5–7 days.
- Alternative regimens: Pentamidine, TMP-SMX plus dapsone, atovaquone.

PROPHYLAXIS

Starting at 6 weeks of age TMP-SMX if CD4 < 15%, or < 200 for age 6–12 years old and < 500 for age 1–5 years old. Risk displacement of bilirubin in neonate.

Rifabutin ↓ serum levels of zidovudine (ZDV) and clarithromycin.

Atypical Mycobacterial Infections

ETIOLOGY

- *Mycobacterium avium* complex (MAC).
- Considered an AIDS-defining illnesses. Patients with CD4 counts < 50/mm³ are at highest risk.

SIGNS AND SYMPTOMS

Disseminated disease:

- Fever.
- Malaise.
- Weight loss.
- Night sweats.
- May have gastrointestinal (GI) symptoms.

DIAGNOSIS

Diagnosis by culture from blood, bone marrow, or tissue.

TREATMENT

Two-drug regimen:
- Either clarithromycin *or* azithromycin
- *Plus* ethambutol, rifabutin, rifampin, ciprofloxacin, *or* amikacin.

PROPHYLAXIS

For CD4 < 50: Azithromycin once a week.

Fluconazole can ↓ the level of rifabutin by 80%.

Rifabutin can color body secretions such as urine, sweat, and tears a bright orange

Cytomegalovirus (CMV)

ETIOLOGY

Member of Herpesviridae family.

PATHOPHYSIOLOGY

Infection is lifelong, as with any other herpesvirus. It may be acquired early in life and stay latent until host becomes immunocompromised, years later. Lung, liver, kidney, GI tract, and salivary glands are most common organs infected.

CMV is the most frequently transmitted virus to a child before birth.

SIGNS AND SYMPTOMS

- Pneumonitis.
- Esophagitis.
- **Retinitis** (can cause blindness).

DIAGNOSIS

- Reactivation may be associated with appearance of IgM in serum.
- Detection of pp65 antigen in white blood cells is used to detect infection in immunocompromised hosts. Quantitative polymerase chain reaction (PCR) (viral load) in blood is available.
- Urine shedding of virus is lifelong. Positive urine CMV culture does not indicate association with current disease.

TREATMENT

- Gancyclovir. Addition of intraocular to systemic for retinitis.
- IV foscarnet in gancyclovir-resistant infection.

Handwritten note in margin: Rash

- **Enanthema:** Lesion(s) on mucosa.
- **Exanthema:** Lesion(s) on the skin, rash.
- **Polymorphous rash:** Consists of various primary elements.
- Primary elements of rash:
  - Macule: Flat, pink blanching spot.
  - Papule: Small, raised spot.
  - Vesicle: Small, round fluid-filled lesion.
  - Pustule: Small, round pus-filled lesion.
  - Petechia: **Pinpoint** nonblanching purplish spot (extravasation).
  - Purpura: Small, raised, purplish nonblanching lesion (extravasation).
  - Erythroderma: Confluent redness of the skin.
  - Excoriation: Crust.
  - Eschar: Dead tissue (or ulcer) covered by dry, dark scab.
- **In order to recognize infection, keep in mind:**
  - Primary element(s) of rash.
  - Distribution and/or pattern of the rash.
  - Sequence (timeline) of events.
  - Associated hallmarks of infection.
  - Vaccine-preventable infection is most likely to develop in an unvaccinated child, for example, in a new immigrant or in an adoptee.
- **Remember: Any** rash may be itchy.
- See Table 10-3.

Rubeola (Measles)

Rubeola classic findings:
- **Coryza**
- **Cough**
- **Conjunctivitis**
- **Koplik spots**

A 6-year-old girl has a 1-day history of a rash. It started on her face and then spread to the trunk. Prior to developing the rash, she had a 4-day history of running nose, pink eyes with crusting, barking cough, and high fever. She was never immunized because of her parents' beliefs. On exam, her temperature is 103°F (39.4°C), and there is a maculopapular rash most prominent on the trunk. There are three tiny whitish round spots on her buccal mucosa. *Think: Measles.*

Measles is characterized by high fever, an enanthem (Koplik's spots), cough, conjunctivitis, and a maculopapular rash. The rash usually begins on the face and appears several days after the initial symptoms. Koplik's spots precede the onset of rash.

Handwritten: paramyovirus

ETIOLOGY

Paramyxovirus (RNA virus).

SIGNS AND SYMPTOMS

- Fever is high and, together with "3Cs" (see Table 10-3), **precedes** rash (3–5 days).
- Conjunctivitis is exudative (yellow discharge).
- Cough is croupy (barking, or "seal-like").
- Rash starts as faint macules on upper lateral neck, behind ears, along hairline, and on cheeks.

Handwritten notes in left margin: coryza cough conjunct. koplick → rash face/ears

TABLE 10-3. Fever and Rash

INFECTION	SEQUENCE OF EVENTS	PRIMARY ELEMENT(S) OF RASH	DISTRIBUTION, PATTERN	HALLMARKS
Measles (rubeola)	Fever and **"3Cs"** × 3–4 days **precede rash:** Coryza, Conjunctivitis, Cough (barking)	Maculopapular	"Shower" from the top down Becomes confluent, also from the top	**Koplik's spots** on buccal mucosa *behind ears*
Rubella	Low-grade fever may start 1–2 days prior to rash	Maculopapular	"Shower" from the top down	Suboccipital lymphatic nodes
Roseola (HHV 6,7) (exanthem subitum)	**High** fever 4–5 days; rash appears **after** fever has resolved *Roseola infantum*	Maculopapular	Discrete, may last just for a few hours	Febrile seizures, suboccipital lymphatic nodes, red eardrums
Erythema infectiosum (Parvovirus B19) (fifth disease)	Fever and malaise prodrome, then red **("slapped") cheeks**	Maculopapular	Lacelike, fluctuates over time with room temperature changes	Rare arthritis, knee; aplastic crisis in sickle cell disease; hydrops fetalis in pregnancy
Scarlet fever (erythrotoxin of group A *Streptococcus*)	Exactly "red fever," often with sore throat, × 7 days; desquamation **(peeling)** in week 2	**Sandpaper-**feeling confluent redness of the skin (erythroderma)	Accentuated in **folds,** where darker **Pastia's lines** are seen	Nasolabial triangle and chin are spared **("circumoral pallor");** high anti-streptolysin O, positive throat culture
Varicella	**Crops** of **"dew drops on a rose petal"** appear over 3–7 days, with fever	Evolution from papule to vesicle to pustule to excoriation	**Rash in the different stages of evolution;** palms and soles spared	May be associated with meningitis or encephalitis
Hand-foot-mouth disease (coxsackievirus A16)	Fever, rash, with or without sore throat, upper respiratory/gastrointestinal infection symptoms	Macules, papules, **vesicles**	**Palms and soles** involved	Enanthema: Erosions on the pharynx, palate, tongue

Children under the age of 6 months do not usually get measles due to passive immunity they still have from mother.

- Lesions become maculopapular and spread quickly downward ("shower distribution"), while the rash becomes confluent (erythrthroderma) starting from the top.
- May have lymphadenopathy or splenomegaly.
- **Koplik spots** (pathognomonic): Irregularly shaped spots with grayish white centers on buccal mucosa (see Figure 10-2).

DIAGNOSIS

- Clinical.
- Laboratory rarely needed.

COMPLICATIONS

- Otitis media.
- Pneumonia: May be fatal in HIV patients.
- Encephalitis.

TREATMENT

Vitamin A for measles.

The World Health Organization recommends vitamin A for all children with measles, regardless of their country of residence.

VACCINE

- Live attenuated vaccine included in measles-mumps-rubella (MMR) vaccine.
- Generally given at 12–15 months with a booster given at 4–6 years.

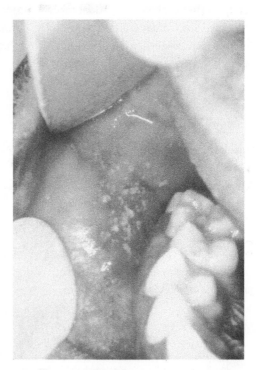

FIGURE 10-2. Koplik spots (rubeola).

(Reproduced, with permission, from Knoop KJ, Stack LB, and Storrow AB. *Atlas of Emergency Medicine*, 1st ed. New York: McGraw-Hill, 1997: 174.)

Rubella

A 3-year-old girl develops a rash. She was recently adopted from Romania, and her immunization history is unknown. She is brought in because of a fever × 1 day. On physical examination, she is not sick-looking, her temperature is 100.4°F (38.0°C), there is a confluent maculopapular rash on her face and discrete rash on her trunk, and the suboccipital and posterior cervical lymph nodes are palpable. WBC 7.2. *Think: Rubella.*

The disease has a prodrome of low-grade fever, sore throat, red eyes, headache, malaise, and anorexia. Suboccipital or postauricular lymphadenopathy is common. Rash is usually the first symptom, which appears on the face and spreads centrifugally to the extremities.

Rubella is contagious from 1 week before the rash appears to 1 week after it fades.

ETIOLOGY
RNA virus.

Lymphedenopathy

SIGNS AND SYMPTOMS
- Mild fever prodrome for 1–2 days.
- Rash begins on face and spreads quickly to trunk ("shower distribution"). As it spreads to trunk, it clears on face.
- Lymphadenopathy: Retroauricular, posterior cervical, and suboccipital.
- Conjunctivitis may be present.
- Polyarthritis common in adolescent females.

COMPLICATIONS
- Progressive panencephalitis (very rare):
  - Insidious behavior change.
  - Deteriorating school performance.
  - Later, dementia and multifocal neurologic deficits.
- Thrombocytopenia (rare).

TREATMENT
- Supportive; usually lasts about 3 days.

Congenital Rubella Syndrome

- The earlier in gestation rubella occurred, the higher is the risk—more than 80% in the first trimester, and 25% at the end of the second trimester.
- Neonatal manifestations:
  - Intrauterine growth retardation.
  - Pneumonitis.
  - Radiolucent bone lesions.
  - Hepatosplenomegaly.
  - Thrombocytopenia.
  - "Blueberry muffin" rash (dermal erythropoiesis).

- Eye: Cataracts, glaucoma, pigmentary retinopathy, microphthalmos.
- Heart: Patent ductus arteriosus (PDA), peripheral pulmonary artery stenosis.
- Sensorineural hearing impairment.
- Neurologic: Meningoencephalitis ↓ mental retardation.

VACCINE

- Live attenuated vaccine included in MMR vaccine.
- Generally given at 12–15 months with a booster given at 4–6 years.

Roseola

Peak age: 6–24 months

An 11-month-old boy has had a fever 103–104°F (39.4–40°C) for 4 days and was seen in ED because of febrile seizures. He had no vomiting, did not look sick, and his neurologic examination was normal. The only finding at the time was small suboccipital lymph nodes. No workup was done. Three days later, the child's fever has resolved, but now he has a maculopapular rash. *Think: Roseola.*

Typical history: Rash appears when the fever disappears. It is associated with high fever, and some children may develop a seizure. Mild cervical or occipital lymphadenopathy may be present.

ETIOLOGY

The **high fever** seen with roseola often triggers **febrile seizures.**

- Human herpesvirus types 6 and 7.
- By the age of 4 years almost all are immune.

SIGNS AND SYMPTOMS

- High fever.
- Mild upper respiratory symptoms.
- Cervical and suboccipital lymphadenopathy.
- Maculopapular rash that spreads to the neck, face and proximal extremities.

TREATMENT

Supportive (antipyretics, ↑ oral fluid intake, rest).

Fifth Disease (Erythema Infectiosum)

parvovirus B19

An 8-year-old girl has a 4-day history of fever and bright red cheeks. Now she has rash everywhere and complains of knee pain. On examination, she is not sick-looking, her temperature is 100.8°F (38.2°C), and she has "slapped"-looking cheeks and a discrete macular rash on the trunk and extremities that looks lacy. **Her joints look intact, with full range of motion.** *Think: Erythema infectiosum, Parvovirus B19.*

Erythema infectiosum is a self-limiting exanthematous illness in children. Slapped-cheek appearance is classic presentation. In addition, lacy, reticulated appearance on the extremities is often present.

ETIOLOGY

Parvovirus B19.

PATHOPHYSIOLOGY

- Attacks red blood cell precursors.
- Transmitted in respiratory secretions.

SIGNS AND SYMPTOMS

- Prodrome: 1 week of low-grade fever, headache, malaise, myalgia, and mild upper respiratory symptoms.
- **"Slapped cheeks,"** circumoral pallor.
- Rash spreads rapidly to trunk and extremities in ornamental **"lacelike"** pattern.
- Arthritis (knee) rare in children.

DIAGNOSIS

- Clinical (serum parvovirus B19 immunoglobulin M is available, eg, for arthritis cases).
- Parvovirus B19 serology may be offered to women of childbearing age to determine their susceptibility to infection (teachers).

COMPLICATIONS

- Transient **aplastic crisis** in patients with chronic hemolysis including sickle cell disease (SCD), thalassemia, hereditary spherocytosis, and pyruvate kinase deficiency.
- Chronic anemia/pure red cell aplasia in immunocompromised hosts.
- **Hydrops fetalis:** Generalized edema due to fetal congestive heart failure (caused by fetal anemia).

TREATMENT

- Supportive (antipyretics, ↑ oral fluid intake, rest).
- Intravenous immune globulin (IVIG) should be considered for immunocompromised patients.

Scarlet Fever

Nose + chin – Ø rash

GaBHS

A 7-year-old boy has a sore throat, fever, and rash. His classmate had similar symptoms 1 week ago. On examination, his temperature is 102°F (38.9°C). He has red tonsils; swollen, tender bilateral anterior cervical lymphatic nodes (2.5 cm); and a confluent red rash that feels "sandpaper-like." He has circumoral pallor (nasolabial triangle and chin are spared). *Think: Scarlet fever.*

Scarlet fever has an abrupt onset, with fever, chills, malaise, and sore throat and a distinctive rash that begins on the chest. Circumoral pallor is often present. The rash has a rough, sandpaper-like texture.

Scarlet fever common findings:
- Sandpaper rash
- Pastia lines
- Desquamation

ETIOLOGY

Erythrogenic exotoxins of group A β-hemolytic *Streptococcus* (GAS).

SIGNS AND SYMPTOMS

- Fever, often sore throat.
- Confluent erythematous (erythroderma) **sandpaper-like rash.**
- Nasolabial triangle and chin are spared: **"Circumoral pallor."**
- Accentuation of rash in a linear pattern in folds (**Pastia lines**).
- Desquamation (**peeling**), starting with fingers, in the second week.

DIAGNOSIS

- Clinical.
- Throat culture, anti-streptolysin O (ASO), and deoxyribonuclease B titers.

COMPLICATIONS

Myocarditis.

TREATMENT

Penicillin.

Varicella (Chickenpox)

 A 5-year-old boy has had a fever for 3 days and an itchy rash that started yesterday. He is a recent immigrant from overseas. On examination, his temperature is 101.8°F (38.8°C) and he does not look sick. There are crops of papules, vesicles, pustules, and crusts on the face, trunk, and extremities. *Think: Varicella.*

Varicella is a highly contagious disease characterized by a generalized vesicular rash. There is centripetal distribution. In a patient with chickenpox, erythematous macules, papules, vesicles, and scabbed lesions are present at the same time.

DEFINITION

Highly contagious, self-limited viral infection characterized by multiple pruritic vesicles (Figure 10-3).

ETIOLOGY

Varicella-zoster virus (VZV), group of herpesviruses.

EPIDEMIOLOGY

- Ninety percent of patients are < 10 years old.
- Often, there is a history of exposure to infected individual.
- Incidence is ↓ with introduction of vaccine.

PATHOPHYSIOLOGY

- Transmitted by respiratory secretions and fluid from the skin lesions.
- Virus replicates in respiratory tract.
- Establishes lifelong infection in sensory ganglia cells.

SIGNS AND SYMPTOMS

- Rash may be preceded by a prodrome of fever, malaise, anorexia, headache, and abdominal pain 24–48 hours before the onset of the rash.

 Herpes zoster (shingles) is the reactivation of VZV and occurs in dermatomal distribution.

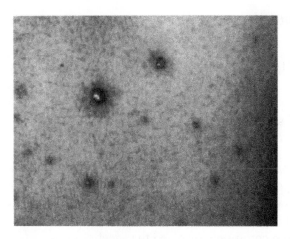

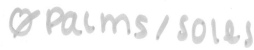

FIGURE 10-3. **Varicella (chickenpox).**

Note dewdrop appearance of lesion and that there are lesions in multiple stages of eruption.

- "**Dew drops on a rose petal**" initially appear on face and spread to trunk and extremities, **sparing palms and soles.**
- Within days, vesicles become turbid and then crusted (see Figure 10-3).

DIAGNOSIS

- Clinical; Tzanck preparation is **not** used anymore.
- PCR test of swab from the vesicle.

COMPLICATIONS

- Skin lesions may be superinfected by bacteria (*Streptococcus pyogenes* or *Staphylococcus aureus*).
- Pneumonia in immunocompromised or pregnant patients.
- Encephalitis.
- **Reye syndrome** (associated with aspirin use).

TREATMENT

- For most immunocompetent children: Symptomatic for fever and pruritus.
- For VZV pneumonia and for immunocompromised individuals: Acyclovir.

Congenital Varicella Syndrome

Caused by maternal varicella infection in **first 20 weeks** of pregnancy.

SYMPTOMS

- **Cicatricial** skin lesions (cutaneous scarring).
- **Limb hypoplasia.**
- Neurologic deficits.
- Eye abnormalities.

VACCINE

Live attenuated vaccine, first dose given between 12 and 18 months of age, second dose age > 4 years.

Smallpox generally presents with all lesions in the same stage (versus chickenpox).

Varicella zoster immune globulin (VZIG) is used for post-exposure prophylaxis in immunocompromised or newborns exposed to maternal varicella

Hand-Foot-Mouth Disease

ETIOLOGY

Enteroviruses: 71, coxsackievirus A16.

EPIDEMIOLOGY

- Fecal-oral and respiratory routes.
- Summer and fall seasonal pattern.

SIGNS AND SYMPTOMS

- GI discomfort.
- Ulcerative mouth lesions (small, superficial, round erosions).
- Hand and foot lesions tender and vesicular.
- Hands more commonly involved than feet.
- May occur on **palms and soles.**

COMPLICATIONS

- Aseptic meningitis
- Encephalitis

Mumps

An unvaccinated 14-year-old boy presented with fever of 100.9°F (38.3°C), bilateral facial swelling, and inability to eat normally because of pain when he tries to chew. On examination, he was active and had trismus (inability to open wide the mouth) and swelling in front of the earlobes. There was no redness or purulent discharge at Stenson duct openings. At follow-up visit 8 days later, parotid swelling is resolved, but now he has a swollen tender left testis. *Think: Mumps orchitis.*

Epididymo-orchitis is a common extra–salivary gland complication of mumps in postpubertal males. Many of these occur during the first week of parotitis. It is characterized by marked testicular swelling and severe pain and may be associated with fever, nausea, and headache. Testicular atrophy may follow, although sterility is not common.

ETIOLOGY

Paramyxovirus (RNA virus).

PATHOPHYSIOLOGY

- Spread via respiratory secretions.
- Incubation period of 14–24 days.

SIGNS AND SYMPTOMS

- Rare viral prodrome.
- Swelling and tenderness in one or both parotid glands.
- Difficult to open mouth.

COMPLICATIONS

- Meningoencephalomyelitis (rare).
- Orchitis/oophoritis common after puberty.
- Pancreatitis.
- Arthritis.
- Thyroiditis.
- Deafness.

VACCINE

- Live attenuated vaccine included in MMR vaccine.
- Generally given at 12–15 months with a booster given at 4–6 years.

BACTERIAL INFECTIONS

Typhoid (Enteric) Fever

An 8-year-old boy returns from Africa, and 5 days later develops fever that gets higher and higher, escalating in the next 7 days. He has abdominal pain and refuses to eat. His last bowel movement was normal and occurred prior to the onset of fever. On examination, his temperature is 103°F (39.4°C), HR 88 beats/min. There are fine pink spots on the abdomen and a palpable spleen (2.5 cm). Abdomen is soft, with mild, nonconstant tenderness and no guarding or rebound. WBC is 11.9, and blood smear shows no parasites. *Think: Typhoid fever.*

Typhoid fever is characterized by prolonged sustained fever, relative bradycardia, splenomegaly, rose spots, and leukopenia. It is due to *S typhi.*

Typhoid fever:
- Relative bradycardia
- Rose spots
- Hepatosplenomegaly

ETIOLOGY

Salmonella typhi.

PATHOPHYSIOLOGY

- Fecal-oral transmission.
- Incubation period of 7–14 days.
- Time of incubation dependent on inoculum size.

SIGNS AND SYMPTOMS

- **Fever:** Gradual rise in the first week, gradual ↓ in the third week.
- Malaise.
- Anorexia.
- Myalgia.
- Headache.
- Abdominal pain.
- Diarrhea is a late symptom.
- **Transient rose-colored spots on trunk.**
- Hepatosplenomegaly.

COMPLICATIONS

- Intestinal hemorrhage
- Intestinal perforation

DIAGNOSIS

- Culture of blood, urine, stool.
- The sensitivity of blood culture is ~60%.

TREATMENT

- Ceftriaxone.
- Severe case with altered mental status: Dexamethasone is to be considered.

VACCINE

Available for travelers to endemic areas (not routinely recommended).

Tick-Borne Infections

LYME DISEASE

Lyme disease:
- Erythema migrans
- Bell's palsy
- Heart block

> A 6-year-old boy developed limping, swelling, and pain in his right knee; there was no fever. Two months ago he was hiking in Wisconsin. Physical examination shows temperature of 98.6°F and no distress. No rash/murmur/organomegaly. The right knee was swollen, warm, but not red, with ↓ range of motion due to pain on passive movement. *Think: Lyme disease.*

> An 11-year-old girl presents with an enlarging erythematous, nonitchy spot on her left shoulder. She was camping in upstate New York 2 weeks ago. On examination, her temperature is 100.3°F (37.9°C), she is not sick-looking, and she has a flat annular lesion 7 cm in diameter on the left shoulder. No regional lymphadenopathy is noted. *Think: Lyme disease.*
>
> Lyme disease is a tick-borne, inflammatory disorder due to the spirochete *Borrelia burgdorferi.* The most common manifestation of Lyme disease in children is erythema migrans rash and arthritis. Most case of Lyme disease are from the following states: New York, Pennsylvania, New Jersey, Massachusetts, Connecticut, Wisconsin, Maryland, Minnesota, and Delaware

DEFINITION

A multisystem disease transmitted by the bite of an *Ixodes* tick infected with a spirochetes.

ETIOLOGY

Borrelia burgdorferi.

EPIDEMIOLOGY

- Patients are often unaware of the tick bite.
- Incubation period: 2–31 days (see Table 10-4).
- Keep in mind geography (presence of a vector) and season (see Table 10-5).

PATHOPHYSIOLOGY

Disseminated Lyme is due to a spirochetemia.

TABLE 10-4. Stages of Lyme Disease

| STAGE | EARLY LOCALIZED | EARLY DISSEMINATED | | | LATE | |
		MULTIPLE EM	CARDITIS	MENINGITIS	ARTHRITIS	POLYRADICULONEUROPATHY
Time after tick bite	2–31 days	3–5 weeks			> 6 weeks	
Clinical features	**EM,** headache, fever, myalgia	Most common	Rare Heart block	Benign CSF: Lymphocytic	Knee, may be relapsing course	Rare Gloves-and-socks: Pain, paresthesias
Diagnosis	Clinical	Serology		Serology, CSF: IgM, PCR	Serology, synovial PCR	Serology
Treatment	Amoxicillin or cefuroxime **Doxycycline: After 8 years of age**	Ceftriaxone or penicillin **IV**			**Acute:** Amoxicillin, doxycycline **Persistent:** Ceftriaxone or penicillin **IV**	Ceftriaxone or penicillin **IV**

CSF, cerebrospinal fluid; EM, erythema migrans; IgM, immunoglobulin M; PCR, polymerase chain reaction.

TABLE 10-5. Epidemiology of Tick-Borne Infections

INFECTION	GEOGRAPHY (UNITED STATES)	TICK (VECTOR)	SEASON
Lyme borreliosis	Upper East Coast: New Hampshire to Virginia Upper Midwest: Wisconsin, Minnesota West Coast: California	*Ixodus scapularis* *Ixodus pacificus*	April–October
Rocky Mountain spotted fever	Western states Southeast: North Carolina, South Carolina South central: Tennessee, Oklahoma Arizona	*Dermacentor andersoni* (wood tick) *Dermacentor variabilis* (American dog tick) *Rhipicephalus sanguineus* (brown dog tick)	May–September

SIGNS AND SYMPTOMS

- See Table 10-4.
- **Erythema migrans (EM):**
  - Begins as a red macule or papule that gradually (over days to weeks) turns into an annular, erythematous lesion of 5–15 cm in diameter (Figure 10-4).
  - Sometimes there is partial central clearing (halo appearance).
  - May have vesicular or necrotic areas in its center and can be confused with cellulitis.
  - The lesion usually is painless and not pruritic.
  - May be located at the axilla or in the groin.
  - May be associated with acute onset of fever, chills, myalgia, weakness, headache, and photophobia.
- **Isolated facial palsy** (CN VII, Bell's palsy): Develops 3–5 weeks after exposure.
  - Treatment has no effect on resolution, but prevents late events (arthritis).
  - Self-limited.

DIAGNOSIS

- Confirmed by serology.
- During the first 4 weeks of infection, serologic tests are negative and therefore not recommended.
- Immunoglobulins M and G (IgM and IgG) peak 4–6 weeks after exposure and are detected by EIA (screening, may be **false positive**) and **Western immunoblot (confirmation).**
- False-positive results with other spirochetal infection and in patients with some autoimmune disorders (systemic lupus erythematosus [SLE], rheumatoid arthritis [RA]).
- An elevated IgG titer in absence of an elevated IgM indicates prior exposure as opposed to recent infection.
- PCR can detect spirochete DNA in CSF and synovial fluid.
- Forty percent of skin biopsies reveal spirochetes.

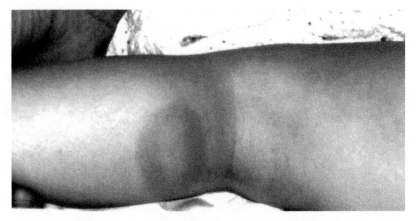

FIGURE 10-4. Erythema chronicum migrans rash characteristic of Lyme disease.

Sixty percent of untreated cases with disseminated infection develop arthritis (mediated by immune complex formation) 6 weeks following tick bite.

TREATMENT

- **Amoxicillin (cefuroxime) or doxycycline:**
  - EM: 14–21days.
  - Multiple EM: 21 days.
  - Isolated facial palsy: 21–28 days.
  - Arthritis: 28 days.
- **Ceftriaxone or Penicillin IV:** Carditis, meningitis, persistent/recurrent arthritis: 14–28 days.

If untreated, lesions fade within 28 days. If delayed diagnosis, may have permanent neurologic or joint disabilities.

If treated adequately, lesions fade within days and the late manifestations are prevented.

ROCKY MOUNTAIN SPOTTED FEVER (RMSF)

An 8-year-old girl from North Carolina presents with fever, severe headache, and myalgia over 3 days in July. She attended a family picnic 1 week ago. On examination, she has a temperature of 102.9°F (39.4°C), HR 134 beats/min. She is complaining of headache and has a macular rash on the wrists, palms, ankles, and soles. There are no other significant findings. Her platelets are 68 and serum sodium is 129. *Think: Rocky Mountain spotted fever.*

RMSF is a systemic tick-borne illness caused by *Rickettsia rickettsii*. Rash is considered the hallmark of this disease, which characteristically involves the palm and soles. Severe frontal headache is common, although it occurs less frequently in children. Abdominal pain, splenomegaly, and conjunctivitis may also be present. RMSF should be considered in the following states: Oklahoma, North and South Carolina, Tennessee, and Pennsylvania. Highest incidence rates for RMSF are in North Carolina and Oklahoma. Since the classic triad of fever, rash, and a history of tick exposure occurs in a few patients, awareness of seasonality and geographic distribution of the disease is important to make the diagnosis. Laboratory abnormalities include hyponatremia, hypoalbuminemia, anemia, and thrombocytopenia.

DEFINITION

A potentially life-threatening disease following a tick bite.

ETIOLOGY

Rickettsia rickettsii.

EPIDEMIOLOGY

Keep in mind geography (presence of a vector) and season (see Table 10-5).

PATHOPHYSIOLOGY

- An **intracellular infection of the endothelial cells** lining the small blood vessels, resulting in vascular necrosis and extravasation of blood.
- Only 60% of patients report a history of a tick bite.
- The **incubation period** is 2–14 days.
- **Rarely** occurs in the Rocky Mountains.
- **Highest incidence in children aged 5–10 years old.**

Outdoor activities in the "tick area"	Sick, fever, myalgia and **severe headache**
Low sodium and platelets	Rash on distal extremities, including **palms and soles,** spreads toward the trunk

SIGNS AND SYMPTOMS

- Sudden onset of high fever, myalgia, severe headache, rigors, nausea, and photophobia.
- Fifty percent develop rash within 3 days. Another 30% develop the rash within 6 days.
- Rash consists of 2- to 6-mm pink initially **blanchable macules** that first appear peripherally on wrists, forearms, ankles, **palms,** and **soles.**
- Within 6–18 hours the exanthem spreads centrally to the trunk, proximal extremities, and face (centrifugal).
- Within 1–3 days the macules evolve to deep red papules, and within 2–4 days the exanthem is hemorrhagic and no longer blanchable.
- **Up to 15% have no rash** ("spotless").
- Many patients have exquisite tenderness of the gastrocnemius muscle.
- Meningitis is common.
- If untreated, myocarditis, disseminated intravascular coagulation (DIC), shock, fatality rate up to 25%.

DIAGNOSIS

- Clinical.
- Rash biopsy would demonstrate necrotizing vasculitis.
- Indirect fluorescent antibody (IFA) assay: Titer > 1:64 is diagnostic.

TREATMENT

- Doxycycline, irrespective of a patient's age.

COMPLICATIONS

- Fulminant infection in glucose-6-phosphate dehydrogenase (G6PD) deficiency.
- Noncardiogenic pulmonary edema.
- Meningoencephalitis.
- Multiorgan damage due to vasculitis.

RMSF is a clinical diagnosis. It is important not to delay treatment.

RMSF is one of the few current indications to use chloramphenicol. It is seldom used anymore due to potential for **gray baby syndrome (aplastic anemia).**

Toxic Shock Syndrome

DEFINITION

An acute, febrile, exanthematous illness that involves multiple systems with potential complications, including shock, renal failure, myocardial failure, and adult respiratory distress syndrome.

PATHOPHYSIOLOGY

- A result of hematogenous dissemination of a toxin.
- Toxins from *Staphylococcus* or *Streptococcus* (Table 10-6) act as superantigens activating T cells, resulting in massive release of cytokines, which has profound physiologic consequences (ie, fever, vasodilation, hypotension, and multisystem organ involvement).

TABLE 10-6. Diagnostic Criteria of Toxic Shock Syndrome (TSS)

STREPTOCOCCAL TSS	STAPHYLOCOCCAL TSS
Isolation of GAS (throat, wound, blood) and hypotension	1. T > 102°F
And > 2 signs:	2. Diffuse erythroderma
▪ **Soft tissue necrosis** (fasciitis, gangrene)	3. Desquamation in **week 2 (hands)**
▪ ARDS	4. Hypotension
▪ Erythroderma, desquamation	**And > 3 signs:**
▪ Renal (creatinine)	▪ **Vomiting/diarrhea at onset**
▪ Liver (transaminases)	▪ Myalgia or elevated CPK
▪ Coagulopathy (thrombocytopenia, DIC)	▪ **Red mucosae** (oropharyngeal, vaginal, conjunctival)
	▪ CNS: altered mental status
	▪ Renal (creatinine)
	▪ Liver (transaminases)
	▪ Thrombocytopenia

ARDS, adult respiratory distress syndrome; CPK, creatine phosphokinase; DIC, disseminated intravascular coagulation; GAS, group A *Streptococcus.*

SIGNS AND SYMPTOMS

- Sick-looking patient—streptococcal TSS (group A *Streptococcus* [GAS]): Usually, there is evidence of soft tissue infection (Table 10-7), classically **necrotizing fasciitis in a patient with varicella.**
- **Less than half of staphylococcal TSS is associated with menstrual tampons.** Source also may be nasal or wound packing, or an abscess.
- Recovery in 7–10 days.

TREATMENT

- Aggressive fluid replacement.
- Eradication of source.
- Parenteral β-lactamase-resistant antibiotic.

TABLE 10-7. Streptococcal versus Staphylococcal

	GROUP A STREPTOCOCCUS	STAPHYLOCOCCUS AUREUS
Prodrome	Flulike	*Vomiting, diarrhea*
Focal infection	Soft tissue	Sometimes—wound
Erythroderma	Rare	Yes
Positive blood culture	60%	Rare

See Table 10-8 for a summary of endemic fungal infections.

TABLE 10-8. Summary of Endemic Fungal Infections

	HISTOPLASMOSIS	COCCIDIOIDOMYCOSIS
Geography	Mississippi, Ohio, and Missouri River valleys	Utah, Arizona, New Mexico, Texas, California
Setting	Gardening, demolition, visiting **caves (bat droppings);** playing in barns, hollow trees with **bird roosts**	Dust storms, earthquakes, **archeologic digging,** picnic in a desert
Focal infection	Pulmonary infiltrates, hilar adenopathy In adolescents: **Erythema nodosum**a	Influenza-like or pneumonia: Fever, cough, headache, malaise, myalgia, and chest pain **Erythema multiforme** **Erythema nodosum**a
Disseminated infection	**Prolonged fever,** pneumonitis, lymphadenopathy, hepatosplenomegaly, failure to thrive or weight loss, meningitis, **pancytopenia**	**Rare** Skin: Papules, nodules **Osteomyelitis,** arthritis Meningitis, pneumonitis
Diagnosis	**Culture** of sputum, blood, bone marrow Histology: **Intracellular yeast** with silver stain	**Serology:** IgM and IgG Histology: **Spherules** in pleural fluid bronchoalveolar lavage, and skin biopsy specimens
Treatment Focal infection Disseminated infection	Itraconazole Amphotericin B	Fluconazole or itraconazole Amphotericin B

a Erythema nodosum is an inflammatory exanthem, an area of tender, red and shiny induration, usually on the shins.

Coccidioidomycosis

A 13-year-old girl develops fever, cough, and chest pain soon after she has visited relatives in Arizona, where they were outing in a desert quite often. On examination, her temperature is 102.5°F (39.2°C), RR 44 breaths/min, no hypoxemia, and rales are heard over her left lower lobe. There are symmetrical tender, red, shiny indurations on both shins. WBC: 16.8. Chest radiograph shows left lower lobe consolidation. *Think: Coccidioidomycosis.*

Coccidioidomycosis is an infectious disease caused by the fungus *Coccidioides immitis*. Also known as San Joaquin Valley fever, coccidioidomycosis should be considered in southwestern U.S. states (Arizona, California, New Mexico, Utah, Nevada, and Texas). Symptoms usually develop 1–3 weeks after exposure. Clinical features include dry cough, chest pain, myalgias, arthralgia, fever, anorexia, and weakness.

ETIOLOGY

Coccidioides immitis, the dimorphic fungus.

EPIDEMIOLOGY

- Southwestern United States.
- Black and Filipino, pregnant women, neonates, and immunocompromised people have higher risk of dissemination.
- Person-to-person transmission **does not occur.**
- Incubation period: 1–3 weeks.
- Transmission: Inhalation of airborne spores.
- Infection produces **lifelong immunity.**

SIGNS AND SYMPTOMS

- Usually asymptomatic or self-limited: Influenza-like or pneumonia, with fever, headache, cough, malaise, myalgia, and chest pain.
- Maculopapular rash, erythema multiforme, or erythema nodosum may be the only manifestations.
- Dissemination is rare, mostly in infants: Skin, bones and joints, central nervous system (CNS), and lungs.
- Night sweats and anorexia.
- Meningitis almost invariably is fatal if untreated.

DIAGNOSIS

- Residual coin-like pulmonary lesions may be present on chest x-ray.
- Spherules with endospores in tissue or body fluid is pathognomonic.
- Cultures are hazardous.
- Elevated erythrocyte sedimentation rate (ESR) and alkaline phosphatase.
- Marked eosinophilia.

TREATMENT

- Same as for histoplasmosis below.
- Surgery for chronic pulmonary coccidioidal disease that is unresponsive to IV azole or amphotericin B therapy.

Histoplasmosis

A 6-year-old boy from Indiana develops fever, chest pain, and cough. He was playing in a cave 10 days ago and got scared of bats. Physical exam shows no distress, temperature of 100.7°F (38.2°C), RR 28 breaths/min, oxygen saturation 95%. Rhonchi are heard over the lung fields bilaterally. WBC: 14.9. Chest x-ray shows diffuse bilateral reticulonodular infiltrates and hilar lymph node. *Think: Histoplasmosis.*

It is the most common endemic mycosis causing human infection. Pneumonia is the most common presentation. Atypical pneumonia is usually the initial diagnosis. Initial chest x-ray may show patchy infiltrate, while diffuse reticulonodular infiltrates are present in a progressive disease. The presence of hilar or mediastinal lymphadenopathy ↑ the suspicion for fungal pneumonia.

ETIOLOGY

Histoplasma capsulatum.

EPIDEMIOLOGY

- **Endemic** infection: Ohio and Mississippi River valleys.
- History of exposure to **bird or bat droppings.**
- Incubation period: 1–3 weeks.
- Transmission: Inhalation of airborne spores.
- Reinfection happens with large inoculum.

SIGNS AND SYMPTOMS

- Generally asymptomatic
- Flulike prodrome.
- The more spores inhaled, the more symptoms.
- Severe acute pulmonary infection: Diffuse nodular infiltrates, prolonged fever, fatigue, and weight loss.
- **Progressive disseminated histoplasmosis (PDH):** In infants < 2 years of age and in immunosuppressed, often starts as prolonged "fever of unknown origin."

DIAGNOSIS

- Mediastinal adenitis or granuloma may be seen on chest x-ray.
- Cultures: Sputum, blood, bone marrow; may be negative.
- *Histoplasma* antigen assay: Cross-reaction with other endemic fungi.

TREATMENT

- Uncomplicated infection in an immunocompetent child is self-limited, and does not require treatment.
- Oral itraconazole for serious focal (pulmonary) infection.
- IV amphotericin B for PDH.

In order to recognize endemic infection, keep in mind:

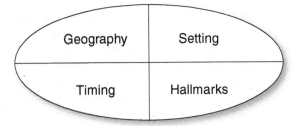

PROTOZOAL INFECTIONS

Schistosomiasis

A 16-year-old male presents with fever, arthralgia, cough, abdominal pain, and rash of 5 days' duration. He went to Puerto Rico for a river rafting trip 3 weeks ago. On examination, his temperature is 102°F (38.9°C), there are scattered urticaria on the trunk and extremities that wax and wane, and his spleen is palpable 3 cm below the costal margin. WBC count is 6.1, with 23% eosinophils. *Think: Schistosomiasis.*

Schistosomiasis is transmitted in tropical and subtropical areas. Clinical presentations are chills, cough, abdominal pain, diarrhea, nausea, vomiting, headache, rash, and lymphadenopathy. Physical examination may show an enlarged, nontender liver and an enlarged spleen. Eosinophilia is often prominent in schistosomiasis.

ETIOLOGY

Caused by trematodes (flukes). See Table 10-9.

TABLE 10-9. Schistosomiasis

	SCHISTOSOMA MANSONI	*SCHISTOSOMA JAPONICUM*	*SCHISTOSOMA HAEMATOBIUM*
Geography	Africa, Arabian Peninsula, Caribbean, Latin America	China, Indonesia, Philippines	Africa, eastern Mediterranean
Target	Mesenteric vessels	Liver	Urinary bladder
Presentation	**Hepatosplenomegaly, portal hypertension,** hematemesis, ascites		**Dysuria, hematuria,** bladder fibrosis, or cancer
Egg emboli	Lungs, spinal cord		Lungs, brain

EPIDEMIOLOGY

- Fecal or urine ova get into the snails and form larvae.
- Larvae leave the snail into the fresh water and penetrate the skin.
- Larvae travel to particular organs and tissues, and there develop into mature forms.

SIGNS AND SYMPTOMS

- "Swimmer's itch" transient, a few hours after water exposure, followed in 1–2 weeks by an intermittent pruritic, papular rash.
- Invasive stage: Within weeks to months of exposure—fever, malaise, cough, abdominal pain, and nonspecific rash.
- Ulceration of intestine and colon, abdominal pain, and bloody diarrhea (*Schistosoma interclatum* and *Schistosoma mekongi*).

DIAGNOSIS

- Eggs in stool or urine.
- Eosinophilia.

TREATMENT

Praziquantel.

Visceral Larva Migrans

ETIOLOGY

Toxocara canis and *Toxocara cati* (roundworms of puppies or kittens).

EPIDEMIOLOGY

- Fecal-oral transmission: Eggs in soil make their way into the mouth by getting onto hands or toys.
- Role of **pica**—eating soil: Ingested eggs hatch and penetrate the GI tract, migrating to the liver, lung, eye, central nervous system, and heart, where they die and calcify.

SIGNS AND SYMPTOMS

- Most individuals are asymptomatic.
- Symptomatic in young children (under 4 years of age).
- The more larvae, the more symptoms.
- **Visceral:** Fever, cough, wheezing (pneumonitis), **hepatomegaly.**
- Rare: Myocarditis, encephalitis (seizures).
- **Ocular:** Endophthalmitis or retinal granulomas, **usually in older children** or adolescents.

DIAGNOSIS

- **Leukocytosis** and **hypereosinophilia.**
- Hypergammaglobulinemia and ↑ titers of isohemagglutinin to the A and B blood group antigens.
- EIA for *Toxocara* antibodies. EIA is more sensitive in visceral than in ocular form of infection.

TREATMENT

Albendazole.

Pay attention to travel history and timing from return (incubation period from weeks to months).

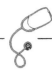

Exposure to fresh water (lake, river) at the endemic area: swimming, fishing, playing.

Differentiate eye lesions of visceral larva migrans from retinoblastoma.

A 4-year-old boy presents with fever and cough of 10 days' duration. On exam, he has a temperature of 101.8°F (38.8°C) and hepatomegaly. He has leukocytosis, with **45% eosinophils.** He likes to play with his **puppy** in a **sandbox.** What is the diagnosis? Visceral larva migrans.

Animal Bites/Scratches

- Cleaning, debridement, and irrigation are most important treatment.
- Antibiotic prophylaxis for human, cat, and dog bites (amoxicillin/clavulanate).
- X-ray to check for bone involvement if deep wound.
- Most wounds should **not** be sutured; if deep wounds, surgical consult is best.
- Assess risk for rabies: Local epidemiological information.
- Ensure **tetanus immunization** is up to date.

Pathogens in bites:
- Human: *Eikenella corrodens*
- Cats: *Pasteurella multocida*
- Dogs: *Capnocytophagia canimorsus*

Abrasions and Lacerations

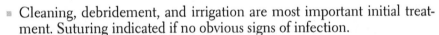

A 10-year-old boy steps on a dirty nail that punctures his foot through his sneaker. Two days later he presents with pain, swelling, and redness of the heel, with purulent drainage from a central pinpoint opening. He has no fever. WBC is 14.6. X-ray: no foreign body, no fracture, no gas in the soft tissue. *Think: Wound likely to become infected with* Pseudomonas. The association of *Pseudomonas* infection with puncture wounds to the foot is well recognized.

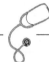

In human bites, consider child abuse and risk for HIV and hepatitis B.

- Cleaning, debridement, and irrigation are most important initial treatment. Suturing indicated if no obvious signs of infection.
- If secondarily infected, debride and drain.
- Initial antibiotic given based on most likely organism; Gram stain and culture to determine best antibiotic in chronic or complex wounds.
- *Staphylococcus* and *Streptococcus* are the most common pathogens, so a first-generation cephalosporin such as cephalexin or clindamycin is commonly given as empiric treatment.

Gastrointestinal Disease

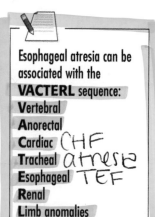

Handwritten margin notes:
MC—
proximal
atresia

distal TE
Fistula

A full-term infant was noted to have copious oral secretions requiring frequent suctioning to prevent choking. Attempts to place a nasogastric tube were unsuccessful, with the tube curling in the esophagus. X-ray is shown in the figure. What is the likely diagnosis and management of this condition?

The nasogastric tube with the tip in the proximal esophagus and failure to advance further signifies an esophageal atresia. The most common type is where the proximal esophagus ends in a blind pouch (as in this case) and there is a distal tracheoesophageal fistula. Also evident are ribs and vertebral anomalies in this case. This could be part of VATER (vertebral anomalies, anal atresia, tracheoesophageal anomalies, renal anomalies) syndrome. Infant was noted to have a single right kidney on renal ultrasound. Management includes surgical repair of the tracheoesophageal fistula.

DEFINITION

- The esophagus ends blindly ~10–12 cm from the nares.
- Occurs in 1/3000–1/4500 live births.
- In 85% of cases the distal esophagus communicates with the posterior trachea (distal tracheoesophageal fistula [TEF]).

SIGNS AND SYMPTOMS

- History of maternal polyhydramnios.
- Newborn with ↑ oral secretions.
- Choking, cyanosis, coughing during feeding (more commonly aspiration of pharyngeal secretions).
- Esophageal atresia with fistula.
- Aspiration of gastric contents via distal fistula—life threatening (chemical pneumonitis).
- Tympanitic distended abdomen.
- Esophageal atresia without fistula.
- Recurrent coughing with aspiration pneumonia (delayed diagnosis).
- Aspiration of pharyngeal secretions common.
- Airless abdomen on abdominal x-ray.

DIAGNOSIS

- Usually made at delivery.
- Unable to pass nasogastric tube (NGT) into stomach (see coiled NGT on chest x-ray).
- May also use contrast radiology, video esophagram, or bronchoscopy.
- Chest x-ray (CXR) demonstrates air in upper esophagus (see Figure 11-1).

TREATMENT

Surgical repair (may be done in stages).

Esophageal atresia can be associated with the **VACTERL** sequence:
Vertebral
Anorectal
Cardiac *CHF*
Tracheal *atresia*
Esophageal *TEF*
Renal
Limb anomalies

Suspect esophageal atresia in a neonate with drooling and excessive oral secretions.

Inability to pass a rigid nasogastric tube from the mouth to the stomach is diagnostic of esophageal atresia.

HIGH-YIELD FACTS

GASTROINTESTINAL DISEASE

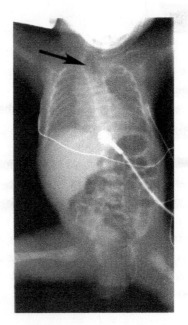

FIGURE 11-1. Esophageal atresia.

Radiograph demonstrating air in the upper esophagus (arrow) and GI tract, consistent with esophageal atresia.

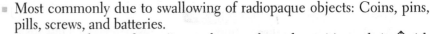

ESOPHAGEAL FOREIGN BODY

- Most commonly due to swallowing of radiopaque objects: Coins, pins, pills, screws, and batteries.
- Preexisting abnormalities (ie, tracheoesophageal repair) result in ↑ risk of having foreign body impaction at site of abnormality.
- Site of impaction:
  - 70%: Thoracic inlet (between clavicles on CXR).
  - 15%: Midesophagus.
  - 15%: Lower esophageal sphincter (LES).

The most common site of esophageal impaction is at the thoracic inlet.

SIGNS AND SYMPTOMS

- Gagging/choking.
- Difficulty with secretions.
- Dysphagia/food refusal.
- Throat pain or chest pain.
- Emesis/hematemesis.

DIAGNOSIS

- History, sometime witnessed event.
- X-ray (AP/lateral CXR, see Figure 11-2).

TREATMENT

- Objects found within the esophagus are generally considered impacted.
- Generally require endoscopic treatment if symptomatic or fail to pass to stomach (below diaphragm on x-ray) within a few hours.

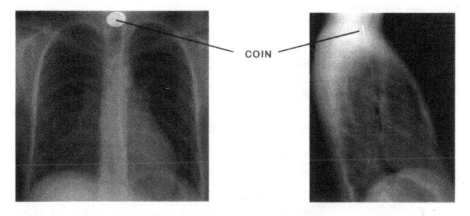

FIGURE 11-2. Esophageal foreign body.

A coin in the esophagus will be seen flat or en face on an AP radiograph, and on its edge on a lateral view. (Photo courtesy of Dr. Julia Rosekrans.)

- Impacted objects, pointed objects, and batteries must be removed immediately.
- Important to assess time of ingestion; > 24 hours can → erosion or necrosis of esophageal wall.

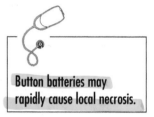

Button batteries may rapidly cause local necrosis.

GASTROESOPHAGEAL REFLUX DISEASE (GERD)

An 8-month-old preterm infant has been hospitalized for 4 months in the neontal care unit. In the past 2 weeks, the nurses have noted that he is regurgitating several times an hour. He makes chewing movements preceding these episodes of regurgitation. *Think: Rumination.*

Gastroesophageal reflux (GER) is common in preterm infants. Transient relaxation of the lower esophageal sphincter is the most common mechanism implicated. Signs and symptoms include apnea, chronic lung disease, poor weight gain, and behavioral symptoms. Frequent regurgitation and feeding difficulties may occur.

DEFINITION

- Passive reflux of gastric contents due to incompetent lower esophageal sphincter (LES).
- Approximately 1 in 300 children suffer from significant reflux and complication.
- Functional gastroesophageal reflux is most common.

RISK FACTORS

- Prematurity.
- Neurologic disorders.
- Incompetence of LES due to prematurity, asthma.
- Medications (theophylline, calcium channel blockers or β-blockers).

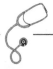

GERD is the etiology for Sandifer syndrome (reflux, back arching, stiffness, and torticollis). Sandifer syndrome is most often confused with a neurologic or apparent life-threatening event.

SIGNS AND SYMPTOMS

- Excessive spitting up in the first week of life (in 85% of affected).
- Symptomatic by 6 weeks (10%).
- Symptoms resolve without treatment by age 2 (60%).
- Forceful vomiting (occasional).
- Aspiration pneumonia (30%).
- Chronic cough, wheezing, and recurrent pneumonia (later childhood).
- Rarely may cause laryngospasm, apnea, and bradycardia.
- Regurgitation.

DIAGNOSIS

- Clinical assessment in mild cases.
- Esophageal pH probe studies and barium esophagography in severe cases.
- Esophagoscopy with biopsy for diagnosis of esophagitis.

TREATMENT

- Positioning following feeds—keep infant upright up to an hour after feeds.
- In older children, mealtime more than 2 hours before sleep and sleeping with head elevated.
- Thickening formula with rice cereal.
- Medications:
  - Antacids, histamine-2 (H$_2$) blockers (ranitidine) and proton pump inhibitors (PPIs; omeprazole).
  - Motility agents such as metoclopramide and erythromycin (stimulate gastric emptying).
  - Surgery—Nissen fundoplication.

PEPTIC ULCER

DEFINITION

Includes primary and secondary (related to stress).

SIGNS AND SYMPTOMS

- **Primary**—pain, vomiting, and acute and chronic gastrointestinal (GI) blood loss.
  - First month of life: GI hemorrhage and perforation.
  - Neonatal–2 months: Recurrent vomiting, slow growth, and GI hemorrhage.
  - Preschool: Periumbilical and postprandial pain (with vomiting and hemorrhage).
  - > 6 years: Epigastric abdominal pain, acute/chronic GI blood loss with anemia.
- **Secondary:**
  - Stress ulcers secondary to sepsis, respiratory or cardiac insufficiency, trauma, or dehydration in infants.
  - Related to trauma or other life-threatening events (older children).
  - Stress ulcers and erosions associated with burns (Curling ulcers).
  - Ulcers following head trauma or surgery usually Cushing ulcers.

- Drug related—nonsteroidal anti-inflammatory drugs (NSAIDs) or steroids.
- Infectious—*Helicobacter pylori*.

DIAGNOSIS

- Upper GI endoscopy.
- Barium meal not sensitive.
- Plain x-rays may diagnose perforation of acute ulcers.
- Angiography can demonstrate bleeding site.
- *H pylori* testing (hydrogen breath test, stool antigen).

TREATMENT

- Antibiotics for eradication of *H pylori*: Triple therapy—PPI + 2 antibiotics (amoxicillin, clarithromycin, PPI).
- Antacids, sucralfate, and misoprostol.
- H_2 blockers and PPIs.
- Give prophylaxis for peptic ulcer when child is NPO or is receiving steroids.
- Endoscopic cautery.
- Surgery (vagotomy, pyloroplasty, or antrectomy) for extreme cases.

Antimicrobials: 14 days
PPIs: 1 month

COLIC

DEFINITION

- Rule of 3's: Crying > 3 hours/day, > 3 days/week for > 3 weeks between the ages of 3 weeks and 3 months.
- Frequent complex of paroxysmal abdominal pain, severe crying.
- Usually in infants < 3 months old.
- Etiology unknown. Can be related to under- or overfeeding, milk protein allergy, parental stress, and smoking.
- Colic is a diagnosis of exclusion. First look for other causes (hair in eye, corneal abrasion, strangulated hernia, otitis media, sepsis, etc.).

SIGNS AND SYMPTOMS

- Sudden-onset loud crying (paroxysms may persist for several hours).
- Facial flushing.
- Circumoral pallor.
- Distended, tense abdomen.
- Legs drawn up on abdomen.
- Feet often cold.
- Temporary relief apparent with passage of feces or flatus.

A head-to-toe examination is essential.
Physical examination MUST be normal.

TREATMENT

- No single treatment provides satisfactory relief.
- Careful exam is important to rule out other causes.
- Improve feeding techniques (burping).
- Avoid over- or underfeeding.
- Resolves spontaneously with time.

Parents and caretakers of children with colic are often very stressed out, putting the child at risk for child abuse.

👤 A 4-week-old male infant has a 5-day history of vomiting after feedings. Physical exam shows a hungry infant with prominent peristaltic waves in the epigastrium. Laboratory evaluation revealed the following: Na 129, Cl 92, HCO$_3$ 28, K 3.1, BUN 24). *Think: Hypertrophic pyloric stenosis.*

Pyloric stenosis is the most common cause of intestinal obstruction in infants. It is more common in males (M:F 4:1). It usually presents during the third to fifth week of life. Initial symptom is nonbilious vomiting. Classic sign of olive mass is not as common since increasing awareness has resulted in ultrasound imaging and early diagnosis. Criteria for diagnosis include pyloric muscle thickness > 4 mm and length of pyloric canal > 14 mm. Hypochloremic, hypokalemic metabolic alkalosis is the classic electrolyte abnormality.

DEFINITION

- Most common etiology is idiopathic.
- Not usually present at birth.
- Associated with exogenous administration of erythromycin, eosinophilic gastroenteritis, epidermolysis bullosa, trisomy 18, and Turner syndrome.
- First-born male.

SIGNS AND SYMPTOMS

- Typical: Projectile vomiting, palpable mass and peristalsis—not always present.
- Nonbilious vomiting (projectile or not).
- Usually progressive, after feeding.
- Usually after 3 weeks of age, may be as late as 5 months.
- Hypochloremic, hypokalemic metabolic alkalosis (rare these days due to earlier diagnosis).
- Palpable pyloric olive-shaped mass in midepigastrium (difficult to find).
- Visible peristalsis: Left to right.

DIAGNOSIS

- Ultrasound (90% sensitivity).
- Elongated pyloric channel (> 14 mm).
- Thickened pyloric wall (> 4 mm).
- Radiographic contrast series (Figure 11-3).
- String sign: From elongated pyloric channel.
- Shoulder sign: Bulge of pyloric muscle into the antrum.
- Double tract sign: Parallel streaks of barium in the narrow channel.

TREATMENT

- Surgery: Pyloromyotomy is curative.
- Must correct existing dehydration and acid-base abnormalities prior to surgery.

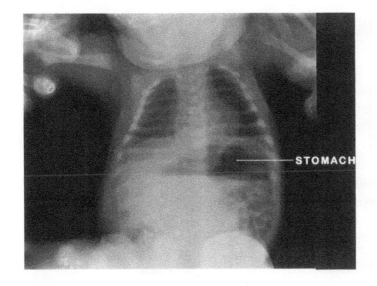 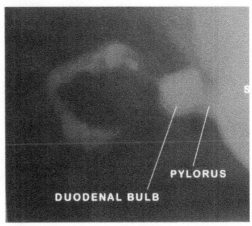

FIGURE 11-3. Abdominal x-ray on the left demonstrates a dilated air-filled stomach with normal caliber bowel, consistent with gastric outlet obstruction.

Barium meal figure on the right confirms diagnosis of pyloric stenosis. The dilated duodenal bulb is the "olive" felt on physical exam. Note how there is a paucity of contrast traveling through the duodenum. (Photo courtesy of Drs. Julia Rosekrans and James E. Colletti.)

DUODENAL ATRESIA

DEFINITION
- Failure to recanalize lumen after solid phase of intestinal development.
- Several forms.

SIGNS AND SYMPTOMS
- Bilious vomiting without abdominal distention (first day of life). Onset of vomiting within hours of birth.
- Can be nonbilious if the defect is proximal to the ampulla of Vater.
- Scaphoid abdomen.
- Placement of orogastric tube typically yields a significant amount of bile-stained fluid.
- History of polyhydramnios in 50% of pregnancies.
- Down syndrome seen in 20–30% of cases.
- Associated anomalies include malrotation, esophageal atresia, and congenital heart disease.

DIAGNOSIS
- Clinical.
- X-ray findings: Double-bubble sign (air bubbles in the stomach and duodenum) proximal to the site of atresia (Figure 11-4).

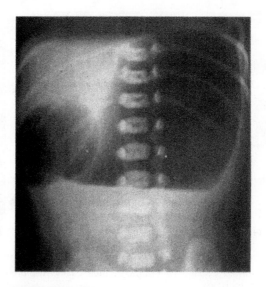

FIGURE 11-4. Duodenal atresia.

Gas-filled and dilated stomach show the classic "double-bubble" appearance of duodenal atresia. Note no distal gas is present. (Reproduced, with permission, from Rudolph CD, et al (eds). *Rudolph's Pediatrics*, 21st ed. New York: McGraw-Hill, 2002: 1403.)

TREATMENT

- Initially, nasogastric and orogastric decompression with intravenous (IV) fluid replacement.
- Treat life-threatening anomalies.
- Surgery.
- Duodenoduodenostomy.

VOLVULUS

DEFINITION

- Gastric and intestinal:
  - Gastric: Sudden onset of severe epigastric pain; intractable retching with emesis.
  - Intestinal: Associated with malrotation (Figure 11-5).
- Volvulus occurs as a consequence of intestinal malrotation—obstruction is complete, and compromise to the blood supply of the midgut has started.

RISK FACTORS

- Embryological abnormalities: Arrest of development at any stage during embryological development of GI tract can → changes in anatomical position of organs and narrowing of mesenteric base, resulting in ↑ risk for volvulus.
- Male-to-female presentation: 2:1.

dlt
malrotation

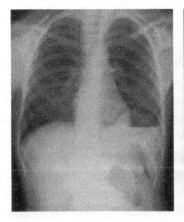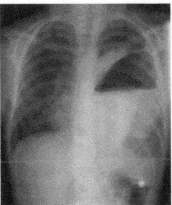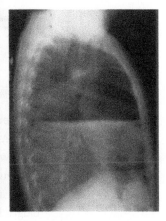

FIGURE 11-5. Volvulus.

First AP view done 6 weeks prior to the second AP and corresponding lateral view. Note the markedly dilated stomach above the normal level of the left hemidiaphragm in the thoracic cavity. Also present is a large left-sided diaphragmatic hernia. (Photo courtesy of Dr. Julia Rosekrans.)

SIGNS AND SYMPTOMS

- Vomiting in infancy.
- Emesis (commonly bilious).
- Abdominal pain → acute abdomen.
- Early satiety.
- Blood-stained stools.
- Distention.
- A neonate with bilious vomiting must be considered at risk for having a midgut volvulus.

DIAGNOSIS

BIRD BEAK

- Plain abdominal films: Characteristic bird-beak appearance.
- May also see air-fluid level without beak.

TREATMENT

- Treatment is surgical correction.
- Gastric: Emergent surgery.
- Intestinal: Surgery or endoscopy.

COMPLICATIONS

- Perforation
- Peritonitis

A 9-month-old female infant was brought to the ED due to vomiting and crying. She had a "cold" 3 days ago. On arrival she was sleepy but arousable. When she woke up, she cried and vomited. Physical examination revealed distended abdomen with an ill-defined mass in the right upper abdomen. What is the cause of her symptoms? Intussusception.

How she should be treated? A contrast enema should be performed to reduce the intussusception. It is both diagnostic and therapeutic. It should be performed in consultation with a pediatric surgeon caring for the child and a pediatric radiologist interpreting the study. It is the most common cause of intestinal obstruction between 5 months and 6 years of age. Most children with intussusception are under 1 year of age. The classic triad of intermittent, colicky abdominal pain; vomiting; and bloody, mucous stools occurs in only 20–40%.

DEFINITION

Invagination of one portion of the bowel into itself. The proximal portion is usually drawn into the distal portion by peristalsis.

EPIDEMIOLOGY

- Incidence: 1–4 in 1000 live births.
- Male-to-female ratio: 2:1 to 4:1.
- Peak incidence: 5–12 months.
- Age range: 2 months to 5 years.
- Most common cause of acute intestinal obstruction under 2 years of age.
- Most common site is ileocolic (90%).

> Intussusception is the most common cause of bowel obstruction in children ages 2 months to 5 years.

ETIOLOGY

- Most common etiology is idiopathic.
- Other causes:
  - Viral (enterovirus in summer, rotavirus in winter).
  - A "lead point" (or focus) is thought to be present in older children 2–10% of the time. These lead points can be caused by Meckel's diverticulum, polyp, lymphoma, Henoch-Schönlein purpura, cystic fibrosis.

SIGNS AND SYMPTOMS

- Classic triad:
  - Intermittent colicky abdominal pain.
  - Bilious vomiting.
  - Currant jelly stool (late finding).
- Neurologic signs:
  - Lethargy
  - Shocklike state
  - Seizure activity
  - Apnea
- Right upper quadrant mass:
  - Sausage shaped.
  - Ill defined.
- Dance's sign: Absence of bowel in right lower quadrant.

> **Intussusception**
> - Classic triad is present in only 20% of cases.
> - Absence of currant jelly stool does not exclude the diagnosis.
> - Neurologic signs may delay the diagnosis.

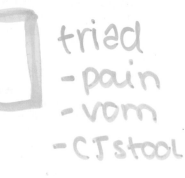

triad
- pain
- vom
- CJ stool

- Abdominal x-ray:
    - X-ray is neither specific nor sensitive. Can be completely normal.
    - Paucity of bowel gas (Figure 11-6).
    - Loss of visualization of the tip of liver.
    - "Target sign": Two concentric circles of fat density.
- Ultrasound:
    - Test of choice.
    - "Target" or "donut" sign: Single hypoechoic ring with hyperechoic center.
    - "Pseudokidney" sign: Superimposed hypoechoic (edematous walls of bowel) and hyperechoic (areas of compressed mucosa) layers.
- Barium enema:
    - Not useful for ileoileal intussusceptions.
    - May note cervix-like mass.
    - Coiled spring appearance on the evacuation film.
    - Contraindications: Peritonitis, perforation, profound shock/hemodynamic instability.
- Air enema:
    - Air enema is preferred (safe, with a lower absorbed radiation).
    - Often provides the same diagnostic and therapeutic benefit of a barium enema without the barium.

Contrast enema for intussusception can be both diagnostic and therapeutic.
Rule of threes:

- Barium column should not exceed a height of 3 feet.
- No more than 3 attempts.
- Only 3 minutes/ attempt.

TREATMENT

- Correct dehydration.
- NG tube for decompression.
- Hydrostatic reduction.
- Barium/air enema (see Figure 11-7).
- Surgical reduction:
    - Failed reduction by enema.
    - Clinical signs of perforation or peritonitis.
- Recurrence:
    - With radiologic reduction: 7–10%.
    - With surgical reduction: 2–5%.

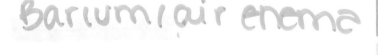

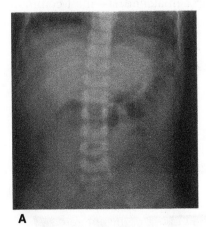

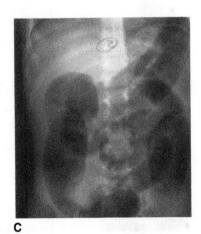

A   **B**   **C**

FIGURE 11-6. **Intussusception.**

Note the paucity of bowel gas in film A. Air enema partially reduces it in film B and then completely reduced it in film C.

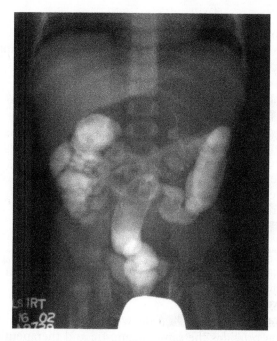

FIGURE 11-7. Abdominal x-ray following barium enema in a 2-month-old boy, consistent with intussusception.

Note paucity of gas in right upper quadrant and near obscuring of liver tip.

MECKEL'S DIVERTICULUM

DEFINITION

Persistence of the omphalomesenteric (vitelline) duct (should disappear by seventh week of gestation).

SIGNS AND SYMPTOMS

- Usually in first 2 years:
  - Intermittent painless rectal bleeding (hematochezia—most common presenting sign).
  - Intestinal obstruction.
  - Diverticulitis.
- Occurs on the antimesenteric border of the ileum, usually 40–60 cm proximal to the ileocecal valve.

DIAGNOSIS

- Meckel's scan (scintigraphy) has 85% sensitivity and 95% specificity. Uptake can be enhanced with cimetidine, glucagons, or gastrin.
- Most common heterotopic mucosa is gastric.

TREATMENT

Surgical: Diverticular resection with transverse closure of the enterotomy.

Meckel's Rules of 2
- 2% of population
- 2 inches long
- 2 feet from the ileocecal valve
- Patient is usually under 2 years of age
- 2% are symptomatic

Meckel's diverticulum may mimic acute appendicitis and also act as lead point for intussusception.

DEFINITION

- Acute inflammation and infection of the vermiform appendix.
- Most common cause for emergent surgery in childhood.
- Perforation rates are greatest in youngest children (can't localize symptoms).
- Occurs secondary to obstruction of lumen of appendix.
- Three phases:
  1. Luminal obstruction, venous congestion progresses to mucosal ischemia, necrosis, and ulceration.
  2. Bacterial invasion with inflammatory infiltrate through all layers.
  3. Necrosis of wall results in perforation and contamination.

SIGNS AND SYMPTOMS

- Classically: Pain, vomiting, and fever.
- Initially, periumbilical pain; emesis infrequent.
- Anorexia.
- Low-grade fever.
- Diarrhea infrequent.
- Pain radiates to right lower quadrant.
- Perforation rate > 65% after 48 hours.
- Rectal exam may reveal localized mass or tenderness.

DIAGNOSIS

- History and physical exam is key to rule out alternatives first.
- Pain usually occurs before vomiting, diarrhea, or anorexia.
- Atypical presentations are common—risk for misdiagnosis.
- Most common misdiagnosis: Gastroenteritis.
- Labs helpful to rule other diagnosis but no laboratory test specific for appendicitis.
- Computed tomographic (CT) scan (Figure 11-8) indicated for patients in whom diagnosis is equivocal—not a requirement for all patients.
- Higher rate of ruptured appendix on presentation in young children.

TREATMENT

- Surgery as soon as diagnosis made.
- Antibiotics are controversial in nonperforated appendicitis.
- Broad-spectrum antibiotics needed for cases of perforation (ampicillin, gentamicin, clindamycin, or metronidazole × 7 days).
- Laparoscopic removal associated with shortened hospital stay (nonperforated appendicitis).

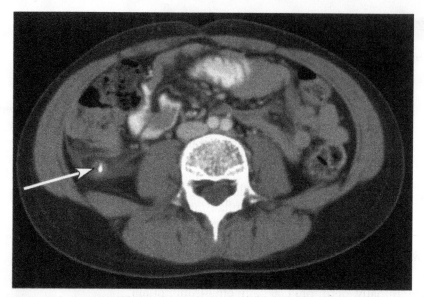

FIGURE 11-8. Abdominal CT of a 10-year-old girl demonstrating enlargement of the appendix, some periappendiceal fluid, and an appendicolith (arrow), consistent with acute appendicitis.

CONSTIPATION

A 4-year-old girl has not had a bowel movement for a week, and this has been a recurring problem. Various laxatives and enemas have been tried in the past. Prior to toilet training, the girl had one bowel movement a day. Physical examination is normal except for the presence of stool in the sigmoid colon and hard stool on rectal examination. After removing the impaction, the next appropriate step in management would be to administer mineral oil or other stool softener.

Constipation is a common problem in children. It is the most common cause of abdominal pain in children. Functional constipation is more common in children, and organic causes are common in neonates. The physical examination often reveals a large volume of stool palpated in the suprapubic region. The finding of rectal impaction may establish the diagnosis.

DEFINITION/SIGNS AND SYMPTOMS

- Common cause of abdominal pain in children.
- Passage of bulky or hard stool at infrequent intervals.
- During the neonatal period usually caused by Hirschsprung, intestinal pseudo-obstruction, or hypothyroidism.
- Other causes include organic and inorganic (eg, cow's milk protein intolerance, drugs).
- May be metabolic (dehydration, hypothyroidism, hypokalemia, hypercalcemia, psychiatric).

TREATMENT

- ↑ oral fluid and fiber intake.
- Stool softeners (eg, mineral oil).
- Glycerin suppositories.
- Cathartics such as senna or docusate.
- Nonabsorbable osmotic agents (polyethylene glycol) and milk of magnesia for short periods only if necessary—can cause electrolyte imbalances.

Osmotic - PEG, MOM

HIRSCHSPRUNG'S MEGACOLON

A full-term male infant was noted to have progressive abdominal distention on the second day of life, with no stool since birth. He was feeding well on demand whether mother's milk or infant formula. He was otherwise healthy, active, and had no signs of infection. Abdominal x-ray and barium enema are shown in the figure. What is the diagnosis and management of this infant?

Abdominal x-ray is consistent with distended loops of bowel with no evidence of free air. Contrast enema is notable for a narrowed segment of the colon leading to a very distended loop. The diagnosis is likely Hirschsprung disease, as there is a narrowed transitional zone followed by distended loop as described. Hirschsprung disease results from absence of ganglion cells in the bowel wall and resultant narrowed segment of the bowel. The proximal normal bowel progressively dilates due to accumulated food. Definitive diagnosis is made by rectal biopsy, which demonstrates absent ganglion cells.

narrow segment of bowel ∅ gang cells (shows LBO)

DEFINITION

- Abnormal innervation of bowel (ie, absence of ganglion cells in bowel).
- ↑ in familial incidence.
- Occurs in males more than females.
- Associated with Down syndrome.

SIGNS AND SYMPTOMS

- Delayed passage of meconium at birth.
- ↑ abdominal distention → ↓ blood flow → deterioration of mucosal barrier → bacterial proliferation → enterocolitis.
- Chronic constipation and abdominal distention (older children).

- Meconium ileus -

DIAGNOSIS

- Rectal manometry: Measures pressure of the anal sphincter.
- Rectal suction biopsy: Must obtain submucosa to evaluate for ganglionic cells.

TREATMENT

Surgery is definitive (usually staged procedures).

IMPERFORATE ANUS

DEFINITION

- Absence of normal anal opening.
- Rectum is blind; located 2 cm from perineal skin.
- Sacrum and sphincter mechanism well developed.
- Prognosis good.
- Can be associated with VACTERL anomalies.

SIGNS AND SYMPTOMS

- First newborn examination in nursery.
- Failure to pass meconium.
- Abdominal distention.

DIAGNOSIS

- Physical examination.
- Abdominal ultrasonography to examine the genitourinary tract.
- Sacral radiography
- Spinal ultrasound: Association with spinal cord abnormalities, particularly spinal cord tethering.

TREATMENT

Surgery (colostomy in newborn period).

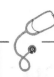

Imperforate anus is frequently associated with Down syndrome and VACTERL.

ANAL FISSURE

A well-nourished 3-month-old infant is brought to the ED because of constipation, blood-streaked stools, and excessive crying on defecation. *Think: Anal fissure.*

Anal fissure is a painful linear tear or crack in the distal anal canal. Constipation may be exacerbated because of fear of pain with defecation. Diagnosis often can be made based on history and physical examination.

DEFINITION

- Painful linear tears in the anal mucosa below the dentate line induced by constipation or excessive diarrhea.
- Tear of squamous epithelium of anal canal between anocutaneous junction and dentate line.
- Often history of constipation is present.
- Predilection for the posterior midline.
- Common age: 6–24 months.

SIGNS AND SYMPTOMS

- Pain with defecation/crying during bowel movement.
- ↑ sphincter tone.
- Visible tear upon gentle lateral retraction of anal tissue.

DIAGNOSIS

Anal inspection.

TREATMENT

Sitz baths, fiber supplements, ↑ fluid intake.

INFLAMMATORY BOWEL DISEASE

DEFINITION

Idiopathic chronic diseases include Crohn disease and ulcerative colitis (UC).

EPIDEMIOLOGY

- Common onset in adolescence and young adulthood.
- Bimodal pattern in patients 15–25 and 50–80 years of age.
- Genetics: ↑ concordance with monozygotic twins versus dizygotic (↑ for Crohn versus UC).

SIGNS AND SYMPTOMS (TABLE 11-1)

- Crampy abdominal pain.
- Extraintestinal manifestations greater in Crohn than UC.
- Crohn: Perianal fistula, sclerosing cholangitis, chronic active hepatitis, pyoderma gangrenosum, ankylosing spondylitis, erythema nodosum.
- UC: Bloody diarrhea, anorexia, weight loss, pyoderma gangrenosum, sclerosing cholangitis, marked by flare-ups.

TREATMENT

- Crohn disease: Corticosteroids, aminosalicylates, methotrexate, azathioprine, cyclosporine, metronidazole (for perianal disease), sitz baths, anti–tumor necrosis factor-α, surgery for complications.
- UC: Aminosalicylates, oral corticosteroids, colectomy.

TABLE 11-1. Crohn Disease versus Ulcerative Colitis

FEATURE	CROHN DISEASE	ULCERATIVE COLITIS (UC)
Depth of involvement	Transmural	Mucosal
Ileal involvement	Common	Unusual
Ulcers	Common	Unusual
Cancer risk	↓	↑
Pyoderma gangrenosum	Slightly ↑	Greatly ↑
Skip lesions	Common	Unusual
Fistula	Common	Unusual
Rectal bleeding	Sometimes	Common

DEFINITION

Abdominal pain associated with intermittent diarrhea and constipation without organic basis; ~10% in adolescents.

SIGNS AND SYMPTOMS

- Abdominal pain.
- Diarrhea alternating with constipation.

DIAGNOSIS

- Difficult to make, exclude other pathology.
- Obtain CBC, ESR, stool occult blood.

TREATMENT

- None specific.
- Supportive with reinforcement and reassurance.
- Address any underlying psychosocial stressors.

ACUTE GASTROENTERITIS AND DIARRHEA

DEFINITION

- **Diarrhea** is the excessive loss of fluid and electrolytes in stool, usually secondary to disturbed intestinal solute transport. Technically limited to lower GI tract.
- **Gastroenteritis** is an inflammation of the entire (upper and lower) GI tract, and thus involves both vomiting and diarrhea.

EPIDEMIOLOGY

- ↑ susceptibility seen in young age, immunodeficiency, malnutrition, travel, lack of breast-feeding, and contaminated food or water.
- Most common cause of diarrhea in children is viral: (1) rotavirus, (2) enteric adenovirus, (3) Norwalk virus.
- Bacterial: (1) *Campylobacter,* (2) *Salmonella* and *Shigella* species and enterohemorrhagic *Escherichia coli.*
- Children in developing countries often also get infected by bacterial and parasitic pathogens:
  - Enterotoxigenic *E coli* number one in developing countries.
  - Parasitic causes: (1) *Giardia* and (2) *Cryptosporidium.*

SIGNS AND SYMPTOMS

- Important to obtain information regarding frequency and volume.
- General patient appearance important (well appearing versus ill appearing).
- Associated findings include cramps, emesis, malaise, and fever.
- May see systemic manifestations, GI tract involvement, or extraintestinal infections.
- Extraintestinal findings include vulvovaginitis, urinary tract infection (UTI), and keratoconjunctivitis.
- Systemic manifestations: Fever, malaise, and seizures.
- Inflammatory diarrhea: Fever, severe abdominal pain, tenesmus. May have blood/mucus in stool.

> Acute diarrhea is usually caused by infectious agents, whereas chronic persistent diarrhea may be secondary to infectious agents, infection of immunocompromised host, or residual symptoms due to intestinal damage.

- Noninflammatory diarrhea: Emesis, fever usually absent, crampy abdominal pain, watery diarrhea.

DIAGNOSIS

- Examine stool for mucus, blood, and leukocytes (colitis).
- Fecal leukocyte: Presence of invasive cytotoxin organisms (*Shigella*, *Salmonella*).
- Patients with enterohemorrhagic *E coli* and *Entamoeba histolytica*: Minimal to no fecal leukocytes.
- Obtain stool cultures early.
- *Clostridium difficile* toxins: Test if recent antibiotic use.
- Proctosigmoidoscopy: Diagnosis of inflammatory enteritis.

TREATMENT

- Rehydration.
- Oral electrolyte solutions (eg, Pedialyte®).
- Oral hydration for all but severely dehydrated (IV hydration).
- Rapid rehydration with replacement of ongoing losses during first 4–6 hours.
- Do not use soda, fruit juices, gelatin, or tea. High osmolality may exacerbate diarrhea.
- Start food with BRAT diet.
- Antidiarrheal compounds are not indicated for use in children.
- See Table 11-2 for antibiotic treatment of enteropathogens (wait for diagnosis via stool culture, empiric antibiotics generally not indicated).

PREVENTION

- Hospitalized patients should be placed under contact precautions (hand washing, gloves, gowns, etc.).

- Diarrhea and emesis — noninflammatory
- Diarrhea and fever — inflammatory process
- Diarrhea and tenesmus — large colon involvement

Diarrhea is a characteristic finding in children poisoned with bacterial toxin of *Escherichia coli, Salmonella, Staphylococcus aureus,* and *Vibrio parahemolyticus,* but not *Clostridium botulinum.*

BRAT Diet for Diarrhea
Bananas
Rice
Applesauce
Toast

TABLE 11-2. Antimicrobial Treatment for Bacterial Enteropathogens

BACTERIA	TREATMENT	COMMENTS
Aeromonas	Trimethoprim-sulfamethoxazole (TMP-SMZ)	Prolonged diarrhea
Campylobacter	Erythromycin	Early in course of illness
Clostridium difficile	Metronidazole or vancomycin	Moderate to severe diagnosis
Escherichia coli		
Enterotoxigenic	TMP-SMZ	Severe or prolonged illness
Enteropathogenic	TMP-SMZ	Nursery epidemics
Enteroinvasive	TMP-SMZ	All cases
Salmonella	Ampicillin or chloramphenicol or TMP-SMZ	Infants < 3 months, immunodeficient patients, bacteremia
Shigella	TMP-SMZ, ceftriaxone	All susceptible organisms
Vibrio cholerae	Tetracycline or doxycycline	All cases

- Education.
- Exclude infected children from child care centers.
- Report cases of bacterial diarrhea to local health department.
- Vaccines for cholera and *Salmonella typhi* are available.

INTESTINAL WORMS

See Table 11-3 for common intestinal worm infestations.

TABLE 11-3. Common Intestinal Worms

Intestinal Nematodes	Mode of Transmission	Disease, Symptoms and Signs	Treatment
Enterobius vermicularis (pinworm)	Hand to mouth	Perianal itching, especially at night	Albendazole or mebendazole or pyrantel pamoate 11 mg/kg (max. dose, 1 g PO × 1)
Trichuris trichuria (whipworm)	Fecal-oral	▪ Usually asymptomatic ▪ Mild anemia ▪ Abdominal pain ▪ Diarrhea, tenesmus ▪ Perianal itching	Albendazole or mebendazole
Ascaris lumbricoides	Fecal-oral	▪ Pneumonia ▪ Loeffler pneumonitis ▪ Intestinal infection/obstruction ▪ Liver failure	Albendazole or mebendazole
Necator americanus (New World hookworm) and *Ancylostoma duodenale* (Old World hookworm)	Skin penetration	▪ Intense dermatitis ▪ Loeffler pneumonitis ▪ Significant anemia ▪ GI symptoms ▪ Developmental delay in children (irreversible)	Albendazole or mebendazole
Strongyloides stercoralis	Skin penetration	Same as for *Necator*, plus: ▪ Diarrhea × 3–6 weeks ▪ Superimposed bacterial sepsis	Ivermectin 200 μg/kg/day × 2 days
Trichinella spiralis	Infected pork	Trichinosis ▪ Myalgias ▪ Facial and periorbital edema ▪ Conjunctivitis ▪ Pneumonia, myocarditis, encephalitis, nephritis, meningitis	Albendazole 400 mg PO bid × 14 days + prednisone 40–60 mg PO qd

Usual albendazole dose is 400 mg PO × 1; usual mebendazole dose is 100 mg PO × 1 for 3 days.

(Adapted, with permission, from Stead L. *BRS Emergency Medicine.* Lippincott Williams & Wilkins, 2000.)

HIGH-YIELD FACTS

GASTROINTESTINAL DISEASE

DEFINITION

- Major cause of iatrogenic diarrhea.
- Rarely occurs without antecedent antibiotics (usually) penicillins, cephalosporins, or clindamycin.
- Antibiotic disrupts normal bowel flora and predisposes to *C difficile* diarrhea.
- Stool should be tested for *C difficile* toxins if there is a recent history of antibiotic use.

SIGNS AND SYMPTOMS

Classically, blood and mucus with fever, cramps, abdominal pain, nausea, and vomiting days or weeks after antibiotics.

DIAGNOSIS

- Recent history of antibiotic use. *clinda/ampacilin*
- *C difficile* toxin in stool of patient with diarrhea.
- Sigmoidoscopy or colonoscopy.

TREATMENT

- Discontinue antibiotics.
- Oral metronidazole or vancomycin × 7–10 days.

Umbilical

DEFINITION

- Occurs because of imperfect closure of umbilical ring.
- Common in low-birth-weight, female, and African-American infants.
- Soft swelling covered by skin that protrudes while crying, straining, or coughing.
- Omentum or portions of small intestine involved.
- Usually 1–5 cm.

TREATMENT

- Most disappear spontaneously by 1 year of age.
- Strangulation rare.
- "Strapping" ineffective. *wnet...*
- Surgery not indicated unless symptomatic, strangulated, or grows larger after age 1 or 2.

Inguinal

DEFINITION

- Most common diagnosis requiring surgery.
- Occurs in 10–20/1,000 live births (50% < 1 year).
- Indirect > direct (rare) > femoral (even more rare).
- Indirect secondary to patent processus vaginalis.

Direct: in triangl
Indirect: patent
process
vaginalis

> The most frequent symptom of infestation with *Enterobius vermicularis* is perineal pruritus. Can diagnose with transparent adhesive tape to area (worms stick).

> In inguinal hernia, processus vaginalis herniates through abdominal wall with hydrocele into canal.

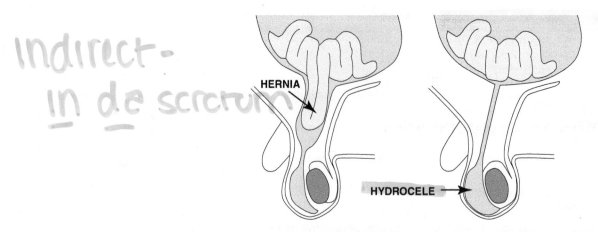

FIGURE 11-9. Inguinal hernia (slippage of bowel through inguinal ring) vs. hydrocele (collection of fluid in scrotum adjacent to testes).

- ↑ incidence with positive family history.
- Embryology: Patent processus vaginalis.
- Incidence: 1–5%.
- Males > females 8–10:1.
- Preemies: 20% males, 2% females.
- Premature infants have ↑ risk for inguinal hernia.
- Sixty percent right (delayed descent of the right testicle), 30% left, 10% bilateral.

SIGNS AND SYMPTOMS

- Infant with scrotal/inguinal bulge on straining or crying.
- Do careful exam to distinguish from hydrocele (see Figure 11-9).
- Bulge in groin ± scrotum, incarceration.

TREATMENT

- Surgery (elective).
- Avoid trusses or supports.
- Contralateral hernia occurs in 30% after unilateral repair.
- Antibiotics only in at-risk children (eg, congenital heart disease).
- Prognosis excellent (recurrence < 1%, complication rate approximately 2%, infection approximately 1%).
- Complications include incarceration.
- Therapy: Incarceration—sedation and manipulation 90–95% reduced. Immediate operation if not reduced. Repair soon after diagnosis especially infants since 60% progress to incarceration by 6 months.

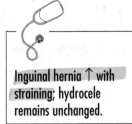

Inguinal hernia ↑ with straining; hydrocele remains unchanged.

PEUTZ-JEGHERS SYNDROME

A 15-year-old girl with spots on her lips has some crampy abdominal pain associated with bleeding. *Think: Peutz-Jeghers syndrome.*

Peutz-Jeghers syndrome is multiple GI hamartomatous polyps + mucocutaneous hyperpigmentation. There is a higher risk of intestinal and extraintestinal malignancies.

DEFINITION

- Mucosal pigmentation of lips and gums with hamartomas of stomach, small intestine, and colon.
- Rare; low malignant potential.

SIGNS AND SYMPTOMS

- Deeply pigmented freckles on lips and buccal mucosa at birth.
- Bleeding and crampy abdominal pain.

DIAGNOSIS

Genetic and family studies may reveal history.

TREATMENT

Excise intestinal lesions if significantly symptomatic.

GARDNER SYNDROME

DEFINITION

Multiple intestinal polyps, tumors of soft tissue and bone (especially mandible).

SIGNS AND SYMPTOMS

- Dental abnormalities.
- Pigmented lesions in ocular fundus.
- Intestinal polyps (usually early adulthood) with high malignant potential.

DIAGNOSIS

- Genetic counseling.
- Colon surveillance in at-risk children.

TREATMENT

Aggressive surgical removal of polyps.

CARCINOID TUMORS

DEFINITION

Tumors of enterochromaffin cells in intestine—usually appendix.

SIGNS AND SYMPTOMS

- May cause appendicitis.
- May cause carcinoid syndrome ($\uparrow$ serotonin, vasomotor disturbances, or bronchoconstriction) if metastatic to the liver.

TREATMENT

Surgical excision.

DEFINITION/ETIOLOGY

- Autosomal dominant.
- Large number of adenomatous lesions in colon.
- Secondary to germ-line mutations in adenopolyposis coli (APC) gene.

SIGNS AND SYMPTOMS

- Highly variable.
- May see hematochezia, cramps, or diarrhea.
- Extracolonic manifestations possible.

DIAGNOSIS

- Consider family history (strong).
- Colonoscopy with biopsy (screening annually after 10 years old if positive family history).

TREATMENT

Surgical resection of affected colonic mucosa.

DEFINITION

- Most common childhood bowel tumor (3–4% of patients < 21 years).
- Characteristically, mucus-filled cystic glands (no adenomatous changes, no potential for malignancy).

EPIDEMIOLOGY

Most commonly between 2 and 10 years; less common after 15 years; rarely before 1 year.

SIGNS AND SYMPTOMS

- Bright red painless bleeding with bowel movement.
- Iron deficiency.

DIAGNOSIS

- Colonoscopy.
- May use barium enema (not best test).

TREATMENT

Surgical removal of polyp.

Short Bowel Syndrome

DEFINITION

- Occurs with loss of at least 50% of small bowel (with or without loss of large bowel).
- ↓ absorptive surface and bowel function.

ETIOLOGY

- May be congenital (malrotation, atresia, etc.).
- Most commonly secondary to surgical resection.

SIGNS AND SYMPTOMS

- Malabsorption and diarrhea.
- Steatorrhea (fatty stools): Voluminous foul-smelling stools that float.
- Dehydration.
- ↓ sodium and potassium.
- Acidosis (secondary to loss of bicarbonate).

TREATMENT

- Total parenteral nutrition (TPN).
- Give small feeds orally.
- Metronidazole empirically to treat bacterial overgrowth.

Celiac Disease

A 5-year-old girl presents with a protuberant abdomen and wasted extremities. *Think: Gluten-induced enteropathy,*

Celiac disease is an autoimmune disorder. The disease primarily affects the small intestine. Gluten is the single major factor that triggers celiac disease. *Gluten-containing foods include* rye, wheat, and barley. Common presentation: diarrhea, borborygmus, abdominal pain, and weight loss. Other systems, including skin, liver, nervous system, bones, reproductive system, and endocrine system, may also be affected. *Serologic marker:* Serum immunoglobulin A (IgA) endomysial antibodies and IgA tissue transglutaminase (tTG) antibodies.

DEFINITION

- Sensitivity to gluten in diet.
- Most commonly occurs between 6 months and 2 years.

ETIOLOGY

- Factors involved include cereals, genetic predisposition, and environmental factors.
- Associated with HLA-B8, -DR7, -DR3, and -DQW2.

SIGNS AND SYMPTOMS

- Diarrhea
- Failure to thrive
- Vomiting
- Pallor
- Abdominal distention
- Large bulky stools

DIAGNOSIS

- Anti-endomysial and anti-tissue transglutaminase antibodies (check total lgH level at the same time).
- Biopsy: Most reliable test.

TREATMENT

- Dietary restriction of gluten (**must** avoid barley, ryes, oats and wheat).
- Corticosteroids used rarely (very ill patients with profound malnutrition, diarrhea, edema, and hypokalemia).

Tropical Sprue

DEFINITION

- Generalized malabsorption associated with diffuse lesions of small bowel mucosa.
- Seen in people who live or have traveled to certain tropical regions—some Caribbean countries, South America, Africa, or parts of Asia.

SIGNS AND SYMPTOMS

- Fever, malaise, and watery diarrhea, acutely.
- After 1 week, chronic malabsorption and signs of malnutrition including night blindness, glossitis, stomatitis, cheilosis, muscle wasting.

DIAGNOSIS

Biopsy shows villous shortening, ↑ crypt depth, and ↑ chronic inflammatory cells in lamina propria of small bowel.

TREATMENT

- Antibiotics × 3–4 weeks.
- Folate.
- Vitamin B_{12}.
- Prognosis excellent.

Lactase Deficiency

DEFINITION

↓ or absent enzyme that breaks down lactose in the intestinal brush border.

ETIOLOGY

- Congenital absence reported in few cases.
- Usual mechanism relates to developmental pattern of lactase activity.
- Autosomal recessive.
- Also ↓ because of diffuse mucosal disease (can occur post viral gastroenteritis).

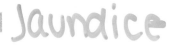

SIGNS AND SYMPTOMS

- Seen in response to ingestion of lactose (found in dairy products).
- Explosive watery diarrhea with abdominal distention, borborygmi, and flatulence.
- Recurrent, vague abdominal pain.
- Episodic midabdominal pain (may or may not be related to milk intake).

TREATMENT

- Eliminate milk from diet.
- Oral lactase supplement (Lactaid) or lactose-free milk.
- Yogurt (with lactase enzyme–producing bacteria tolerable in such patients).

HYPERBILIRUBINEMIA

Physiology: See Gestation and Birth chapter.

DEFINITION

Elevated serum bilirubin.

EPIDEMIOLOGY

- Common and in most cases benign.
- If untreated, severe indirect hyperbilirubinemia neurotoxic (kernicterus).
- Jaundice in first week of life in 60% of term and 80% of preterm infants—results from accumulation of unconjugated bilirubin pigment.

SIGNS AND SYMPTOMS

- Jaundice at birth or in neonatal period.
- May be lethargic and feed poorly.

DIAGNOSIS

- Direct and indirect bilirubin fractions.
- Hemoglobin.
- Reticulocyte count.
- Blood type.
- Examine peripheral smear.

TREATMENT

- Goal is to prevent neurotoxic range.
- Phototherapy.
- Exchange transfusion.
- Treat underlying cause.

Gilbert Syndrome

Benign condition caused by missense mutation in transferase gene resulting in low enzyme levels with unconjugated hyperbilirubinemia.

- Indirect hyperbilirubinemia, reticulosis, and red cell destruction suggest hemolysis.
- Direct hyperbilirubinemia may indicate hepatitis, cholestasis, inborn errors of metabolism, cystic fibrosis, or sepsis.
- If reticulocyte count, Coombs', and direct bilirubin are normal, then physiologic or pathologic indirect hyperbilirubinemia is suggested.

Children with cholestatic hepatic disease need replacement of vitamins A, D, E, and K (fat soluble).

Crigler-Najjar I Syndrome

DEFINITION

- Autosomal recessive, secondary to mutations in glucuronyl transferase gene.
- Parents of affected children show partial defects but normal serum bilirubin concentration.
- Complete absence of the enzyme uridine diphosphate glycosyltransferase.
- Much rarer than Gilbert syndrome.

SIGNS AND SYMPTOMS

- In homozygous infants, will see unconjugated hyperbilirubinemia in first 3 days of life.
- Kernicterus common in early neonatal period.
- Some treated infants survive childhood without sequelae.
- Stools pale yellow.
- Persistence of ↑ levels of indirect bilirubin after first week of life in absence of hemolysis suggests this syndrome.

DIAGNOSIS

- Based on early age of onset and extreme level of bilirubin in absence of hemolysis.
- Definitive diagnosis made by measuring glucuronyl transferase activity in liver biopsy specimen.
- DNA diagnosis available.

TREATMENT

- Maintain serum bilirubin < 20 mg/dL for first 2–4 weeks of life.
- Repeated exchange transfusion.
- Phototherapy.
- Treat intercurrent infections.
- Hepatic transplant.

Crigler-Najjar II Syndrome

DEFINITION

- Autosomal dominant with variable penetrance.
- May be caused by homozygous mutation in glucuronyl transferase isoform I activity.
- ↓ enzyme uridine diphosphate glycosyltransferase.

SIGNS AND SYMPTOMS

- Unconjugated hyperbilirubinemia in first 3 days of life.
- Concentration remains ↑ after third week of life.
- Kernicterus unusual.
- Stool normal.
- Infants asymptomatic.

DIAGNOSIS

- Concentration of bilirubin nearly normal.
- ↓ bilirubin after 7- to 10-day treatment with phenobarbital may be diagnostic.

TREATMENT

Phenobarbital for 7–10 days.

Alagille Syndrome

DEFINITION

- Absence or reduction in number of bile ducts.
- Results from progressive destruction of the ducts.

SIGNS AND SYMPTOMS

- Variably expressed.
- Unusual facies (broad forehead, wide-set eyes, underdeveloped mandible).
- Ocular abnormalities.
- Cardiovascular abnormalities (peripheral pulmonic stenosis).
- Tubulointerstitial nephropathy.
- Vertebral defect.

PROGNOSIS

Long-term survival good but may have pruritis, xanthomas, and ↑ cholesterol and neurologic complications.

Zellweger Syndrome

DEFINITION

- Rare autosomal-recessive condition causing progressive degeneration of liver and kidneys.
- Occurs in 1 in 100,000 births.

SIGNS AND SYMPTOMS

- Usually fatal within 6–12 months.
- Severe generalized hypotonia.
- Impaired neurologic function with psychomotor retardation.
- Abnormal head and unusual facies.
- Hepatomegaly.
- Renal cortical cysts.
- Ocular abnormalities.
- Congenital diaphragmatic hernia.

DIAGNOSIS

- Absence of peroxisomes in hepatic cells (on biopsy).
- Genetic testing available.

Extrahepatic Biliary Atresia

DEFINITION

Distal segmental bile duct obliteration with patent extrahepatic ducts up to porta hepatis.

EPIDEMIOLOGY

- Most common form (85%): Obliteration of entire extrahepatic biliary tree at/above porta.
- Occurs in 1 in 10,000 to 1 in 15,000 live births.

SIGNS AND SYMPTOMS

- Acholic stools (stools are very light in color, almost beige).
- ↑ incidence of polysplenia syndrome with heterotaxia, malrotation, levocardia, and intra-abdominal vascular anomalies.

DIAGNOSIS

- Ultrasound.
- Hepatobiliary scintigraphy.
- Liver biopsy.

TREATMENT

- Exploratory laparotomy and direct cholangiography to determine presence and site of obstruction.
- Direct drainage if lesion is correctable.
- Surgery if lesion is not correctable (liver transplant, Kasai procedure).

HEPATITIS

- Continues to be major problem worldwide.
- Six known viruses cause hepatitis as their primary manifestation—A (HAV), B (HBV), C (HCV), D (HDV), E (HEV), and G (HGV).
- Many others cause hepatitis as part of their clinical spectrum—herpes simplex virus (HSV), cytomegalovirus (CMV), Epstein-Barr virus (EBV), rubella, enteroviruses, parvovirus.
- HBV is a DNA virus, whereas HAV, HCV, HDV, HEV, and HGV are RNA viruses.
- HAV and HEV are not known to cause chronic illness, but HBV, HCV, and HDV cause important morbidity and mortality through chronic infection.
- HAV causes most cases of hepatitis in children.
- HBV causes one-third of all cases; HCV found in 20%.

Hepatitis A
MC

DEFINITION

- RNA-containing member of the Picornavirus family.
- Found mostly in developing countries.
- Causes acute hepatitis only.
- Two thirds of children are asymptomatic.
- Transmission by person-to-person contact; spread by fecal-oral route.
- Percutaneous transmission rare, maternal-neonatal not recognized.
- ↑ risk in child care centers, contaminated food or water, or travel to endemic areas.
- Mean incubation 4 weeks (15–50 days).

SIGNS AND SYMPTOMS

- Abrupt onset with fever, malaise, nausea, emesis, anorexia, and abdominal discomfort.
- Diarrhea common.
- Almost all recover but may have relapsing course over several months.
- Jaundice.

DIAGNOSIS

- Consider when history of jaundice in family contacts or child care playmates or travel history to endemic region.
- Serologic criteria:
  - Immunoglobulin M (IgM) anti-HAV present at onset of illness and disappears within 4 months. May persist for > 6 months (acute infection). IgG is detectable at this point.
  - ↑ alanine transaminase (ALT), aspartate transaminase (AST), bilirubin, and gamma-glutamyl transpeptidase (GGT).

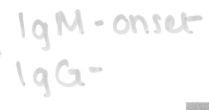

IgM - onset
IgG -

TREATMENT

- Careful hand washing.
- Vaccines available (preferred over immunoglobulin in children > 2 years).

Hepatitis B

DEFINITION

- DNA virus from the Hepadnaviridae family.
- Most important risk factor for infants is perinatal exposure to hepatitis B surface antigen (HbsAg)-positive mother.

SIGNS AND SYMPTOMS

- Many cases asymptomatic.
- ↑ ALT prior to lethargy, anorexia, and malaise (6–7 weeks post exposure).
- May be preceded by arthralgias or skin lesions and rashes.
- May see extrahepatic conditions, polyarteritis, glomerulonephritis, aplastic anemia.
- Jaundice: Icteric skin and mucous membranes.
- Hepatosplenomegaly and lymphadenopathy common.

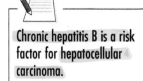

Chronic hepatitis B is a risk factor for **hepatocellular carcinoma.**

DIAGNOSIS

- Routine screening requires assay of two serologic markers: HbsAg (all infected persons, ↑ when symptomatic) and hepatitis B core antigen (HbcAg) (present during acute phase, highly infectious state).
- HbsAg falls prior to symptom resolution; IgMAb to HbcAg also required because it is ↑ early after infectivity and persists for several months before being replaced by immunoglobulin G (IgG) anti-HbcAg.
- HbcAg most valuable; it is present as early as HbsAg and continues to be present later when HBsAg disappears.
- Only anti-HbsAg detected in persons immunized with hepatitis B vaccine, whereas anti-HbsAb and anti-HbcAg are seen in persons with resolved infection.

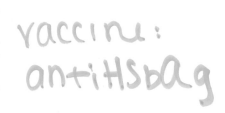

vaccine:
antiHsbAg

PREVENTION

- Screening blood donors.
- Screening pregnant women to prevent vertical transmission.

TREATMENT

- No available medical treatment effective in majority of cases.
- Interferon-α is approved treatment in children.
- Liver transplant for patients with end-stage HBV.

Hepatitis C

DEFINITION

- Single-stranded RNA virus.
- Perinatal transmission described but uncommon except with high-titer HCV.

SIGNS AND SYMPTOMS

- Acute infection similar to other hepatitis viruses.
- Mild and insidious onset.
- Fulminant liver failure rare.
- After 20–30 years, 25% progress to cirrhosis, liver failure, or primary hepatocellular carcinoma.
- May see cryoglobulinemia, vasculitides, and peripheral neuropathy (extrahepatic).

DIAGNOSIS

- Detection of antibodies to HCV or direct testing for RNA virus.
- Polymerase chain reaction (PCR) detection possible.
- ↑ ALT.
- Confirmed by liver biopsy.

TREATMENT

- Treat to prevent progression to future complications.
- INF-α_{2b} for patients with compensated liver disease (response rate long term ~25%).
- May use with ribavirin for higher frequency of sustained response.

Hepatitis D (Delta Agent)

DEFINITION

- Smallest known animal virus.
- Cannot produce infection without HBV infection (coinfective or superinfection).
- Transmission by intimate contact.

SIGNS AND SYMPTOMS

- Similar to but more severe than other hepatitis viruses.
- In coinfection, acute hepatitis is more severe, risk of developing chronic hepatitis low; in superinfection, risk of fulminant hepatitis is highest.

DIAGNOSIS

Detect IgM antibody to HDV (2–4 weeks after coinfection, 1 week after superinfection).

PREVENTION

No vaccine for hepatitis D, but can minimize against hepatitis B (needs hepatitis B to infect).

Hepatitis E

DEFINITION

- RNA virus with nonenveloped sphere shape with spikes (similar to caliciviruses).
- Non-A, non-B hepatitis.

SIGNS AND SYMPTOMS

- Similar to HAV, but more severe.
- No chronic illness.
- High prevalence of fulminant hepatic failure and death in pregnant women.

DIAGNOSIS

- Antibody to HEV exists.
- IgM and IgG assays available.
- Can detect viral RNA in stool and serum by PCR.

PREVENTION

No vaccines available.

Hepatitis G

DEFINITION

- Single-stranded RNA virus of Flaviviridae family.
- Virus not yet isolated.
- Reported in all population groups in ~1.5% U.S. blood donors.
- One percent transmission through transfusions but also by organ transplant.
- Vertical transmission occurs.

SIGNS AND SYMPTOMS

- Symptoms associated with hepatic inflammation.
- Coinfection does not worsen course of HBV or HCV.

DIAGNOSIS

Only PCR assays available for testing.

TREATMENT

No method available.

Neonatal Hepatitis

DEFINITION

- Hepatic inflammation of unknown etiology.
- Most result from systemic disease (eg, sepsis).
- Also caused by CMV, HSV, human immunodeficiency virus (HIV).
- Nonviral causes include congenital syphilis and toxoplasmosis.
- HBV results in asymptomatic infection.

SIGNS AND SYMPTOMS

- Jaundice.
- Vomiting.
- Poor feeding.
- ↑ liver enzyme levels.
- Fulminant hepatitis.

TREATMENT

- Antibiotics for bacteria-associated hepatitis.
- Acyclovir for HSV.
- Ganciclovir and foscarnet for CMV.

Autoimmune (Chronic) Hepatitis

DEFINITION

- Hepatic inflammatory process manifested by ↑ serum aminotransferase and liver-associated autoantibodies.
- Variable severity.
- Fifteen to twenty percent of cases associated with HBV.
- Clinical constellation that suggests immune-mediated disease process responsive to immunosuppressive treatment.

SIGNS AND SYMPTOMS

- Variable.
- May mimic acute viral hepatitis.
- Onset insidious.
- May be asymptomatic or may have fatigue, malaise, anorexia, or amenorrhea.
- Extrahepatic signs include arthritis, vasculitis, and nephritis.
- Mild to moderate jaundice.

DIAGNOSIS

- Detection of autoantibodies (anti-smooth muscle, anti-liver-kidney-microsome, anti-soluble live antigen).
- Liver biopsy.
- Exclude other disease.

TREATMENT

- Corticosteroid
- Azathioprine

DEFINITION

- Acute encephalopathy and fatty degeneration.
- Hepatic dysfunction (> 3-fold ↑ in ALT, AST, and/or ammonia levels).
- No other explanation for cerebral edema or hepatic abnormality.
- ↓ incidence secondary to awareness about association with the use of aspirin during the illness relation to acetylsalicylic acid (ASA) ingestion.
- Many other "Reye-like" syndromes exist (medium-chain fatty-acid oxidation defect or urea-cycle defects).

SIGNS AND SYMPTOMS

- Stereotypic, biphasic course.
- Usually see prodromal illness, upper respiratory infection (URI), influenza, or varicella chickenpox initially, followed by a period of apparent recovery, then see abrupt onset of protracted vomiting 5–7 days after illness onset.
- May see delirium, combative behavior, and stupor.
- First neurologic manifestation: Lethargy.
- Neurologic symptoms including seizures, coma, or death.
- Slight to moderate liver enlargement.

DIAGNOSIS

- Based on clinical staging.
- Liver biopsy may show yellow to white color because of high triglyceride content.

TREATMENT

- Airway, breathing, circulation (ABC) is the priority.
- Bedside glucose (provide dextrose to manage hypoglycemia).
- No specific treatment.
- Control intracranial pressure (ICP) secondary to cerebral edema.
- Supportive management depending on clinical stage.

DEFINITION

- α_1-Antitrypsin is a major protease inhibitor (PI).
- A small percentage of homozygous patients have neonatal cholestasis, and later in childhood cirrhosis.
- Present in > 20 codominant alleles; only a few associated with defective PI.
- PI ZZ usually predisposes to clinical deficiency (< 20% develop neonatal cholestasis).

The most likely clinical manifestation of α_1-antitrypsin deficiency in the newborn is jaundice (neonatal cholestasis).

SIGNS AND SYMPTOMS

- Variable course.
- Jaundice, acholic stools, and hepatomegaly in first week of life; jaundice clears by second to fourth month.
- May have complete resolution, persistent liver disease, or cirrhosis.
- Older children may present with chronic liver disease.

DIAGNOSIS

- Determination of α_1-antitrypsin phenotype.
- Confirmed by liver biopsy.

TREATMENT

- Liver transplant curative.
- No other effective treatment.

WILSON DISEASE

DEFINITION

- Autosomal-recessive disease characterized by excessive copper deposition in brain and liver.
- Worldwide incidence: 1/30,000.

SIGNS AND SYMPTOMS

- Variable manifestations, including:
  - Asymptomatic in early stages.
  - Jaundice, abdominal pain.
  - Hepatomegaly, subacute/chronic hepatitis or fulminant liver failure.
  - Portal hypertension, ascites, edema, esophageal bleeding.
  - Delayed puberty, amenorrhea, or coagulation defect.
  - Psychosis.
  - Tremors.
- Kayser-Fleischer rings are greenish-brown rings of pigment seen at the limbus of the cornea, reflecting deposits of copper in Descemet membrane. They can be seen with the naked eye in patients with blue eyes. In patients with dark eyes, a slit lamp is often needed to identify them. Ninety percent of patients with Wilson disease have Kayser-Fleischer rings.

Consider ordering serum ceruloplasmin for any patient with an unexplained elevation of liver function tests (LFTs).

DIAGNOSIS

Copper indices reveal:

- Low serum ceruloplasmin.
- High serum copper level.
- Liver biopsy for histochemistry and copper quantification.
- Genetic testing, including siblings.

TREATMENT

- Disease is always fatal if left untreated.
- Zinc: Newest Food and Drug Administration (FDA)-approved agent; works by blocking absorption of copper in GI tract.
- Copper-chelating agents to ↓ deposition (eg, penicillamine and trientine).
- Restrict copper intake. Foods high in copper include (Source: *Mayo Clinic Diet Manual*):
  - Lamb, pork, pheasant, quail, duck, goose, squid, salmon, all organ meats (liver, heart, kidney, brain), all shellfish (oysters, scallops, shrimp, lobster, clams, crab), meat gelatin, soy protein meat substitutes, tofu, all nuts and seeds, dried beans (soybeans, lima beans, baked beans, garbanzo beans, pinto beans), dried peas, and lentils.

- Soy milk, chocolate milk, cocoa, chocolate.
- Nectarines, commercially dried fruits (okay if dried at home).
- Mushrooms, sweet potatoes, vegetable juice cocktail.
- Barley, bran breads and bran cereals, cereals with > 0.2 mg of copper per serving (check label), millet, soy flour, soy grits, wheat germ, brewer's yeast.
- Patients with hepatic failure require liver transplant.

Hepatoblastoma

DEFINITION

- Rare in children.
- Fewer than 65% of malignant tumors are hepatoblastomas.
- Associated with Beckwith-Wiedemann syndrome.
- Usually arises from the right lobe of the liver and is unifocal.
- Two histologic types—epithelial and mixed.

SIGNS AND SYMPTOMS

- Generally present in first 18 months of life.
- Large, asymptomatic abdominal mass.
- Abdominal distention and ↑ liver size.
- Weight loss, anorexia, vomiting, and abdominal pain (as disease progresses).
- May spread to regional lymph nodes.

DIAGNOSIS

- α-Fetoprotein (AFP) level helpful as marker.
- Diagnostic imaging includes ultrasound to detect mass, CT, or magnetic resonance imaging (MRI).

TREATMENT

- Complete resection of tumor.
- Cisplatin and doxorubicin adjuvant chemotherapy.
- More than 90% survival with multimodal treatment (surgery with chemotherapy).

Echinococcus

DEFINITION

- Most widespread cestode.
- Transmitted from domestic and wild canine animals.
- Two species: *Echinococcus granulosus* and the more malignant *Echinococcus multilocularis*.
- Hosts are dogs, wolves, coyotes, and foxes that eat infected viscera.
- Humans are infected by ingesting contaminated food or water.

SIGNS AND SYMPTOMS

- Majority of cysts in liver; most never symptomatic.
- Early, nonspecific symptoms; later on, ↑ abdominal girth, hepatomegaly, vomiting, or abdominal pain.
- Anaphylaxis secondary to rupture and spillage of contents.
- Second most common site is lungs; symptoms include chest pain and coughing or hemoptysis.

DIAGNOSIS

- Clinical.
- Ultrasound.
- Serologic studies have high false-negative rate.

TREATMENT

- Surgery.
- May be CT guided.
- If not amenable to surgery, may be treated with albendazole.

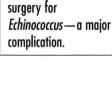

Avoid spillage during surgery for *Echinococcus*—a major complication.

Amebic Abscess

DEFINITION

A very serious manifestation of disseminated infection.

SIGNS AND SYMPTOMS

Abdominal pain, distention, and liver enlargement with tenderness.

DIAGNOSIS

- May see slight leukocytosis.
- Moderate anemia.
- ↑ ESR.
- Nonspecific ALT ↑.
- Stool exam negative in > 50% of patients.
- CT or MRI.

TREATMENT

- Metronidazole.
- Chloroquine.
- Aspiration of left lobe abscesses if rupture is imminent.

Respiratory Disease

TABLE 12-1. Normal Respiratory Rates in Children

Age	Birth–6 Weeks	6 Weeks–2 Years	2–6 Years	6–10 Years	Over 10 Years
Respiratory Rate	45–60/min	40/min	30/min	25/min	20/min

RESPIRATORY DISTRESS

A common reason to visit emergency department (10% of ED visits).

- Intercostal retractions.
- Nasal flaring (indicates ↑ effort is needed to breathe).
- Use of accessory muscles for breathing (eg, abdominals, sternocleido-mastoids).
- Restlessness, agitation.
- Somnolence or lethargy may be due to severe hypoxia or hypercarbia.
- Pallor, cyanosis.
- Wheezing may or may not be present.
- **Stridor** is an inspiratory sound that localizes respiratory distress to the upper airway
- **Grunting:**
  - Due to exhalation against a partially closed glottis.
  - Occurs during expiration.
  - Indicates moderate to severe hypoxia.
- See Table 12-1 for normal respiratory rates by age.

COMMON COLD (UPPER RESPIRATORY INFECTION, NASOPHARYNGITIS)

 A 7-year-old girl is well when she leaves for school, but arrives home afterwards with a sore throat and runny nose. She is also complaining of cough, sneezing, and facial heaviness. *Think: Rhinovirus.* Rhinovirus colds frequently start as a sore or "scratchy" throat with runny nose.

A 17-year-old adolescent has acute onset of fever, cough, conjunctivitis, and pharyngitis. *Think: Adenovirus.* Characteristic presentation: Pharyngitis, rhinitis, and conjunctivitis. Conjunctivitis is typically follicular.

DEFINITION

Multi-etiology illness with a constellation of symptoms including cough, congestion, and rhinorrhea. Upper respiratory infections (URIs) are the most common pediatric ED presentation.

ETIOLOGY

- > **200 viruses**—especially rhinoviruses (one-third), parainfluenza, respiratory syncytial virus (RSV), adenovirus.

- Risk factors: Child care facilities, smoking, passive exposure to smoke, low income, crowding, and psychological stress.

EPIDEMIOLOGY

- Most frequent illness of childhood (three to eight episodes per year).
- Most common medical reason to miss school.
- Occurs in fall and winter especially.

SIGNS AND SYMPTOMS

- Nasal and throat irritation.
- Sneezing, nasal congestion, rhinorrhea.
- Sore throat, postnasal drip.
- Low-grade fever, headache, malaise, and myalgia.
- Possible complications include otitis media, sinusitis, and trigger asthma.
- Infants have a variable presentation—feeding and sleeping are difficult due to congestion, vomiting may occur after coughing, may have diarrhea.

TREATMENT

- Supportive.
- Avoid aspirin and over-the-counter cough suppressants or decongestants.
- Direct therapy toward specific symptoms.

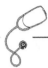

Mucopurulent rhinitis may accompany a common cold and doesn't necessarily indicate sinusitis; it is not an indication for antibiotics.

The best treatment for the common cold is to ↑ oral fluids, *not* pharmacologic treatment.

INFLUENZA

DEFINITION

Viral respiratory illness.

ETIOLOGY

- Influenza A and B—epidemic disease: H1N1 (influenza A).
- Influenza C—sporadic.

EPIDEMIOLOGY

Common over the winter months.

SIGNS AND SYMPTOMS

- Incubation period: 1–3 days.
- Sudden onset of fever, frequently with chills, headache, malaise, diffuse myalgia, and nonproductive cough.
- Conjunctivitis, pharyngitis.
- Typical duration of febrile illness is 2–4 days.
- Complications include otitis media, pneumonia, myositis, and myocarditis.
- Diarrhea and vomiting (H1N1).

DIAGNOSIS

- Nasal swab or nasal washing.
- During epidemic, clinical signs can be used to save on test costs.

Aspirin is avoided in young children due to theoretical risk of Reye syndrome.

Influenza is an orthomyxovirus.

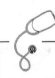

Diagnosis of influenza depends on epidemiologic and clinical consideration.

TREATMENT

- Symptomatic treatment is appropriate for healthy children—fluids, rest, acetaminophen.
- For children at risk, see Table 12-2 for drug options.
- Pregnant patients with H1N1 should receive a 5-day course of antiviral treatment.
- Oseltamivir is preferred during pregnancy.

VACCINE

tamiflu

Influenza can be severe in children with congenital heart disease, bronchopulmonary dysplasia (BPD), asthma, cystic fibrosis, and neuromuscular disease.

Intramuscular

- Now recommended for all children over age 6 months, with priority given to high-risk groups.
- High-risk groups include children with chronic diseases such as asthma, renal disease, diabetes, and any other form of immunosuppression.
- Best administered mid-September to mid-November since the peak of the flu season is late December to early March.
- Antibodies take up to 6 weeks to develop in children. Consider prophylaxis in high-risk children during this period.
- Since composition of influenza virus changes, the flu vaccine needs to be administered every year.
- Vaccine is a killed virus and therefore cannot cause the flu.
- Not approved for children < 6 months of age.

Intranasal

- Live, attenuated vaccine available for children > 5 years old.
- Not licensed for children with reactive airway disease.
- Contraindicated in immunosuppressed individuals.

TABLE 12-2. Drug Treatments for Influenza (All Pregnancy Category C)

	INDICATIONS	AGE GROUPS	RX DOSE	ADVERSE EFFECTS
Amantadine	For type A only Both prophylaxis and treatment	Age > 1 year	200 mg PO bid × 7 days	Central nervous system and gastrointestinal effects
Rimantadine	For type A only	Px: Age > 12 years	100 mg PO bid × 7 days	Same as for amantadine, but less frequent and less severe
	Both prophylaxis and treatment	Tx: Age > 1 year		
Zanamivir	For types A and B Treatment only	Age > 5 years	Two inhalations bid × 5 days	Wheezing in patients with asthma, sinusitis, nausea, diarrhea
Oseltamivir	For types A and B Treatment only	Age > 1 year	Weight based dosing × 5 days	Nausea, vomiting, diarrhea, abdominal pain, bronchitis, dizziness, headache

Tx, treatment; Px, prophylaxis.

H1N1 VACCINE

- Monovalent, inactivated influenza A virus vaccine.
- 6–35 months: 0.25 mL IM. Two doses 4 weeks apart.
- 3–9 years: 0.5 mL IM. Two doses 4 weeks apart.
- Intranasal:
  - Monovalent live virus vaccine.
  - 2–9 years: 0.2 mL/dose (0.1 mL per nostril). Two doses 4 weeks apart.

PARAINFLUENZA

ETIOLOGY

- Type 1 and 2—seasonal.
- Type 3—endemic.
- See Table 12-3.

Parainfluenza is a paramyxovirus.

SIGNS AND SYMPTOMS

- Incubation period: 2–6 days.
- Causes:
  - Colds
  - Pharyngitis
  - Otitis media
  - Croup
  - Bronchiolitis
- Can be severe in immunocompromised patients

Parainfluenza types 1 and 2 cause croup; type 3 causes bronchiolitis and pneumonia; type 4 is a cause of the common cold.

TREATMENT

Specific antiviral therapy is not available.

TABLE 12-3. Respiratory Infections and Pathogens

RESPIRATORY INFECTION	MOST COMMON PATHOGEN	PARTICULAR SIGNS AND SYMPTOMS
Croup	Parainfluenza virus	Barking cough, steeple sign
Epiglottitis	*S pneumoniae, H influenzae* type B	Tripod position, thumb sign
Tracheitis	*S aureus, H influenzae* type B	Rapidly progressive
Bronchiolitis	Respiratory syncytial virus	Paroxysmal wheezing
Bronchitis	Viral	Productive cough
Pharyngitis	Viral, group A strep	Sore throat, tonsillar involvement
Bacterial pneumonia	*S pneumoniae*	Productive cough, lobar consolidation
Pulmonary abscess	*S aureus*	Cavity with air-fluid level

Croup is the most common cause of stridor in a febrile child.

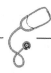

Croup is the most common infectious cause of acute upper airway obstruction.

Most common cause of stridor in children is croup.

Stridor and distress at home and calm and free of stridor in ED: Think croup.

Constant stridor and distress both at home and ED despite treatment: Think tracheitis.

Minimum observation of child brought in with croup is 3 hours.

Infectious Croup (Acute Laryngotracheobronchitis)

An 18-month-old boy with inspiratory stridor and a barking cough and agitation when lying down is brought at night to the emergency department (ED) by parents. He has had a sore throat and cough for 2 days. On examination, he has hoarseness, high-pitched barking cough, and stridor. In addition, tachypnea, retractions, and nasal flaring was noted. Steeple sign is seen on x-ray. *Think: Croup.*

DEFINITION

Viral infection of upper respiratory tract.

ETIOLOGY

Parainfluenza virus types 1 and 2.

EPIDEMIOLOGY

Occurs in children 3 months to 3 years of age in fall and winter months.

SIGNS AND SYMPTOMS

- Inspiratory stridor.
- Seal-like, barking cough with retractions and nasal flaring.
- May have coryza and fever.
- Can progress to agitation, hypoxemia, hypercapnia, tachypnea, and tachycardia.
- Most cases are mild and last 3–7 days.
- Symptoms worse at night, and typically worse on second day of illness.

DIAGNOSIS

- X-ray usually not necessary. Consider only if diagnosis is in doubt.
- Steeple sign—narrowing of tracheal air column just below the vocal cords (see Figure 12-1).
- Ballooning—distention of hypopharynx during inspiration.
- Differentiate croup from epiglottitis.

TREATMENT

- Position of comfort.
- Mild—symptomatic care, cool air, nonsteroidal anti-inflammatories (NSAIDs), consider corticosteroids.
- Moderate—racemic epinephrine (0.25 mL in 3–5 mL of normal saline [NS]), admit, early corticosteroids.
- Severe—racemic epinephrine, intensive care unit (ICU), early use of corticosteroids.
- Dexamethasone 0.6 mg/kg (lower dose [0.15 mg/kg] has also shown be effective).
- Maximum: 10 mg/dose.
- Admission criteria:
  - Persistent stridor (especially at rest).
  - Respiratory distress.

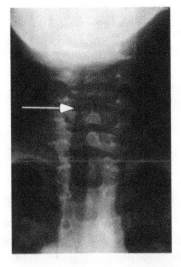

Steeple sign

FIGURE 12-1. Radiograph demonstrating steeple sign of croup.

Note narrowing of airway (arrow). (Courtesy of Dr. Gregory J. Schears.)

- Multiple doses of racemic epinephrine.
- Possibility of alternate diagnosis.

CORTICOSTEROIDS IN RESPIRATORY PROBLEMS

- Dexamethasone (IM or PO 0.6 mg/kg).
- Side effects associated with short-term steroid use are minimal.

Spasmodic Croup (Laryngismus Stridulus, Midnight Croup)

DEFINITION

- Recurrent, sudden onset of barking cough and inspiratory stridor without preceding respiratory tract infection.
- Well known to physicians but still defies definition of pathogenesis.
- Familial predisposition: Family history of allergies.

ETIOLOGY

- Probable viral etiology.
- Other considerations—allergic, psychological, gastroesophageal (GE) reflux.

EPIDEMIOLOGY

- Usually at night.
- Aggravated by excitement.
- Winter months.
- Occurs in children 1–3 years of age.

SIGNS AND SYMPTOMS

- Recurrent episodes of acute-onset barking cough and inspiratory stridor.
- No symptoms of infection.

Reconsider diagnosis of croup if child is hypoxic.

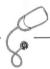

Stridor at rest is an indication for hospital admission.

Give corticosteroids to febrile child with stridor for:
- Croup
- Epiglottitis
- Retropharyngeal abscess
- Bacterial tracheitis

Diagnosis of spasmodic croup can be made only on resolution of the symptoms.

Steroids are not indicated in spasmodic croup.

DIAGNOSIS

Subglottic, noninflammatory edema.

TREATMENT

- Reassurance and cool mist.
- Spontaneous recovery.

EPIGLOTTITIS

A 4-year-old boy brought to the ED is flushed, making high-pitched noises on forced inspiration, leaning forward in his mother's lap, and drooling. His illness started with fever and sore throat and rapidly progressed to difficulty swallowing, drooling, restlessness, and stridor or air hunger. He appeared toxic and anxious. Lateral neck x-ray shows thumb sign. *Think: Epiglottitis,* and get him to an operating room (OR) to intubate and treat!

The classic presentation: "three Ds" (drooling, dysphagia, and distress).

See Figure 12-2.

HFlu (B)

DEFINITION

Acute, life-threatening infection of supraglottic tissues.

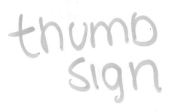

Minutes count in acute epiglottitis.

ETIOLOGY

- *Haemophilus influenzae* type B.
- Other possible pathogens—*Streptococcus pyogenes, Streptococcus pneumoniae, Staphylococcus aureus.*

thumb sign

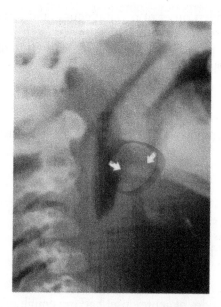

FIGURE 12-2. **Radiograph of lateral soft tissue of neck demonstrating epiglottitis.**

Note the thickening of the epiglottic and ariepiglottic folds (arrows). (Reproduced, with permission, from Schwartz DT, Reisdorff BJ. *Emergency Radiology.* New York: McGraw-Hill, 2000: 608.)

PATHOPHYSIOLOGY

Acute inflammation and edema of epiglottis, aryepiglottic folds, and arytenoids.

EPIDEMIOLOGY

- ↓ incidence due to *H influenzae* type B vaccine (HiB).
- Usually 2–6 years of age, but can occur at any age.
- Suspect in unvaccinated children.
- *H influenzae* immunization has practically eliminated epiglottitis in young children.

SIGNS AND SYMPTOMS

- Sudden onset of inspiratory stridor and respiratory distress.
- Muffled voice ("hot potato" voice).
- High fever (usually the first symptom).
- Toxic appearing.
- Tripod position—hyperextended neck, leaning forward, mouth open.
- Three Ds: Dysphagia, drooling, and distress.
- Cough (less frequent symptom)
- Tachycardia is a constant feature.
- Severe respiratory distress develops within minutes to hours.
- May progress to restlessness, pallor/cyanosis, coma, death.

DIAGNOSIS

- Laryngoscopy—swollen, cherry-red epiglottis.
- Lateral neck x-ray to confirm (portable x-ray should be obtained).
- Swollen epiglottis (thumbprint sign).
- Thickened aryepiglottic fold.
- Obliteration of vallecula.

TREATMENT

- **True medical emergency**—potentially lethal airway obstruction.
- Comfort.
- Anticipate.
- Secure airway (endotracheal intubation in OR).
- Ceftriaxone (100 mg/kg/day) 7–10 days.
- Rifampin prophylaxis for close contacts.

Ceftriaxone

TRACHEITIS/LARYNGITIS

DEFINITION

Rapidly progressive upper airway obstruction due to infection of the trachea and/or larynx.

ETIOLOGY

- *S aureus* and *H influenzae* type b.
- Also *Moraxella catarrhalis*.
- High association with preceding influenza A infection.

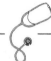

In doubtful cases, radiograph alone should not be used to diagnose epiglottitis.

Epiglottitis is a true medical emergency. If suspected, do not:

- Examine the throat
- Use narcotics or sedatives, including antihistamines
- Attempt venipuncture or other tests
- Place patient supine

SIGNS AND SYMPTOMS

- Often present with croup symptoms. Differentiation can be made by the presence of:
  - High fever
  - Toxicity
  - Inspiratory stridor (constant)
  - Purulent sputum
- A toxic-appearing child with croupy symptoms who responds poorly to croup management should be evaluated for tracheitis.
- Tracheitis has features of both croup (stridor and croupy cough) and epiglottitis (high fever and toxic appearance).

DIAGNOSIS

- X-ray—may be normal or identical to croup. Look for **pseudomembrane** on lateral view.
  - Epiglottis size normal
  - Tracheal narrowing
  - Pseudomembrane
- Endoscopy.
- Copious purulent secretion distal to glottis.
- Secretions should be obtained for Gram stain and culture.

TREATMENT

- Secure an adequate airway (endotracheal intubation):
  - Should be performed in an operating room under anesthesia.
  - Suction endotracheal tube of purulent material.
- Specialty consultation: Ear, nose, and throat (ENT), and anesthesia.
- Ceftriaxone 100 mg/kg/day.
- Ampicillin-sulbactam 200 mg/kg/day.
- ICU admission.

Bacterial tracheitis has a slower onset than epiglottitis.

BRONCHIOLITIS

A previously healthy 4-month-old who had rhinorrhea, cough, and a low-grade fever develops tachypnea, mild hypoxemia, and hyperinflation of lungs. *Think: RSV bronchiolitis.*

Classic presentation: Acute onset of cough, wheezing, and ↑ respiratory effort after an upper respiratory tract prodrome (fever and runny nose), during the winter season.

DEFINITION

Viral infection of upper and lower respiratory tract (medium and small airways).

ETIOLOGY

- RSV—most common cause.
- Adenovirus.
- Parainfluenza 3.
- Influenza.

Bronchiolitis is the most common serious respiratory infection in children < 2 years.

RSV

- Human metapneumovirus (hMPV): First recognized in 2001 and now increasingly implicated.
- *Mycoplasma pneumoniae* (rare).

PATHOPHYSIOLOGY

- Inflammatory obstruction (edema and mucus) of the bronchioles secondary to viral infection.
- Alterations in gas exchange are most frequently the result of mismatching of pulmonary ventilation and perfusion.

EPIDEMIOLOGY

- Occurs in first 2 years of life.
- Reinfection is common.
- Ninety percent are aged 1–9 months.
- Occurs in winter and early spring.
- Risks: Crowded conditions, not breast-fed, mothers who smoke, male gender.
- High-risk infants:
  - Cardiac disease
  - Pulmonary disease
  - Neuromuscular disease
  - Premature infants
  - Immunocompromised

< 2 years old

RSV causes more than 50% of cases of bronchiolitis.

Humans are the only source of RSV infection.

SIGNS AND SYMPTOMS

- Starts with mild respiratory illness.
- Respiratory distress gradually develops.
- Paroxysmal wheezing—common but may be absent, cough, dyspnea.
- Apneic spells—young infants should be monitored.
- Frequent complications include bacteremia, pericarditis, cellulitis, empyema, meningitis, and suppurative arthritis.
- Most common complication is hypoxia.
- Dehydration is the most common secondary complication.

Symptoms of asthma can be identical to bronchiolitis. Suspect asthma if:
- Family history
- Prior episodes
- Response to bronchodilator

DIAGNOSIS

- Viral detection in nasopharyngeal secretions via culture, polymerase chain reaction (PCR), or antigen detection.
- Chest x-ray (rule out pneumonia or foreign body)—hyperinflation of lungs, ↑ anteroposterior (AP) diameter of rib cage.
- Oxygen saturation is the single best objective predictor.

TREATMENT

- Low threshold for hospitalization for high-risk infants.
- Humidified oxygen.
- Trial of nebulized albuterol (only 20–50% are responders, discontinue if no objective benefit).
- **Hypertonic saline**—potential to reduce airway edema and mucous plugging.
- Steroids not indicated.
- Respiratory isolation.
- Ribavirin (aerosol form) if high-risk patients such as immunocompromised, need for mechanical ventilation, or < 6 weeks old.
- RSV intravenous immune globulin (RSV-IVIG) or palivizumab given prior to and during RSV season in high-risk infants < 2 years old.

Indications for rapid antigen detection in suspected RSV bronchiolitis: cohorting RSV-positive patient or to confirm RSV in high-risk patient.

A 7-year-old boy presents with an upper respiratory infection (URI) with productive cough (with purulent sputum). On examination, localized rales on the right side of his chest were noted. X-ray shows two discrete densities located in the right upper lobe of the lungs. *Think: Bronchiectasis.* Predisposition: Cystic fibrosis and ciliary dyskinesia.

DEFINITION

Abnormal and permanent dilatation of bronchi.

ETIOLOGY

- Viruses: Adenovirus, influenza virus.
- Bacteria: *S aureus*, *Klebsiella*, anaerobes.
- Primary ciliary dyskinesia.
- Kartagener syndrome.
- Cystic fibrosis: *Pseudomonas aeruginosa.*
- α_1-antitrypsin deficiency.

PATHOPHYSIOLOGY

Consequence of inflammation and destruction of structural components of bronchial wall.

SIGNS AND SYMPTOMS

- Physical exam quite variable.
- Persistent or recurrent cough.
- Purulent sputum.
- Hemoptysis.
- Dyspnea.
- Wheezing.
- Clubbing.

DIAGNOSIS

- Chest x-ray.
- Bronchography.
- Computed tomographic (CT) scan.
- Sputum culture.

TREATMENT

- Elimination of underlying cause.
- Clearance of secretion.
- Chest physiotherapy.
- Mucolytic agents.
- Control of infection—antibiotics.
- Reversal of airflow obstruction—bronchodilators.

DEFINITION

Infection of conductive airways of lung.

ETIOLOGY

- Viruses: Influenza A and B, adenovirus, parainfluenza, rhinovirus, RSV, coxsackievirus.
- Bacteria: *Bordetella pertussis*, *M pneumoniae*, *Chlamydia pneumoniae*, *S pneumoniae*.

SIGNS AND SYMPTOMS

- Acute productive cough (< 1 week).
- Rhinitis.
- Myalgia.
- Fever.
- No evidence of sinusitis, pneumonia, or chronic pulmonary disease.
- Normal arterial oxygenation.

TREATMENT

- Mostly self-limited.
- Bronchodilators may help.
- Antibiotics for high-risk patients.

Cough is the most common symptom of chronic bronchitis.

PHARYNGITIS

DEFINITION

Infection of the tonsils and/or the pharynx.

ETIOLOGY

SIGNS AND SYMPTOMS

- Viral pharyngitis: MC
  - Gradual onset.
  - Fever, malaise, throat pain.
  - Conjunctivitis, rhinitis, coryza, viral exanthem, diarrhea.
- Streptococcal pharyngitis (> 2 years) (see Figure 12-3):
  - Headache, abdominal pain, and vomiting.
  - Fever (> 104°F [40°C]).
  - Tonsillar enlargement with exudates.
  - Fetid odor.
  - Cervical adenopathy.
  - Palatal petechiae and uvular edema.
- It is not possible to distinguish clinically viral from bacterial pharyngitis, though high fever, cervical adenopathy, and absence of URI symptoms suggest bacterial etiology.

Pharyngitis is the second most common diagnosis in children aged 1–15 years in the pediatric clinic.

Viruses (most common cause of pharyngitis): Rhinovirus, adenovirus, coxsackievirus.

Acute rheumatic fever occurs more after throat than skin infections and in children who have had acute rheumatic fever before.

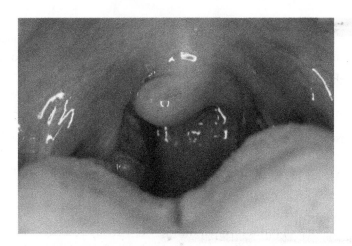

FIGURE 12-3. **Streptococcal pharyngitis.**

Note white exudates on top of erythematous swollen tonsils. (Reproduced, with permission, from Knoop KJ, Stack LB, Storrow AB, et al. *Atlas of Emergency Medicine*, 3rd ed. New York: McGraw-Hill, 2010: 115.)

DIAGNOSIS

Rapid (DNase) antigen detection test (sensitivity 95–98%):

- Culture if negative.
- Treat if positive.

TREATMENT

- Oral penicillin (25–50 mg/kg/day) for 10 days.
- Alternatively, intramuscular (IM) benzathine and procaine penicillin can be used (single dose, weight based).
- Macrolides or clindamycin for penicillin-allergic patients for 10 days.
- Tetracycline and sulfonamides should not be used to treat group A beta-hemolytic streptococci (GABHS).
- Antibiotics are not indicated for pharyngitis negative for GABHS.

COMPLICATIONS

- Suppurative:
  - Peritonsillar abscess
  - Retropharyngeal abscess
  - Cervical adenitis
  - Otitis media
  - Sinusitis
- Nonsuppurative:
  - Acute glomerulonephritis
  - Acute rheumatic fever

Penicillin remains the drug of choice for GABHS.

The more mucous membranes involved, the more likely an infection is viral.

PNEUMONIA

A 2-month-old with fever, tachypnea, and mottled skin has a chest x-ray showing infiltrate of the right upper lung lobe, a pneumatocele, and a pleural effusion. *Think:* S aureus *pneumonia.*

A previously healthy 9-year-old boy has a 7-day history of increasing cough, low-grade fever, and fatigue on exertion. Chest x-ray shows widespread diffuse perihilar infiltrates. *Think:* Mycoplasma *pneumonia.*
Initially, nonproductive cough and no fever. Later, productive cough with fever, headache, coryza, otitis media, and malaise.

DEFINITION

Inflammation of lung parenchyma.

ETIOLOGY

- Viruses: RSV, influenza, parainfluenza, adenovirus.
- Bacteria: Less common, but more severe—*S pneumoniae, S pyogenes, S aureus, H influenzae* type B, *M pneumoniae.*

SIGNS AND SYMPTOMS

- Tachypnea, dyspnea.
- Fever and feeding difficulty (infant).
- Productive cough, chest pain (children).
- *Chlamydia trachomatis* (pneumonitis syndrome).
- Occurs in children 1–3 months of age.
- Staccato cough, tachypnea, progressive respiratory distress.
- Lack of fever and other systemic signs.
- Conjunctivitis.

DIAGNOSIS

- Chest x-ray (Figure 12-4):
  - Viral (hyperinflation, perihilar infiltrate, hilar adenopathy, and atelectasis).
  - Bacterial (alveolar consolidation).
  - *Mycoplasma* (interstitial infiltrates).
  - Tuberculosis (hilar adenopathy).
  - *Pneumocystis* (reticulonodular infiltrates).
- Blood culture (positive in 10–30% of bacterial cases).

 Round pulmonary infiltrate on chest x-ray. *Think:* S pneumoniae *pneumonia.*

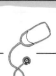 Pneumonia with hilar adenopathy on chest x-ray. *Think: Adenovirus.* However, it is difficult to make an accurate etiologic diagnosis only on the basis of clinical presentation.

 The most reliable sign of pneumonia is tachypnea.

 Consider pneumonia in children with neck stiffness or acute abdominal pain.

In young children, auscultation may be normal with impressive x-ray findings.

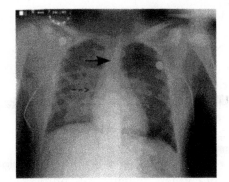

FIGURE 12-4. Chest x-ray demonstrating diffuse bilateral pulmonary infiltrates.

Note tip of endotracheal tube (arrow) is in good position.

HIGH-YIELD FACTS

RESPIRATORY DISEASE

TREATMENT

- **Inpatient:**
    - 1–3 months old: Macrolide (pneumonitis syndrome) or third-generation cephalosporin.
    - ≥ 3 months and older: Third-generation cephalosporin.
- **Outpatient:**
    - Patients should have normal O$_2$ saturation and be able to take oral fluids in order to be outpatients.
    - Amoxicillin or erythromycin.

PERTUSSIS

DEFINITION

- "Whooping cough."
- Highly infectious form of bronchitis.

ETIOLOGY

- *Bordetella pertussis* gram-negative coccobacilli.
- Humans are the only known host.
- Whooping cough syndrome also may be caused by:
    - *Bordetella parapertussis*
    - *M pneumoniae*
    - *C trachomatis*
    - *C pneumoniae*
    - Adenoviruses

PATHOPHYSIOLOGY

- Pertussis toxin is a virulence protein that causes lymphocytosis and systemic manifestations.
- Aerosol droplet transmission.

EPIDEMIOLOGY

- Endemic, but epidemic every 3–4 years.
- 60 million cases/year worldwide.
- 500,000 deaths/year worldwide.
- July to October.
- Occurs in 1- to 5-year-olds worldwide, 50% < 1-year-olds in United States.

SIGNS AND SYMPTOMS

- Incubation period 1–2 weeks.
- Three stages: Catarrhal, paroxysmal, and convalescent.
- Duration: 6 weeks.
- Catarrhal stage: Congestion and rhinorrhea.
- Paroxysmal stage (2–4 weeks):
    - Paroxysmal cough, with characteristic whoop following (chin forward, tongue out, watery, bulging eyes, purple face).
    - Fever is typically absent.
    - Post-tussive emesis and exhaustion.

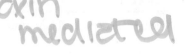
toxin mediated

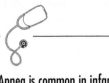

Pertussis means "intense cough."

Despite having "whooping cough," most patients with pertussis do not whoop.

With pertussis, fever may be absent or minimal; cough may be only complaint.

Apnea is common in infants with pertussis.

- Convalescent stage: Number and severity of paroxysms plateaus.
- Each stage lasts ~2 weeks; shorter if immunized.
- Complications include apnea, physical sequelae of forceful coughing, brain hypoxia/hemorrhage, secondary infections (bacterial pneumonia is the cause of death).

DIAGNOSIS

- Diagnosis is primarily clinical:
  - Inspiratory whoop
  - Post-tussive emesis
  - Lymphocytosis
- Chest x-ray—perihilar infiltrate or edema (butterfly pattern).
- Positive immunofluorescence test or PCR on nasopharyngeal secretions.

TREATMENT

- Goal—to ↓ spread of organism. Antibiotics do not affect illness in paroxysmal stage, which is toxin mediated.
- Macrolide antibiotic for patient and household contacts.
- Isolation until 5 days of therapy.
- Admit if:
  - Infant < 3 months.
  - Apnea.
  - Cyanosis.
  - Respiratory distress.
- DTP (diphtheria, tetanus, pertussis)/DTaP (diphtheria, tetanus, acellular pertussis) vaccine.

Macrolide

Suspect pertussis if paroxysmal cough with color change.

No single serologic test is diagnostic for pertussis.

There is a risk of hypertrophic pyloric stenosis in infants younger than 6 weeks treated with oral erythromycin.

DIPHTHERIA

DEFINITION

Membranous nasopharyngitis or obstructive laryngotracheitis.

ETIOLOGY

- *Corynebacterium diphtheriae.*
- Humans are the only reservoir.

SIGNS AND SYMPTOMS

- Incubation period: 2–7 days.
- Erosive rhinitis with membrane formation.
- Tonsillopharyngeal—sore throat, membranous exudate.
- Cardiac symptoms.
- Tachycardia out of proportion to fever.

DIAGNOSIS

- Culture (nose, throat, mucosal, or cutaneous lesion).
- Material should be obtained from beneath the membrane or a portion of membrane.
- All *C diphtheriae* isolates should be sent to diphtheria laboratory.

For treatment of diphtheria, antibiotics are not a substitute for antitoxin.

Most tuberculosis infections in children are asymptomatic with positive PPD.

A patient may develop TB despite prior bacillus Calmette-Guérin (BCG) vaccination.

A positive PPD skin test results from infection, not from exposure.

Asymptomatic children with a positive PPD should be considered infected and get treatment.

All cases of active TB should be referred to public health department.

Persons with TB should be tested for HIV.

TREATMENT

- Antitoxin—dose depends on:
  - Site of membrane
  - Degree of toxic effects
  - Duration of illness
- Antibiotics:
  - Erythromycin or penicillin G for 14 days.
  - Elimination of organism should be documented by two consecutive cultures.

TUBERCULOSIS (TB)

DEFINITION

- Signs and symptoms and/or radiographic manifestations caused by *M tuberculosis* are apparent.
- May be pulmonary, extrapulmonary, or both.

ETIOLOGY

Mycobacterium tuberculosis.

PATHOPHYSIOLOGY

Primary portal of entry into children is lung.

EPIDEMIOLOGY

- Children are never the primary source (look for adult contacts).
- Risk factors:
  - Urban living
  - Low income
  - Recent immigrants
  - HIV

SIGNS AND SYMPTOMS

- Chronic cough (nonproductive)
- Hemoptysis
- Fever
- Night sweats
- Weight loss
- Anorexia
- Lymphadenopathy
- Present to ED with:
  - Primary pneumonia
  - Miliary TB (may mimic sepsis)

DIAGNOSIS

- When to suspect TB:
  - Hilar adenopathy.
  - Pulmonary calcification.
  - Pneumonia with infiltrate and adenopathy.
  - Pneumonia with pleural effusion.
  - Painless unilateral cervical adenopathy (scrofula).
  - Meningitis of insidious onset.

- Bone or joint disease.
- When any of the above are unresponsive to antibiotics.
- PPD test (Mantoux test).
- QuantiFERON®-TB Gold test.
- Culture (gastric aspirates, sputum, pleural fluid, cerebrospinal fluid, urine, or other body fluids).
- Look for the adult source.
- Acid-fast stain or PCR.

TREATMENT

- Two to four or more drugs (isoniazid, rifampin, pyrazinamide, ethambutol, streptomycin) for a minimum of 6 months for active disease.
- Isoniazid for 9 months for latent disease.

TB in children < 4 years of age is much more likely to disseminate; prompt and vigorous treatment should be started when the diagnosis is suspected.

CYSTIC FIBROSIS (CF)

A 3-year-old child presents with constant cough with sputum. He has had six episodes of pneumonia, with *Pseudomonas* being isolated from sputum; loose stools; and is at the 20th percentile for growth. *Think: CF.*
CF is an inherited multisystem disorder resulting in chronic lung disease, exocrine pancreatic insufficiency, and failure to thrive.

DEFINITION

Disease of exocrine glands that causes viscous secretions:

- Chronic respiratory infection
- Pancreatic insufficiency
- ↑ electrolytes in sweat

ETIOLOGY

- Defect of cyclic adenosine monophosphate (cAMP)-activated chloride channel of epithelial cells in pancreas, sweat glands, salivary glands, intestines, respiratory tract, and reproductive system.
- Autosomal recessive.

PATHOPHYSIOLOGY

- Chloride does not exit from cells.
- ↑ osmotic pressure inside cells attracts water and → thick secretions.

EPIDEMIOLOGY

- Most common cause of severe, chronic lung disease in children.
- One in 2000–3000 live births (Caucasians).

SIGNS AND SYMPTOMS

- Respiratory:
  - Cough—most common pulmonary symptom.
  - Wheezing, dyspnea, exercise intolerance.
  - Bronchiectasis, recurrent pneumonia.
  - Sinusitis, *nasal polyps*.
  - Reactive airway disease, hemoptysis.

Cystic fibrosis is the most common lethal inherited disease of Caucasians.

The gene for cystic fibrosis is CFTR; the mutation is delta F508.

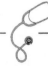

A patient with severe CF breathing room air can have an arterial blood gas (ABG) showing ↓ chloride and ↑ bicarbonate.

- ↑ AP chest diameter.
- Hyperresonant lungs.
- Clubbing of nails.
- Gastrointestinal (GI):
  - **Failure to thrive.**
  - Meconium ileus (10%).
  - Constipation, rectal prolapse.
  - Intestinal obstruction.
  - Pancreatic insufficiency:
    - **Malabsorption.**
    - Fat-soluble vitamin deficiencies.
    - Glucose intolerance.
  - Biliary cirrhosis (uncommon): Jaundice, ascites, hematemesis from esophageal varices
- Reproductive tract: ↓/absent fertility—female, thick cervical secretions; male, azoospermic.
- Sweat glands:
  - Salty skin.
  - Hypochloremic alkalosis in severe cases.
- Complications may include pneumothorax, chronic pulmonary hypertension, cor pulmonale, atelectasis, allergic bronchopulmonary aspergillosis, respiratory failure, gastroesophageal reflux.

DIAGNOSIS

- Sweat test—chloride concentration > 60 mEq/L (gold standard).
- Genetic studies.
- *In utero* screen available.
- Pulmonary function tests (PFTs): Obstructive and restrictive abnormalities.
- Prenatal diagnosis via gene proves CF mutations or linkage analysis.

TREATMENT

- Multidisciplinary team approach—pediatrician, physiotherapist, dietitian, nursing staff, teacher, child, and parents.
- Respiratory:
  - Chest physical therapy.
  - Exercise.
  - Coughing to move secretions and mucous plugs.
  - Bronchodilators.
  - Normal saline aerosol.
  - Anti-inflammatory medications.
  - Dornase-alpha nebulizer (breaks down DNA in mucus).
- Pancreatic/digestive:
  - Enteric coated pancreatic enzyme supplements (add to all meals).
  - Fat-soluble vitamin supplements.
  - High-calorie, high-protein diet.
- Antibiotics—sputum cultures used to guide antibiotic choice. Pseudomonal infections are especially common.
- Lung transplant.
- Gene therapy is being aggressively studied.

PROGNOSIS

Advances in therapy have ↑ life expectancy into adulthood.

False-positive sweat test (not CF):
- Nephrogenic diabetes insipidus
- Myxedema
- Mucopolysaccharidosis
- Adrenal insufficiency
- Ectodermal dysplasia

Features of CF: CF PANCREAS
Chronic cough
Failure to thrive
Pancreatic insufficiency
Alkalosis
Nasal polyps
Clubbing
Rectal prolapse
Electrolytes ↑ in sweat
Absence of vas
Sputum mucoid

Ninety-nine percent of cases of meconium ileus are due to CF.

Tonsillitis/Adenoiditis

DEFINITION

Inflammation of:

- Tonsils—two faucial tonsils.
- Adenoids—nasopharyngeal tonsils.

SIGNS AND SYMPTOMS

- Sore throat.
- Pain with swallowing.
- May have whitish exudate on tonsils.
- Chronic tonsillitis:
  - Seven in past year.
  - Five in each of the past 2 years.
  - Three in each of the past 3 years.

TREATMENT

- < 2–3 years old: Tonsillectomy is performed for obstructive sleep symptoms.
- Large size alone is not an indication to remove tonsils.

Enlarged Adenoids

DEFINITION

Nasopharyngeal lymphoid tissue.

SIGNS AND SYMPTOMS

- Mouth breathing
- Persistent rhinitis
- Snoring

DIAGNOSIS

- Digital palpation
- Indirect laryngoscopy

TREATMENT

- Adenoidectomy:
  - Persistent mouth breathing.
  - Hyponasal speech.
  - Adenoid facies.
  - Recurrent otitis media or nasopharyngitis.
- Tonsillectomy should not be performed routinely unless separate indication exists.

Peritonsillar Abscess

DEFINITION

Walled-off infection occurring in the space between the superior pharyngeal constrictor muscle and tonsils.

Fat-soluble vitamin deficiencies:
A—night blindness
D—↓ bone density
E—neurologic dysfunction
K—bleeding

Tonsils and adenoids are part of Waldeyer's ring that circles the pharynx.

It can be normal for tonsils to be relatively large during childhood.

HIGH-YIELD FACTS

RESPIRATORY DISEASE

ETIOLOGY

- GABHS
- Anaerobes

EPIDEMIOLOGY

Usually preadolescent.

augmentin

SIGNS AND SYMPTOMS

- Preceded by acute tonsillopharyngitis.
- Severe throat pain.
- Trismus.
- Refusal to swallow or speak.
- "Hot potato voice."
- Markedly swollen and inflamed tonsils.
- Uvula displaced to opposite side.

TREATMENT

- Antibiotics covering staph and strep. Typically, ampicillin—sulbactam.
- Incision and drainage.

Trismus is limited opening of the mouth.

RETROPHARYNGEAL ABSCESS

DEFINITION

Potential space between the posterior pharyngeal wall and the prevertebral fascia. Commonly occurs in children < 5 years old.

ETIOLOGY

Usually a complication of pharyngitis:

- GABHS
- Oral anaerobes
- *S aureus*

Lymph nodes in the retropharyngeal space usually disappear by the third to fourth year of life.

SIGNS AND SYMPTOMS

- Sudden onset of high fever with difficulty in swallowing.
- Refusal of feeding.
- Throat pain.
- Hyperextension of the head.
- Toxicity is common.
- May cause meningismus—extension of the neck causes pain.

DIAGNOSIS

Lateral neck x-ray: Normal retropharyngeal space should be less than one-half of width of adjacent vertebra (see Figure 12–5).

TREATMENT

Clindamycin or ampicillin-sulbactam.

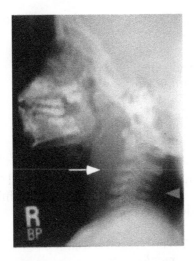

FIGURE 12-5. Lateral radiograph of the soft tissue of the neck.

Note the large amount of prevertebral edema (solid arrow) and the collection of air (dashed arrow). Findings are consistent with retropharyngeal abscess. (Courtesy of Dr. Gregory J. Schears.)

ASTHMA

 A 5-year-old boy with a history of sleeping problems presents with a non-productive nocturnal cough and shortness of breath and cough during exercise. *Think: Asthma.*

Start on a trial of a bronchodilator, which is helpful in confirming the diagnosis by the demonstration of reversible airways obstruction ($\uparrow$ in forced expiratory volume in 1 second [FEV_1]). Asthma is an inflammatory disease. Diagnosis of asthma should be considered in the presence of recurrent wheezing in a child with a family history of asthma.

DEFINITION

Respiratory hypersensitivity, inflammation, and reversible airway obstruction.

ETIOLOGY

Hyperresponsiveness to a variety of stimuli:

- Respiratory infection
- Air pollutants
- Allergens
- Foods
- Exercise
- Emotions

PATHOPHYSIOLOGY

- Bronchospasm (acute).
- Mucus production (acute).

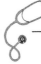

Asthma is the most common chronic lung disease in children.

Lack of wheezing does not exclude asthma.

- Inflammation and edema of the airway mucosa (chronic).
- Two types:
  - Extrinsic:
    - Immunologically mediated
    - Develop in childhood
  - Intrinsic:
    - No identifiable cause
    - Late onset
    - Worsen with age
- Underlying abnormalities in asthma include ↑ pulmonary vascular pressure, diffuse narrowing of airways, ↑ residual volume and functional residual capacity, and ↑ total ventilation maintaining normal or reduced PCO_2 despite ↑ dead space.

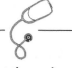

Asthma is the most common cause of cough in school-age children.

SIGNS AND SYMPTOMS

- Cough, wheezing, dyspnea.
- ↑ work of breathing (retractions, use of accessory muscles, nasal flaring, abdominal breathing).
- ↓ breath sounds.
- Prolongation of expiratory phase.
- Acidosis and hypoxia may result from airway obstruction.
- See Table 12-4 for classification of severity.

Classic trilogy of asthma:
- Bronchospasm
- Mucus production
- Inflammation and edema of the airway mucosa

DIAGNOSIS

- Clinical diagnosis, usually.
- Peak expiratory flow rate (PEFR):
  - Maximal rate of airflow during forced exhalation after a maximal inhalation.
  - Normal values depend on age and height:
    - Mild (80% of predicted).
    - Moderate (50–80% of predicted).
    - Severe (< 50% of predicted).

Respiratory drive is not inhibited in asthma.

TABLE 12-4. Asthma Severity Classification

CLASSIFYING SEVERITY OF ASTHMA EXACERBATIONS IN THE URGENT OR EMERGENCY CARE SETTING	
Mild	Dyspnea only with activity
	PEFR > 70% predicted personal best
Moderate	Dyspnea interferes with or limits usual activity
	PEFR 40–69% predicted personal best
Severe	Dyspnea at rest, interferes with conversation
	PEFR < 40% predicted personal best
Life threatening	Too dyspneic to speak
	PEFR < 25% predicted personal best

PEFR, peak expiratory flow rate.

(Adapted from National Asthma Education & Prevention Program Expert Panel Report 3: Guidelines for the Diagnosis & Management of Asthma NHLBI guidelines. *Summary Report* 2007: 54.)

- Chest x-ray will demonstrate hyperinflation and can be useful to look for pneumonia.
- Pulse oximetry may demonstrate hypoxia.
- Fever and focal lung exam—think pneumonia.
- Unresponsive to usual URI therapy.
- ABG—hypoxia in severe exacerbations; hypercapnia suggestive of impending respiratory failure.
- Bloodwork should not be routinely ordered in the evaluation of asthma.

All wheezing is not caused by asthma; all asthmatics do not wheeze.

TREATMENT

Goals: Improve bronchodilation, avoid allergens, ↓ inflammation, educate patient.

First-Line Agents
1. Oxygen.
2. Inhaled β₂ agonist:
   - Albuterol (2.5 mg) (nebulized).
   - Short-acting/rescue medication—treats only symptoms, not underlying process.
   - Bronchial smooth-muscle relaxant.
   - Side effects: Tachycardia, tremors, hypokalemia.
3. Corticosteroids (sooner is better):
   - For treatment of chronic inflammation.
   - Oral prednisone (2 mg/kg, max 60 mg) or IV methylprednisolone 2 mg/kg max 125 mg).
   - Contraindication: Active varicella or herpes infection.
4. Anticholinergic agents:
   - Ipratropium bromide (nebulized).
   - Act synergistically with albuterol.
   - Bind to cholinergic receptors in the medium and large airways.

Asthmatic patient in severe respiratory distress may not wheeze.

Second-Line Agents
1. Magnesium sulfate—bronchodilation via direct effect on smooth muscle.
2. Epinephrine or terbutaline.
3. No role in acute asthma for theophylline; not recommended.

Spirometry is the most important study in asthma.

Others
1. Heliox—mixture of 60–70% helium and 30–40% oxygen:
   - ↓ work of breathing by improving laminar gas flow (nonintubated patient).
   - Improves oxygenation and ↓ peak airway pressure (intubated patients).
2. Mechanical ventilation indications:
   - Failure of maximal pharmacologic therapy.
   - Hypoxemia.
   - Hypercarbia.
   - Change in mental status.
   - Respiratory fatigue.
   - Respiratory failure.
3. Leukotriene modifiers:
   - Inflammatory mediators.
   - Improve lung function.
   - No role in acute asthma.
4. Cromolyn and nedocromil:
   - Effective in maintenance therapy.
   - Exercise-induced asthma.
   - May reduce dosage requirements of inhaled steroid.

O₂ is indicated for all asthmatics to keep O₂ saturation > 95%.

Long-acting β₂ agonist (salmeterol) should not be used for acute asthma exacerbation.

Asthmatic child's ability to use inhaler correctly should be regularly assessed.

Inhaled corticosteroids are recommended as the first-line prophylactic therapy.

Most important risk factor for morbidity is failure to diagnose asthma from recurrent wheezing.

↑ white blood cell (WBC) count does not always signify infection in status asthmaticus.

Dehydration may be present in status asthmaticus, but overhydration should be avoided (risk for syndrome of inappropriate antidiuretic hormone secretion [SIADH]).

Admit if:

- Respiratory failure requiring intubation.
- Status asthmaticus.
- Return ED visit in 24 hours.
- Complete lobar atelectasis.
- Pneumothorax/pneumomediastinum.
- Underlying cardiopulmonary disease.

Status Asthmaticus

DEFINITION

- Life-threatening form of asthma.
- Condition in which a progressively worsening attack is unresponsive to usual therapy.

SIGNS AND SYMPTOMS

Look for:

- Pulsus paradoxus > 20 mm Hg.
- Hypotension, tachycardia.
- Cyanosis.
- One- to two-word dyspnea.
- Lethargy.
- Agitation.
- Retractions.
- Silent chest (no wheezes—poor air exchange).

FOREIGN BODY ASPIRATION

A 2-year-old boy is brought to the ED with a history of a choking or gagging episode, followed by a coughing spell. In the ED, he was noted to have wheezing. His respiratory rate is 24, and he has mild intercostal retractions. His babysitter found him playing in his room. *Think: Foreign body aspiration.*

A previously healthy 12-year-old boy presented with cough for almost a year. He had a persistent dry cough during the day and night that was occasionally productive. His parents reported a history of pneumonia with consolidation of the right lower lobe on three different occasions in 6 months. On physical examination, no nasal congestion is noted. ↓ air entry and wheezing is noted on the right side of his chest. *Think: Foreign body aspiration.*

However, this classic triad (sudden onset of paroxysmal coughing, wheezing, and diminished breath sounds on the ipsilateral side) may not be present in all children with foreign body aspiration.

PATHOPHYSIOLOGY

Cough reflex usually protects against aspiration.

EPIDEMIOLOGY

- Twice as likely to occur in males, particularly 6-month-olds to 3-year-olds.
- Most common age: 1–2 years.

SIGNS AND SYMPTOMS

- Determined by nature of object, location, and degree of obstruction.
- Narrowest portion of the pediatric airway is at the cricoid ring.
- Foreign body in the upper airway: Respiratory distress with severe retractions and stridor.
- Foreign body in the lower airway (most foreign bodies lodge in the lower airways [80%]). Symptoms may be subtle.
- Initial respiratory symptoms may disappear for hours to weeks after incident.
- Vegetal/arachidic bronchitis due to vegetable (usually peanut) aspiration causes cough, high fever, and dyspnea.
- Most common aspirated foreign body: Peanut.
- Most common foreign body aspirations resulting in death: Balloons.
- Complications if object is not removed include pneumonitis/pneumonia, abscess, bronchiectasis, pulmonary hemorrhage, erosion, and perforation.

DIAGNOSIS/TREATMENT

Larynx
- Croupy cough; may have stridor, aphonia, hemoptysis, cyanosis.
- Lateral x-ray.
- Direct laryngoscopy—confirm diagnosis and remove object.

Trachea
- Stridor, audible slap, and palpable thud due to expiratory impaction.
- Chest x-ray (see Figure 12-6), bronchoscopy.

Bronchi
- Initial choking, gagging, wheezing, coughing.
- Latent period with some coughing, wheezing, possible hemoptysis, recurrent lobar pneumonia, or intractable asthma.

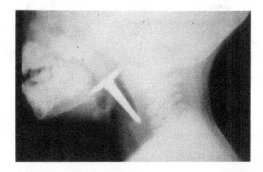

FIGURE 12-6. Radiograph of lateral soft tissue of the neck demonstrates a foreign body (nail) in the pharynx.

(Courtesy of Dr. Gregory J. Schears.)

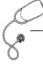

Prevention is key! Keep small food and objects away from young children.

Caution! Do not try to remove foreign bodies causing partial upper airway obstruction because these attempts may result in complete glottic obstruction.

Foreign Body Aspiration
- Toddlers: R = L mainstem
- Adults: R mainstem predominates

Percussion of Lung Fields
- Hyperresonant = overinflation
- Dull = atelectasis

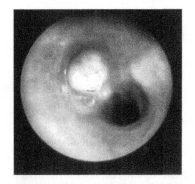

FIGURE 12-7. Foreign body (peanut) in the right mainstem bronchus visualized by bronchoscopy.

Foreign bodies tend to lodge most commonly in the right mainstem bronchus due to the larger anatomic angle that makes traveling down right mainstem easier. (Courtesy of Dr. Gregory J. Schears.)

- Tracheal shift, ↓ breath sounds.
- Midline obstruction can cause severe dyspnea or asphyxia.
- → chronic bronchopulmonary disease if not treated.
- Direct bronchoscopic visualization (Figure 12-7).
- Antibiotics for secondary infection if prolonged exposure.
- Emergency treatment of local upper airway obstruction if necessary.
- If the child can cough and verbalize:
    - Provide supplemental oxygen.
    - Maintain position of comfort.
    - Immediate consultation with ENT and anesthesia.
- If the child cannot cough or verbalize, initiate basic life support.

TRACHEOESOPHAGEAL FISTULA (TEF)

DEFINITION

Connection between the trachea and esophagus (see Figure 12-8).

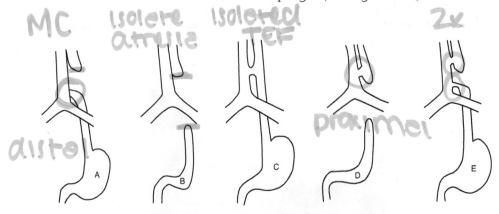

FIGURE 12-8. Types of tracheoesophageal fistulas (TEFs).

Type A, esophageal atresia (EA) with distal TEF (87%). Type B, isolated EA. Type C, isolated TEF. Type D, EA with proximal TEF. Type E, EA with double TEF.

ETIOLOGY

- Congenital
- Acquired

SIGNS AND SYMPTOMS

- Suspect esophageal atresia.
- Maternal polyhydramnios.
- Inability to pass catheter into stomach.
- ↑ oral secretions—drooling.
- Choking, cyanosis, or coughing with an attempt to feed.
- Tachypnea.

DIAGNOSIS

- X-ray: Radiopaque feeding tube passes no further than proximal esophagus.
- Barium swallow: Aspiration of barium into the tracheobronchial tree.

TREATMENT

Esophageal atresia is a surgical emergency.

There is an association of tracheoesophageal fistulae with esophageal atresia.

H-type tracheoesophageal fistula is the least common but the most likely to be seen in ED.

TRACHEOMALACIA/LARYNGOMALACIA

DEFINITION

- Floppy epiglottis and supraglottic aperture.
- Disproportionately small and soft larynx.

SIGNS AND SYMPTOMS

- Usually begins within first month.
- Noisy breathing.
- Stridor—laryngomalacia is the most frequent cause of stridor in children.
- Symptoms can be intermittent.
- Hoarseness or aphonia (laryngeal crow).
- Feeding difficulty.
- Symptoms worse when crying or lying on back.

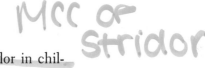

MCC of stridor

DIAGNOSIS

- Direct laryngoscopy.
- Collapse of laryngeal structures during inspiration especially arytenoid cartilages.

TREATMENT

- Reassurance.
- No specific therapy required.
- Usually resolves spontaneously by 18 months.

CONGENITAL LOBAR EMPHYSEMA (INFANTILE LOBAR EMPHYSEMA)

DEFINITION

Overexpansion of the airspaces of a segment or lobe of the lung.

EPIDEMIOLOGY

Most common congenital lung lesion.

PATHOPHYSIOLOGY

No significant parenchymal destruction.

SIGNS AND SYMPTOMS

- Normal at birth.
- Cough, wheezing, dyspnea, and cyanosis within a few days.

DIAGNOSIS

- Chest x-ray.
- Radiolucency.
- Mediastinal shift to opposite side.
- Flattened diaphragm.

TREATMENT

- Remove bronchial obstruction (foreign bodies, mucous plug).
- Lobectomy.

CYSTIC ADENOMATOID MALFORMATION

DEFINITION

- Developmental anomaly of the lower respiratory tract.
- Excessive overgrowth of bronchioles.
- ↑ in terminal respiratory structure.
- Hamartomatous lesions.

EPIDEMIOLOGY

Second most common congenital lung lesion.

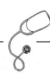

In patients with cystic adenomatoid malformation, avoid attempted aspiration or chest tube placement, as there is the risk of spreading infection.

SIGNS AND SYMPTOMS

- Neonatal respiratory distress.
- Recurrent pneumonia in same location.
- Pneumothorax.
- May be confused with diaphragmatic hernia in neonatal period.

DIAGNOSIS

- Chest x-ray (posteroanterior [PA], lateral, and decubitus).
- Cystic mass (multiple grapelike sacs) and mediastinal shift.
- Air-fluid level.
- CT scan.

Cystic adenomatoid malformation ↑ the risk for pulmonary neoplasia.

TREATMENT

Surgical excision of affected lobe.

Cardiovascular Disease

Normal Heart Sounds

- S1 may split.
- S2 normally splits with respiration.
- S3 can represent normal, rapid ventricular refilling.
- P2 should be soft after infancy.

EPIDEMIOLOGY

- Up to 90% of children have a murmur at some point in their lives.
- Two to seven percent of murmurs in children represent pathology.

DESCRIPTION AND GRADING

Murmurs are graded for intensity on a six-point system:

- **Grade I:** Very soft murmur detected only after very careful auscultation.
- **Grade II:** Soft murmur that is readily heard but faint (equal to S1/S2).
- **Grade III:** Moderately intense murmur not associated with a palpable precordial thrill (louder than S1 or S2).
- **Grade IV:** Loud murmur; a palpable precordial thrill is not present or is intermittent.
- **Grade V:** Loud murmur associated with a palpable precordial thrill; the murmur is not audible when the stethoscope is lifted from the chest.
- **Grade VI:** Loud murmur associated with a palpable precordial thrill. It can be heard even when the stethoscope is lifted slightly from the chest.

The difference between grade I and II murmur: A grade I can be heard only in a quiet room with a quiet child.

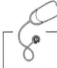

Murmur grading is usually written as "Grade [#]/6."

SITES OF AUSCULTATION

See Figure 13-1 to correlate the following points:

1. This site corresponds to the location of the **carotid arteries.** Common murmurs heard here: carotid bruit, aortic stenosis (AS). AS is usually louder at the right upper sternal border and often has an associated ejection click.
2. **Aortic valve.** Right upper sternal border. Common murmurs: aortic valve stenosis (supravalvular, valvular, and subvalvular). Valvular stenosis will often have an ejection click, whereas the others will not.

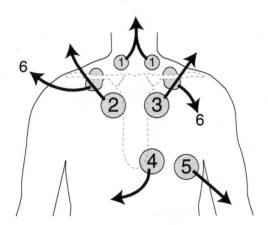

FIGURE 13-1. **Sites of auscultation.**

3. **Pulmonic valve.** Left upper sternal border. Common murmurs: pulmonary valve stenosis, atrial septal defect (ASD), pulmonary flow murmur, pulmonary artery stenosis, AS, coarctation of the aorta, patent ductus arteriosus (PDA), total anomalous pulmonary venous return (TAPVR).

4. **Tricuspid valve.** Left lower sternal border. Common murmurs: ventricular septal defect (VSD), Still's murmur, hypertrophic obstructive cardiomyopathy (HOCM), tricuspid regurgitation, endocardial cushion defect.

5. **Mitral valve.** Apex. Common murmurs: mitral regurgitation, mitral valve prolapse, Still's murmur, aortic stenosis, HOCM.

6. This site correlates with areas of **venous confluence.** Common murmurs: venous hum or subclavian bruit.

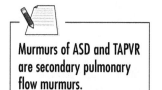

Murmurs of ASD and TAPVR are secondary pulmonary flow murmurs.

Accentuation Maneuvers

Various positions and activities can diminish and intensify a murmur (see Table 13-1). The following section also reiterates the positions that aid in diagnosing innocent murmurs.

TABLE 13-1. Accentuation Maneuvers for Pathologic Murmurs

MURMUR	INCREASED WITH	DECREASED WITH
Patent ductus arteriosus	Supination	
Atrial septal defect	(Valsalva can cause a temporary middiastolic murmur)	(Occasional crescendo-decrescendo systolic ejection murmur heard with ASD will not ↓ in intensity with the Valsalva maneuver like the pulmonary murmur)
Aortic stenosis	Valsalva release, sudden squatting, passive leg raising	Valsalva maneuver, handgrip, standing
Subaortic stenosis	Valsalva maneuver, standing	
Hypertrophic obstructive cardiomyopathy	Valsalva maneuver, standing	Handgrip, squatting, leg elevation
Mitral valve prolapse	(Click and murmur occur earlier and the murmur is longer [not louder] with inspiration, when upright, and during the Valsalva maneuver)	
Mitral regurgitation	Sudden squatting, isometric handgrip	Valsalva maneuver, standing
Pulmonic stenosis	Valsalva release	Valsalva maneuver, expiration
Tricuspid regurgitation	Inspiration, passive leg raising	Expiration
Aortic regurgitation	Sudden squatting, isometric handgrip	
Mitral stenosis	Exercise, left lateral position, isometric handgrip, coughing	
Tricuspid stenosis	Inspiration, passive leg raising	

TABLE 13-2. **Innocent Murmurs**

MURMUR	CAUSE	EPIDEMIOLOGY	LOCATION	SOUND	CHARACTERISTICS
Pulmonary flow murmur	Turbulent flow through a normal pulmonary valve	Most common between 8 and 14 years	Mid to upper left sternal border	Midfrequency, crescendo–decrescendo, systolic	Louder when patient is supine than upright
Still's (vibratory) murmur	Possibly turbulent flow in the left ventricular outflow tract region	Most common between 3 and 6 years; uncommon < 2 years	Lower left sternal border	Musical or vibratory with midsystolic accentuation	Louder supine, may disappear with Valsalva, softer during inspiration
Venous hum	Turbulent flow of systemic venous return in the jugular veins and superior vena cava	Most common between 3 and 6 years	Infra- and supraclavicular, base of neck	High frequency, best heard with diaphragm, during systole and diastole	More prominent on right than left, can be accentuated or eliminated with head position, disappears supine or digital compression of jugular vein
Carotid bruit or subclavian bruit	Turbulent flow from abrupt transition from large-bore aorta to smaller carotid and brachiocephalic arteries	Any age	Over carotid arteries with radiation to head	Systolic	Rarely, a faint thrill is palpable over the artery
Physiologic pulmonary branch stenosis (PPS)	Turbulent flow as blood enters right and left pulmonary arteries that are relatively hypoplastic at birth due to patent ductus arteriosus predominance	Newborns, especially low birth weight (usually disappears by 3–6 months)	Upper left sternal border, axillae, and back	Crescendo-decrescendo, systolic	Louder supine
Patent ductus arteriosus	Turbulent flow as blood is shunted left to right from the aorta to the pulmonary artery	Can be innocent in newborns, abnormal if persists	Upper left sternal border	Continuous, machinery-like, louder in systole	

Reminders for a systematic cardiac exam:

1. Assess the child's appearance, color, etc.
2. Palpate the precordium.
3. Listen in a quiet room, during systole and diastole.
4. Listen first for heart sounds, then repeat your "sweep" of the chest for murmurs.
5. Don't forget to listen to the back and in the axillae.
6. Move the patient in different positions.
7. Feel the pulses and assess capillary refill.
8. Palpate the liver.

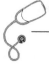

Any murmur > grade III is likely pathologic.

Cardiology consultation is indicated with any "noninnocent" murmur.

INNOCENT MURMURS

- **Pulmonary flow murmurs, physiologic pulmonary branch stenosis, and Still's murmurs** can all be heard best when the patient is supine versus upright.
- A Still's murmur may disappear with the Valsalva maneuver.
- Pulmonary flow murmurs are augmented by full exhalation, diminished by inhalation.
- **Venous hum** can be extinguished or accentuated with head and neck movement. It disappears in the supine position, and can also be eliminated with digital compression of the jugular vein.

PATHOLOGIC MURMURS

See Table 13-1.

Innocent Murmurs

- Common to all innocent murmurs are:
  - Absence of structural heart defects.
  - Normal heart sounds (S1, S2).
  - Normal peripheral pulses.
  - Normal chest radiographs and electrocardiogram (ECG).
  - Asymptomatic.
  - Usually systolic and graded less than III.
  - **No association with cardiovascular disease.**
  - **Accentuate in high-output states (fever and anemia).**
- See Table 13-2.

INTERPRETATION OF PEDIATRIC ECGs

- Always approach an ECG systematically:
  1. Measure atrial and ventricular rates.
  2. Define the rhythm (sinus, or other).
  3. Measure the P-R interval, QRS duration, and Q-T interval.
  4. Measure the axes of the P waves, QRS complexes, and T waves.
  5. Look for abnormalities of wave patterns and voltages.
- **Pediatric considerations:**
  - The interpretation is age dependent.
  - Heart rate varies with age—higher in infants and children.
  - The QRS duration is shorter in children.
  - PR interval is shorter.
  - QT_c is longer in infants than in older children (QT interval varies with heart rate).
  - Right axis deviation alone not enough as a criterion for right ventricular hypertrophy (RVH).

Expiration Rate

Age-dependent—see Table 13-3.

TABLE 13-3. Heart Rate by Age

Age	Normal Range (Average)
< 1 day	93–154 bpm (123)
1–2 days	91–159 bpm (123)
3–6 days	91–166 bpm (129)
1–3 weeks	107–182 bpm (148)
1–2 months	121–179 bpm (149)
3–5 months	106–186 bpm (141)
6–11 months	109–169 bpm (134)
1–2 years	89–151 bpm (119)
3–4 years	73–137 bpm (108)
5–7 years	65–133 bpm (100)
8–11 years	62–130 bpm (91)
12–15 years	80–119 bpm (85)
> 16 years	60–100 bpm

ECG Paper

- Speed = 25 mm/s.
- Small box = 0.04 sec = 1 mm.
- Large box = 0.20 sec = 5 mm.

Atrial Rate

- Look for P wave count that exceeds QRS complex count.
- If P wave number is greater than QRS complex number, an atrial dysrhythmia may be present.
- Premature atrial contractions (PACs) are common in infancy.

Ventricular Rate

- Count number of small boxes between 2 R waves, then divide into 1500.
- Count R-R cycles in six large divisions, then multiply by 50 (use with irregular or fast rate).

Bradycardia

Found in sleep, sedation, vagal stimulation (stooling, cough, or gag), hypothyroid, hyperkalemia, hypothermia, **hypoxia**, athletic heart, second- or third-degree atrioventricular (AV) block, junctional rhythm, ↑ intracranial pressure, medicine (ie, digitalis, β blockers). Hypoxemia is the most common cause of bradycardia.

Tachycardia

Found in fever, anxiety, hypovolemia, sepsis, congestive heart failure (CHF), hyperthyroidism, supraventricular tachycardia (SVT), ventricular tachycardia, atrial flutter and fibrillation, medicine (ie, theophylline, stimulants).

Sinus Arrhythmia

Normal variation in heart rate, due to inspiration and expiration (commonly seen in childhood).

Rhythm

Check for sinus rhythm:

- Verify a P wave before every QRS complex.
- Verify a QRS complex after every P wave.
- All P waves should look the same.
- Normal P wave axis (0° to +90°).
- Upright P waves in leads I and aVF.
- Normal P wave:
  - < 0.10 sec in children.
  - < 0.08 sec in infant.

P-R INTERVAL

- Beginning of P to beginning of QRS.
- Prolonged P-R (first-degree AV block): Found in myocarditis, digitalis, hyperkalemia, ischemia, ↑ vagal tone, hyperthyroidism.
- Short P-R: Found in ectopic atrial pacemaker, preexcitation syndromes (Wolff-Parkinson-White syndrome [WPW], Lown-Ganong-Levine syndrome), and glycogen storage disease. It may show patient is at risk for SVT.

QRS DURATION

Prolonged: Found in right bundle branch block (RBBB), left bundle branch block (LBBB), WPW, premature ventricular contractions (PVCs), mechanical pacemaker rhythms.

QT — Congenital Syndromes
WPW
Ischemic heart disease
Drugs
Torsades
Hypokalemia,
  Hypomagnesemia,
  Hypocalcemia

QT AND QTc

- QTc — corrected QT.
- Normal: < 0.45 (< 6 months), < 0.44 (> 6 months).
- Beginning of Q to end of T.
- QTc = QT interval (sec) divided by the square root of the R-R interval (sec).
- Long QT predisposes to ventricular tachycardia and is associated with sudden death.

Abnormal Rhythms

Premature Atrial Contraction (PAC)

- Preceded by a P wave, followed by a normal QRS.
- The length of two cycles (R-R) including a PAC is usually shorter than the length of two normal cycles.
- No hemodynamic significance.

Premature Ventricular Contraction (PVC)

- Premature and wide QRS, no P wave, T wave opposite to QRS:
  - **Multifocal PVCs:** Different-shaped PVCs in same strip.
  - **Bigeminy:** Coupled beat (sinus, PVC, sinus, PVC).
  - **Trigeminy** (sinus, sinus, PVC, sinus, sinus, PVC).
  - **Couplets** (sinus, sinus, PVC, PVC, sinus, sinus).
- May be normal if they are uniform and ↓ with exercise.

Atrial Flutter

- A rapid atrial rate (~300 bpm) with a varying ventricular rate, depending on degree of block (ie, 2:1, 3:1).
- Sawtooth pattern (II, III, aVF, V1).
- Normal QRS.
- Usually suggests significant pathology (atrial enlargement).

Atrial Fibrillation

- Very fast atrial rate (350–600 bpm).
- Irregularly irregular ventricular response.
- No P waves; normal QRS.
- Usually suggests significant pathology.

Ventricular Tachycardia

- Series of 3++ PVCs with a heart rate between 120 and 200 bpm.
- Wide, unusually shaped QRS complexes.
- T waves in opposite direction of QRS complex.
- Usually suggests significant pathology.

Ventricular Fibrillation

- Very irregular QRS complexes.
- The rate is rapid and irregular.
- This is a terminal arrhythmia because the heart cannot maintain effective circulation.

Supraventricular Tachycardia (SVT)

- Typically narrow QRS complex, no variability in R-R internal.
- Reentrant tachycardia that utilizes the AV node in reentrant circuit.
- Sudden onset and resolution.
- Absent P waves.
- Usually associated with structurally normal hearts.
- SVT with aberrant conduction producing wide QRS may look like V-tach.

Axis

QRS Axis

- Examine leads I and aVF.
- In lead I, count all forces above the baseline by the number of boxes (mm) and subtract all forces below baseline. If the total is +[+], the axis range is between ++90° and –90°.
- Do the same in aVF. If the total is +[+], the QRS is also between 0° and ++180°.
- Superimpose the ranges. Region of overlap is quadrant QRS lies in.
- Find lead with isoelectric QRS complex. The axis points perpendicular to that lead.
- If all leads are equiphasic, the axis is perpendicular to all leads and perpendicular to that plane. It is directed anterior or posterior and called indeterminate.

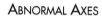

Axis Summary
0 to ++90: I++/aVF ++
0 to –90: I+/aVF–
+90 to 180: I–/aVF +
90 to 180: I–/aVF–

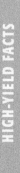

Abnormal Axes

- Right axis deviation (RAD): Caused by severe pulmonary stenosis with RVH, pulmonary hypertension (HTN), conduction disturbances (RBBB). RAD is normal in a newborn because of right ventricular dominance.
- Left axis deviation (LAD) with RVH is highly suggestive of AV canal. Consider especially with Down syndrome.
- Mild LAD with left ventricular hypertrophy (LVH) in a cyanotic infant suggests tricuspid atresia.

Quick Way to QRS Axis

Normal = [+] in lead I, [+] in aVF:

- I–, aVF– = Extreme axis deviation (direction based on Q wave).
- I+, aVF– = LAD.
- I, aVF+ = RAD.

P Axis

- Normal defines sinus rhythm and normally related atria (atrial situs solitus).
- A P axis between 0 and –90° may result from an ectopic low right atrial pacemaker (in absence of sinus node dysfunction, it is not significant).
- A P axis > +90° suggests atrial inversion or misplaced leads.

T Axis

- If differs by > 60 to 90° from QRS axis in presence of ventricular hypertrophy, it is called a "strain pattern" and may be a sign of ischemia.
- If strain is present, examine left precordial leads (V5, V6) for abnormal repolarization (indicated by T-wave inversion).
- LVH with strain in patients with aortic stenosis or hypertrophic cardiomyopathy is an ominous finding indicating severe disease.
- Varies depending on age.

Abnormal Wave Patterns and Voltages

ABNORMAL Q WAVES

- If no narrow Q waves in inferior (II, III, aVF) and leftward leads (I, V5, V6), suspect congenital heart disease (CHD) with ventricular inversion.
- Q waves of new onset or of ↑ duration of previous Q waves, with or without notching of Q, may represent myocardial infarction (MI). Uncommon.
- ST elevation or prolonged QTc is also supportive of MI.
- Causes of ischemia and infarction: Anomalous origin of left coronary artery from pulmonary artery, coronary artery aneurysm and thrombosis in Kawasaki disease, asphyxia, cardiomyopathy, severe aortic stenosis, myocarditis, cocaine use.
- A deep, wide Q wave in aVL is a marker for LV infarction. Suspect anomalous origin of left coronary artery, particularly in a child < 2 months old.

ST-T SEGMENT

- End of S to beginning of T.
- Causes of ST displacement: Pericarditis, cor pulmonale, pneumopericardium, head injury, pneumothorax, early ventricular repolarization, and normal atrial repolarization.
- Elevation may result from ischemia or pericarditis; depression is consistent with subendocardial ischemia or effects of digoxin.

T WAVE

- Peaked, pointed T waves occur with hyperkalemia, LVH, and head injury.
- Flattened T waves are seen in hypokalemia and hypothyroidism.

RIGHT ATRIAL ENLARGEMENT

- Peaked P waves (leads II and V1): P = > 2.5 mm (> 6 months) or > 3 mm (< 6 months).
- Causes include cor pulmonale (pulmonary hypertension, RVH), anomalous pulmonary venous connection, large ASD (uncommon), Ebstein's anomaly.

LEFT ATRIAL ENLARGEMENT

- Wide P wave (notched in II, deep terminal inversion in V1): P = > 0.08 sec (< 12 months old) or > 0.10 sec (> 12 months old).
- Causes include VSD, PDA, mitral stenosis.
- The wider and deeper the terminal component, the more severe the enlargement.

RIGHT VENTRICULAR HYPERTROPHY (RVH)

- R wave > 98% in V1 or S wave > 98% in I or V6.
- ↑ R/S ratio in V1 or ↓ R/S in V6.
- RSR' in V1 or V3R in the absence of complete RBBB. RSR' with R > 15 mm (> 1 year) is characteristic of RVH secondary to right ventricular overload.

- In newborns, a pure R wave in V1 > 10 mm = pressure-type RVH.
- Upright T wave in V1 (> 3 days).
- Presence of a Q wave in V1, V3R, V4R.
- Adult pattern may occur as early as 6 years.
- A qR pattern of Q wave in V1 suggests severe RVH.
- Causes include ASD, TAPVR, pulmonary stenosis, tetralogy of Fallot (TOF), large VSD with pulmonary HTN, coarctation in the newborn.
- **Caution!** The diagnosis of RVH via ECG should be made cautiously in newborns. Consider right-sided obstructive lesions (tetralogy of Fallot) in children > 6 months.

LEFT VENTRICULAR HYPERTROPHY (LVH)

- R > 98% in V6, S > 98% in V1.
- ↑ R/S ratio in V6 or ↓ R/S in V1.
- Q > 5 mm in V6 with peaked T (occurs with LV diastolic overload and denotes septal hypertrophy).
- Flat or inverted T waves in lead I or V6, in presence of LVH, suggests severe LVH.
- Excessive LAD supports LVH but is not sufficient to make the diagnosis.
- Causes include VSD, PDA, anemia, complete AV block, aortic stenosis, systemic HTN, obstructive and nonobstructive hypertrophic cardiomyopathies.

COMBINED VENTRICULAR HYPERTROPHY (CVH)

- If criteria for RVH exist and left ventricular forces exceed normal mean values for age, the patient has CVH.
- If LVH present, similar reasoning may apply to the diagnosis of RVH.
- In the presence of RVH, dominant RV forces diminish apparent LV forces, causing lower LV voltages (small R in V6 and small S in V1).
- Large equiphasic voltages in limb leads and midprecordial leads are called Katz-Wachtel phenomenon and suggest biventricular hypertrophy.
- Causes include left-to-right shunts with pulmonary HTN (large VSD) and complex structural heart disease.
- Cannot diagnose ventricular hypertrophy in the absence of normal conduction (RBBB).

DECREASED QRS VOLTAGE

- < 5 mm in limb leads.
- Causes include pericardial effusion, pericarditis, hypothyroidism.
- Sometimes normal newborns have ↓ voltages—not a concern.

WOLFF-PARKINSON-WHITE SYNDROME

- Ventricular preexcitation via accessory conduction pathway through the Bundle of Kent.
- Accessory pathway conducts more rapidly (than the normal AV node) but takes longer to recover.
- Shortened PR interval, widened QRS caused by slurred upstroke of the delta wave.
- Associated with Ebstein's anomaly.
- ↑ risk of SVT and sudden death.
- **Treatment:** Surgical ablation of accessory pathway.

Causes of Sudden Cardiac Deaths in Young Athlete
- Hypertrophic cardiomyopathy
- Arrhythmogenic right ventricular cardiomyopathy
- Congenital coronary artery anomalies
- Aortic rupture with Marfan syndrome
- Wolff-Parkinson-White syndrome
- Congenital long QT syndrome

- There are four basic cross-sectional views taken of the heart with **transthoracic echocardiography (TTE):**
  - Parasternal (long and short axis).
  - Apical.
  - Subcostal (taken in the midline below the xiphoid process).
  - Suprasternal.
- **Transesophageal echocardiography** employs a transducer introduced down the esophagus for enhanced imaging during cardiac surgery or catheterization.

2-D Echocardiography

- Cross-sectional images of the heart are seen via this method.
- **Parasternal views:**
  - Long axis: Left ventricular inflow and outflow tracts.
  - Short axis: Aortic valve, pulmonary valve, pulmonary artery and branches, right ventricular outflow tract, atrioventricular valves, right side of heart.
- **Apical views:** Atrial and ventricular septa, atria and ventricles, atrioventricular valves, pulmonary veins.
- **Subcostal views:** Atrial and ventricular septa, atrioventricular valves, atria and ventricles, and pulmonary venous drainage.
- **Suprasternal views:** Ascending and descending aorta, pulmonary artery size, systemic and pulmonary veins.

In infants and children, coronary arteries can be evaluated nicely using TTE.

Color-Flow Doppler Echocardiography

- Blood flow and direction can be seen via this method.
  - Red indicates blood flowing toward the transducer.
  - Blue indicates blood flowing away from the transducer.
- When blood flow velocity exceeds a certain limit (called the Nyquist limit), the color signal is often yellow. This is indicative of high velocities that may be seen in VSDs, ASDs, and valvar regurgitation and stenosis.

M Mode Echocardiography

- In this mode, the information from one scan point is measured over time.
- Motion creates a graph of depth of structures (ie, valves, ventricular wall, etc.) versus time.
- This modality is used to determine cardiac chamber dimension, valve annuli size, fractional shortening and ejection fraction, left ventricular mass.

Fetal Echocardiography

- For the prenatal diagnosis of congenital heart diseases.
- Allows for improved counseling and better understanding of the postnatal prognosis.
- Screen at > 16 weeks.

- Indications:
  - Fetal:
    - Abnormal screening obstetric ultrasound.
    - Extracardiac anomalies.
    - Chromosomal abnormalities.
    - ↑ first-trimester nuchal translucency measurement (trisomy 21 and Turner syndrome).
  - Maternal (diabetes, phenylketonuria).

INTERPRETATION OF PEDIATRIC CHEST X-RAYS

Heart Size

Cardiothoracic ratio:

- Measure largest width of the heart and divide by the largest diameter of the chest. A normal ratio is < 0.5.
- The CXR must have a good inspiratory effort. For this reason, newborns and infants are difficult to evaluate by this method.
- Cardiomegaly on CXR is most suggestive of volume overload; ECG better reflects ↑ pressure.

Cardiac Chamber Enlargement

- **Left atrial enlargement (LAE):**
  - May produce a "double density" on the PA CXR.
  - More severe LAE can elevate the left mainstem bronchus.
- **Right atrial enlargement (RAE):** RAE is noted most at the right lower cardiac border; however, it is difficult to diagnose by CXR alone.
- **Left ventricular enlargement:**
  - The apex is seen further to the left and downward.
  - On lateral CXR, the posterior cardiac border is further displaced posteriorly.
- **Right ventricular enlargement:**
  - VH is not seen well on PA CXR because it does not make up the cardiac silhouette.
  - On lateral CXR, it is noted by filling the retrosternal space.

Pulmonary Vascular Markings

INCREASED PULMONARY VASCULAR MARKINGS

- Noted by the visualization of pulmonary vasculature in the lateral one-third of the lung field.
- In an **acyanotic** child this could be ASD, VSD, PDA, endocardial cushion defect, or partial anomalous pulmonary venous return.
- In a **cyanotic** child this could be transposition of the great arteries, TAPVR, hypoplastic left heart syndrome, persistent truncus arteriosus, or single ventricle.

In newborns and small infants, the upper aspects of the heart are obscured by a large "boat sail–shaped" opacity — the thymus. This organ will involute after puberty. It is often not seen in premature newborns.

DECREASED PULMONARY VASCULAR MARKINGS

- The lung fields are dark, with small vessels.
- Seen in pulmonary stenosis and atresia, tricuspid stenosis and atresia, tetralogy of Fallot.

PULMONARY VENOUS CONGESTION

- Manifested as hazy lung fields.
- Kerley B lines are often present.
- Caused by LV failure or obstruction of the pulmonary veins.
- Seen in mitral stenosis, TAPVR, cor triatriatum, hypoplastic left heart syndrome, or any left-sided obstructive lesion with heart failure.

Abnormal Cardiac Silhouettes

TETRALOGY OF FALLOT

- A "boot-shaped" heart with ↓ pulmonary vascular markings is sometimes seen. The boot is due to the hypoplastic main pulmonary artery.
- RVH is noted.
- About 25% will have a right aortic arch.

Transposition of the Great Arteries

- An "egg-shaped" heart is sometimes seen.
- The narrow superior aspect of the cardiac silhouette is due to the absence of the thymus and the irregular relationship of the great arteries.

TOTAL ANOMALOUS PULMONARY VENOUS RETURN

- A "snowman" shape is sometimes seen.
- The left vertical vein, left innominate vein, and dilated superior vena cava create the "snowman's" head.

RHEUMATIC FEVER

DEFINITION

- Rheumatic fever is a delayed immunologic sequela of a previous group A streptococcal infection of the pharynx (not of the skin).
- Cutaneous streptococcal infection is a precursor of glomerulonephritis.
- Affects the brain, heart, joints, and skin.

EPIDEMIOLOGY

- Although an uncommon disease in the United States, small outbreaks occur in various regions.
- Peak age range: 6–15 years.
- A positive family history of rheumatic fever ↑ risk.
- Incidence: 0.3–3% in developed countries.
- Risk of RF after untreated strep pharyngitis is 1–3%.
- Patients with the infection < 3 weeks have a 0.3% risk.
- Follows pharyngitis by 1–5 weeks (average: 3 weeks).
- Rate of recurrent RF with subsequent strep infection may approach 65%.
- Recurrence rate ↓ to < 10% over 10 years.

Jones Criteria (Modified)

2 major or 1 major + 2 minor

Major—J♥NES:
- **Joints**—polyarthritis
- **♥**—carditis
- **Nodules**, subcutaneous
- **Erythema marginatum**
- **Sydenham's chorea**

Minor:
- Arthralgia
- Fever
- Elevated erythrocyte sedimentation rate (ESR) or C-reactive protein (CRP)
- Prolonged P-R interval

Plus
- Laboratory evidence of antecedent group A strep infection (ASO titer)

Absence of tachycardia or murmur usually excludes the diagnosis of myocarditis.

Rheumatic fever can cause long-term valvular disease, both stenosis and insufficiency.

DIAGNOSIS

- To diagnose acute rheumatic fever you must fulfill the following combination of the Jones criteria:
  - Two major manifestations *or*
  - One major and two minor manifestations
- In addition to the major and minor manifestations, patients may appear pale and complain of abdominal pain and epistaxis.
- Aschoff bodies (found in atrial myocardium) are diagnostic.

CARDITIS

- Incidence: 50% of patients.
- Clinical presentation:
  - Tachycardia is common.
  - Heart murmur, most commonly due to valvulitis of the following (in order of decreasing frequency):
    - Mitral valve regurgitation
    - Aortic valve regurgitation
    - Tricuspid valve regurgitation—less common.
  - Pericarditis (a friction rub may be heard).
  - Cardiomegaly.
  - CHF (a gallop may be heard).

ARTHRITIS

- Most common manifestation, affecting 70%.
- Usually affects the large joints, but can affect the spine and cranial joints.
- Migratory in nature, affecting a new joint as other affected joints resolve (can affect more than one joint at a time).
- Joints are red, warm, swollen, and very tender, particularly if moved.
- Responds well to aspirin therapy (give once diagnosis is confirmed).
- Duration is usually < 1 month, even without treatment.

CHOREA

- Incidence: 15% of patients; most commonly prepubertal girls.
- Movements last on average 7 months before slowly diminishing (can last up to 17 months).
- Characteristics:
  - Initial emotional lability: Behaviors characteristic of attention deficit/hyperactivity disorder (ADHD) and obsessive-compulsive disorder (OCD) have been noted to precede the movement disorder.
  - Loss of motor coordination.
  - Spontaneous, purposeless movement.
  - Motor weakness.

ERYTHEMA MARGINATUM

- Incidence: < 10% of patients.
- Pink, erythematous macular rash.
- Often has a clear center and serpiginous outline.
- Nonpruritic.
- Evanescent and migratory.
- Disappears when cold.
- Reappears when warm.
- Found primarily on the trunk and proximal extremities.

Subcutaneous Nodules

- Incidence: 2–10% of patients.
- Hard, painless, small (0.5–1 cm) swellings over bony prominences, primarily the extensor tendons of the hand.
- Can also be found on the scalp and along the spine.
- Not transient, lasting for weeks.

Diagnosis

- Streptococcal antibody tests are the most reliable evidence of preceding group A strep infection → acute rheumatic fever.
- Antistreptolysin O (ASO) titer is the most commonly used. It is elevated in 80% of patients with acute rheumatic fever (ARF) and 20% of normal individuals.
- Other antibody tests exist (antihyaluronidase, antistreptokinase, antideoxyribonuclease B) wherein at least one will be positive in 95% of patients with ARF.
- Positive throat cultures and "rapid strep tests" are less reliable because they do not differentiate acute infection versus chronic carrier state.

Treatment

- Upon diagnosis, the patient should receive benzathine penicillin G 1.2 million units IM to eradicate the streptococci (if < 27 kg = 600,000 U).
- Patients allergic to penicillin can receive 4 days of erythromycin 40 mg/kg/day.
- Prophylaxis should be initiated:
  - Benzathine penicillin G 1.2 million units IM every 3–4 weeks *or*
  - Penicillin 200,000 units PO three times per day *or*
  - Sulfadiazine 1 g PO once per day
- Length of prophylaxis is undetermined but often advocated at least throughout adolescence, if not indefinitely. Obviously, compliance becomes a difficult issue.
- Seventy-five percent of patients recover within 6 weeks, and less than 5% are symptomatic beyond 6 months. Seventy percent of those with carditis recover without permanent cardiac damage.

If a patient's arthritis doesn't improve within 48 hours of therapeutic aspirin therapy, he or she probably does not have rheumatic fever.

The chorea of rheumatic fever is known as Syndenham's chorea or St. Vitus' dance.

Erythema marginatum is never found on the face.

ENDOCARDITIS

A 6-year-old girl with PDA develops fever and anorexia. Her Hgb is 9; she has hematuria, ↑ ESR, positive rheumatoid factor (RF), and immune complexes are present. *Think: Bacterial endocarditis.*

Predisposition: Congenital heart disease. Greatest risk: Systemic-pulmonary arterial communications such as patent ductus arteriosus. Chronic anemia, microscopic hematuria, elevated ESR, positive rheumatoid factor, circulating immune complexes, and low complement levels *are* all may be present in infective endocarditis.

Etiology

- α-Hemolytic streptococci are most common (70%).
- *Streptococcus viridans.*

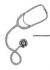
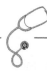

Subcutaneous nodules are also found in connective tissue diseases such as systemic lupus erythematosus (SLE) and rheumatoid arthritis.

Subcutaneous nodules in rheumatic fever have a significant association with carditis.

A history of sore throat or scarlet fever is insufficient evidence for rheumatic fever without a positive strep test.

Carditis is the only manifestation of rheumatic fever that can cause permanent cardiac damage. Therefore, once definitively diagnosed, anti-inflammatory therapy (with prednisone in extreme cases, or aspirin) should be started.

- *Staphylococcus aureus* is also common, accounting for 20% of cases.
- If felt to be secondary to cardiac surgery complications, *Staphylococcus epidermidis*, gram-negative bacilli, and fungi should be considered.
- Culture-negative endocarditis: *Coxiella burnetii* or *Bartonella*.
- Most endocarditis is left-sided.
- Right-sided endocarditis is associated with IV drug use.

PATHOPHYSIOLOGY

Most likely to occur on congenitally abnormal valves, valves damaged by rheumatic fever, acquired valvular lesions, prosthetic replacement valves, and any cardiac defect → turbulent blood flow.

SIGNS AND SYMPTOMS

- Fever is most common.
- New or changing heart murmur.
- Chest pain, dyspnea, arthralgia, myalgia, headache.
- Embolic phenomena:
  - Hematuria with red cell casts.
  - Acute brain ischemia.
  - Roth spots, splinter hemorrhages, Osler nodes, Janeway lesions (less common in children).

PREDISPOSING CONDITIONS

- High risk:
  - Prosthetic cardiac valves.
  - Previous bacterial endocarditis (due to scar formation on valve).
  - Congenital heart disease—complex cyanotic types.
  - Surgical pulmonary-systemic shunts.
- Moderate risk:
  - Congenital cardiac diseases not in high and low risk.
  - Acquired valvular dysfunction.
  - Rheumatic heart disease, Libman-Sacks valve, antiphospholipid syndrome–associated valve disease.
  - Hypertrophic cardiomyopathy.
  - Complicated mitral valve prolapse (valvular regurgitation, thickened valve leaflets).
- Low risk:
  - Isolated ASD, secundum type.
  - Surgically repaired cardiac defects > 6 months postoperative (ASD, VSD, PDA).
  - Heart murmurs with normal echocardiogram (physiologic or functional, flow murmurs).
  - Systemic diseases without cardiac valve involvement:
    - Kawasaki disease: Normal echo only.
    - Rheumatic heart disease: Normal echo only.
  - Cardiac pacemakers and implantable defibrillators.

DIAGNOSIS

- Four sets of blood cultures over 48 hours from different sites.
- Most common findings:
  - Positive blood cultures
  - Elevated ESR

- Hematuria
- Anemia
- Echocardiographic evidence of vegetations or thrombi is diagnostic.

TREATMENT

- Four to eight weeks of organism-specific antibiotic therapy.
- Surgery is necessary when endocarditis is refractory to medical treatment. Also considered in cases of prosthetic valves, fungal endocarditis, and hemodynamic compromise.
- Antibiotic prophylaxis is necessary for children with structural heart disease and other predisposing conditions.

PROPHYLAXIS RECOMMENDATIONS

- Prophylaxis is recommended with:
  - Most dental and periodontal procedures.
  - Tonsillectomy or adenoidectomy.
  - Rigid bronchoscopy or surgery involving gastrointestinal (GI) or upper respiratory mucosa.
  - Gallbladder surgery.
  - Catheterization in setting of urinary tract infection, cystoscopy, urethral dilation.
  - Urinary tract surgery.
  - Incision and drainage of infected tissues.
- Prophylaxis is *not* usually recommended with:
  - Intraoral injection of local anesthetic.
  - Shedding of primary teeth.
  - Tympanostomy tube insertion.
  - Endotracheal tube insertion.
  - Bronchoscopy with flexible bronchoscope.
  - Transesophageal echo.
  - Cardiac catheterization.
  - Cesarean section (only when no infection present).
  - GI endoscopy, with or without biopsy (prophylaxis for high-risk patients).
  - Genitourinary (GU) procedures with no infection present (except those above).
  - Circumcision.

Janeway lesions — painless
Osler nodes — painful

Risk Factors for Endocarditis
- Previous endocarditis
- Dental procedures
- Gastrointestinal and genitourinary procedures
- IV drug use (usually affects the tricuspid valve)
- Indwelling central venous catheters
- Prior cardiac surgery

MYOCARDITIS

ETIOLOGY

- Most often caused by viruses. Coxsackieviruses and echoviruses are most common. Recent evidence suggests adenovirus as a common etiology.
- Immune-mediated diseases (eg, acute rheumatic fever, Kawasaki disease).
- Collagen vascular diseases.
- Toxic ingestions.

EPIDEMIOLOGY

Clinically recognizable myocarditis is rare in the United States.

SIGNS AND SYMPTOMS

- Presentation depends on the degree of myocardial injury.
- Ranges from asymptomatic to fulminant CHF.
- Common symptoms are fever, dyspnea, upper respiratory symptoms, vomiting, and lethargy.
- CHF should be considered if patient is tachycardic and tachypneic and has a gallop on auscultation.

DIAGNOSIS

- ECG findings: Low voltages, S-T changes, prolonged QT interval, premature beats.
- Radiology: Chest radiographs will show cardiomegaly.
- Echocardiography: Chamber enlargement is present with impaired ventricular function.

TREATMENT

- First, treat the underlying cause (ie, antibiotics if bacterial).
- Since it is most often viral, treatment is largely supportive. Rest and activity limitation is important.
- Treatment of CHF may be necessary (ie, diuretics, inotropic agents if severely ill). Gamma globulin also has been effective.

PERICARDITIS

ETIOLOGY

- Viral (most common).
- Bacterial infection (also common): acute rheumatic fever, *S aureus*, *Haemophilus influenzae*, *Neisseria meningitidis*, streptococci, tuberculosis.
- Complications from heart surgery.
- Collagen vascular diseases.
- Uremia.
- Medications (ie, dantrolene, oncology agents).

SIGNS AND SYMPTOMS

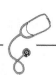

Digitalis is typically not given in pericarditis, as this blocks the compensatory tachycardia the heart utilizes to overcome ↓ venous return.

- Precordial pain with radiation to the shoulder and neck (often relieved by standing).
- **Pericardial friction rub** on auscultation.
- Signs of cardiac tamponade:
  - Distant heart sounds.
  - Tachycardia.
  - Pulsus paradoxus.
  - Hepatomegaly and venous distention.

DIAGNOSIS

- CXR: A pear- or water bottle–shaped heart indicates a large effusion.
- Echocardiography is diagnostic (can also detect tamponade).

TREATMENT

- Treat the underlying disease process.
- Supportive treatment for viral etiologies.

- Pericardiocentesis is indicated if effusion is present.
- Urgent drainage is indicated when symptoms of tamponade are present.

CONGESTIVE HEART FAILURE (CHF)

ETIOLOGY

- Caused from either congenital heart disease (CHD) or acquired heart disease.
- CHD: Most common cause is from volume or pressure overload.
- VSD, PDA, and endocardial cushion defects are the most common causes of CHF in the first 6 months of life.
- ASD can cause CHF in adulthood if unrepaired.
- Acquired heart disease: Potential causes of CHF are metabolic abnormalities (ie, hypoxia, acidosis, hypoglycemia, hypocalcemia), myocarditis, rheumatic fever with carditis, cardiomyopathy, and drug toxicity.

SIGNS AND SYMPTOMS

- Often similar symptoms to those found in respiratory illnesses: tachycardia, tachypnea, shortness of breath, rales and rhonchi, intercostal retractions.
- Poor weight gain/poor feeding.
- Cold sweat on forehead.
- Older children develop peripheral edema.
- Gallop on auscultation.
- Hepatomegaly, jugular venous distention (JVD).

DIAGNOSIS

- CXR: Cardiomegaly, evidence of pulmonary edema.
- Echo: Enlarged ventricular chamber, impaired ventricular function.

TREATMENT

- Treat the underlying cause (ie, surgical correction of CHD, correction of metabolic defects).
- Oxygen can be used if patient is hypoxic or in respiratory distress.
- Medication:
  - **Digitalis** is used to improve ventricular function. Contraindicated in complete heart block and hypertrophic cardiomyopathy.
  - **Diuretics** are used to ↓ volume overload and pulmonary edema. Most common are the "loop diuretics" (ie, furosemide).
  - **Afterload-reducing agents** (ie, angiotensin-converting enzyme [ACE] inhibitors, calcium channel blockers, nitroglycerin) are used to dilate peripheral vasculature and thus ↓ the work on the heart.

VASCULITIDES

Henoch-Schönlein Purpura

- Immune-mediated vasculitis that affects the GI tract, joints, and kidneys and causes a characteristic rash (see Chapter 20).
- Palpable purpura.

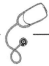

Onset of CHF is dependent on the fall of pulmonary vascular resistance and the subsequent ↑ left-to-right shunting.

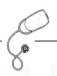

A left-to-right shunt usually takes about 6 weeks to become significant enough to stress the left ventricle.

Use of diuretics in CHF is preferred to salt and fluid restriction.

Watch out for hypokalemia, as ↑ potassium is lost with some diuretic use.

Hypokalemia can precipitate digitalis toxicity.

- Most often occurs in winter months, following a group A streptococcal upper respiratory infection (URI).
- GI involvement is most significant, → vomiting and upper and lower GI bleeding.
- Renal involvement, in the form of glomerulonephritis, with RBC casts, can progress to acute renal failure. More common is chronic proteinuria, which can be a late sequelae.
- Treatment is supportive, with full recovery within 4–6 weeks.

Kawasaki Disease

A 2-year-old boy with fever for 7 days, often reaching 104°F (40°C), develops nonexudative conjunctival injection bilaterally; intensely erythematous lips, palms, and soles; generalized erythema multiforme; and an enlarged, tender anterior cervical lymph node. Blood cultures are sterile, and platelets are ↑. *Think: Kawasaki disease.*

Beware of his risk for coronary aneurysms and MI. Fever lasting for 5 or more days is the hallmark that must be present with at least four of the following features: conjunctival injection, oropharyngeal mucous membrane changes, extremity changes, polymorphous rash, and cervical lymphadenopathy.

DEFINITION

- Also known as mucocutaneous lymph node syndrome.
- Most common acquired heart disease in children.

ETIOLOGY

Acute vasculitis of unknown etiology.

EPIDEMIOLOGY

- Affects infants and young children (> 80% under age 4 years).
- More common in Asians than other racial groups.
- More common in males than females (ratio 1.5:1).
- Most common in winter/spring months.

SIGNS AND SYMPTOMS

- Sterile pyuria.
- Aseptic meningitis.
- Thrombocytosis.
- Desquamation of fingers and toes.
- Elevated ESR or CRP.
- Most significant sequelae:
  - Coronary aneurysms (usually resolve within 12 months of adequate therapy).
  - Pericardial effusion.
  - CHF.

PLTS ↑

RISK MI
aneurysm

DIAGNOSIS

- Diagnostic criteria: Fever for > 5 days plus ≥ 4 of the following:
    1. Bilateral conjunctivitis (without exudate).
    2. Mucocutaneous lesions ("strawberry" tongue; dry, red, cracked lips; diffuse erythema of oral cavity).
    3. Changes in upper and lower extremities (erythema and/or edema of hands/feet).
    4. Polymorphic rash (usually truncal).
    5. Cervical lymphadenopathy (> 1.5 cm in diameter), usually unilateral.
- Echocardiogram: Initial study at diagnosis to establish baseline and to evaluate for early coronary aneurysms; follow-up echo to establish presence or absence.

TREATMENT

- Used to prevent cardiac sequelae.
- Intravenous immune globulin (IVIG): Usually one dose of IVIG, 2 g/kg over 10–12 hr. Reduces incidence of coronary artery dilation (< 3%).
- High-dose aspirin (80–100 mg/kg/day divided in four doses) until 48–72 hr after defervescence.
- If no coronary artery abnormality, low-dose aspirin (3–5 mg/kg/day as a single daily dose) for 6–8 weeks or until platelet count and ESR are normal.
- If coronary artery abnormality, continue indefinitely in consultation with a pediatric cardiologist. Aspirin is reduced after the patient is afebrile for 48 hours.
- Use of steroids remains controversial and typically reserved for cases refractory to repeat doses of IVIG.

Polyarteritis Nodosa

DEFINITION

A necrotizing inflammation of the small and medium-sized muscular arteries.

SIGNS AND SYMPTOMS

- Prolonged fever, weight loss, malaise, subcutaneous nodules on extremities.
- Various rashes can be associated with this condition.
- Respiratory symptoms: Rhinorrhea, congestion.
- Often waxes and wanes.
- Gangrene of distal extremities is found in severe disease.

DIAGNOSIS

- No diagnostic tests.
- Associated with abnormal cell counts (thrombocytosis, leukocytosis), abnormal urine analysis, elevated acute-phase reactants, perinuclear antineutrophil cytoplasmic antibody (p-ANCA).
- Conclusive with findings of medium-sized artery aneurysms.
- Echocardiographic evidence of coronary artery aneurysms is diagnostic if other clinical evidence is present.

Hypertension and abdominal pain can be important clues in polyarteritis nodosa.

TREATMENT

- Corticosteroids suppress the clinical manifestations.
- Cyclophosphamide or azathioprine may be required to induce remission.

Takayasu's Arteritis

DEFINITION

- Also known as aortoarteritis.
- Chronic inflammatory disease involving:
  - Aorta.
  - Arterial branches from the aorta.
  - Pulmonary vasculature.

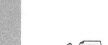

Takayasu arteritis is also known as "pulseless disease."

PATHOPHYSIOLOGY

- Lesions are segmental and often obliterative.
- Aneurysmal and saccular dilation also occur.
- Thoracoabdominal aorta is the predominantly affected site in the pediatric population.

EPIDEMIOLOGY

Most patients are female, aged 4–45 years.

SIGNS AND SYMPTOMS

- A significant number of patients experience LV dysfunction and CHF (even in the absence of coronary artery involvement, HTN, or valvular abnormalities).
- A lymphocytic infiltration consistent with myocarditis is present in about 50% of patients.
- Other symptoms include fever, polyarthralgias, polyarthritis, and loss of radial pulsations.

Essentially, Takayasu arteritis is giant cell arteritis of the aorta (and large branches).

TREATMENT

Corticosteroids may induce remission.

Wegener's Granulomatosis

DEFINITION

A rare vasculitis of both arteries and veins → widespread necrotizing granumolas.

EPIDEMIOLOGY

Most common in adults, although occurrence in children has been described.

Children with cyanotic heart disease are at ↑ risk for strokes and scoliosis.

SIGNS AND SYMPTOMS

- Rhinorrhea, nasal mucosa ulcers, sinusitis.
- Hematuria.
- Cough, hemoptysis, pleuritis.
- Heart involvement: Granulamatous inflammation of cardiac muscle causing arrhythmias.

DIAGNOSIS

- Antineutrophil cytoplasmic antibodies (c-ANCA) are present.
- ESR is greatly elevated.
- Organ biopsy (kidney and/or lung) may be essential to establish early diagnosis.

TREATMENT

- Corticosteroids alone may be unsuccessful.
- Cyclophosphamide or azathioprine is recommended (have changed a once uniformly fatal disease into an excellent prognosis).

Central Cyanosis versus Acrocyanosis

- Central cyanosis:
  - Involves mucous membranes.
  - Always pathologic in a newborn.
  - Cyanosis in neonates is almost always due to either pulmonary or cardiac disease.
  - > 5 mg/dL of deoxyhemoglobin.
- Acrocyanosis:
  - Involves distal extremities.
  - Normal in newborns.
  - Peripheral cyanosis is the result of acrocyanosis, exposure to cold, and ↓ peripheral perfusion.

CYANOTIC HEART DEFECTS

See Figure 13-2.

Tetralogy of Fallot (TOF)

The most common form of cyanotic CHD in the postinfancy period.

DEFINITION

Four anomalies constitute the tetralogy:

1. Right ventricular outflow tract obstruction (RVOTO). (PS)
2. VSD.
3. Aortic override.
4. RVH.

ETIOLOGY

Prenatal factors associated include maternal rubella or viral illness.

PATHOPHYSIOLOGY

RVOTO dictates degree of shunting:
- **Minimal obstruction:** → ↑ pulmonary blood flow as pulmonary vascular resistance (PVR) ↓, → CHF.
- **Mild obstruction:** Hemodynamic balance pressure between right and left ventricles is equal, thus no net shunting ("pink tet").
- **Severe obstruction:** ↓ pulmonary blood flow, → cyanosis.

Cyanotic Heart Defects
Five T's and a P
Tetralogy of Fallot
Transposition of the great vessels
Truncus arteriosus
Tricuspid atresia
Total anomalous pulmonary venous return (obstructive)
Pulmonic atresia

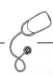

Two key features are required for diagnosis of TOF:
- **VSD** (typically large enough to equalize pressures in right and left ventricles).
- **RVOTO** (eg, pulmonary stenosis).
- **Aortic override** is variable.
- **RVH** is secondary to the RVOTO.

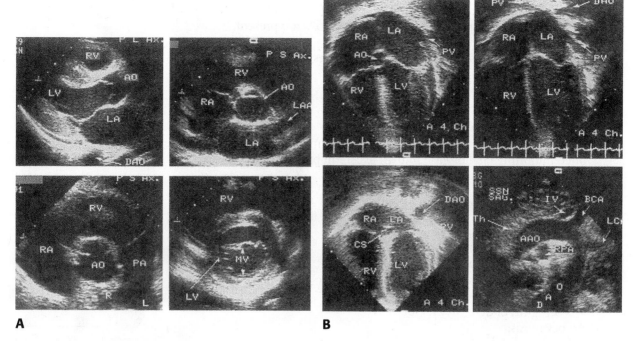

FIGURE 13-2. Basic echocardiography views.

A. *Top left*: This frame, taken from a normal subject, is a parasternal long-axis (P L Ax) view taken slicing the heart from a parasternal location at the fourth left interspace, subtending a sector with the right ventricle (RV) anteriorly. The sound beams then pass through the ventricular septum and the aorta (AO), the left ventricular cavity (LV), and the left ventricular posterior wall. Behind the ascending aortic root is the left atrium (LA). Posterior to the heart behind the pericardium, the descending aorta (DAO) can be seen running in its cross-section, indicating how far from the sagittal body plane this image is as the descending aorta runs on the left of the spine. *Bottom left*: From the same normal subject in the parasternal short-axis (P S Ax) view from the third intercostal space. The sector subtends the right side of the heart as it winds around the aortic root (AO) in the center of image. The right atrium (RA) is separated from the right ventricle (RV) by the tricuspid valve. The pulmonary artery (PA) is separated from the right ventricle by the pulmonary valve. The cusps of the aortic valve can also be identified in this figure. The pulmonary artery bifurcates into its left (L) and right branches. *Top right, bottom right*: These parasternal short-axis (P S Ax) views taken from the same normal subject are sequential scans through the heart from the top to the bottom (from the cranial-to-caudal direction). The *top frame* represents a short-axis view of the entire right heart. In the center, the aortic valve (AO) cusps are seen in their open position, demonstrating a tri-leaflet aortic valve. Posteriorly, the left atrium (LA), with the left atrial appendage (LAA) extending to the left side of the heart, is observed. The interatrial septum separates the left atrium from the right atrium (RA). The tricuspid valve separates the right atrium from the right ventricle (RV). In the *bottom frame* with the caudal scan, the right (RV) and left (LV) ventricles are seen. The ventricular septum is seen between the two ventricles. The mitral valve (MV) is seen in its open position with the anterior cusp (arrow) at the top and the posterior cusp (arrow) at the bottom.

B. This is a series of apical four-chamber views (A 4 Ch) from a normal subject, demonstrating the scan from the anterior to the posterior aspect of the heart (from the apex to base). The electrocardiogram shown on the bottom indicates the timing within the cardiac cycle. The *top frame* is taken in systole. A left pulmonary vein (PV) can be seen entering the left atrium (LA). The right atrium (RA) is separated from the left atrium (LA) by the faint echo of the interatrial septum. The aortic root (AO) can be seen to be arising out of the heart, and the left and right ventricles (LV, RV) can be seen separated from their respective atria by the tricuspid and mitral valves in the closed position, and from each other by the ventricular septum. The *second frame*, taken with more caudal scanning, demonstrates the descending aorta in cross-section, the pulmonary veins (PV) from the left and the right (arrows), the atria, and the ventricles. This is an end-systolic frame, as seen from the electrocardiogram. The *third frame*, taken with most caudal scanning, demonstrates the descending aorta (DAO) posteriorly, and a small portion of the left atrium (LA) with a coronary sinus (CS) running inferiorly at the crux of the heart. The other labels are as for the previous panels. The *fourth frame* shows the aortic arch from the suprasternal notch sagittal view (SSN, SAG) in a normal infant. The scan comes from the suprasternal notch area, and the sector subtends the innominate vein (IV) superiorly, as it crosses in front of the ascending aorta (AAO). The whole arch is seen from the ascending aorta to the descending aorta (DAO). The brachiocephalic artery (BCA) and left carotid artery (LCA) can be seen arising from the aortic arch. The circular right pulmonary artery can be seen running under the arch (RPA). The label obscures the area of the right bronchus, lying between the aortic arch and the right pulmonary artery. Anteriorly, the thymus (Th) is identified.

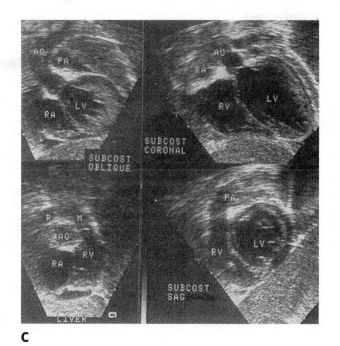

C

FIGURE 13-2. **Basic echocardiography views. (continued)**

C. These images from a normal subject are taken with the subcostal transducer position in coronal and sagittal (SAG) planes. The scans pass from the subcostal region through the liver and diaphragm, and into the heart. *Right panels:* In the *top right panel* with posterior angulation, the left ventricle (LV) and right ventricle (RV) are identified. The aorta (AO) arises from the left ventricle, separated from it by the aortic valve; the right atrium (RA) and right ventricle (RV) can be identified. The *bottom right panel,* taken in an orthogonal cut in the sagittal plane, demonstrates the left ventricle (LV) cut in cross-section with its papillary muscles; the right ventricle (RV) and pulmonary artery (PA) can be seen wrapping around the left ventricle. *Left panels:* These subcostal oblique cuts demonstrate the exit of the aorta (AO) and the pulmonary artery (PA) from their respective ventricles, the left ventricle (LV) and the right ventricle (RV). In the *upper left panel,* the aorta (AO) can be seen arising from the left ventricle (LV) and arching toward the left side over the main pulmonary artery (PA). In the *bottom left panel,* taken with an orthogonal view and more anterior angulation, the right-sided structures, right atrium (RA), right ventricle (RV), main (M) pulmonary artery, and right (R) pulmonary artery can be seen as they surround the aortic valve (AO). (Reproduced, with permission, from *Rudolph's Pediatrics,* 20th ed. Appleton & Lange, 1996.)

EPIDEMIOLOGY

Most common cyanotic heart defect in children who survive infancy.

SIGNS AND SYMPTOMS

- Failure to thrive (FTT) (if diagnosed late).
- "Conotruncal facies."
- Variable cyanosis (clubbing later if unrepaired).
- RV impulse; occasional thrill; single S2, systolic ejection murmur at the upper left sternal border with or without ejection click.
- Squatting is a common posture in older, unoperated children with TOF:
    - Often occurs after exercise.
    - Causes trapping of desaturated blood in the lower extremities and ↑ systemic vascular resistance (SVR) while the RVOTO remains fixed. Thus, it:
        - ↓ right-to-left shunting.
        - ↑ pulmonary blood flow.
        - ↑ arterial saturation.

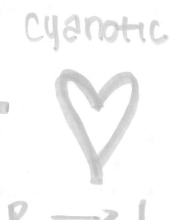

"TET SPELLS"

- Most common: 2–6 months of age.
- Occur in the morning or after a nap when SVR is low.
- Precipitating factors:
  - Stress
  - Drugs that ↓ SVR
  - Hot baths
  - Fever
  - Exercise
- Mechanism: Unknown, but likely due to ↑ cardiac output with fixed RVOT, → ↑ right-to-left shunting, which ↑ cyanosis
- If prolonged or severe: Syncope, seizures, cardiac arrest.

DIAGNOSIS

- CXR (Figure 13-3).
- "Boot-shaped heart."
- ↓ pulmonary vascular markings.
- Right aortic arch (25%).

TREATMENT

- Patient's clinical status may prevent definitive repair initially.
- Shunting (ie, Blalock-Taussig shunt) is often used when pulmonary stenosis is severe and an alternative route for blood to reach the lungs is necessary.
- Complete repair entails:
  - VSD closure.
  - Relief of RVOTO.
  - Ligation of shunts.
  - ASD/patent foramen ovale (PFO) closure.

CXR with the boot shape, ↓ pulmonary vascular markings, and a right aortic arch. *Think: Tetralogy of Fallot.*

Without repair of TOF, mortality is:
- 50% by 3 years
- 90% by 20 years
- 95% by 30 years

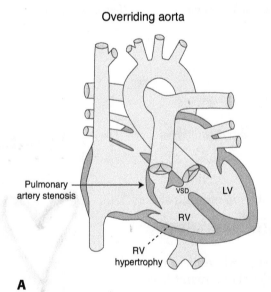

Overriding aorta

Pulmonary artery stenosis

VSD

LV

RV

RV hypertrophy

A

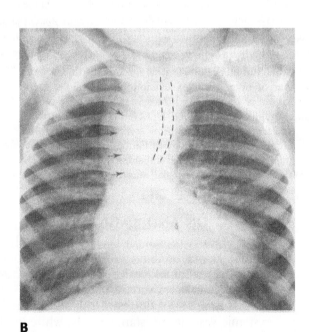

B

FIGURE 13-3. Chest x-ray in tetralogy of Fallot.

Arrows indicate right-sided aortic arch and upper thoracic aorta. Dashed lines indicate right-sided aortic indentation on the air bronchogram. (X-ray reproduced, with permission, from Rudolph CD, et al (eds). *Rudolph's Pediatrics*, 21st ed. New York: McGraw-Hill, 2002: 1821.)

Transposition of the Great Vessels

The most common cyanotic heart lesion in the newborn period.

PATHOPHYSIOLOGY

This lesion occurs when, in the development of the heart, the primitive heart loops to the left instead of the right and the following result (see Figure 13-4):

- Aorta originates from the RV.
- Pulmonary artery originates from LV.
- Aorta is anterior; pulmonary trunk is posterior.
- Right and left hearts are in parallel:
  - Pulmonary venous return goes to the pulmonary artery via left ventricle.
  - Systemic venous return goes to the aorta via the right ventricle.
- The presence of a VSD, ASD, or PDA is essential to survival.
- A PDA alone is usually not sufficient to allow adequate mixing in the extrauterine environment.
- Cyanosis becomes more prevalent with the closure of the PDA.
- Presentation: CHF in the first week of life.
- CXR: Egg-shaped heart with a narrow mediastinum. Cardiomegaly with ↑ pulmonary vascular marking.

EPIDEMIOLOGY

Most common cyanotic congenital heart defect presenting in the neonatal period.

Intact Ventricular Septum (with no valve abnormality)	With VSD (a large VSD allows adequate mixing)

SIGNS AND SYMPTOMS

- Early cyanosis, a single S2, and no murmur.
- An intact atrial septum or very restrictive PFO is a medical emergency.

- Symptoms are related to ↑ pulmonary blood flow, with CHF sometimes occurring early.
- May have little cyanosis.

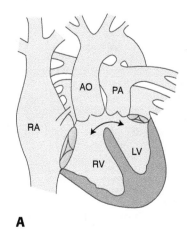 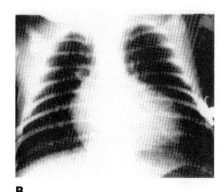

FIGURE 13-4.   Transposition of the great vessels.

"Egg on a string"—spinal column serving as the string and the globular presentation of the heart as the egg. (X-ray reproduced, with permission, from Moller JH, Neal WA. *Fetal, Neonatal, and Infant Cardiac Disease*, 2nd ed. Appleton & Lange, 1992: 532.)

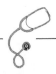

Transposition of the great vessel: "Big blue baby" as intrauterine growth is normal.

DIAGNOSIS

- ECG will be normal initially, but will demonstrate right ventricular hypertrophy by 1 month.
- CXR: "Egg on a string."

TREATMENT

- Patient is "ductal dependent" and will require prostaglandin E_1 (PGE_1) to keep the PDA patent.
- Early **balloon atrial septostomy** (BAS) is necessary to allow mixing of oxygenated and deoxygenated blood.
- Arterial switch procedure is definitive.

- ECG: Right or biventricular hypertrophy.
- BAS if VSD does not allow adequate mixing.

- PA band to control ↑ pulmonary blood flow.
- Arterial switch with VSD closure is definitive.

Truncus Arteriosus

DEFINITION

- A persistent truncus is a single arterial trunk that emerges from the ventricles, supplying the coronary, pulmonary, and systemic circulations (see Figure 13-5).
- Association: DiGeorge syndrome.

TYPES

- **I:** Short common pulmonary trunk arising from right side of common trunk, just above truncal valve.
- **II:** Pulmonary arteries (PAs) arise directly from ascending aorta, from posterior surface.
- **III:** Similar to type II, with PAs arising more laterally and more distant from semilunar valves.

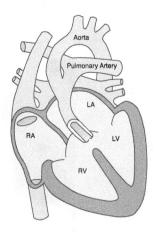

FIGURE 13-5. Truncus arteriosus.

PATHOPHYSIOLOGY

- The valve has two, three, or four leaflets and is usually poorly functioning.
- The truncus overrides a VSD.

SIGNS AND SYMPTOMS

- Presentation: CHF and cyanosis in first week.
- Initial left-to-right shunt symptoms:
  - Dyspnea.
  - Frequent respiratory infections.
  - FTT.
- If pulmonary vascular resistance ↑, cyanosis ↑.
- Second heart sound is prominent and single due to the single semilunar valve.
- Peripheral pulses are strong, often bounding.
- Often, a systolic ejection click can be appreciated.

DIAGNOSIS

CXR shows cardiomegaly and ↑ pulmonary vascular markings.

TREATMENT

- Surgery must occur before patient develops significant pulmonary vascular disease (usually 3–4 months of age).
- VSD is surgically closed, leaving the valve on the LV side.
- The pulmonary arteries are freed from the truncus and are connected to a valved conduit (Rastelli procedure), which will serve as the new pulmonary trunk.

Hypoplastic Left Heart Syndrome (HLHS)

DEFINITION

The syndrome consists of the following (see Figure 13-6):

- Aortic valve hypoplasia, stenosis, or atresia with or without mitral valve stenosis or atresia.

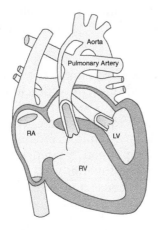

FIGURE 13-6. Hypoplastic left heart syndrome.

Note small size of left ventricle.

- Hypoplasia of the ascending aorta.
- LV hypoplasia or agenesis.
- Mitral valve stenosis or atresia.
- The result is a single (right) ventricle that provides blood to the pulmonary system, the systemic circulation via the PDA, and coronary system via retrograde flow after crossing the PDA.
- In utero:
  - All systemic blood flow is ductus dependent.
  - Pulmonary resistance > systemic vascular resistance.
  - Normal perfusion pressure is maintained with right-to-left shunt through PDA and pulmonary resistance.
- At birth:
  - PDA closes.
  - Systemic vascular resistance > pulmonary resistance.
  - PDA closure + hypoplastic LV = ↓ cardiac output and ↓ aortic pressure → circulatory death and metabolic acidosis.
  - PDA dependent until intervention is undertaken.

EPIDEMIOLOGY

The second most common congenital heart defect, presenting in the first week of life (and the most common cause of death from CHD in the first month).

SIGNS AND SYMPTOMS

- Pulses range from normal to absent (depending on ductal patency).
- Hyperdynamic RV impulse.
- Single S2 of ↑ intensity.
- Gallop at apex due if there is heart failure.
- Nonspecific systolic murmur at left sternal border (LSB).
- Skin may have a characteristic grayish pallor.

DIAGNOSIS

- CXR: Cardiomegaly with globular-shaped heart; ↑ pulmonary vascular markings, pulmonary edema.
- Echocardiogram is diagnostic.

TREATMENT

- No intervention: Due to the high mortality and complicated surgical course of this disease, ethical dilemmas are frequent as to how far physicians should intervene.
- Three-stage surgery:
  - **Norwood procedure:** The pulmonary trunk is used to reconstruct the hypoplastic aorta, and the right ventricle subsequently becomes the functional left ventricle. This leaves the pulmonary arteries connected but separated from the heart. The pulmonary blood flow is then reestablished via systemic to pulmonary conduits from the subclavian arteries to the pulmonary arteries.
  - **Glenn procedure:** The superior vena cava is connected to the right PA, restoring partial venous return to the lungs.

- **Fontan procedure:** The inferior vena cava is anastamosed to the PAs, resulting in complete venous diversion from the systemic circulation to the lungs.
- **Heart transplant:** This alternative occurs either as a primary intervention (if an organ is available) or after any of the previous palliative surgeries have provided maximal but ultimately insufficient benefit.

Left-to-right shunt (see Figure 13-7).

Subendocardial Cushion Defect

PATHOPHYSIOLOGY

Related to the ostium primum ASD, this defect results from abnormal development of the AV canal (endocardial cushions) resulting in:

- A VSD.
- An ostium primum ASD.
- Clefts in the mitral and tricuspid valves.

EPIDEMIOLOGY

- Association: Down syndrome (30% of patients with this defect have trisomy 21).
- Also frequently found with asplenia and polysplenia syndromes.

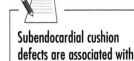

Subendocardial cushion defects are associated with Down syndrome.

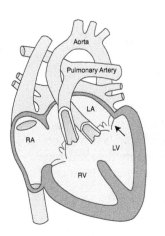
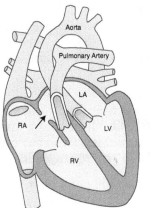
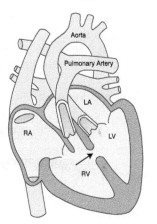
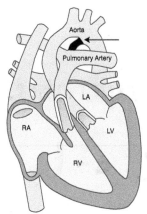

Subendocardial cushion defect   Atrial septal defect   Ventricular septal defect   Patent ductus arteriosus

FIGURE 13-7. Acyanotic heart defects.

SIGNS AND SYMPTOMS

- Often the result of the specific components of the accumulated defects:
  - Holosystolic murmur from the VSD, if restrictive.
  - Systolic murmur from mitral and tricuspid valve insufficiency.
- High risk of developing Eisenmenger syndrome.
- ECG: Superior QRS axis with RVH, right bundle branch block (RBBB), and LVH, along with a prolonged PR interval.

TREATMENT

- Surgical correction is sometimes the only option (despite high risk) when patient has an unbalanced AV canal.
- Some benefit from PA banding if shunting is predominantly at the ventricular level (rare).

Children with trisomy 21 often have more favorable anatomy for surgical intervention.

Atrial Septal Defect (ASD)

Ten percent of all congenital heart disease.

DEFINITION

Three types:

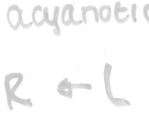

ASD is the most common congenital heart lesion recognized in adults.

- **Secundum defect** (most common—50–70%): Located in the central portion of the atrial septum.
- **Primum defect** (about 30% of ASDs):
  - Located at the atrial lower margin.
  - Associated with abnormalities of the mitral and tricuspid valves.
- **Sinus venosus defect** (about 10% of ASDs): Located at the upper portion of the atrial septum and often extends into the superior vena cava.

EPIDEMIOLOGY

- A common "co-conspirator" in CHD.
- As many as 50% of patients with congenital heart defects have an ASD as one of the defects.
- More common in females (male-to-female ratio 1:2).

SIGNS AND SYMPTOMS

- Children with ASDs are typically asymptomatic.
- Widely split and fixed S2. Murmurs are uncommon, but may occur as patient gets older. Murmur is a secondary pulmonary flow murmur.
- Symptoms of CHF and pulmonary HTN occur in adults (second and third decades).

DIAGNOSIS

- ECG: The left-to-right shunt may produce right atrial enlargement and RVH.
- CXR: Cardiomegaly with ↑ pulmonary vascular markings.

TREATMENT

- Nearly 90% will close spontaneously.
- One hundred percent close if < 3 mm.
- ASDs > 8 mm are unlikely to close spontaneously.
- Surgical or catheter closure (via a "clamshell" or "umbrella" device) are used when indicated.

acyanotic

R ← L

Patent Foramen Ovale (PFO)

- The foramen ovale is used prenatally to provide oxygenated blood from the placenta to the left atrium.
- It normally functionally closes when ↑ left atrial pressure causes the septa to press against each other (many remain "probe-patent" into adulthood).
- In some children, the tissue of the foramen ovale is insufficient to cover the foramen (either from insufficient growth or becoming stretched from ↑ pressure or volume).
- Some CHDs require a PFO for patient survival after birth (eg, tricuspid and mitral atresia, TAPVR).

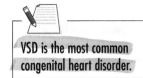

VSD is the most common congenital heart disorder.

Ventricular Septal Defect (VSD)

A 2-month-old male born at term appeared well until 3 weeks ago, when he became dyspneic and had difficulty feeding. A loud pansystolic murmur is heard at the left lower sternal border, and ECG shows LVH and RVH. *Think: VSD.*

Small VSD causes no symptoms. Large VSD may result in left-to-right shunt and pulmonary HTN. Left-sided volume overload and RVH are suggestive of a large VSD.

EPIDEMIOLOGY

- The most common form of recognized congenital heart disease (30–60% of all patients with CHDs).
- Usually membranous, as opposed to in the muscular septum.
- Occurs in 2 per 1000 live births.

SIGNS AND SYMPTOMS

Dependent on defect size:

- Small VSDs:
  - Usually asymptomatic.
  - Normal growth and development.
  - High-pitched, holosystolic murmur.
  - No ECG or CXR changes.
- Large VSDs:
  - Can → CHF and pulmonary HTN.
  - May have FTT.
  - Lower-pitched murmur; intensity dependent on the degree of shunting.

DIAGNOSIS

- ECG: LVH.
- CXR: Cardiomegaly with ↑ pulmonary vascular markings.

Spontaneous closure occurs in 30–50% of VSDs.

TREATMENT

- Spontaneous closure:
  - Muscular defects are most likely to close (up to 50%), with closure occurring during the first year of life.
  - Inlet and infundibular defects do not reduce in size or close.

- Intervention is based on the development of CHF, pulmonary HTN, and growth failure.
- Initial management with diuretics and digitalis.
- Surgical closure is indicated when therapy fails.
- Catheter-induced closure devices are less commonly used with VSDs than ASDs.
- Endocarditis prophylaxis.

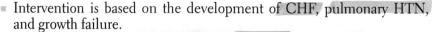

PATENT DUCTUS ARTERIOSUS (PDA)

PATHOPHYSIOLOGY

- Most often a problem in premature neonates:
  - Left-to-right shunts are handled poorly by premature infants.
  - Many develop idiopathic respiratory distress syndrome.
  - Some progress to develop left ventricular failure.
- Failure of spontaneous closure:
  - Premature infants: Due to ineffective response to oxygen tension.
  - Mature infants: Due to structural abnormality of ductal smooth muscle.

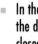
EPIDEMIOLOGY

- PDA is more common in females (male-to-female ratio 1:3).
- Incidence is higher at higher altitudes due to lower atmospheric oxygen tension.
- Maternal rubella in the first trimester has also been implicated in PDA.

SIGNS AND SYMPTOMS

- Small PDAs usually are asymptomatic.
- Large PDAs ↑ incidence of lower respiratory tract infections and CHF.
- Machinery-like murmur.
- Bounding peripheral pulses and wide pulse pressure.
- If Eisenmenger syndrome results, patient may have cyanosis restricted to the lower extremities.

TREATMENT

- Indomethacin: Used in premature infants. Inhibits prostaglandin synthesis, → closure.
- Catheter closure via devices such as double-umbrella devices and coils in older children.
- Surgical ligation and division via a left lateral thoracotomy.
- An occasional complication is recurrent laryngeal nerve injury → hoarseness.
- Eisenmenger syndrome is a contraindication to surgery.

PDA-Dependent Congenital Heart Abnormalities

- PDA-dependent congenital heart abnormalities include:
  - Tetralogy of Fallot
  - Tricuspid atresia
  - TAPVR with obstruction
  - Aortic coarctation (severe)

- Pulmonic atresia
- Hypoplastic left heart
- Prostaglandin E_1 (PGE_1) can be potentially lifesaving in a cyanotic newborn with PDA-dependent congenital heart abnormalities.
- CHD presenting in first 2–3 weeks of life are usually due to ductal-dependent lesions.

INDICATIONS FOR PGE_1 ADMINISTRATION

- Critically ill newborn with:
  - Suspected ductal-dependent lesion.
  - Suspected LV outflow tract obstruction.
- Dose:
  - 0.05 to 0.1 μg/kg/min (to reopen the ductus).
  - 0.01 μg/kg/min (to maintain ductal patency).
- Side effects:
  - Apnea: Endotracheal intubation prior to transport.
  - Fever, hypotension, and seizures.
- **Do not delay PGE_1 administration** in critically ill neonates with suspected ductal-dependent lesion pending definitive cardiac diagnosis.

Eisenmenger Syndrome

- Can occur in unrepaired left-to-right shunts (ie, VSD) that cause an ↑ pressure load on the pulmonary vasculature.
- Pressure overload on the pulmonary vasculature can result in irreversible changes in the arterioles.
- This develops into pulmonary vascular obstructive disease, usually over several years.
- The pulmonary HTN reduces the left-to-right shunt and previous LVH often resolves.
- Persistent HTN maintains an enlarged right ventricle and can dilate the main pulmonary segment (this becomes evident on CXR).
- Avoidance of this condition via surgical correction of CHD is essential, as it causes irreversible changes.

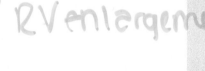

RV enlargement

CONGENITAL VALVULAR DEFECTS

See Figure 13-8.

Tricuspid Atresia

DEFINITION

RV inlet is absent or nearly absent:

- Eighty-nine percent have no evidence of tricuspid valve tissue, only dimple.
- Seven percent have a membranous septum forming part of the right atrial floor.
- Three percent are Ebstein's.
- One percent have a tiny, imperforate valvelike structure.

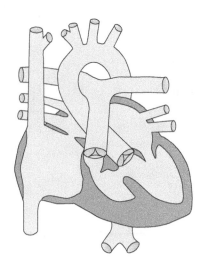

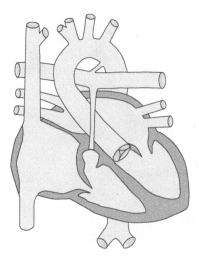

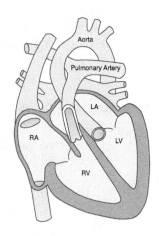

Tricuspic atresia   Pulmonary atresia   Aortic insufficiency

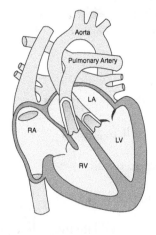

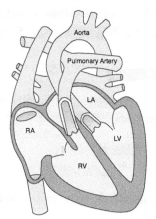

Mitral stenosis   Mitral valve prolapse

FIGURE 13-8.   Congenital valvular defects.

Bicuspid aortic valve is the most common congenital heart defect, occurring in 1–2% of the population. This defect goes largely unrecognized.

EPIDEMIOLOGY

- ASD and/or VSD is usually present.
- Seventy-five percent will present with cyanosis within the first week.

SIGNS AND SYMPTOMS

LV impulse displaced laterally.

DIAGNOSIS

ECG: LVH, prominent LV forces (due to ↓ RV voltages).

TREATMENT

- PGE₁ to maintain ductal patency.
- Surgical intervention.
- Modified Blalock-Taussig (BT) shunt.
- Glenn procedure, followed by Fontan procedure.

Pulmonary Atresia (with Intact Ventricular Septum)

SIGNS AND SYMPTOMS

- Cyanosis within hours of birth (PDA closing).
- Hypotension, tachypnea, acidosis.
- Single S2, with a holosystolic murmur (tricuspid regurgitation).

DIAGNOSIS

- ECG: ↓ RV forces and occasionally RVH.
- CXR: Normal to enlarged RV with ↓ pulmonary vascular markings.

TREATMENT

- PGE₁ to maintain ductal patency.
- Balloon atrial septostomy (sometimes).
- Reconstruction of RVOT with transannular patch or pulmonary valvotomy.
- ASD left open to prevent systemic venous HTN.

Aortic Stenosis

A 4-year-old boy with recurrent episodes of syncope while playing has a harsh systolic murmur radiating to the carotids, diminished cardiac pulses, and severe LVH. *Think: Congenital aortic stenosis.*

Angina, syncope, and congestive heart failure are the presentation of aortic stenosis. Syncope during exertion occurs due to the reduced cerebral perfusion when arterial pressure declines. However, many patients now are diagnosed before the development of these symptoms on the basis of the finding of a systolic murmur followed by echocardiography.

EPIDEMIOLOGY

Eighty-five percent of congenitally stenotic aortic valves are bicuspid.

SIGNS AND SYMPTOMS

- Severe stenosis generally presents shortly after birth.
- Older children may complain of chest or stomach pain (epigastric).
- Patients with untreated severe aortic stenosis are at risk for syncope and sudden death.
- The characteristic murmur is a **crescendo-decrescendo systolic murmur.**

- A **systolic ejection click** is also common (particularly if bicuspid aortic valve).
- In severe disease, paradoxical splitting of S2 occurs (split narrows with inspiration).

DIAGNOSIS

- Clinical findings, including ECG findings, and symptoms can be deceiving.
- Echo or catheterization to evaluate pressure differences between the aorta and left ventricle is essential.

TREATMENT

- Surgical or interventional balloon.
- Valvotomy is most common intervention:
  - Indication is usually if the measured catheterization gradient is > 50 mm Hg.
  - High incidence of recurrent stenosis.
- Valve replacement: Deferred, when possible, until patient completes growth.

Aortic Insufficiency

EPIDEMIOLOGY

Uncommon and usually associated with mitral valve disease or aortic stenosis.

SIGNS AND SYMPTOMS

- A diastolic, decrescendo murmur is present at the left upper sternal border.
- Presentation with symptoms indicates advanced disease.
- Chest pain and CHF are ominous signs.

DIAGNOSIS

CXR: LV enlargement, dilated ascending aorta.

TREATMENT

- Surgery or balloon valvuloplasty to treat aortic stenosis may worsen the insufficiency.
- Aortic valve replacement is the only definitive therapy.

Mitral Stenosis

EPIDEMIOLOGY

- Rare in children; usually a sequela of acute rheumatic fever.
- Congenital forms are generally severe.

SIGNS AND SYMPTOMS

- When symptomatic, dyspnea is the most common symptom.
- Weak peripheral pulses with narrow pulse pressure.
- An **opening snap** is heard on auscultation; also, a **presystolic murmur** may be heard.

Supravalvular aortic stenosis is associated with idiopathic hypercalcemia.

People with Marfan syndrome frequently have aortic insufficiency as well.

- Pulmonary venous congestion occurs, →:
  - CXR evidence of interstitial edema.
  - Hemoptysis from small bronchial vessel rupture.

TREATMENT
- Balloon valvuloplasty
- Surgical:
  - Commissurotomy
  - Valve replacement

Mitral Valve Prolapse

PATHOPHYSIOLOGY
Caused by thick and redundant valve leaflets that bulge into the mitral annulus.

EPIDEMIOLOGY
- Usually occurs in older children and adolescents.
- Has a familial component (autosomal dominant).
- Nearly all patients with Marfan syndrome have it.

SIGNS AND SYMPTOMS
- Auscultation: Midsystolic click and late systolic murmur.
- Often asymptomatic with some history of palpitations and chest pain.

TREATMENT
Management is symptomatic (eg, β blocker for chest pain).

Coarctation of the aorta is associated with Turner syndrome.

OTHER CONGENITAL CARDIOVASCULAR DEFECTS

Coarctation of the Aorta

PATHOPHYSIOLOGY
- Most commonly found in the juxtaductal position (where the ductus arteriosus joins the aorta).
- Development of symptoms may correspond to the closure of the ductus arteriosus (the patent ductus provides additional room for blood to reach the postductal aorta).

The presence of ↓ pulses in the lower extremities is the clue for diagnosis of coarctation.

EPIDEMIOLOGY
- More common in males than females (male-to-female ratio 2:1).
- Association: Seen in one-third of patients with Turner syndrome.

SIGNS AND SYMPTOMS

Clinical Presentation of Symptomatic Infants
- FTT, respiratory distress, and CHF develop in the first 2–3 months of life.
- Lower extremity changes: ↓ pulses in the lower extremities.
- Acidosis may develop as the lower body receives insufficient blood.
- Usually, a murmur is heard over the left back.

Comparison of the right upper extremity blood pressures and pulse oximeter readings with the lower extremity should be performed with a possible diagnosis of coarctation.

Clinical Presentation of Asymptomatic Infants or Children

- Normal growth and development.
- Occasional complaint of leg weakness or pain after exertion.
- ↓ pulses in the lower extremities.
- Upper-extremity HTN (or at least greater than in the lower extremities).

DIAGNOSIS

CXR: "3 sign," dilated ascending aorta that displaces the superior vena cava to the right (see Figure 13-9).

TREATMENT

- Resection of the coarctation segment with end-to-end anastomosis is the intervention of choice for initial treatment.
- Allograft patch augmentation can also be used.
- Catheter balloon dilation can be used:
  - Has a higher restenosis rate than surgery.
  - Has an ↑ risk of producing aortic aneurysms.
  - Balloon dilation is more frequently used when stenosis occurs at the surgical site of a primary reanastamosis.

Ebstein's Anomaly

DEFINITION

Components of the defect (see Figure 13-10):

- The tricuspid valve is displaced apically in the right ventricle.
- The valve leaflets are redundant and plastered against the ventricular wall, often causing functional tricuspid atresia.
- The right atrium is frequently the largest structure.

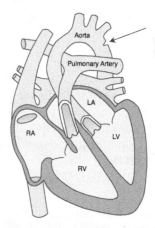

FIGURE 13-9.   Coarctation of the aorta.

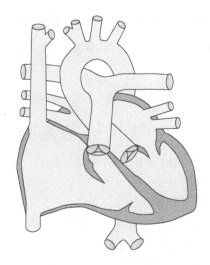

FIGURE 13-10. Ebstein's anomaly.

EPIDEMIOLOGY

Without intervention:

- CHF in first 6 months.
- Nearly 50% mortality.

SIGNS AND SYMPTOMS

- Growth and development can be normal depending on severity of the lesion.
- Older patients usually complain of dyspnea, cyanosis, and palpitations.
- Widely split S1, fixed split S2, variable S3 and S4 (characteristic triple or quadruple rhythm).
- Holosystolic murmur at left lower sternal border.
- Opening snap.
- Cyanosis from atrial right-to-left shunt.

DIAGNOSIS

- ECG: Right axis deviation, right atrial enlargement, RBBB; WPW is present in 20%.
- CXR: Cardiomegaly ("balloon-shaped") "wall-to-wall heart" in severely affected infants.
- Echocardiogram is diagnostic.

TREATMENT

Intervention (87% do well):

- Glenn procedure to ↑ pulmonary blood flow.
- Severely affected infants may require aortopulmonary shunt.
- Tricuspid valve replacement or reconstruction.
- Right atrial reduction surgery.
- Ablation of accessory conduction pathways.

Total Anomalous Pulmonary Venous Return (TAPVR)

The pulmonary veins bring the blood from the lungs to the right atrium (instead of the left atrium).

PATHOPHYSIOLOGY

- See Figure 13-11A and B.
- No communication exists between the pulmonary veins and the left atrium.
- All pulmonary veins drain to a common vein.
- The common vein drains into the:
  - Right superior vena cava (50%).
  - Coronary sinus or right atrium (20%).
  - Portal vein or inferior vena cava (20%).
  - Combination of the above types (10%).
- An ASD is needed for survival.

EPIDEMIOLOGY

Dramatically more common in males (male-to-female ratio 4:1).

SIGNS AND SYMPTOMS/DIAGNOSIS/TREATMENT

Presence or absence of obstruction of pulmonary venous return changes the clinical presentation.

TAPVR with Obstruction
- Obstruction → ↑ pulmonary artery pressure (and subsequent pulmonary edema) that ↑ pulmonary then right atrial and ventricular pressures. This causes a right-to-left shunt and resultant cyanosis.
- Presents with early, severe respiratory distress and cyanosis, no murmur, and hepatomegaly.
- CXR: Normal-size heart, pulmonary edema.
- Echocardiogram is diagnostic.
- Management: Baloon atrial septostomy or immediate corrective surgery.

TAPVR Without Obstruction
- Free communication between right atrium and left atrium.
- Large right-to-left shunt ("large ASD").
- Presents later during first year of life, with mild FTT, recurrent pulmonary infections, tachypnea, right heart failure, and rarely cyanosis.
- CXR: Cardiomegaly, large PAs; ↑ pulmonary vascular markings ("snowman" or "figure eight" sign) is found in infants > 4 months old.
- Management: Surgical movement of pulmonary veins to the left atrium.

Hypertrophic Obstructive Cardiomyopathy

- Autosomal dominant 60%, sporadic 40%.
- Sudden death: 4% to 6% incidence.
- Asymmetrical septal hypertrophy or idiopathic hypertrophic subaortic stenosis (IHSS) is the most common form.
- Outflow obstruction potentially caused by leaflet of mitral valve.
- ECG: LVH and left atrial enlargement, large Q wave (indicates septal hypertrophy).
- Echo: Asymmetrical septal hypertrophy, outflow obstruction (which predict the severity of disease).

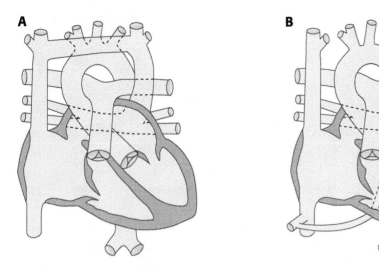

FIGURE 13-11. **Total anomalous pulmonary venous return.**

A. Supracardiac view. **B.** Infracardiac view.

TREATMENT

- Moderate restriction of physical activity.
- β blocker or calcium channel blocker to improve filling.
- Endocarditis prophylaxis.

Renal, Gynecologic, and Urinary Disease

Normal Acid-Base Balance

pH, 7.4; P_{CO_2}, 40; O_2 sat, 98–100%.

DIAGNOSIS

Diagnose acid-base disorders by obtaining an arterial blood gas (ABG—pH and P_{CO_2}) and an electrolyte panel (HCO_3^-).

- Assess the acid-base disorder step by step:
  - Is the primary disorder an acidosis (pH < 7.4) or alkalosis (pH > 7.4)?
  - Is the disorder respiratory (pH and P_{CO_2} move in opposite directions)?
  - Is the disorder metabolic (pH and P_{CO_2} move in the same direction)?
  - Is the disorder a simple or mixed disorder?

The notation commonly used for blood gases whether arterial or venous is: **pH/P_{CO_2}/PO_2/ calculated HCO_3/ calculated Sao_2—** bicarbonate may also be included.

Acidosis

- Acidosis induces ion shifts at the cellular level that cause hyperkalemia and hypercalcemia. This can manifest clinically as a cardiac arrhythmia.
- There is a right shift of the O_2-Hg dissociation curve, which means ↓ affinity resulting in ↑ oxygen release of oxygen to the tissues
- ↑ cerebral blood flow, but ↓ pulmonary blood flow.

ABG = 7.35–7.45/35–45/80–100/18–23
VBG = 7.25–7.35/41–51/35–40/18–23

METABOLIC ACIDOSIS

- ↓ serum pH caused by a ↓ in plasma HCO_3^-. It is important to identify the underlying cause of metabolic acidosis by calculating the anion gap (AG).
- AG = $[Na^+]$ – $([Cl^-] + [HCO_3^-])$. Normal AG = 8–16 mEq/L, and reflects unmeasured serum ions (organic acids, phosphates, etc.).
- Normal AG metabolic acidosis results when the low HCO_3^- levels are balanced by a compensatory ↑ in renal Cl^- reabsorption, keeping the AG in range. This is also commonly referred to as a hyperchloremic metabolic acidosis.
- Diarrhea is the most common cause of normal AG metabolic acidosis, and is due to excessive gastrointestinal HCO_3^- loss. Renal tubular acidosis is another metabolic disturbance caused by ineffective reabsorption of HCO_3^- (proximal), or excretion of H^+ (distal).
- ↑ AG metabolic acidosis can be due to ↑ serum H^+ from exogenous sources (MUDPILES), or ↑ endogenous production (lactic acidosis/ketoacidosis/renal failure).
- Treat metabolic acidosis by correcting the underlying disorder. Severe metabolic acidosis (pH < 7.2) results in compensatory hyperventilation (Kussmaul's breathing), and diminished responsiveness to catecholamines that results in ↓ cardiac output and tissue perfusion. Treat patients with pH < 7.15 with $Na^+HCO_3^-$.

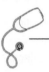

Although bicarbonate levels can be calculated from ABGs, the level obtained from electrolyte panels (venous CO_2) is a measured value, more reliable, and necessary for interpretation.

RESPIRATORY ACIDOSIS

- ↓ serum pH due to pulmonary retention of CO_2 (Pa_{CO_2} > 40 mmHg).
- Renal compensation consists of increasing reabsorption of HCO_3^-.
- Acute compensation occurs at a rate of 1 mmol/L per 10 mmHg ↑ in Pa_{CO_2}.

Causes of ↑ anion gap metabolic acidosis:
MUDPILES
Methanol
Uremia
Diabetic ketoacidosis (DKA)
Paraldehyde
Isoniazid
Lactate
Ethylene glycol
Salicylates

PaCO_2 is expected to ↓ as a result of compensatory hyperventilation in metabolic acidosis.

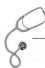

Expected PaCO_2 should be calculated with **Winter's formula** and compared with measured PCO_2 to see if compensation is appropriate.

$$Expected\ PCO_2 = 1.5\ (measured\ HCO_3^-) + 8 \pm 2$$

Failure of compensation is indicative of an additional primary acid-base disorder.

Watch for the possibility of two concurrent primary disturbances. In salicylate toxicity, both primary respiratory alkalosis and metabolic acidosis exist.

If an asthmatic has respiratory distress that is expected to have respiratory alkalosis, has a normal pH and normal PCO_2, beware of impending respiratory failure.

- Chronic compensation occurs at a rate of 4 mmol/L per 10 mmHg ↑ in PaCO_2.
- Make sure the airway is patent.
- Correct potential reversible causes.

Alkalosis

- Alkalosis induces ion shifts at the cellular level that cause hypokalemia and hypocalcemia.
- There is a left shift of the O_2-Hg dissociation curve, resulting in ↓ oxygen delivery to the tissue.
- ↓ cerebral blood flow.

METABOLIC ALKALOSIS

A 6-week-old child has a 2-week history of projectile vomiting that is not bile-stained. He is dehydrated and slightly jaundiced. *Think: Pyloric stenosis.*

The initial symptom of pyloric stenosis is nonbilious vomiting. Progressive vomiting results in hypochloremic hypokalemic metabolic alkalosis. Most likely lab findings: Na 138, K 3.0, Cl 88, HCO₃ 35, pH 7.52. Jaundice due to ↓ level of glucuronyl transferase may be present, which resolves after relief of the obstruction. ↑ awareness has resulted in earlier diagnosis.

- ↑ serum pH due to an ↑ plasma HCO_3^-.
- Mechanism relies on fact that the renal system cannot excrete excess HCO_3^-.
- In children, metabolic alkalosis is caused by excessive loss of H^+ (vomiting).
- Urinalysis (UA) is the best initial step in evaluation to determine if the extracellular fluid (ECF) volume is contracted or expanded:
  - If urine Cl⁻ is < 10 mEq/L, ECF contraction, hypokalemia, and is saline sensitive.
  - If urine Cl⁻ is > 20 mEq/L, ECF expansion, hypertension, and is saline resistant.
- PaCO_2 is expected to ↑ as a result of compensatory hypoventilation in metabolic alkalosis.
- Failure to compensate indicates an additional underlying primary respiratory alkalosis.
- Treat the underlying cause.
- Volume repletion in cases of ECF volume contraction will correct the alkalosis, and diuretics should be used when ECF volume is expanded.

RESPIRATORY ALKALOSIS

- ↑ serum pH due to ↓ plasma CO_2.
- Caused by hyperventilation (anxiety, asthma, pulmonary embolism, pneumonia, hypoxia).
- Renal compensation (excretion of HCO_3^-) occurs over a period of several hours:
  - Acute compensation ↓ HCO_3^- 2 mEq/L, for every 10 mmHg ↓ in PaCO_2.

- Chronic compensation ↓ HCO_3^- 6 mEq/L, for every 10 mmHg ↓ in $PaCO_2$.
- Treat respiratory alkalosis by treating the underlying disorder. Breathing into a paper bag can be useful in cases of psychogenic hyperventilation.

A 1-year-old child is brought into the emergency department (ED) with vomiting, constipation, and ↓ urine production. The child is found to have normal anion gap metabolic acidosis. A renal ultrasound reveals medullary nephrocalcinosis. *Think: Renal tubular acidosis.*

Renal tubular acidosis is characterized by normal anion gap metabolic acidosis. A urine pH < 5.5 suggests proximal RTA, whereas in distal RTA urine pH > 6.0. Presence of nephrocalcinosis and hypercalciuria are suggestive of distal RTA.

DEFINITION

- A renal tubular disorder resulting in normal anion gap hyperchloremic acidosis, due to impaired urinary acidification.
- Presence of acidemia and alkaline urine, with preserved glomerular function.
- Hyperchloremic metabolic acidosis with a high urinary pH.
- RTA type 1 is the most common form.

ETIOLOGY

Three types: 1, 2, and 4. Type 3 RTA is exceedingly rare.

- **Type 1—distal RTA:**
  - Hyperchloremic metabolic acidosis with a high urinary pH.
  - Inability to secrete H^+ by the distal tubule and collecting duct (bicarbonate cannot be generated) → metabolic acidosis with alkaline urine (> 5.5).
  - Compensatory ↑ in excretion of other cations causing hypokalemia and hypercalciuria.
  - Can be complicated by rickets, secondary to phosphate wasting.
  - Type 1 RTA is the only type associated with renal stones.
- **Type 2—proximal RTA:**
  - Caused by ↓ proximal tubular reabsorption of bicarbonate.
  - The mechanisms of H^+ secretion in the distal tubule are overwhelmed → HCO_3 loss in urine.
  - The bicarbonate is replaced in the circulation by Cl → hyperchloremia.
  - ↑ sodium delivery to the distal tubule ↑ aldosterone secretion → hypokalemia.
  - Isolated disorder.
  - Generalized defect in proximal tubular transport (Fanconi syndrome). Nephrocalcinosis and nephrolithiasis do not occur despite ↑ urinary calcium (urinary citrate levels are not reduced).
  - Plasma HCO_3^- remains at 15–20 mEq/L.

- Type 4—mineralocorticoid deficiency RTA.
  - Aldosterone deficiency or resistance.
  - ↓ aldosterone production by the adrenal gland (Addison disease, congenital adrenal hyperplasia, primary hypoaldosteronism).
  - ↓ production of renin by the juxtaglomerular apparatus (interstitial damage).
  - Nephrocalcinosis and nephrolithiasis are rarely seen.
  - Characteristic features: Hyperkalemia, acidic urine—urinary pH < 5.5 (distal tubule H^+ pump functions normally).

SIGNS AND SYMPTOMS

- Polyuria, dehydration, anorexia, vomiting, constipation, and hypotonia.
- Children often present with growth failure.

TREATMENT

- Correct acidosis:
  - Sodium bicarbonate (alkalinize the urine, correct the sodium defect, lower aldosterone, and raise the potassium).
  - Potassium citrate (augments urinary citrate and inhibits stone formation).
  - Caution! $NaHCO_3$ in Type II can correct the condition but can → further hypokalemia, and potassium supplements may also be required.
- Correct electrolyte abnormalities to maintain bicarbonate and potassium levels: Potassium citrate therapy is able to correct the metabolic acidosis and hypokalemia in distal renal tubular acidosis.

PROGNOSIS

- Distal RTA can be a lifelong disease and may → renal failure.
- Proximal RTA and mineralocorticoid RTA usually resolve within 12 months.

The primary defect in distal renal tubular acidosis is a defect in secretion of hydrogen ions.

ACUTE RENAL FAILURE (ARF)

A 4-year-old boy develops oliguria 12 hours after operation for a ruptured appendix. Creatinine (Cr) is 0.5 mg/dL, blood urea nitrogen (BUN) is 23 mg/dL, urine sodium is 12 mEq/L. *Think: Prerenal azotemia.*

Oliguria is most often due to dehydration. Historical features are vomiting, diarrhea, and poor oral intake. A BUN-to-serum creatinine ratio of > 20:1 is suggestive of prerenal azotemia. Other features are ↓ concentration of urinary sodium, ↑ urinary excretion of creatinine, and a high urine osmolality. The precipitating event for prerenal azotemia is renal hypoperfusion. Give physiologic saline for blood volume expansion. Reversibility with treatment of the underlying cause is the hallmark.

A 2-year-old boy develops bloody diarrhea a few days after eating in a fast-food restaurant. A few days later, he develops facial edema, pallor, lethargy, and ↓ urine output. Blood work shows a low hematocrit and platelet count. A UA reveals blood and protein in the urine. *Think: HUS secondary to* Escherichia coli *O157:H7 infection.*

This infection is commonly acquired by eating undercooked red meat (hamburgers). It is usually preceded by either gastroenteritis (usually diarrheal) or an upper respiratory tract infection. Sudden onset of pallor, lethargy, and oliguria suggest HUS. Microangiopathic hemolytic anemia and thrombocytopenia support the diagnosis of HUS. The peripheral smear may show helmet cells, burr cells, and fragmented red cells.

A 5-year-old patient with ARF has an electrocardiogram (ECG) that shows peaked T waves and a widened QRS complex. *Think: Hyperkalemia.*

Hyperkalemia occurs due to impaired renal excretion. As K^+ levels rise, peaked T waves are the first ECG changes. Further rise results in widening of the QRS complex. All patients with suspected hyperkalemia should be placed on a cardiac monitor. The initial treatment includes administration of calcium chloride or gluconate to treat hemodynamic instability, and initiation of measures to lower serum K^+.

DEFINITION

- ARF develops when renal function is diminished to the point where body fluid homeostasis can no longer be maintained.
- Acute rise in BUN, serum creatinine, or both.
- Three main types: prerenal, renal, and postrenal.
- ARF results in azotemia (elevated BUN).
- May present with symptoms of oliguria, anuria, or insidiously without oliguria.

PATHOPHYSIOLOGY

- Prerenal:
  - Caused by hypoperfusion of the kidneys secondary to hemorrhage, sepsis, heart failure, or salt/protein-wasting disease.
  - This is the most common cause of ARF.
  - Potentially reversible if blood flow is restored prior to progression to acute tubular necrosis (ATN).
  - Oliguria is always present.
  - Gastroenteritis is the most common cause of hypovolemia.
- Renal:
  - Caused by renal parenchyma damage, usually from tubular disease (most commonly ATN), glomerular disease (Wegener, Goodpasture, systemic lupus erythematosus [SLE]), vascular disease (HUS or renal vein thrombosis), and interstitial disease (medications).

The most common cause of ARF in toddlers is hemolytic-uremic syndrome (HUS).

Nephritic syndrome: Hematuria, edema, and hypertension.

Normal urinary output: 2–4 ml/kg/hr

Oliguria: < 0.5 mL/kg/hr urine production

Children with renal failure may have a normal urinary output.

Patients with ARF could be either volume overloaded or volume depleted. Always assess a patient's hydration status.

- The kidneys are unable to concentrate urine effectively.
- Usually presents with edema.
- Consider poststreptococcal glomerulonephritis in a child presenting with hypertension, edema, hematuria, and renal failure.
  - **Postrenal:**
  - Caused by any significant obstruction of the urinary tract (posterior urethral valves, bilateral uretropelvic or uretrovesical obstruction).
  - Almost always associated with infection.

SIGNS AND SYMPTOMS

- Oliguria.
- Edema (salt and water overload).
- Hypertension (HTN).
- Congestive heart failure (CHF).
- Seizures.

DIAGNOSIS

- Find out the duration, and attempt to get a baseline Cr level.
- Obtain a careful history to determine the cause of renal failure.
- Serum and urine chemistry are useful tests for differentiating the cause.
  - Prerenal: BUN:Cr > 20:1 with FeNa < 1%.
  - Renal: BUN:Cr < 20:1 and FeNa > 2–3%.
- In children with postrenal ARF, a renal ultrasound will show dilation of the renal pelvis and collecting system.

TREATMENT

- Catheterize the patient to monitor urine output and relieve obstruction.
- Treat patients with hypovolemia with volume replacement.
- Treat patients who fail to produce adequate urine output with fluid restriction.
- Avoid drugs that can precipitate prerenal failure (such as nonsteroidal anti-inflammatories [NSAIDs]) in patients with ↓ renal perfusion.

COMPLICATIONS OF UNTREATED ARF

- **Hyperkalemia** can develop secondary to impaired renal tubule function and ion shifts due to acidosis. A serum potassium level > 7 mEq/L must be treated emergently. Give calcium gluconate to stabilize the myocardium, bicarbonate, glucose and insulin, Kayexalate (sodium polystyrene), and albuterol. Cardiac arrest from hyperkalemia is a life-threatening complication of untreated ARF.
- **Hypocalcemia** and **hyperphospatemia** may result from parathyroid hormone (PTH) resistance and loss of ability to hydroxylate vitamin D into an active form. Severe hypocalcemia manifests as tetany, and is treated by lowering phosphate and replacing active vitamin D.
- **Anemia** is often caused by lowered erythropoietin levels. Erythropoietin can be supplemented.
- **Hyponatremia** secondary to excessive administration of hypotonic fluids to oliguric patients. Patients with a serum sodium < 120 are at risk for developing cerebral edema and central nervous system (CNS) hemorrhage. Partial correction should be undertaken to raise the Na level to at least 120 mEq Na.

$$\text{Required} = (\text{Desired Na concentration} - \text{Observed Na concentration}) \times \text{Body weight (Kg)} \times 0.6$$

Treat patients with water restriction.
- **Metabolic acidosis** is due to ↓ excretion of hydrogen and ammonia.
- **Infection** is a common and serious complication.

CHRONIC RENAL FAILURE (CRF)

On a routine exam, a 10-year-old girl has HTN that is confirmed by repeated measurements. Her blood pressure (BP) is 160/90 in the right arm and similar in the left arm and right leg. *Think: Renal disease.*

BP should be measured at least twice with appropriate cuff size. A short or narrow cuff may artificially ↑ BP measurement. Renal parenchymal disease and coarctation of the aorta are common causes of hypertension in children 1–10 years of age. BP should be obtained in all four extremities to determine the presence of coarctation of the aorta. The most appropriate next diagnostic test is UA.

DEFINITION

CRF is a result of irreversible kidney damage → end-stage renal failure.

ETIOLOGY

- CRF in children under age 5 is most often due to anatomic abnormalities, such as renal hypoplasia, dysplasia, or malformations.
- After age 5, CRF usually results from glomerular diseases such as HUS or glomerulonephritis, hereditary diseases such as Alport syndrome, or cystic diseases.

SIGNS AND SYMPTOMS

- The development of uremic symptoms in chronic renal disease is usually insidious and nonspecific.
- Patients may present with headache, fatigue, lethargy, anorexia, vomiting, polydipsia, polyuria, and growth failure.
- Most patients with CRF are weak and have HTN, as the renin-angiotensin-aldosterone system is stimulated by diminished GFR regardless of actual volume status.
- See Table 14-1 for a listing of symptoms of uremia.

Patients will often present with bleeding due to defective platelets secondary to uremia. Uncontrolled bleeding can be treated with dialysis and desmopressin.

DIAGNOSIS

- Serum Cr measurement will give a good estimate of glomerular filtration rate (GFR) as the two vary with an inverse relation.
- GFR < 20% of normal is typical for CRF.

	GFR Range (mL/min)
Mild CRF	70–120
Moderate CRF	30–70
Severe CRF	< 30
ESRD	< 10

Always attempt to obtain a baseline Cr level to differentiate between ARF, CRF, and acute-on-chronic renal insufficiency/failure.

TREATMENT

- Dialysis and renal transplant are indicated for patients when serum Cr is > 10 mL/dL.

TABLE 14-1. Symptoms of Uremia

Azotemia (accumulation of nitrogen products)

Acidosis

Sodium wasting

Sodium retention

Urinary concentrating defect

Hyperkalemia

Renal osteodystrophy

Growth retardation

Anemia

Bleeding tendency

Infection

Neurologic (fatigue, poor concentration, headache, drowsiness, muscle weakness, seizures, coma)

Gastrointestinal ulceration

Hypertension

Hypertriglyceridemia

Pericarditis and cardiomyopathy

Glucose intolerance

Absolute indications for emergent dialysis:
AEIOU
Acidosis
Electrolyte abnormalities
Toxic **I**ngestion
Fluid **O**verload
Uremia

- **Diet:** Children with CRF are growth retarded. Children should be given adequate caloric intake. Nasogastric (NG) tube feeds and recombinant human growth hormone therapy has been shown to improve linear growth. Water-soluble vitamins, zinc, and iron should be supplemented.
- **Renal osteodystrophy:** Children with CRF are unable to excrete phosphate. The resulting hyperphosphatemia and hypocalcemia stimulate PTH. The ensuing secondary hyperparathyroidism → fibrosis of the bone marrow space (osteitis fibrosis cystica). Symptoms of renal osteodystrophy include muscle weakness, bone pain, and growth retardation. Treatment includes normalization of the serum calcium and phosphorus levels.
- **Anemia:** Anemia results from inadequate erythropoietin production by the kidneys. Children with Hgb < 6 should be transfused with packed red blood cells (RBCs). Erythropoietin can also be administered subcutaneously.
- **Hypertensive emergencies:** HTN should be treated with salt restriction and a combination of angiotensin-converting enzyme (ACE) inhibitors and β blockers.

An 8-year-old patient receiving peritoneal dialysis for ESRD develops abdominal pain and fever. *Think: Peritonitis.*

The most serious complication of peritoneal dialysis is peritonitis. It should be suspected in the presence of abdominal pain and fever in a patient who is on peritoneal dialysis. Clinical manifestations include fever and abdominal pain and tenderness. Common causative organisms are coagulase-negative staphylococci, *S aureus*, streptococci, *Escherichia coli*, *Pseudomonas*, and other gram-negative organisms.

DEFINITION

ESRD occurs when a patient's renal function has been irreversibly compromised and failed (the serum Cr is typically > 10 mg/dL).

CAUSES

Congenital anatomic abnormalities are the most common cause in children < 5 years old, and glomerulonephritis is the most common culprit in children > 5 years old.

TREATMENT

- **Dialysis:** Peritoneal dialysis is the standard technique for infants and children. However, dialysis patients remain uremic, which restricts normal growth and development.
- **Renal transplant:** Renal transplantation is the preferred mode of treatment of most children with ESRD. Preparation for transplantation from living donors or listing for cadaver donor transplant should begin for all children with ESRD. The contraindications for transplant include children with human immunodeficiency virus (HIV) and children with metastatic malignancy.

High BUN/Cr levels are not an absolute indication for dialysis.

The most common causes of HTN in children are secondary causes—renal (75%), infection, glomerulonephritis, HUS, obstructive uropathy.

A previously healthy 2-year-old boy has a left-sided flank mass discovered by his mother. His physical examination reveals a BP of 110/70 and a large mass arising in his left flank. A UA shows 5–10 erythrocytes and 2–3 leukocytes. *Think: Wilms tumor.*

The usual presentation of Wilms tumor is an abdominal mass, and it is not uncommon for the parent to discover this mass. Other features may include abdominal pain, fever, anemia, hematuria, and HTN. The most appropriate next diagnostic test is an ultrasound of the abdomen and urinary tract. Because Wilms tumor metastasizes to the lungs, a chest radiograph should be obtained.

DEFINITION

- Nephroblastoma.
- Embryonal neural crest cell origin.
- It most commonly presents between the ages of 1 and 4 years (median age at diagnosis: 3.5 years).
- The most common type of renal tumor in children.

ETIOLOGY

Wilms tumors are associated with mutations of the p53 tumor suppressor gene on chromosome 11.

SIGNS AND SYMPTOMS

- Abdominal/flank mass (typically asymptomatic):
  - The most common presentation.
  - Rarely crosses the midline, as opposed to neuroblastoma.
- Vomiting.
- May present with gross hematuria, fever, and HTN due to obstruction of renal artery.
- Associated with aniridia, genitourinary malformation (cryptorchidism), mental retardation, hemihypertrophy, and Beckwith-Wiedemann syndrome (macroglossia, omphalocele, visceromegaly).
- Can be bilateral (5–10%).

PATHOLOGY

- **Stage 1:** Tumor limited to kidneys and can be removed with an intact capsule.
- **Stage 2:** Grows beyond the kidney but can be completely removed.
- **Stage 3:** Nonhematogenous extension into the abdomen.
- **Stage 4:** Hematogenous metastases.
- **Stage 5:** Bilateral renal metastasis.

SPREAD

- Contiguous invasion of adjacent organs.
- Extension into the renal vein and inferior vena cava.
- Distant spread: Lung and liver.

DIAGNOSIS

- Renal ultrasound (US): Echogenic intrarenal masses that may contain cystic areas.
- Computed tomography (CT): To determine the origin and extent of spread.
- Biopsy: To determine cell type.

TREATMENT

- Stage 1–3 tumors are treated with nephrectomy and chemotherapy with or without radiation.
- Stage 4 tumors are treated with pulmonary irradiation and three-drug combination chemotherapy in addition to above.

An 8-month-old girl has an easily palpable kidney. US shows cystic kidneys, hepatic fibrosis, and portal HTN. *Think: Autosomal-recessive polycystic kidney disease.*

Classic presentation: Bilateral flank masses during the neonatal period or early infancy. Ultrasound may show uniformly hyperechogenic kidneys. Presence of hepatic fibrosis supports this diagnosis. Associations: oligohydramnios, pulmonary hypoplasia, respiratory distress, and spontaneous pneumothorax.

DEFINITION

- Bilateral renal cysts without dysplasia.
- Congenital malformation of the urinary tract resulting in cysts within the kidneys.

PATHOPHYSIOLOGY

- **Autosomal-recessive PKD** (ARPKD; previously known "infantile polycystic disease"): Cysts are a dilation of the collecting ducts. Many patients also have cysts in the liver, cirrhosis, and portal HTN.
- **Autosomal-dominant PKD** (ADPKD; previously known "adult polycystic disease"): Cortical and medullary cysts that are primarily dilated tubules. Although most patients are identified between 30 and 50 years of age, the condition has been recognized in newborn.
- Currently, the nomenclature of infantile versus adult is no longer used.

SIGNS AND SYMPTOMS

ARPKD

- ↓ urine formation by the fetus → oligohydramnios, Potter syndrome (flat nose, recessed chin, epicanthal folds, low-set abnormal ears, limb abnormalities), and pulmonary hypoplasia.
- At birth, infants may present with renal insufficiency or HTN. Children will also present with bilateral flank masses at birth.

ADPKD

- Commonly presents in the fourth or fifth decade of life with hematuria, bilateral flank pain or masses, and HTN.
- Also associated with hepatic cysts and aneurysms of the cerebral circulation.

ARPKD—innumerable tiny cysts
ADPKD—large cysts

DIAGNOSIS

US of the kidneys reveals enlarged and hyperechogenic kidneys.

TREATMENT

Treatment is supportive. PKD results in ESRD. Treat patients with ESRD with dialysis and kidney transplant.

HIGH-YIELD FACTS

RENAL, GYNECOLOGIC, AND URINARY DISEASE

RENAL DYSPLASIA

DEFINITION

Abnormal metanephric differentiation resulting in nonrenal components affecting all or part of the kidney. A dysplastic kidney can contain nonrenal elements such as cartilage.

RENAL HYPOPLASIA

A 1-week-old male newborn has a wrinkled abdomen that lacks anterior abdominal musculature. He also has clubfeet and is in respiratory distress. His bladder is distended and easily palpable, and neither testis is in his scrotum. Lab findings include BUN 30, Cr 2, and HCO₃ 15. *Think: Prune belly syndrome.*

Triad: Absent abdominal wall muscles, undescended testes, and renal dysplasia. The renal collecting system is dilated. The bladder usually enlarged with a pseudodiverticulum at the urachus. Respiratory distress may be related to pulmonary hypoplasia due to severe oligohydramnios.

DEFINITION

- Nondysplastic small kidney that has decreased calyces and nephrons.
- Children with bilateral hypoplasia usually present with chronic renal failure.
- This is the leading cause of ESRD during the first decade of life.

FANCONI SYNDROME

DEFINITION

Rare disorder characterized by wasting of variable amounts of phosphate, glucose, amino acid, and bicarbonate by the proximal renal tubule.

ETIOLOGY

- Inherited.
- Cystinosis (defect of cystine metabolism that results in deposition of cystine in major organs of body, especially kidney, liver, eye, and brain).
- Galactosemia.
- Fructosemia.
- Lowe syndrome (X-linked disorder with congenital cataracts, mental retardation, and Fanconi syndrome).
- Tyrosinemia.
- Wilson disease.
- Acquired secondary to exposure to:
  - Chemotherapeutic/immunosuppressive agents (ifosfamide, tacrolimus, cyclosporine).
  - Heavy metals.
  - Gentamicin or outdated tetracycline.

Cystinosis is the most common cause of Fanconi syndrome.

Fanconi syndrome is one of the causes of proximal RTA.

SIGNS AND SYMPTOMS

- Growth retardation
- Rickets
- Polyuria
- Dehydration
- Anorexia
- Vomiting

DIAGNOSIS

- Elevated levels of glucose and electrolytes (phosphate, sodium, potassium, bicarbonate) in the urine.
- Evidence of renal insufficiency.

TREATMENT

- Bicarbonate therapy is mainstay.
- Replacement of phosphate.

It is important to distinguish Fanconi *syndrome* from Fanconi *anemia*. Fanconi anemia is an inherited disorder of bone marrow failure, whereas Fanconi syndrome is a disorder of renal tubules.

HORSESHOE KIDNEY

DEFINITION

Midline fusion of the lower kidney poles.

EPIDEMIOLOGY

- Seven percent of horseshoe kidneys are associated with Turner syndrome and are four times more common in children with Wilms' tumor.
- Horseshoe kidneys occur in 1 in 500 births.

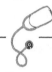

The major pathologic finding in congenital nephrotic syndrome is dilation of the proximal tubules.

NEPHROTIC SYNDROME

A 2-year-old boy has a 1-week history of edema. On examination, his BP is 100/60 and he has generalized edema and ascites. Lab values show Cr 0.4, albumin 1.4 g/dL, and cholesterol 569 mg/dL. A UA shows 4+ protein and no blood. *Think: Nephrotic syndrome.*

The common age of presentation is 2–6 years. Minimal change disease is the most common pattern of nephrotic syndrome in children. Typical presentation: periorbital and peripheral edema. Additional findings may include HTN and microscopic hematuria. Histopathologic examination shows no glomerular abnormalities on light microscopy in minimal change disease.

Nephrotic range proteinuria = Protein excretion of > 40 mg/m^2/hr. Random urine protein/ creatinine ratio > 3.0.

DEFINITION

Nephrotic syndrome is characterized by proteinuria, hypoalbuminemia, edema, and hyperlipidemia.

Patients can develop a hypercoagulable state due to nephrotic loss of antithrombin III.

Renal Biopsy

- Age < 1 year or > 8 years
- Recurrent gross hematuria
- Family history of kidney disease
- Laboratory findings suggestive of secondary nephrotic syndrome:
  - Sustained elevation in serum creatinine levels
  - Low C3/C4 levels
  - Positive antinuclear antibody (ANA) findings
  - Positive anti-double-stranded DNA antibody

Urine dipstick is not an accurate measure of protein excretion.

ETIOLOGY

- Eighty-five percent of nephrotic syndrome in children is caused by minimal change disease.
- Other causes of nephrotic syndrome include mesangial proliferation and focal segmental glomerulosclerosis.

PATHOPHYSIOLOGY

A loss of negatively charged glycoproteins in the capillary walls causes an ↑ in basement membrane permeability.

EPIDEMIOLOGY

- More common in boys than girls (2:1).
- Most common in children between 2 and 6 years of age, and commonly follows a viral illness.

SIGNS AND SYMPTOMS

- Pitting edema (most common clinical finding).
- Periorbital edema.
- Oliguria.
- Anasarca.

DIAGNOSIS

- The diagnosis is usually made clinically, with supportive laboratory values.
- Proteinuria > 3.5 g/24 hr.
- Serum albumin < 2.5 g/dL.
- Hyperlipidemia.
- A confirmatory renal biopsy shows fusion of the epithelial foot process by electron microscopy.

TREATMENT

- Most children will respond to steroids (4–6 weeks of prednisone).
- Relapses can be treated with steroids or alternative agents like cyclophosphamide or cyclosporine if steroid resistant.
- Salt/fluid restriction to ↓ edema.
- The majority of children will have ↓ relapses with age, most resolving by the end of the second decade.

COMPLICATIONS

- Infection is most common, especially spontaneous bacterial peritonitis. Two organisms: *Streptococcus pneumoniae* and *Escherichia coli*.
- Thromboembolism:
  - Higher in secondary nephrotic syndrome and membranous nephrotic syndrome.
  - Renal vein thrombosis, deep vein thrombosis, and pulmonary embolism.

A 4-year-old girl presents with malaise, periorbital edema, and smoky-colored urine. She had a strep throat infection 2 weeks prior. A serum complement level is ↓, and an antistreptolysin O (ASO) titer is ↑. *Think: PSGN.*

PSGN occurs after an infection of the throat or skin by group A β-hemolytic streptococci. It is manifested as an acute nephritic syndrome or as isolated hematuria and proteinuria. It is mediated by immune complexes, which is suggested by low complement level. The ASO is elevated. Urinalysis shows red blood cells and RBC casts.

DEFINITION

- Immune complex disease caused by group A β-hemolytic streptococcus types 12 and 49.
- Typically occurs 10–14 days following strep pharyngitis or a skin infection (impetigo).

DIAGNOSIS

- Positive throat cultures or ↑ antibody titers to streptococcal antigen.
- UA: RBC casts, RBCs, protein.
- **Light microscopy:** Enlarged glomeruli with mesangial proliferation and exudation of neutrophils.
- **Immunofluorescent microscopy:** Granular pattern of immunoglobulin deposition.
- **Electron microscopy:** Electron microscopy reveals electron-dense humps (immune complexes) on the epithelial side of the glomerular basement membrane (GBM).

TREATMENT

- Treat with penicillin for 10 days to prevent spread of nephrogenic strain of group A β-hemolytic streptococci.
- Treat renal and cardiac failure with peritoneal dialysis.
- Microscopic hematuria may take up to 1 year to resolve.

DEFINITION

- Acute glomerulonephritis = hematuria, proteinuria, and HTN.
- Severe glomerulonephritis that rapidly progresses to acute renal failure if left untreated.
- The underlying abnormality is the presence of crescent-shaped scars in the majority of the glomeruli.

Proteinuria

Normal protein excretion = ≤ 4 mg/m²/hr

Normal urine protein/creatinine ratio =
< 0.5 (< 2 year)
< 0.2 (> 2 year)

Transient
- Fever
- Dehydration
- Exercise

Orthostatic proteinuria (most common cause):
- Obtain two samples of urine (one in recumbent and the other in ambulatory position).
- Practically first morning urine and another sample later in the day.
- 24-hour urinary protein excretion < 1000 mg/day.
- Persistent (> 1+ on > 1 occasion).
- Requires further evaluation.

HIGH-YIELD FACTS

RENAL, GYNECOLOGIC, AND URINARY DISEASE

Causes of gross hematuria:
OUCH RED URINE HURTS
- **Oncologic agents**
- **Urethrorrhagia** (secondary to squamous metaplasia of urethra)
- **Coagulopathy**
- **Hydronephrosis**
- **Renal vein thrombosis**
- **Exercise**
- **Dead papillae** (papillary necrosis)
- **Urolithiasis**
- **Renal contusion**
- **Infections**
- **Neoplasm**
- **External manipulation** (masturbation)
- **Hypercalciuria**
- **Urethral injury**
- **Renal custs**
- **Trauma**
- **Sickle cell**

SIGNS AND SYMPTOMS

- RPGN presents like nephritic syndrome with nephrotic range proteinuria and rapidly progresses to ARF within weeks to months after onset.
- Gross hematuria and/or edema is the most common presentation.

DIAGNOSIS

- Complement C3 and C5 are usually decreased. The complement levels generally return to normal after 6–8 weeks.
- Light, immunofluorescent, and electron microscopy reveal presence of crescents on the inside of Bowman's capsule. The crescents are composed of the proliferative epithelial cells of the capsule, fibrin, and macrophages.

TREATMENT

Although some patients respond to corticosteroids or cyclophosphamide, prognosis is generally very poor, with most patients requiring dialysis.

MEMBRANOPROLIFERATIVE GLOMERULONEPHRITIS

A patient presents with hemoptysis, sinusitis, and glomerulonephritis. *Think: Wegener granulomatosis.*

Wegener granulomatosis involves the upper and lower airways and kidneys. Triad: Necrotizing granulomatous lesions in the respiratory tracts, necrotizing vasculitis, and focal glomerulonephritis. It is rare before adolescence. Most patients present with respiratory symptoms. The radiographic findings may include nodular infiltrates, pulmonary nodule, cavitation, and diffuse alveolar hemorrhage.

DEFINITION

Most common cause of chronic glomerulonephritis in older children.

SIGNS AND SYMPTOMS

- Nephrotic syndrome
- Hematuria
- HTN

DIAGNOSIS

- **Light microscopy:** Glomeruli arranged in a lobular pattern, often appearing duplicated with a "tram tracking" appearance.
- **Immunofluorescent microscopy:** Lobular deposits of C3 and immunoglobulins.
- **Electron microscopy:** Immune complex deposits in mesangial and subendothelial regions.

TREATMENT AND PROGNOSIS

- Poor prognosis. Fifty percent of patients will develop chronic renal failure within 10 years.
- There is no definitive therapy, although some patients respond to prednisone.

HIGH-YIELD FACTS

RENAL, GYNECOLOGIC, AND URINARY DISEASE

314

A patient presents with dyspnea, hemoptysis, and ARF. *Think:* Goodpasture syndrome.

Goodpasture syndrome is an antiglomerular basement membrane disease. Triad: glomerulonephritis, pulmonary hemorrhage, and antibody to basement membrane antigens. Respiratory manifestations: cough, dyspnea, and hemoptysis associated with pulmonary hemorrhage. Renal manifestations: acute nephritic syndrome with hematuria, proteinuria, and HTN. UA may show active sediment with RBCs and RBC casts.

DEFINITION

Membranous glomerulonephritis is an immune complex disease of the kidney.

EPIDEMIOLOGY

- It is the most common cause of nephrotic syndrome in adults and is uncommon in children.
- Can be idiopathic or secondary (SLE 10–20% of lupus nephritis).

SIGNS AND SYMPTOMS

- Presents as a nephrotic syndrome.
- Some patients have microscopic hematuria.

DIAGNOSIS

- **Light microscopy:** Diffuse thickening of the GBM without proliferative changes.
- **Immunofluorescent microscopy:** Granular deposits of immunoglobulin G (IgG) and C3.
- **Electron microscopy:** Deposits of IgG and C3 located on the epithelial side of the membrane.

TREATMENT

- Most cases resolve spontaneously in children, although some children will have persistent proteinuria.
- Nephrotic syndrome is best controlled with salt restriction and diuretics.

The most common cause of gross hematuria in children is IgA nephropathy.

Electron microscopy of membranous glomerulonephritis shows a "spike-and-dome" pattern on the epithelial side of the GBM.

DEFINITION

- Proteinuria up to 150 mg/day may be normal.
- Proteinuria consists of plasma, albumin, and Tamm-Horsfall proteins.
- **Postural proteinuria:** Proteinuria is ↑ from lying in supine to upright position due to unknown cause.
- **Febrile proteinuria:** Proteinuria caused by fever > 101°F (41.1°C). Febrile proteinuria will normalize after fever resolves.

■ **Exercise proteinuria:** Proteinuria following vigorous exercise. Usually resolves after 48 hours of rest.
■ Persistent proteinuria = glomerular lesion.
■ The most common cause of proteinuria in children is orthostatic proteinuria.

INTERSTITIAL NEPHRITIS—ACUTE AND CHRONIC

DEFINITION

Inflammation in the interstitium between the glomeruli in the areas surrounding the tubules.

RISK FACTORS

■ **Acute:** Allergy to medications (penicillin, cephalosporins, sulfonamides, rifampin, phenytoin, thiazides, furosemide, allopurinol, amphotericin B, NSAIDs) is the most common cause. Infections (especially in children), sarcoidosis, glomerulonephritis, and transplant rejection are also risk factors.
■ **Chronic:** Drugs (analgesics, lithium), infections, vesicoureteral reflux, urinary tract obstruction.

PATHOPHYSIOLOGY

Interstitial nephritis is often associated with tubular damage, edema, and necrosis between tubules.

SIGNS AND SYMPTOMS

■ **Acute:** Most patients present with ARF of generalized tubular dysfunction. Recent infections, new medications, fever, malaise, and signs of ARF should be investigated.
■ **Chronic:** Children usually present with symptoms of CRF such as nausea and vomiting, headache, fatigue, HTN, and growth failure.

DIAGNOSIS

■ **Acute:** Eosinophils in the urine suggest the diagnosis. A renal biopsy demonstrates an interstitial infiltrate of lymphocytes, plasma cells, eosinophils, and neutrophils and may help to differentiate acute interstitial nephritis (AIN) and ATN. Edema is present, and the glomeruli are typically normal.
■ **Chronic:** In chronic interstitial nephritis, the inflammatory cells consist of lymphocytes and plasma cells. Tubular fibrosis is present and the glomeruli are sclerosed secondary to ischemia. Renal papillary necrosis may be present.

TREATMENT

■ Treat renal failure.
■ Children with AIN may recover completely after withdrawal of the inciting agents. Children with chronic interstitial nephritis progress to ESRD.

DEFINITION

- A systemic autoimmune disease characterized by fever, weight loss, rash, hematologic abnormalities, and arthritis.
- Lupus nephritis is the most common manifestation of SLE in childhood.

PATHOPHYSIOLOGY

- Immune complexes deposit into the glomeruli, causing characteristic kidney diseases.
- See Table 14-2 for classification.

EPIDEMIOLOGY

- Most common in adolescent females.
- Uncommon in children < 8 years old.

SIGNS AND SYMPTOMS

- See Table 14-2.
- Renal disease is more frequent in children.

DIAGNOSIS

- Elevated serum levels of anti-Smith antibodies and anti-double-stranded DNA antibodies (anti-dsDNA antibodies) are highly specific for SLE.
- Markers of disease activity:
  - Anti-double-stranded DNA.
  - Complement levels C3 and C4.

TABLE 14-2. SLE Nephritis—World Health Organization (WHO) Classification and Symptoms

CLASSIFICATION	HISTOPATHOLOGY	SYMPTOMS
Class I	No histologic abnormalities detected.	No symptoms
Class II	Mesangial lupus nephritis. Glomeruli have mesangial deposits containing immunoglobulin and complement.	Hematuria Normal renal function Proteinuria of < 1 g/24 hr
Class III	Focal segmental lupus glomerulonephritis. Mesangial deposits in all glomeruli and subendothelial deposits in some.	Hematuria ± Proteinuria ± Reduced renal function ± Nephrotic syndrome
Class IV	Diffuse proliferative lupus nephritis. All glomeruli contain massive mesangial and subendothelial deposits of immunoglobulin and complement.	Hematuria ± Proteinuria ± Reduced renal function ± Nephrotic syndrome
Class V	Membranous lupus nephritis. Resembles idiopathic membranous glomerulopathy.	Nephrotic syndrome

TREATMENT

Immunosuppressive therapy (eg, prednisone, azathioprine) is used to help reduce/prevent flare-ups but cannot cure the disease.

RENAL VEIN THROMBOSIS (RVT) IN INFANCY

DEFINITION

- Thrombus formation in the renal vein.
- In infants, RVT is associated with dehydration, shock, and sepsis.
- Occurs in infants born to mothers with diabetes mellitus.
- In older children, RVT is associated with nephrotic syndrome (membranous nephropathy), cyanotic heart disease, hypercoagulable states, and contrast agents.

SIGNS AND SYMPTOMS

- Acute gross hematuria
- Oliguria
- Flank masses
- Flank pain

DIAGNOSIS

- US shows enlarged kidneys.
- Doppler flow studies show impaired (little) renal function.
- UA shows proteinuria and/or hematuria.

TREATMENT

- Correction of fluid and electrolyte abnormalities.
- Prophylactic anticoagulation with heparin.

COMPLICATIONS

- ARF (especially if bilateral).
- Systemic HTN.

Sudden onset of gross hematuria and unilateral or bilateral flank masses. *Think: Renal vein thrombosis.* **Must** evaluate for hypercoagulable states.

NEUROGENIC BLADDER

DEFINITION

Abnormal innervation to the bladder and sphincter muscles, associated with spinal abnormalities such as CNS tumors, spina bifida, teratomas, and myelodysplasia.

SIGNS AND SYMPTOMS

- Urinary incontinence.
- Urinary retention.
- Urinary tract infections (UTIs).
- Renal dysfunction caused by urinary reflux from bladder to kidneys (upper tract deteriorations).

TREATMENT

- Intermittent catheterization.
- Anticholinergic medication (oxybutinin).
- Surgical correction.

UROLITHIASIS

 An 8-year-old boy presents with left flank pain radiating to his left testicle. The pain does not change with movement or positioning and is colicky in nature. Urine dip is positive for blood. *Think: Urolithiasis.*

The pain begins in the flank, extends around the abdomen, and may radiate into the groin. Ipsilateral costovertebral tenderness may be present. Children with a history of multiple UTIs may be at risk of renal stones. UA typically shows hematuria, but absence of hematuria does not exclude the diagnosis of urolithiasis. Metabolic evaluation should include measurement of uric acid, electrolytes, creatinine, calcium, phosphorus, and bicarbonate. Serum PTH level should be obtained in the presence of hypercalciuria, hypercalcemia, or hypophosphatemia.

DEFINITION

Accumulation of urinary calculi in the urinary tract.

EPIDEMIOLOGY

- More common in boys than girls (2:1), children with metabolic abnormalities, urinary tract abnormalities, neuropathic bladder, enterocystoplasty.
- Only 7% of stones occur in children < 16 years of age.

ETIOLOGY

- Most stones are made of calcium, struvite, uric acid, or cystine that accumulates in the calyx or bladder.
- **Calcium stones:** Radiopaque stones due to ↑ intestinal calcium absorption or ↓ renal absorption.
- **Struvite stones:** Radiopaque stones composed of magnesium, ammonium, and phosphate. Most commonly secondary to chronic UTIs by urea-splitting bacteria such as *Proteus*.
- **Uric acid stones:** Radiolucent stones associated with high serum uric acid levels, such as hyperuricosuria, Lesch-Nyhan syndrome, after chemotherapy, myeloproliferative disorders, and inflammatory bowel disease.
- **Cystine stones:** Radiopaque stones associated with cystinuria, an autosomal-recessive disorder causing decreased absorption of dibasic amino acids (cystine, lysine, arginine, and ornithine) by the renal epithelial cells.

Metabolic disorders are often the cause of pediatric stones.

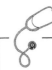

Hypercalciuria is the most common metabolic cause of stones.

SIGNS AND SYMPTOMS

- Microscopic or gross hematuria.
- Urinary tract obstruction.
- Abdominal/flank pain radiating to the genitalia (renal colic).
- Recurrent UTIs.

The most sensitive test for identifying stones in the urinary system is a noncontrast helical CT scan.

DIAGNOSIS

- Plain abdominal x-ray will show radiopaque stones (calcium and struvite). Ninety percent of stones are radiopaque.
- Abdominal CT can be better at detecting stones and will also yield information on the presence of hydronephrosis.

TREATMENT

- Pain management: NSAIDs are mainstay; opiates occasionally needed.
- IV hydration.
- Remove calculi if they are > 5–6 mm via urethral stent or lithotripsy, especially if they are associated with obstruction and hydronephrosis.
- **Calcium stones:** Treat with thiazide diuretic to reduce renal calcium excretion or potassium citrate, an inhibitor of calcium stones.
- **Struvite stones:** Treat with antibiotics to prevent recurrence of bacterial infections.
- **Uric acid stones:** Treat with allopurinol and urine alkalization.
- **Cystine stones:** Treat with D-penicillamine to chelate cystine.

URINARY TRACT INFECTION (UTI)

A 2-month-old male infant presents with fever, vomiting, and ↓ fluid intake. A UA reveals 100 WBCs. *Think: E coli UTI.*

The initial manifestations may be nonspecific and may include irritability, fever, and vomiting. *E coli* is the most common organism in children of all ages. Urinalysis may show positive urinary leukocyte esterase, positive urinary nitrite, pyuria (> 5 WBC/hpf) and bacteriuria.

A 7-year-old girl presents with urinary urgency, frequency, suprapubic pain, and no flank pain or mass. UA shows many leukocytes, 2–5 RBCs, and no protein or casts. *Think: Next step—urine culture.*

Older children with UTI are more likely to develop localizing symptoms such as frequency, dysuria, and abdominal or flank pain. The definitive diagnosis of UTI requires a positive urine culture from a specimen obtained with sterile techniques. An appropriately collected urinary specimen is critical to make the diagnosis of UTI.

A hospitalized 6-month-old infant with a UTI remains febrile after adequate IV antibiotic treatment. *Think: The next most appropriate diagnostic procedure is a renal US.*

The classic clinical manifestations of upper UTI include fever and flank pain. The persistence of fever despite antibiotics is suggestive of upper UTI (pyelonephritis). Febrile UTI in children may indicate either an underlying anatomic abnormality or vesicoureteral reflux (VUR). Ultrasound evaluation may detect underlying condition that predisposes the infant or child to infection.

DEFINITION

- Infection of the urinary system by bacterial pathogens. UTIs are often ascending infections from fecal/colonic flora.
- The most common bacteria are *E coli*, followed by *Klebsiella*, *Proteus*, enteroccci, and *Staphylococcus saprophyticus* (among female adolescents).
- UTIs are more common in males in the first year of life and more common in females afterwards.
- UTI occurs in 3–8% of girls and 1–2% of boys.

PREDISPOSING FACTORS

- Female.
- Uncircumcised male.
- Vesicoureteral reflux/anatomic abnormalities.
- Toilet training (wiping from back to front).
- Tight clothing.
- Bubble baths.
- Nylon panties, bathing suit.

CLASSIFICATION OF UTIs

- **Pyelonephritis:** Infection of the kidney characterized by abdominal or flank pain, fever, malaise, nausea, vomiting, and diarrhea.
- **Cystitis:** Infection of the bladder. Common symptoms include dysuria, urgency, frequency, suprapubic pain, incontinence, and malodorous urine. Cystitis does not cause fever.
- **Asymptomatic bacteriuria:** Presence of > 100,000/mL of a single bacterial organism on two successive urine cultures in a patient without any UTI-like symptoms.

SIGNS AND SYMPTOMS

Symptoms vary with age:

- Neonates: Failure to thrive, feeding irregularities, diarrhea, vomiting, fever, hyperbilirubinemia.
- 1 month–2 years: Colic, irritability, gastrointestinal (GI) complaints.
- > 2 years: Urgency, frequency, dysuria, abdominal and flank pain.

DIAGNOSIS

- Gold standard: **Urine culture.** If child is not toilet trained, specimen should be obtained via suprapubic tap or catheterization.
- Presence of > 100,000 colonies of a single bacteria or > 10,000 colonies in a symptomatic child or any bacterial growth from a properly obtained specimen.
- Leukocytes > 5/hpf.
- Hematuria.
- White cell casts.

TREATMENT

Treatment varies depending on the age of the child:

- Consider sepsis < 3 months of age with UTI.
- 2 months–2 years: UTIs are often associated with bacteremia in this age group, and 10–14 days of parenteral antibiotics is the treatment of

Consider nosocomial UTIs with *Pseudomonas* and methicillin-resistant *Staphylococcus aureus* in institutionalized or recently hospitalized patients.

choice. Trimethoprim-sulfamethoxazole, fluoroquinolones, and amino-penicillins are effective.
- Older children: 5–7 days of oral antibiotics.
- Pyelonephritis: 14-day therapy of β-lactam/cephalosporin. Antibiotics given intravenously initially, then switched to oral when clinical improvement is seen.
- Further investigations:
  - All children under the age of 5 and all male children should have a renal US to identify anatomic abnormalities including hydronephrosis, dilation of distal ureters, or bladder hypertrophy and to rule out pyelonephritis.
  - Voiding cystourethrogram (VCUG) is performed by placing a catheter through the urethra into the bladder and instilling a radionuclide testing agent until the bladder is full and the child voids. Images are taken to record reflux disease. Indications for VCUG:
    - Females < 5 years old with UTI.
    - Females > 5 years old presenting with second UTI.
    - All males.
    - Febrile UTI.
    - Some experts recommend waiting 4–6 weeks after febrile UTI is treated to obtain VCUG.
- Indications for admission:
  - Toxic-appearing child.
  - Pyelonephritis.
  - Child cannot tolerate oral antibiotics.

Perform a Gram stain on urine after obtaining a clean-catch specimen. A delay of 1–2 hours after receiving the specimen may cause bacterial multiplication and false positives.

VESICOURETERAL REFLUX

DEFINITIONS

- Retrograde flow of urine from the bladder to the ureter and renal pelvis.
- Reflux predisposes to (renal infections) pyelonephritis by facilitating the transport of bacterial from the bladder to the upper urinary tract.
- Recurrent pyelonephritis can result in renal scarring and ESRD.
- See Table 14-3 for grading of vesicoureteral reflux.

TABLE 14-3. Grading of Vesicoureteral Reflux

GRADE	ASSOCIATED SYMPTOM
I	Reflux into a nondilated ureter
II	Reflux into the upper collecting system without dilation
III	Reflux into dilated ureter and blunting of calyces
IV	Reflux into a grossly dilated ureter
V	Massive reflux, with significant ureteral dilation and tortuosity and loss of the papillary impression

EPIDEMIOLOGY

- VUR is seen in up to 50% of children with pyelonephritis.
- Eighty percent of children with reflux are female.
- Average age of diagnosis: 2–3 years.

SIGNS AND SYMPTOMS

Most reflux is diagnosed by VCUG during a workup for a UTI.

DIAGNOSIS/GRADING

VCUG or radionuclide cystogram.

TREATMENT

- The goal of treatment is to prevent pyelonephritis and renal injury.
- Children with low-grade reflux are managed medically with low-dose antibiotic prophylaxis (one-fourth to one-third dose of trimethoprim-sulfamethoxasole or nitrofurantoin) and UA and cultures every 3–4 months.
- Surgical therapy is performed in children with breakthrough UTI on antibiotic prophylaxis, unresolving reflux, and bilateral grade IV or V reflux.

OVARIAN/TESTICULAR TORSION

A 15-year-old boy presents with severe pain in his right testicle. This occurred suddenly while he was playing basketball. A physical exam reveals a tender, swollen, firm testicle with a transverse lie. There is no cremasteric reflex on the right. *Think: Testicular torsion.*

Diagnosis is made mainly by clinical suspicion. Classical presentation includes nausea, vomiting, and severe acute testicular pain. An absent or decreased cremasteric reflex is the most sensitive physical sign for diagnosing testicular torsion. However, its presence does not exclude the diagnosis. Abnormal testicular orientation such as transverse lie is another clue. Doppler ultrasound is helpful in making the diagnosis and would show no blood flow. Immediate surgical exploration should be performed if the suspicion is high.

A 16-year-old previously healthy boy experiences a sudden onset of abdominal and scrotal pain. A physical examination shows severe tenderness in the inguinal canal on the right, and the right side of scrotum is empty. A UA is within normal limits. *Think: Testicular torsion of an undescended testicle.*

Most undescended testes are found either in or just distal to the inguinal canal. Torsion may occur in an undescended testis. Torsion of testicle should be considered in a boy with inguinal pain and/or swelling with an undescended testis. The most effective management is an immediate operation. Early management of the undescended testes may avoid these complications.

> A 16-year-old boy presents with lower left abdominal pain and left testicular pain for 2 weeks. Palpation of the testes is normal except for isolated tenderness of the epididymis. Cremasteric reflex is normal. *Think: Epididymitis.*
>
> Patients with epididymitis experience scrotal pain of gradual onset and the tenderness is localized to the epididymis. However, history and physical findings may not reliably differentiate torsion from epididymitis. Urinalysis may show pyuria. Congenital genitourinary anomalies may be present which predispose to recurrent infection.

DEFINITION

Twisting of the ovary or testicle on its respective vascular pedicle.

EPIDEMIOLOGY

Testicular torsion is the most common cause of testicular pain in boys > 12 years and is most often due to poor fixation of the testis inside the scrotum (bell clapper deformity) due to redundancy of the tunica vaginalis.

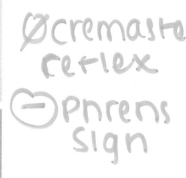

SIGNS AND SYMPTOMS

- **Ovarian torsion:** Acute unilateral intermittent sharp lower abdominal pain.
- **Testicular torsion:** Acute pain and swelling of the scrotum, absent cremasteric reflex. Testicle with horizontal lie.

DIAGNOSIS

Doppler US shows low blood flow but diagnosis should be made clinically to avoid delay in treatment.

TREATMENT

- Manual detorsion, followed by surgical fixation (orchiopexy). Torsion is a surgical emergency.
- Time is of the essence. The longer the ovary or testis remains torsed, the less the chance of salvaging it. Ninety percent of gonads survive if detorsion and fixation take place within 6 hours of symptom onset.
- Often a bilateral condition, so opposite testes is also fixed to the posterior scrotal envelope during surgery.

POLYCYSTIC OVARIAN (PCO) SYNDROME/OVARIAN CYSTS

DEFINITION

- PCO syndrome is the most commonly diagnosed ovarian cause of hirsutism.
- Other causes of ovarian cysts include ovarian hyperthecosis.

PATHOPHYSIOLOGY

- Anovulation:
  - Lack of characteristic hormonal fluctuations result in chronic anovulation and ↓ levels of progesterone due to the absence of a corpus luteum.

- Unopposed estrogen results in irregular shedding of a hyperplastic endometrium.
- Endometrial hyperplasia predisposes PCOS patients to endometrial carcinoma.
- Elevated testosterone: ↑ levels of LH stimulate ovarian follicular theca cells to produce androgens, resulting in hirsutism.

SIGNS AND SYMPTOMS

Hirsutism, amenorrhea, anovulatory infertility, obesity, insulin resistance.

DIAGNOSIS

- Elevated LH-to-FSH ratio of 3:1 (normal LH:FSH is 1.5:1)
- US shows multicystic ovaries (20–100 cystic follicles in each ovary) resembling a "pearl necklace."

TREATMENT

- Ovarian suppression with combined estrogen/progestin oral contraceptive pills. The progestin component will help reduce endometrial hyperplasia.
- Hirsutism can be treated with oral contraceptives, spironolactone, and electrolysis.

UNDESCENDED TESTES

DEFINITION

- Failure of one or both testes to descend into the scrotum. The undescended testes are usually found in the inguinal canal, but some may be ectopic.
- Cryptorchidism is the failure of the testes to descend by 6 months of age.

6mo old

SIGNS AND SYMPTOMS

- Cryptorchidism is associated with infertility, malignancy especially seminomas, hernias, and testicular torsion.
- The risk of malignancy is ↑ even if the testes are surgically placed into the scrotum; however, repositioning the testes makes them accessible for periodic examinations.
- Orchiopexy also helps to decrease the risk of testicular torsion by decreasing the mobility of the testis. Usually performed between 9 and 15 months of age.

TREATMENT

- **If testes are not palpated in the inguinal canal:** Orchiopexy after age 12 months.
- **If testes are palpated in the inguinal canal:** Hormonal therapy with luteinizing hormone–releasing hormone (LHRH) is controversial.

Orchiopexy at 12 mo.

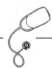

PainFUL ulcers:
Chancroid
Herpes
PainLESS ulcers:
Lymphogranuloma
   venereum (LGV)
Syphilis

Urethral discharge:
Gonorrhea
Chlamydia
Trichomonas

"Whiff test": Two drops of KOH mixed with the discharge and heated onto a slide produces a fishy smell. This is characteristic of both *Trichomonas* and bacterial vaginosis.

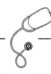

Due to the high rate of concurrent gonorrhea infection with chlamydia infection (60%), treatment for gonorrhea should always be included with that for chlamydia (and vice versa).

A 15-year-old female presents to the ED with a fever for 1 day, dyspareunia, and vaginal discharge. She had unprotected sexual intercourse with a new male partner 2 weeks ago. Physical exam reveals adnexal tenderness, cervical motion tenderness, and a friable cervix. *Think: Pelvic inflammatory disease.*

Acute PID is a condition of young females. Risk factors include younger age at first intercourse and unprotected sex. The most common clinical features are lower abdominal pain, ↑ vaginal discharge, and adnexal tenderness. Empiric treatment for PID is recommended in sexually active young women with pelvic or lower abdominal pain if any one of the following minimum criteria is present (cervical motion tenderness, adnexal tenderness, or uterine tenderness).

A 3-year-old girl presents with malodorous bloody vaginal discharge. *Think: Foreign body.*

Presentation: foul-smelling discharge or vaginal bleeding. Most common vaginal foreign body in children is toilet paper. A gentle examination should be performed. Complete history and focused physical examination are usually sufficient to make this diagnosis.

See Table 14-4.

EPIDEMIOLOGY

- Sexually transmitted diseases affect ~25% of adolescents.
- In infants and children, detection of an STD is an important clue to sexual abuse.

RISK FACTORS

- Sexual contact with person(s) with a history of STD.
- Multiple sexual partners.
- More than two sexual partners during previous 12 months.
- Intercourse with new partner during last 2 months.
- No contraception or use of nonbarrier methods.
- Street involvement (eg, homelessness).
- Injection drug use.
- "Survival sex" (eg, exchanging sex for money, drugs, shelter, or food).
- Men who have sex with men.

SCREENING AND PREVENTION

- All women should receive a Papanicolaou smear annually to screen for cervical dysplasia within the three years of first sexual experience or at the age of 21. In addition, screen all asymptomatic sexually active patients annually for HIV, herpes simplex virus (HSV), hepatitis B, and chlamydia.

- Educate all children how to ↓ the risk of contracting STDs, such as limiting number of sexual partners, using condoms, having regular check-ups, and engaging in open discussions about STDs.
- If sexual abuse is suspected, social services and law enforcement agencies must be contacted to ensure the child's protection.

TABLE 14-4. **Sexually Transmitted Diseases in Children**

	URETHRITIS AND CERVICITIS	EPIDIDYMITIS	VULVOVAGINITIS	PELVIC INFLAMMATORY DISEASE	CONDYLOMA ACUMINATA	GENITAL ULCERS
Definition	Inflammation of the urethra or cervix with mucopurulent discharge	Inflammation of the epididymis with mucopurulent discharge	Infectious causes of vaginal discharge, vulvar itching, and irritation	Inflammation of the upper female genital tract	Anogenital warts caused by human papillomavirus (HPV)	Ulcerative lesions on vagina, vulva, or penis
Symptoms	Urethral discharge Dysuria Possible proctitis or pharyngitis Women are symptomatic half as often as men Complications can include PID in women and Reiter syndrome in men, disseminated infection in both	Scrotal swelling Tenderness of the epididymis	Pruritus Vaginal discharge	Abdominal pain Fever Vomiting Cervical motion tenderness Adnexal tenderness Peritonitis Long-term complications result from scarring of the fallopian tubes, including infertility, ectopic pregnancy, and perihepatitis (Fitz-Hugh–Curtis syndrome)	Large, fleshy warts around anus	Lesion can be painful or painless, depending on etiology Inguinal lymphadeno-pathy Urethritis

(continues)

TABLE 14-4. Sexually Transmitted Diseases in Children (continued)

	URETHRITIS AND CERVICITIS	EPIDIDYMITIS	VULVOVAGINITIS	PELVIC INFLAMMATORY DISEASE	CONDYLOMA ACUMINATA	GENITAL ULCERS
Pathogens	*Chlamydia trachomatis* *Neisseria gonorrhoeae*	*C trachomatis* *N gonorrhea* *N gonorrhoeae*	*Trichomonas vaginalis* *Gardnerella vaginalis* (causes bacterial vaginosis [BV]) *Candida albicans*	*C trachomatis*	**HPV:** Types 6 and 11 are most frequently in genital warts, and types 16 and 18 are most common in cervical dysplasia	PAINFUL: Herpes simplex virus (HSV) *Haemophilus ducreyi* *Treponema pallidum* PAINLESS: *T pallidum* Lympho-granuloma venereum (LGV)
Diagnosis	Gram stain of urethral/vaginal discharge Polymerase chain reaction (PCR)/ enzyme-linked immunosorbent assay (ELISA) Culture (gonorrhea on Thayer–Martin agar)	UA shows pyuria (> 10 WBC/high-power field)	**Trichomoniasis:** Flagellated protozoan on wet preparation **BV:** Fishy odor of vaginal discharge; "clue cells" and pH > 4.5 on wet prep ***Candida:*** Cottage cheese discharge without odor; yeast or pseudohyphae with KOH stain present	Diagnosis is made clinically A positive culture for *N gonorrhoeae* or *C trachomatis* seen ~75% of the time	Acetic acid whitening is used to indicate the extent of infection (colposcopy) Pap smears detect cervical abnormalities	**HSV:** Tzanck smear **Syphilis:** *T pallidum* on darkfield microscopy **Chancroid:** Gram stain reveals gram-positive cocci arranged in boxcar formation **LGV:** Elevated Ab titers on complement fixation and microimmuno-fluorescence tests

TABLE 14-4. Sexually Transmitted Diseases in Children (continued)

	URETHRITIS AND CERVICITIS	EPIDIDYMITIS	VULVOVAGINITIS	PELVIC INFLAMMATORY DISEASE	CONDYLOMA ACUMINATA	GENITAL ULCERS
Treatment	**Chlamydia:** Single-dose oral azithromycin or doxycycline, erythromycin, levofloxacin, or ofloxacin for 7 days **Gonorrhea:** IM ceftriaxone or oral cefixime, ciprofloxacin, or ofloxacin If patient has gonorrhea, then treat for chlamydia as well (Treat for both bugs and treat both partners)	Scrotal supporter for comfort Trimethoprim-sulfamethoxazole	**Trichomoniasis and BV:** Metronidazole **Candida:** Topical azoles	Doxycycline for 2 weeks	Posodilox Cryotherapy Surgical removal	**HSV:** Acyclovir ***T pallidum:*** Penicillin **Chancroid + LGV:** Azithromycin

PHIMOSIS/PARAPHIMOSIS

DEFINITION

- **Phimosis:** Inability to retract the prepuce (foreskin) over the glans penis. Phimosis is normal in (boys) males younger than 3 years of age. In older males, phimosis is considered pathologic and may be due to the inflammation at the tip of the foreskin.
- **Paraphimosis:** Inability to reduce to foreskin due to venous congestion of the distal foreskin. Paraphimosis can progress to arterial compromise → penile infarction/necrosis and gangrene.
- Risk factors for phimosis/paraphimosis:
  - Poor hygiene → recurrent balanitis.
  - Repeated catheterization.
  - Forceful retraction of the foreskin resulting in scarring/phimosis.
  - Penile piercing.

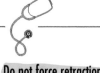

Do not force retraction of the foreskin in phimosis. This may → paraphimosis.

SIGNS AND SYMPTOMS

- Phimosis may cause urinary retention secondary to pain or obstruction of the urethra.
- The most acute complication of phimosis is paraphimosis.

TREATMENT

- **Phimosis:** Steroid cream applied to the foreskin or manual stretching to loosen the phimotic ring. Circumcision is recommended for chronic phimosis in children > 10 years old.
- **Paraphimosis:** Lubrication and manual compression of the foreskin and glans. Superficial vertical incision of the ligating band may be needed in refractory cases. Treatment is directed at reducing penile edema and restoring the foreskin to its original position as paraphimosis is a urologic emergency.

HYPOSPADIAS

It is important to not circumcise children with hypospadias, as the foreskin is used in the repair.

DEFINITION

- Ventral opening of the urethra on the penile shaft due to incomplete development of the foreskin "dorsal hood."
- Hypospadias is sometimes associated with in vivo exposure to estrogens or antiandrogens.
- Associated with cryptorchidism and chordee (congenital malformation in which the head of the penis curves downward or upward).

TREATMENT

Surgical repair at 6–12 months.

EPISPADIAS

- Dorsal opening of the urethra on the penile shaft.
- Associated with more serious congenital abnormalities such as bifid phallus, bladder, and/or cloacal exstrophy.

TREATMENT

Surgical repair recommended within first 2 months of life.

Hematologic Disease

TABLE 15-1. Normal Hemoglobin and Mean Corpuscular Volume (MCV) by Age

AGE	HGB (G/DL)	MCV (FL)
Birth	13.5–24.0	95–121
< 2 month	10.0–20.0	
2–6 months	9.5–14.0	
6 months–2 years	10.5–13.5	70–86
2–12 years	11.5–15.5	
12–18 years	12.0–16.0	78–102

NORMAL HEMOGLOBIN BY AGE

Normal values of hemoglobin and red cell parameters vary with age (see Table 15-1).

ANEMIA

DEFINITION

Reduced circulating red blood cell (RBC) mass.

CLASSIFICATION

- Size and hemoglobin content (mean corpuscular volume [MCV], mean corpuscular hemoglobin concentration [MCHC]) (see Table 15-2).
- Mechanism—loss/sequestration, ↑ destruction, ↓ production.

PATHOPHYSIOLOGY

- Less oxygen transport.
- ↓ blood volume.
- ↑ cardiac output.

SIGNS AND SYMPTOMS

- Somnolence, light-headedness, headache.
- Angina, dyspnea, palpitations, flow murmur.
- Fatigue, claudication, edema.
- Pallor—conjunctiva, palmar creases.
- Hepatosplenomegaly in some cases.
- Irritability.
- Pica: Desire to eat unusual things (eg, clay).

DIAGNOSIS

- Family history.
- Exposure history.
- Past medical history, including medications.

TABLE 15-2. Anemias

MCV	MCHC	ANEMIA	RDW	SMEAR	LABS
Microcytic < 80 (↓ Hgb production)	Hypochromic	Iron deficiency	↑	Elliptocytes Nucleated/Target RBCs	↓ ferritin, ↓ TIBC ↑ platelets
		Thalassemia	+/– Nl		↑ Red cell count
		Lead toxicity		Stippled RBCs	
	Normochromic	Neoplastic			
Normocytic 80–100	Normochromic	Acute blood loss		Schistocytes	Bilirubin/LDH
		Hemolytic (microangiopathic)	Nl		
		Anemia of chronic disease	Nl		↓ TIBC
		Hemoglobinopathy	Nl	Target cell	
		Renal disease		Acanthocyte	BUN/creatinine
Macrocytic > 100 (defective DNA synthesis)	Normochromic	Hemolytic (autoimmune)	↑	Spherocytes	Bilirubin/LDH Direct Coombs' test
		Alcohol	Nl	Round	
		Liver disease	Nl	Round, target, echinocyte, acanthocyte	
		Aplastic anemia	Nl		
		Hypothyroidism	↑	Round	T$_4$/TSH
		Drug effect (eg, hydroxyurea)		Oval	
		Myelodysplasia		Oval, dacrocyte	
Megaloblastic > 110 (defective DNA synthesis)		Folate deficiency	↑	Oval PMN segmented	↓ reticulocytes ↓ serum folate ↑ homocysteine
		B$_{12}$ deficiency/pernicious anemia	↑	Oval PMN segmented	↓ serum cobalamin Schilling test ↓ reticulocytes ↑ serum methylmalonic acid and homocysteine

BUN, blood urea nitrogen; LDH, lactic dehydrogenase; MCV, mean corpuscular volume; MCHC, mean corpuscular hemoglobin concentration; PMN, polymorphonuclear neutrophil; RBC, red blood cell; RDW, red cell distribution width; T$_4$, thyroxine; TIBC, total iron-binding capacity; TSH, thyroid-stimulating hormone.

- Physical exam.
- Complete blood count (CBC): See Table 15.2.
- Peripheral blood smear: See Table 15-3.
- Platelet and white blood cell (WBC) size, morphology.
- Possible bone marrow aspirate/biopsy—cellularity, morphology, stroma.

TABLE 15-3. Some Erythrocyte Morphology and Inclusion Bodies

CELL	SPHEROCYTE	TARGET CELL	ECHINOCYTE (BURR)	ACANTHOCYTE	DACROCYTE
Description	Round, no central clearing	Concentric circles	Evenly spaced projections (spikes)	Irregularly spaced projections	Teardrop shape
Mechanism	Defective RBC membrane	↑ in membrane to Hgb ratio	Spiculed, crenated	Excess lipid in membrane	Extramedullary hematopoiesis
Etiologies	Hereditary spherocytosis Autoimmune hemolytic anemia	Liver disease Hemoglobinopathies (eg, Hgb C, S) Postsplenectomy Thalassemia	Liver disease Postsplenectomy Azotemia/uremia Gastric carcinoma	Liver disease Renal failure Splenic disease DIC Pyruvate kinase deficiency	Myelofibrosis

CELL	SCHISTOCYTE	SICKLE CELLS	BASOPHILIC STIPPLING	HOWELL-JOLLY BODY	HEINZ BODIES
Description	"Bite cell"	Pointed	Round, dark-blue granules in the cell	Densely blue cytoplasmic inclusions	Round protuberances deforming the cell
Mechanism	Mechanical damage		Aggregated ribosomes	Nuclear fragments	Oxidized/ denatured Hgb
Etiologies	G6PD deficiency DIC HUS Vasculitis	Sickle cell disease	Sideroblastic anemia Myelodysplastic syndrome Heavy metal poisoning	Hemolytic anemia Megaloblastic anemia Hyposplenism Postsplenectomy	Oxidative medications, chemicals Abnormal Hgb (H, Köln) Enzyme deficiencies (G6PD)

DIC, disseminated intravascular coagulation; G6PD, glucose-6-phosphate dehydrogenase; HUS, hemolytic-uremic syndrome; RBC, red blood cell.

- Chemistry—liver function tests (LFTs), lactic dehydrogenase (LDH), creatinine (Cr), uric acid.
- Imaging as appropriate.
- Other special tests—serum ferritin, B_{12}, folate, reticulocyte count, Coombs' test, osmotic fragility, etc.

TREATMENT

- Supplement or remove causative factor.
- Support hemodynamics as appropriate.

HIGH-YIELD FACTS

HEMATOLOGIC DISEASE

Coombs test: Direct—detects auto-IgG bound RBCs (autoimmune hemolysis); indirect—detects unbound autoantibodies to RBCs (antenatal, pretransfusion testing).

Schilling test: Radiolabeled B$_{12}$ used to investigate B$_{12}$ deficiency

Normal newborn Hgb is 14–20 g/dL.

Physiologic Anemia of Infancy

- Normal newborns have higher hemoglobin until third week.
- ↓ to 9–11 g/dL at 8–12 weeks.
- Decline in hemoglobin level is both more extreme and more rapid in premature infants: 7–9 g/dL by 3–6 weeks.

ETIOLOGY

- Abrupt cessation of erythropoiesis with the onset of respiration.
- ↓ survival of fetal RBCs.
- Expansion of blood volume in first 3 months.
- No therapy needed.
- Transient erythroblastopenia of childhood (TEC).
- The most common acquired red cell aplasia in children.
- Age 6 months to 3 years (most children > 12 months).

Transient Erythroblastopenia of Childhood

A previously healthy 1-year-old male infant had a cold 8 weeks ago. He now is pale and irritable and refuses to eat. A CBC shows Hgb 5.0, Hct 10%, MCV 80, reticulocyte count 0%, WBC 9, platelets 400K. *Think: Transient erythroblastopenia of childhood (TEC).*

TEC occurs in previously healthy children and is often preceded by a viral infection. Classic history is gradual onset of pallor between the ages of 1 and 4 years. Characteristic features include normocytic anemia, severe reticulocytopenia, transient neutropenia, and ↑ platelet counts. It is often confused with Diamond-Blackfan anemia. TEC is a self-limited condition and has an excellent prognosis.

Diamond-Blackfan should be differentiated from transient erythroblastopenia of childhood based on the features listed.
- Age (average age of diagnosis = 3 months)
- Macrocytic (↑ MCV)
- Reticulocytopenia

DEFINITION

Transient failure of the bone marrow to produce RBCs usually at 18–26 months; may occur at < 6 months and up to 10 years.

ETIOLOGY

Possible link to parvovirus B19.

SIGNS AND SYMPTOMS

Gradual pallor and fatigue; appearance better than expected for Hgb level.

DIFFERENTIAL DIAGNOSIS

- Diamond-Blackfan anemia.
- Etiology: Genetic.

- Age: During first year.
- ↑ MCV.
- ↑ Red cell adenosine deaminase (ADA).
- ↑ Hemoglobin F.
- ↑ i Antigen.

DIAGNOSIS

- CBC: Hgb 5–7, clinically insignificant neutropenia.
- Normochromic, normocytic anemia (MCV normal for age).
- Reticulocyte count initially < 1%, ↑ with recovery (↑ MCV during recovery).
- Any child with presumed TEC who requires more than one transfusion should be considered for alternate diagnoses.

TREATMENT

- Supportive until RBC production returns; should occur spontaneously in 30–60 days.
- If continues, different causes of the anemia must be investigated.

NUTRITIONAL ANEMIAS

Iron Deficiency Anemia   MICRO

 A 9-month-old child who has been fed whole milk from early infancy presents with the following lab values: Hgb 7.5 g, MCV 62, RBC 3.2. *Think: Iron deficiency anemia.*

Consumption of large amounts of cow's milk is the most common dietary pattern in children with iron deficiency anemia. Cow's milk has poor iron bioavailability, especially in infants < 12 months. In the first year, full-term infants need to absorb 1.2 mg of elemental iron. Since only up to 10% of dietary iron is absorbed, daily intake of iron should exceed 12 mg. Characteristic findings are microcytic, hypochromic anemia, low mean corpuscular volume (MCV) and mean corpuscular hemoglobin (MCH), ↑ red cell distribution width (RDW), and ↓ reticulocyte count. Depletion of iron stores is the earliest finding.

ETIOLOGY

- Inadequate intake (whole cow's milk has no iron).
- Loss of iron.
- Bleeding.
- Rapid growth spurts (early infancy and adolescence).
- Prematurity (↓ iron stores).
- Chronic diseases (juvenile rheumatoid arthritis [JRA], cystic fibrosis [CF]).

EPIDEMIOLOGY

- Most common anemia in children.
- Especially 6 months to 3 years old.
- Rare in infants under 6 months.

Mentzer Index
MCV/RBC
≥ 13 Iron deficiency
≤ 13 Thalassemia trait

SIGNS AND SYMPTOMS

- Usual symptoms of anemia.
- Cheilosis/angular stomatitis, glossitis.
- Koilonychia (spoon nails).
- Esophageal web.
- Blue sclera.
- Splenomegaly.

DIAGNOSIS

- ↓ serum ferritin (< 10 ng/mL).
- ↓ serum iron.
- ↑ iron-binding capacity.
- Microcytic and hypochromic, ↑ RDW.
- Low reticulocyte count.
- ↑ platelet count (> 600,000/mm³).
- Hypercellular marrow with erythroid hyperplasia.
- ↓ stainable iron.

TREATMENT

- Ferrous sulfate 3 mg/kg/day for at least 8 weeks after a normal Hgb level is obtained.
- Retic response to oral iron within 4 days.

Remember: Ferritin is an acute phase reactant. A normal or high ferritin does not exclude iron deficiency during an acute infection.

Lead Poisoning 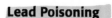 MICRO

A 2½-year-old boy with hyperactivity lives in old apartment building with peeling paint on the walls. His gait has become ataxic and his speech has regressed. His Hgb is 8.5 g. *Think: Lead poisoning.*

Lead poisoning is usually caused by exposure to dust and paint chips from interior surfaces of homes. The initial signs and symptoms may be nonspecific. Laboratory screening should be considered for children at risk for lead poisoning and should be screened routinely starting at age 1 year. A blood lead level of ≥ 10 μg/dL is considered abnormal. To avoid contamination, a venous sample should be obtained for confirmation. Other features are anemia and basophilic stippling on peripheral smear and elevated free erythrocyte protoporphyrin level.

Chronic lead poisoning interferes with iron utilization and hemoglobin synthesis.

DEFINITION

Variant of iron deficiency anemia.

ETIOLOGY

- Environmental (aerosolized and oral).
- Lead-containing paint.

Screening for lead poisoning occurs at 10–14 months and at 2 years of age.

PATHOPHYSIOLOGY

- Irreversible binding with sulfhydryl group of proteins.
- Inhibits enzymes involved in heme production.
- Impairs iron utilization.

SIGNS AND SYMPTOMS

- Acute encephalopathy.
- Lead lines—thick transverse radiodense lines in the metaphyses of growing bones on radiographs.

DIAGNOSIS

- Microcytic hypochromic anemia, basophilic stippling.
- ↑ serum lead and free erythrocyte protoporphyrin (FEP) level. Lead level < 9 is considered acceptable.
- ↑ urine coproporphyrin.

TREATMENT

- Environment control, education, level dependent.
- 70 μg/dL—medical emergency: Dimercaprol (BAL) followed by ethylenediaminetetraacetic acid (EDTA)—5 days' treatment.
- 45–69 μg/dL: Both medical and environmental intervention including chelation (EDTA or DMSA).
- 20–45 μg/dL: Environmental evaluation + pharmacologic treatment such as EDTA provocative chelation test.
- 10–19 μg/dL: Education.
- Prevention: Banning of lead-based paint in 1978.

Folate Deficiency *MACRO*

DEFINITION

Megaloblastic anemia.

ETIOLOGY

- Deficient intake or absorption. *alcoholics*
- Pregnancy (↑ requirement).
- Very-low-birth-weight (VLBW) infants.
- Drugs (phenytoin, methotrexate).
- Vitamin C deficiency.

EPIDEMIOLOGY

Peak age 4–7 months.

SIGNS AND SYMPTOMS

- Features of anemia.
- Failure to gain weight.
- Chronic diarrhea.

DIAGNOSIS

- Macrocytic anemia, thrombocytopenia, neutropenia (hypersegmented PMNs).
- Low reticulocyte count.
- ↑ LDH.
- Bone marrow hypercellular and megaloblastic changes.
- Serum and RBC folate levels.

Lead paint remains the most common cause of lead poisoning.

Goat's milk is folate deficient.

Green vegetables, fruits, liver, and kidneys contain folate.

RBC folate is the best indicator of chronic deficiency.

TREATMENT

- Parenteral folic acid only after confirmation.
- Folic acid is contraindicated in vitamin B$_{12}$ deficiency, because it will mask anemia, yet B$_{12}$ deficiency neurologic symptoms will progress.

Vitamin B$_{12}$ Deficiency

DEFINITION

Megaloblastic anemia.

ETIOLOGY

- Inadequate intake (strict vegetarians).
- Pernicious anemia.
- Surgery of stomach or terminal ileum.

PATHOPHYSIOLOGY

Deficiency of intrinsic factor due to autoimmunity or gastric mucosal atrophy prevents adequate B$_{12}$ absorption.

SIGNS AND SYMPTOMS

- Juvenile pernicious anemia.
- Red, beefy tongue.
- Premature graying, blue eyes, vitiligo.
- Myxedema, gastric atrophy.
- Weakness, irritability, anorexia.
- Neurologic (ataxia, paresthesias, hyporeflexia, Babinski response, clonus).

Subacute combined systems disease in B$_{12}$ deficiency — demyelination of dorsal and lateral columns of spinal cord:
- ↓ vibration sense
- ↓ proprioception
- Gait apraxia
- Spastic paraparesis
- Paresthesias
- Incontinence
- Impotence

DIAGNOSIS

- Macrocytic anemia, large hypersegmented neutrophils.
- ↑LDH.
- Methylmalonic acid in urine.
- Anti-intrinsic factor antibody.
- Schilling test.

TREATMENT

- Vitamin B$_{12}$ IM monthly.
- Oral therapy is contraindicated.

Copper Deficiency

PATHOPHYSIOLOGY

Copper is essential for production of red blood cells, transferrin, and hemoglobin.

SIGNS AND SYMPTOMS

- Refractory anemia, pancytopenia.
- Osteoporosis.
- Ataxia, spasticity.
- Menke disease in newborns — X linked.

ETIOLOGY

- Copper-deficient total parenteral nutrition (TPN).
- Persistent infantile diarrhea.
- Post gastric bypass surgery.
- Zinc supplementation ($\downarrow$ copper absorption).

DIAGNOSIS

- Hypochromic anemia unresponsive to iron supplementation.
- Neutropenia.
- Impaired bone calcification.
- Serum copper and ceruloplasmin levels.

TREATMENT

Treat underlying cause.

Dietary copper is found in liver, oysters, meat, fish, whole grains, nuts, and legumes.

Anemia of Chronic Disease

ETIOLOGY

- JRA, systemic lupus erythematosus (SLE), ulcerative colitis.
- Malignancies.
- Renal disease.

DIAGNOSIS

- Can be normochromic and normocytic or hypochromic and microcytic.
- Hgb ranges 7–10 g/dL.
- Low serum iron with normal or low total iron-binding capacity (TIBC).
- Elevated serum ferritin.

TREATMENT

- Treat underlying cause.
- Iron if concomitant iron deficiency is present.

See Figure 15-1.

SIGNS AND SYMPTOMS

- Can vary from asymptomatic to generalized symptoms to severe pain crises.
- Icterus, fever, splenomegaly.
- $\uparrow$ products of RBC destruction.
- Compensatory $\uparrow$ in hematopoiesis-reticulocytosis.
- See Table 15-4.

DIAGNOSIS

- $\uparrow$ direct bilirubin.
- $\downarrow$ haptoglobin (intravascular especially).
- $\uparrow$ hemoglobinuria/hemosiderinuria (intravascular).
- $\uparrow$ LDH.

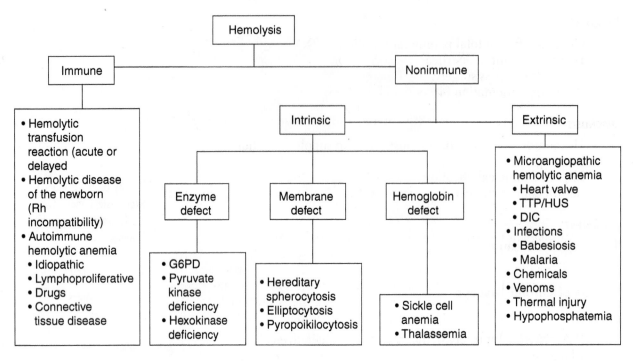

FIGURE 15-1. Hemolytic anemias.

TABLE 15-4. Hemolysis

FEATURE	EXTRAVASCULAR	INTRAVASCULAR
RBC morphology	Abnormal	Normal
Hemoglobinemia/uria	–	+
Hemosiderinuria	–	+
Serum haptoglobin	Normal	↓
Splenomegaly	+	–
Examples		Transfusion reactions
		Microangiopathic hemolytic
		Infections: babesiosis, malaria
		G6PD deficiency
		Paroxysmal nocturnal hemoglobinuria

G6PD, glucose-6-phosphate dehydrogenase; RBC, red blood cell.

Hemolytic Disease of the Newborn

DEFINITION

Erythroblastosis fetalis.

ETIOLOGY

Maternal sensitization to Rh, ABO, or other blood system antigens (Kell, Duffy).

PATHOPHYSIOLOGY

- Paternal heterozygosity allows an Rh-positive (or other alloantibody) infant to be carried by an Rh-negative mother.
- Maternal blood comes into contact with fetal blood cells.
- Maternal antibodies are produced against the Rh antigen.
- During a subsequent pregnancy with an Rh-positive infant, maternal antibodies cross the placenta and bind to fetal RBCs, → hemolysis.
- Destruction of RBCs causes ↑ unconjugated bilirubin, becoming clinically apparent only after delivery as the placenta effectively metabolizes it.
- Severe anemia → ↑ extramedullary erythropoiesis, with potential replacement of hepatic parenchyma.

EPIDEMIOLOGY

- Severe Rh disease is rare in the United States nowadays.
- Rh sensitization occurs in 11 of 10,000 pregnancies.
- < 1% of births are associated with significant hemolysis.
- Approximately 50% of affected newborns do not require treatment, 25% are term but die or develop kernicterus, and 25% become hydropic in utero.

SIGNS AND SYMPTOMS

- Hemolytic anemia.
- Fetal hydrops:
  - Large placenta.
  - ↑ unconjugated hyperbilirubinemia—rapidly progressive jaundice after birth, kernicterus.
  - Abdominal distention—hepatosplenomegaly, ascites, hepatic dysfunction.
  - Abduction of limbs, loss of flexion.
  - Scalp edema.
  - Purpura.
  - Cyanosis.

DIAGNOSIS

Positive direct Coombs' test.

TREATMENT

- Know blood types of both parents early in the pregnancy.
- Prophylaxis (RhoGam) during and immediately after delivery for mothers at risk for alloimmunization
- Exchange transfusion to infant of Rh-negative blood.

Mutation causing sickle cell disease: Glu-6-val.

Sickle Cell Disease (SCD)

A 16-month-old African-American boy is brought to the ED because of crying and refuses to stand. He has no fever, vomiting, or diarrhea. His parents denied trauma or fall. On examination, he is afebrile. He cries when his right leg is touched. X-ray of his right leg showed no fracture. *Think: Sickle cell disease.*

Acute sickle cell painful episode (painful crisis) is the most common presentation in children with SCD. Newborn screening has resulted in detection in early infancy. CBC shows chronic hemolytic anemia with low hematocrit and hemoglobin levels and a reticulocytosis. Peripheral smear may show sickled forms, target cells, and polychromasia suggestive of reticulocytosis.

As part of a routine genetic screening, a term African-American newborn has Hgb F, A, and S. Possible diagnoses on quantitative testing could be HgbAS trait or HgbS-thalassemia.

DEFINITION

Chronic hemolytic anemia due to premature destruction of red cells.

ETIOLOGY

Defect in β-globin–hemoglobin S (HgbS)—substitution of glutamic acid at sixth position of β chain by valine.

PATHOPHYSIOLOGY

- Unusual solubility problem in the deoxygenated state.
- HgbS is a low-affinity hemoglobin.

EPIDEMIOLOGY

- Autosomal recessive.
- One in 500 African-Americans.
- Eight percent of African-Americans are carriers.

Four sickle cell crises:
- Vaso-occlusive crisis
- Aplastic crisis (parvovirus)
- Sequestration crisis
- Hemolytic crisis

SIGNS AND SYMPTOMS

- Appears after 6 months of age (when HbF is ↓).
- Anemia (due to hemolysis).
- Vaso-occlusive: Leg ulcers, stroke, priapism, pain crises.
- Hand-foot syndrome (swollen hands and feet).
- Infection (encapsulated organisms):
  - *Streptococcus pneumoniae* (30%)
  - *Haemophilus influenzae*
  - *Salmonella* osteomyelitis
- Splenomegaly.
- Cardiac enlargement.
- Short stature, delayed puberty.
- Gallstones/jaundice.

The most common cause of fatal sepsis in patients with sickle cell disease is *Streptococcus pneumoniae.*

DIAGNOSIS

- Newborn screening.
- Hgb electrophoresis (definitive test).
- HgbS 90%.
- HgbF 2–10%.
- No HgbA.

- Hgb ranges 5–9 g/dL.
- Peripheral smear—target cells and sickled cells.
- ↑ WBCs and platelets.

TREATMENT

- Pneumococcal vaccine (at 2 and 5 years).
- Prophylactic penicillin by 4 months of age.
- Painful crisis—hydration and analgesics. *hydroxurea*
- Priapism—exchange transfusion.

There now exists universal newborn screening for sickle cell disease.

Thalassemia

A 2-year-old boy has required transfusion since early infancy. *Think: β-Thalassemia major.*

Children with β-thalassemia usually become symptomatic in early infancy because of progressive hemolytic anemia and cardiac decompensation. Severe hypochromia and microcytosis is the characteristic of β-thalassemia. The hemoglobin level declines progressively in the first year and may be as low as 3–4 g/dL, requiring transfusion.

DEFINITION

Hereditary hemolytic anemia.

ETIOLOGY

Total or partial deletions of globin chain.

- **α-Thalassemia (gene deletion):**
  - Hgb Bart's (four-gene deletion).
  - HgbH (three-gene deletion).
  - α-Thalassemia minor (two-gene deletion).
  - Silent carrier (one-gene deletion).
- **β-Thalassemia:**
  - Homozygous (β-thalassemia major).
  - Heterozygous (β-thalassemia minor).

β-thalassemia major is fatal without regular transfusion.

SIGNS AND SYMPTOMS

- Severe hemolytic anemia.
- Hepatosplenomegaly.
- Extramedullary hematopoiesis (classic facies—maxillary overgrowth and skull bossing).

DIAGNOSIS

- Hypochromic, microcytic anemia.
- Hgb < 5 g/dL.
- Reticulocytopenia.
- Markedly ↑ LDH (ineffective erythropoiesis).
- Hgb electrophoresis:
  - HgbA: ↓ or absent
  - ↑ HgbA$_2$
  - HgbF: Marked elevation

TREATMENT

- Monthly transfusion of packed RBCs to maintain Hgb > 10 g/dL.
- Splenectomy if requiring > 240 mL/kg of packed RBCs/year.

Hemosiderosis:
- Cardiomyopathy
- Cirrhosis
- Diabetes

HEMOLYTIC ENZYMOPATHIES

Glucose-6-Phosphate Dehydrogenase (G6PD) Deficiency

A previously well 2-year-old African-American male child is treated with sulfonamide. Two days later, he develops fever, back pain, dark urine, and anemia. Blood smear shows fragmented erythrocytes. *Think: G6PD deficiency.*

The highest prevalence of G6PD deficiency is in Africans and people of Mediterranean descent. It is a recessive X-linked trait; therefore, males are at higher risk. Episodic hemolysis is the characteristic of G6PD deficiency. It is caused by exposures that cause oxidant stress such as infection or drugs. Sulfonamides and antimalarial drugs (primaquine and chloroquine) are the common agents.

A male child has sudden onset of dark urine, pallor, and jaundice after an exposure to an oxidant stress. *Think: G6PD deficiency.*

Most patients are asymptomatic unless exposed to an oxidant stress that results in a hemolytic crisis. Jaundice and splenomegaly may be present during an acute crisis. Heinz bodies, indicative of denatured hemoglobin, are typically present and can be detected by a methyl violet stain. G6PD levels can be deceptively normal during an acute crisis because of an elevated reticulocyte count. Therefore, G6PD levels should be obtained weeks to months later to obtain an actual baseline measurement.

DEFINITION

- Enzyme defect of hexose monophosphate (HMP) pathway, resulting in hemolysis when exposed to stresses such as infection or certain drugs.
- Develops 24–48 hours after the exposure of an oxidizing agent.

ETIOLOGY

Hereditary ↓ of G6PD that normally maintains adequate level of glutathione in a reduced state in RBCs.

PATHOPHYSIOLOGY

- Oxidized glutathione complexes with Hgb, forming Heinz bodies.
- RBC less deformable.
- Splenic macrophages "bite out" RBCs.

EPIDEMIOLOGY

- Most common hemolytic enzymopathy.
- X-linked.
- Higher incidence in African-American, Middle Eastern, and Mediterranean populations.

Parents of a child with G6PD deficiency should be provided a list of drugs and foods to avoid.

infection
Depsone
Bactrim
Flava beans

SIGNS AND SYMPTOMS

- Episodic intravascular hemolysis secondary to oxidant stress (drugs, fava beans, etc.).
- Spontaneous chronic nonspherocytic hemolytic anemia.
- Jaundice, dark urine.
- Splenomegaly.

DIAGNOSIS

- Reduced G6PD activity in RBCs.
- Anemia, Heinz bodies, and bite cells on peripheral smear.
- Reticulocytosis.
- Elevated serum bilirubin and LDH.
- ↓ serum haptoglobin.
- Hemoglobinuria.

TREATMENT

- Removal of oxidant stressor.
- Oxygen.
- Transfusion of packed RBC for Hgb < 6, hemodynamic instability, ongoing hemolysis.

Pyruvate Kinase (PK) Deficiency

DEFINITION

Congenital hemolytic anemia (↓ RBC PK).

PATHOPHYSIOLOGY

Pyruvate kinase catalyzes the final step in the glycolytic pathway.

EPIDEMIOLOGY

- Second most common hemolytic enzymopathy.
- Autosomal recessive.

SIGNS AND SYMPTOMS

- Chronic hemolytic anemia.
- Hyperbilirubinemia/failure to thrive (FTT) in newborn.
- ↓ reticulocytes (selective destruction).

DIAGNOSIS

↓ RBC PK activity.

TREATMENT

- Avoid oxidant stresses.
- Exchange transfusion (hyperbilirubinemia).
- Transfusion of packed RBCs if severe anemia or aplastic crisis.
- Splenectomy (after 5–6 years of age), if persistently severe anemia or frequent transfusion requirement, will ↑ reticulocyte count.
- Folate supplementation.

Suspect G6PD deficiency when G6PD activity is within low normal range in the presence of high reticulocyte count.

G6PD deficiency protects against parasitism of erythrocytes (such as malaria).

Drugs causing hemolysis in G6PD deficiency:
- Aspirin
- Sulfonamides *Bactrim*
- Ciprofloxacin
- Antimalarials *Dapsone*

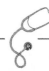

Ingestion of fava beans can cause hemolysis in patients with G6PD deficiency ("favism").

Hereditary Spherocytosis

A 4-year-old boy has pallor and a family history of gallstone surgery. His Hgb is 8 g, retics 11, bili 2. *Think: Hereditary spherocytosis.*

Hereditary spherocytosis is a common inherited hemolytic anemia that is transmitted as an autosomal dominant. The characteristic feature is spherocytic red cells that are intrinsically defective. Hemolysis results in reticulocytosis and indirect hyperbilirubinemia. Splenomegaly and gallstones are common. Spherocytes are present in the peripheral blood smear. Splenectomy is helpful in reducing the rate of hemolysis.

DEFINITION

Red cell membrane defect → abnormally shaped erythrocytes and hemolysis.

ETIOLOGY

Genetic defect in erythrocyte membrane proteins, such as ankyrin.

PATHOPHYSIOLOGY

- Abnormal proteins cause destabilized RBC membrane—spherocytes.
- Abnormal RBCs become sequestered in the spleen and hemolyze.

EPIDEMIOLOGY

Autosomal dominant.

SIGNS AND SYMPTOMS

- Commonly asymptomatic.
- Evidence of hemolysis.
- Aplastic/hemolytic crisis.
- Splenomegaly.
- Gallstones.
- Leg ulcers.
- Positive family history.

DIAGNOSIS

- ↑ osmotic fragility.
- Spherocytes on peripheral film.
- Reticulocytosis.
- Hyperbilirubinemia.

TREATMENT

- Splenectomy (avoid or at least delay until > 5 years old).
- Pneumococcal, meningococcal, and *Haemophilus influenzae* (Hib) vaccines before splenectomy.
- Treatment does not fix underlying RBC defect.

Hereditary spherocytosis has the following characteristics: ↑ osmotic fragility, ↑ reticulocyte count, positive family history, and splenomegaly. Coombs' test is *not* positive.

Paroxysmal Nocturnal Hemoglobinuria

DEFINITION

- Complement-induced hemolytic anemia caused by acquired defect in RBC membrane.
- Red urine (intravascular hemolysis worse with relative hypoxia at night vs. more concentrated urine at night).
- Thrombosis.

SIGNS AND SYMPTOMS

- Hemolysis worse during sleep → morning hemoglobinuria.
- Marrow failure.
- Intermittent or chronic hemolytic anemia.
- Leukopenia, thrombocytopenia.
- Complications can include thromboembolic phenomenon and acute myelogenous leukemia.

DIAGNOSIS

- ↑ LDG, ↓ haptoglobin, direct Coombs' is negative since hemolysis is not antibody directed.
- Sucrose lysis test, Ham's acid hemolysis test.
- Flow cytometry.

TREATMENT

- Prednisone.
- Bone marrow transplantation for severe disease.
- Splenectomy is not indicated.
- Eculizumab (humanized antibody which inhibits the activation of terminal complement components).
- Iron supplementation unless frequently transfused.
- Folic acid supplementation.

Splenectomy predisposes patients to overwhelming postsplenectomy infections (OPSIs) caused by encapsulated organisms:
- *Streptococcus pneumoniae*
- *Neisseria meningitidis*
- *Haemophilus influenzae*

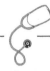

Onset of paroxysmal nocturnal hemoglobinuria is in late childhood.

APLASTIC ANEMIA

DEFINITION

Rare group of closely related disorders → ↓ numbers of blood cells in each of the lines—RBCs, WBCs, and platelets.

ETIOLOGY

- Exact cause is unknown.
- Chemical exposure.
- Viral infection.
- Genetic causes (eg, Fanconi anemia).

SIGNS AND SYMPTOMS

- Fatigue (fewer RBCs).
- Infections (fewer WBCs).
- Bleeding (fewer platelets).
- ↑ risk of leukemia.

DIAGNOSIS

- CBC—suspicious if at least two of the three cell lines are ↓.
- Bone marrow biopsy is definitive.

TREATMENT

- Platelet and RBC transfusions.
- Immunosuppressive drugs—antilymphocyte globulin (ALG), antithymocyte globulin (ATG), cyclosporine.
- Growth factors—erythropoietin (EPO), granulocyte colony-stimulating factor (G-CSF), granulocyte macrophage colony stimulating factor (GM-CSF).
- Stem cell transplantation is definitive cure but requires chemotherapy and/or radiation in preparation.

THROMBOTIC THROMBOCYTOPENIC PURPURA (TTP)

DEFINITION

Hemolytic anemia that results from deposition of abnormal VWF multimers into microvasculature.

SIGNS AND SYMPTOMS

- Fever.
- Microangiopathic hemolytic anemia.
- Thrombocytopenia.
- Abnormal renal function.
- Neurologic signs.

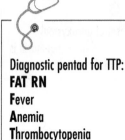

Diagnostic pentad for TTP:
FAT RN
Fever
Anemia
Thrombocytopenia
Renal dysfunction
Neurologic abnormality

DIAGNOSIS

- Normal prothrombin time (PT) and activated partial thromboplastin time (aPTT).
- Microangiopathic hemolytic anemia.
- Abnormal red cell morphology with schistocytes, spherocytes, helmet cells.
- ↑ reticulocyte count.
- Thrombocytopenia.

TREATMENT

- Plasmapheresis
- Corticosteroids
- Splenectomy

Ten days after an episode of viral diarrhea, a 2-year-old boy has pallor and icterus and petechiae of the skin and mucous membranes. His mother reports that he has not urinated for 24 hours. Characteristic lab findings include fragmented erythrocytes on smear, ↑ blood urea nitrogen (BUN), ↑ reticulocyte count, indirect hyperbilirubinemia, and normal platelet count. *Think: HUS.*

HUS is a common cause of renal failure in children. Triad: microangiopathic hemolytic anemia, thrombocytopenia, and uremia. Onset is usually preceded by gastroenteritis. It may be epidemic during summer months. Platelet count is usually low, but may be normal early in the course of illness.

ETIOLOGY

Acute gastroenteritis caused by *Escherichia coli* O157:H7 (produces a shiga-like toxin).

SIGNS AND SYMPTOMS

- Hemolytic anemia
- Thrombocytopenia
- Acute renal failure (ARF)

DIAGNOSIS

- History of bloody diarrhea.
- Abnormal red cell morphology.
- Thrombocytopenia with normal megakaryocytes in marrow.
- Urine—protein, RBCs, and casts.

TREATMENT

- Fluid management.
- Dialysis.
- Plasmapheresis (for neurologic complications).
- Antibiotics not indicated.

Immune Thrombocytopenic Purpura (ITP)

A 4-year-old previously healthy girl with purple skin lesions had a visit to the ED with an upper respiratory infection (URI) a month ago. CBC is normal except for low platelets. *Think: ITP.*

Typical presentation: Sudden onset of generalized petechiae and purpura in a previously healthy child. Often, there is a history of a viral infection weeks before the onset. Physical examination is usually normal except petechiae and purpura. Complete remission occurs in most children.

ITP is the most common thrombocytopenia of childhood.

Purpuric lesions do not blanch.

Primary ITP is a diagnosis of exclusion.

Don't give prednisone in ITP without a marrow examination.

DEFINITION

- Acquired hemorrhagic disorder that results from excessive destruction of platelets—typically benign.
- Acute (remission within 6 months).
- Chronic (> 6 months).
- Also called autoimmune thrombocytopenic purpura.

ETIOLOGY

- Unknown.
- Associated with antecedent viral illnesses (varicella, rubella, mumps, infectious mononucleosis) in 50–65% of cases.

PATHOPHYSIOLOGY

- Immune mechanism—autoantibodies.
- Sensitization.

DIAGNOSIS

- Diagnosis of exclusion.
- WBC and Hgb levels normal.
- Normal peripheral smear except thrombocytopenia.
- Bone marrow (not always indicated).
- Normal erythrocytic and granulocytic series.
- Normal or ↑ megakaryocytes.

TREATMENT

- Treatment based on severity of bleeding.
- Admit if platelet count is < 20.
- > 80% recover within several months without treatment.
- Intravenous immune globulin (IVIG) or anti-Rho antibodies.
- Intravenous methylprednisolone.
- Splenectomy.
- Older children (> 4 years).
- Severe ITP.
- Chronic ITP (> 1 year).
- Platelet transfusion generally not helpful.

DISSEMINATED INTRAVASCULAR COAGULATION (DIC)

DEFINITION

↑ fibrinogenesis and fibrinolysis.

ETIOLOGY

- Sepsis.
- Incompatible transfusion.
- Rickettsial infection.
- Snake bite.
- Acute promyelocytic leukemia.

PATHOPHYSIOLOGY

- Hypoxia
- Acidosis
- Tissue necrosis
- Shock
- Endothelial damage

DIC is frequently associated with purpura fulminans and acute promyelocytic leukemia.

SIGNS AND SYMPTOMS

- Bleeding
- Petechiae and ecchymoses
- Hemolysis

DIAGNOSIS

- ↑ PT and aPTT.
- ↓ fibrinogen and platelets.
- ↑ fibrin degradation products and D-dimer.

TREATMENT

- Treat underlying cause.
- Replacement therapy:
  - Platelets (thrombocytopenia).
  - Cryoprecipitate (hypofibrinogenemia).
  - Fresh frozen plasma (FFP) (replacement of coagulation factors).
- Heparin prevents consumption of coagulation factors.

COAGULATION DISORDERS

- Bleeding due to platelet problems usually occurs immediately and is mucocutaneous.
- Bleeding due to factor deficiencies is often "deeper" bleeding (intra-articular, intramuscular).
- See Table 15-5.

von Willebrand Disease

A child presents with epistaxis, prolonged bleeding time, and a normal platelet count. *Think: von Willebrand disease.*

von Willebrand disease is the most common inherited bleeding disorder. A family history of an established bleeding disorder should be sought. Typical presentation: Mucocutaneous bleeding (excessive bruising, epistaxis, and menorrhagia). The evaluation involves qualitative and quantitative measurements of von Willebrand factor (vWF).

DEFINITION

Most common hereditary bleeding disorder, seen in up to 1% of population, resulting from deficiency of vWF (qualitative or quantitative).

TABLE 15-5. Coagulation Tests

TEST	PURPOSE	
PT (INR)	Extrinsic system	Elevated in DIC, warfarin use, liver failure, myelofibrosis, vitamin K deficiency, fat malabsorption, circulating anticoagulants, factor deficiencies
aPTT	Intrinsic	Elevated in factor deficiencies, circulating anticoagulants, heparin use, higher doses of warfarin
Bleeding time	Surgical	Related to platelet count
		If lengthened and platelet count is normal, consider qualitative platelet defect
Platelet count	Related to bleeding time	< 100,000/mm³—mild prolongation of bleeding time
		< 50,000—easy bruising
		< 20,000—↑ incidence of spontaneous bleeding
Platelet aggregation	Qualitative	May be abnormal even with normal platelet count—qualitative platelet disorders (Glanzmann's thrombasthenia), von Willebrand factor deficiency
Fibrin degradation products	Fibrin activation	Elevated in DIC, trauma, inflammatory disease
D-dimer	Intravascular fibrinolysis	Present in most individuals, especially with cancer, trauma
		Sensitive for active clotting, but not specific
Assays for specific factors	Quantitative	Hemophilia A (VIII), hemophilia B (IX), von Willebrand factor deficiency (VIII, vWF)

aPTT, activated partial thromboplastin time; DIC, disseminated intravascular coagulation; INR, International Normalized Ratio; PT, prothrombin time.

ETIOLOGY

- Autosomal dominant—chromosome 12.
- Deficiency of factor VIII-R.

PATHOPHYSIOLOGY

Defective platelet function due to ↓ in level or function of von Willebrand cofactor.

SIGNS AND SYMPTOMS

- Easy bruising.
- Heavy or prolonged menstruation.
- Frequent or prolonged epistaxis.
- Prolonged bleeding after injury, surgery (circumcision), or invasive dental procedures.

DIAGNOSIS

- ↑ aPTT and bleeding time.
- Abnormal factor VIII clotting activity.
- Quantitative assay for vWF antigen.
- Reduced ristocetin cofactor activity.
- Abnormal platelet aggregation tests.
- Normal platelet count.

TREATMENT

- Usually no therapy necessary.
- Avoid unnecessary trauma.
- Desmopressin (DDAVP), factor VIII for surgery if needed.
- Cryoprecipitate recommended only in life-threatening emergencies due to the risk of human immunodeficiency virus (HIV) and hepatitis infection.

Avoid aspirin and nonsteroidal anti-inflammatory drug (NSAID) use in patients with von Willebrand disease.

FACTOR VIII REPLACEMENT

Bleeding Time	Desired Level (%) VIII
Hematoma	20–40%
Dental extraction	50%
Head injury	100%
Major surgery	100%

Hemophilia

DEFINITION

- Inherited coagulation defects.
- Hemophilia A: Factor VIII deficiency.
- Hemophilia B: Factor IX deficiency.

PATHOPHYSIOLOGY

Slowed rate of clot formation.

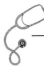

Patients with hemophilia may lose large amounts of blood into an iliopsoas hematoma.

SIGNS AND SYMPTOMS

- Easy bruising.
- Intramuscular hematomas.
- Hemarthroses (ankles, then knees and elbows) → joint destruction if untreated.
- Spontaneous hemorrhaging if levels < 5%.

DIAGNOSIS

- Family history.
- aPTT 2–3 times upper limit of normal.
- Specific factor assays.

Only 30% of male infants with hemophilia bleed at circumcision.

TREATMENT

- Early diagnosis.
- Prevent trauma.
- Recombinant factors.
- Cryoprecipitate.
- Beware of transfusion complications, including disease transmission.

- 1 unit of VIII/ kg — ↑ 2%
- 1 unit of IX/kg — ↑ 1%

DEFINITION

Predisposition to thrombosis.

PATHOPHYSIOLOGY

Primary (inherited) or secondary (acquired) disturbances in the three areas of Virchow's triad:

- Endothelial damage (eg, inflammation, trauma, burns, infection, surgery, central lines, artificial heart valves).
- Change in blood flow (eg, immobilization, local pressure, congestive heart failure [CHF], hypovolemia, hyperviscosity, pregnancy).
- Hypercoagulability (eg, factor release secondary to surgery, trauma, malignancy); antiphospholipid antibodies, lupus, oral contraceptive use; genetic predispositions such as deficiencies of protein S, protein C, antithrombin III, or factor V Leiden; nephrotic syndrome, polycythemia vera, sickle cell anemia, homocystinemia, fibrinogenemia.

SIGNS AND SYMPTOMS

- Deep vein thrombosis (DVT)
- Pulmonary embolism (PE)
- Myocardial infarction (MI)
- Stroke
- Recurrent pregnancy loss

DIAGNOSIS

- Family history.
- Patient history of recurrent, early, unusual, or idiopathic thromboses.
- Appropriate screening.
- Risk factor assessment.

TREATMENT

- Reduce risk factors—mobilize patients, encourage to quit smoking and alcohol, hydrate.
- Aspirin, heparin, warfarin, etc., as appropriate.

MALARIA

 An 8-year-old American-born boy of Somali parents presents with fever for 1 week after returning from his vacation. On examination he has splenomegaly. *Think: Malaria.*

Malaria should be considered in any child who presents with fever and has traveled or resided in a malaria-endemic area. It is characterized by fever, chills, sweats, fatigue, anemia, and splenomegaly. The diagnosis is established by identification of organisms on peripheral smear.

356

DEFINITION

Blood-borne parasite infection.

ETIOLOGY

- Transmitted by female *Anopheles* mosquito.
- Four species of *Plasmodium:*
  - *P falciparum*
  - *P malariae*
  - *P ovale*
  - *P vivax*

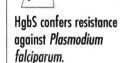

HgbS confers resistance against *Plasmodium falciparum.*

EPIDEMIOLOGY

Most frequent cause of hemolysis worldwide.

SIGNS AND SYMPTOMS

- Fever
- Chills
- Jaundice
- Splenomegaly
- Sweats

DIAGNOSIS

- Traditional method: Identification of organisms on thick and thin peripheral blood smears obtained when patient is acutely febrile.
- Newer methods include polymerase chain reaction (PCR) and immunoassays.

TREATMENT

- See CDC Web site for specific guidelines—usually dependent on resistance in geographic location.
- Chloroquine is used for *P ovale*, *P vivax*, *P malariae*, and chloroquine-sensitive *P falciparum.*
- Significant areas of chloroquine-resistant *P falciparum* exist. In these places, mefloquine or atovaquone-proguanil should be used.

TRANSFUSION REACTIONS

EPIDEMIOLOGY

- Approximately 4% of transfusions are associated with some form of adverse reaction.
- Most are febrile nonhemolytic or urticarial.
- See Table 15-6.

INDICATIONS FOR TRANSFUSION OF BLOOD PRODUCTS

- Packed RBCs: Hgb < 8 or 8–10 if symptomatic.
- Platelets: < 10,000/µL; 10,000–50,000 if bleeding; < 75,000 in preparation for surgery.
- FFP: Treatment of bleeding from vitamin K deficiency, ↑ International Normalized Ratio (INR), liver disease, or during plasma exchange for TTP.

TABLE 15-6. Transfusion Reactions

Type	Etiology	Signs and Symptoms	Treatment	Prevention
Acute hemolytic (1 in 15,000–36,000) (fatal 1 in 630,000)	RBC incompatibility	Fever, chills, nausea	Stop transfusion	Pretransfusion testing
	Damaged RBCs	Chest/arm/back pain	Manage blood pressure and renal perfusion	Accurate labeling, unit inspection
	Hypotonic solution	Hemoglobinuria, oliguria Shock, hypotension DIC Dyspnea	Control DIC	Proper patient identification
Delayed hemolytic	Antibodies to minor blood group antigens during prior transfusion (Kidd, Duffy, Rh, Kell)	3–10 days post-transfusion	Usually self-limited	Chronically transfused patients should received leukocyte reduced products
		Falling hematocrit, fever, hyperbilirubinemia/uria	Supportive	
Allergic (1 in 30–100)	Antibodies to plasma proteins	Hives, itching, local erythema	Antihistamines	Pretransfusion antihistamines Washed cellular blood products
Anaphylactic (1 in 18,000–170,000)	Antibodies to IgA	Cough, respiratory distress, bronchospasm Nausea, vomiting, abdominal cramps, diarrhea Shock, vascular instability, loss of consciousness	Stop transfusion Epinephrine Supportive care	IgA-deficient plasma products Washed cellular blood products
Febrile nonhemolytic (1 in 50–100)	Antibodies to granulocytes	Fever, chills	Stop transfusion	Pretransfusion antipyretics
		Dyspnea, anxiety	Demerol	
	Cytokines in plasma		Antipyretics	Leukocyte-reduced blood products

TABLE 15-6. Transfusion Reactions (continued)

Type	Etiology	Signs and Symptoms	Treatment	Prevention
Transfusion-related acute lung injury (TRALI) (1 in 5000–10,000)	Antigranulocyte antibodies in donor product	Bilateral pulmonary edema Cyanosis, hypoxemia Respiratory distress, cough Hypotension, normal central venous pressure ARDS-like picture Fever, chills	Supportive	Do not use plasma products from implicated donor
Circulation overload	Hypervolemia Rapid infusion CHF	Dyspnea, cyanosis, hypoxemia Tachycardia, hypertension Pulmonary edema, cough	Diuretics Oxygen Phlebotomy	Pretransfusion diuretics Slow infusion Limit volume

ARDS, adult respiratory distress syndrome; CHF, congestive heart failure; DIC, disseminated intravascular coagulation; IgA, immunoglobulin A; RBC, red blood cell.

- Cryoprecipitate: Hypofibrinogenemia, hemophilia A, vWF deficiency, factor XIII deficiency.

COMPLICATIONS

- Hemolytic, febrile, and allergic reactions.
- Transfusion-related acute lung injury (TRALI).
- Disease transmission (eg, HIV, hepatitis B virus [HBV], hepatitis C virus [HCV], human T-lymphotropic virus [HTLV], cytomegalovirus [CMV], parvovirus).
- Iron overload, electrolyte disturbances.
- Fluid overload, hypothermia.

Children rarely have febrile reactions to initial transfusion unless they are immunoglobulin A (IgA) deficient.

METHEMOGLOBINEMIA

ETIOLOGY

- Inherited:
  - Deficiency of cytochrome b5 reductase.
  - Hgb M disease—inability to convert methemoglobin back to hemoglobin.
- Acquired—↑ production of methemoglobin: Nitrites (contaminated water), xylocaine/benzocaine (teething gel), sulfonamides, benzene, aniline dyes, potassium chlorate.

Life-threatening transfusion reactions are nearly always due to clerical errors (wrong ABO blood type).

PATHOPHYSIOLOGY

- Hgb iron in ferrous form.
- Methemoglobin iron is in ferric form (< 2%) and is unable to transport oxygen.

SIGNS AND SYMPTOMS

Depends on the concentration:

- 10–30%: Cyanosis.
- 30–50%: Dyspnea, tachycardia, dizziness.
- 50–70%: Lethargy, stupor.
- > 70%: Death.

DIAGNOSIS

Methemoglobin level—co-oximetry studies.

TREATMENT

- Concentration dependent.
- < 30%: Treatment not needed.
- 30–70%: IV methylene blue.
- Hyperbaric O_2.
- Oral ascorbic acid (200–500 mg).

Suspect methemoglobinemia if:
- Oxygen-unresponsive cyanosis
- Chocolate brown blood

PORPHYRIA

DEFINITION AND ETIOLOGY

Porphyria refers to a group of disorders (inherited and acquired) characterized by an inherited deficiency of the heme biosynthetic pathway.

SIGNS AND SYMPTOMS

- Acute (hepatic) porphyria: Abdominal pain, vomiting, neuropathy, mental disturbances, seizures, autonomic nervous system dysfunction, cardiac arrythmias, tachycardia; ↑ risk of hepatocellular carcinoma over lifetime.
- Cutaneous (erythropoietic) porphyria: Edema, blister formation, ↑ hair growth, photosensitivity, red urine.
- Precipitated by drugs, infection.

DIAGNOSIS

- Spectroscopy: Blood, urine, stool.
- Hyponatremia/syndrome of inappropriate antidiuretic hormone secretion (SIADH).
- Renal insufficiency.
- Serum/urine porphyrin levels.

TREATMENT

- For acute attacks: Analgesia, hydration, maintain electrolytes, IV hematin especially if low serum sodium or status epilepticus, high-carbohydrate diet, glucose 10% infusion.
- Long-term management:
  - Avoid alcohol and all drugs that can precipitate an attack.
  - Sunscreen.

Neutropenia

DEFINITION

Absolute neutrophil count (ANC) < 1500/mm³:

- Mild: 1000–1500
- Moderate: 500–1000
- Severe: < 500

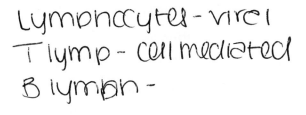

neutrophils-bacterial

ANC = Total WBC × (Segs + Bands).

Lymphocytes - viral
T lymp - cell mediated
B lymph -

ETIOLOGY

- Congenital.
- Kostmann syndrome.
- Schwachman syndrome.
- Fanconi syndrome.
- Acquired.
- Infection.
- Immune.
- Hypersplenism.
- Drugs.
- Aplastic anemia.
- Vitamin B_{12}, folate, or copper deficiency.

SIGNS AND SYMPTOMS

- ↑ susceptibility to bacterial infection.
- Stomatitis, gingivitis, recurrent otitis media, cellulitis, pneumonia, and septicemia.

LEUKEMIA

 A 3-year-old girl has had fever, anorexia, and fatigue for the past month. She has lost 5 kg. She has pallor, cervical adenopathy, splenomegaly, skin ecchymoses, and petechiae. *Think: Acute leukemia.*

Typical presentation: Pancytopenia—anemia (pallor and fatigue), thrombocytopenia (epistaxis, ecchymoses, and petechiae) and white cell may be low (sepsis) or high. Initial presentation may be nonspecific and subtle and develop over weeks to months. Final diagnosis depends on the results of bone marrow aspirate and biopsy.

EPIDEMIOLOGY

Leukemia is the most common malignancy, followed by brain tumors.

RISK FACTORS

- Trisomy 21
- Fanconi anemia
- Bloom syndrome
- Immune deficiency
- Wiskott-Aldrich syndrome
- Agammaglobulinemia
- Ataxia–telangiectasia

SIGNS AND SYMPTOMS

- Fever
- Pallor
- Bleeding
- Bone pain
- Abdominal pain
- Lymphadenopathy
- Hepatosplenomegaly

Acute Lymphoblastic Leukemia (ALL)

DEFINITION

Malignant disorder of lymphoblasts.

EPIDEMIOLOGY

- Most common malignancy in children.
- Eighty percent of leukemia in children.

SIGNS AND SYMPTOMS

- Fatigue, anorexia, lethargy, pallor.
- Bone pain.
- Fever.
- Bleeding, bruising, petechiae.
- Lymphadenopathy.
- Hepatosplenomegaly.
- Bone tenderness.
- Testicular swelling.
- Septicemia.

DIAGNOSIS

- CBC: Anemia, abnormal white count, low platelet count.
- Electrolytes, calcium, phosphorus, uric acid, lactic dehydrogenase (LDH).
- Chest x-ray (mediastinal mass).
- Bone marrow—hypercellular, ↑ lymphoblasts.
- Cerebrospinal fluid (CSF)—blasts.

Marrow exam is essential to confirm the diagnosis of ALL.

TREATMENT

- Four phases:
  - Remission induction: Cytoxan, vincristine, prednisone, L-asparaginase, and/or doxorubicin.
  - Consolidation: May add 6MP, 6TG, or cytosine arabinoside.
  - Maintenance therapy: 2 years—methotrexate and 6MP, may add vincristine and prednisone.
  - CNS prophylaxis: Methotrexate to CSF, may have radiation to the head.
- Infection prevention—antibiotics, isolation if necessary

Acute Myelogenous Leukemia (AML)

DEFINITION

Malignant proliferation of immature granular leukocytes.

EPIDEMIOLOGY

- Fifteen to twenty percent of leukemia cases.
- Occurs primarily in children < 1 year old.
- One in 10,000 people.

ETIOLOGY

Predisposing factors:

- Trisomy 21
- Diamond–Blackfan syndrome
- Fanconi anemia
- Bloom syndrome
- Kostmann syndrome
- Toxins such as benzene
- Immunosuppression
- Polycythemia vera

SIGNS AND SYMPTOMS

- Manifestations of anemia, thrombocytopenia, or neutropenia, including fatigue, bleeding, and infection.
- Chloroma—localized mass of leukemic cells.
- Bone/joint pain.
- Hepatosplenomegaly.
- Lymphadenopathy.

DIAGNOSIS

- > 25% myeloblasts in the bone marrow, hypercellular.
- Abnormal white count, platelet count, and anemia.
- Bone destruction and periosteal elevation on x-ray.

TREATMENT

- Two phases:
  - Remission induction: 1 week—anthracycline (daunorubicin) and cytosine arabinoside (cytarabine).
  - Postremission therapy: Several more courses of high-dose cytarabine chemotherapy, allogenic stem cell transplant, or autologous stem cell transplant.
- Infection prevention—isolation, antibiotics.
- RBC transfusions for anemia.
- Platelet transfusions for bleeding.
- Complete remission in 70–80%.

CLL - MC leukemia

Chronic Myelogenous Leukemia (CML)

DEFINITION

Clonal disorder of the hematopoietic stem cell with Philadelphia chromosome translocation—t(9;22)(q34;q11).

EPIDEMIOLOGY

Tends to occur in middle-aged people.

SIGNS AND SYMPTOMS

- Insidious onset.
- Splenomegaly (massive).
- Fever, bone pain, sweating.

TREATMENT

- Hydroxyurea
- α-Interferon
- Bone marrow transplant
- Radiation

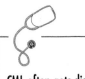

CML often gets diagnosed when CBC shows elevated WBCs.

Juvenile Chronic Myelogenous Leukemia (JCML)

DEFINITION

- Clonal condition involving pluripotent stem cell.
- < 2 years.

Neurofibromatosis is associated with an ↑ incidence of JCML and leukemia.

EPIDEMIOLOGY

Ninety-five percent diagnosed before age 4.

SIGNS AND SYMPTOMS

- Skin lesions (eczema, xanthoma, café au lait spots).
- Lymphadenopathy.
- Hepatosplenomegaly.

DIAGNOSIS

- Monocytosis.
- ↑ marrow monocyte precursors.
- Philadelphia chromosome absent.
- Blast count.
- < 5% (peripheral blood).
- < 30% (marrow).

TREATMENT

- Complete remissions have occurred with stem cell transplant.
- Majority relapse, with overall survival of 25%.

Congenital Leukemia

DEFINITION

Serious neonatal malignancy.

EPIDEMIOLOGY

- Rare.
- AML more common, unlike the predominance of ALL in later childhood.

Lymphoma

DEFINITION

- Lymphoid malignancy arising in a single lymph node or lymphoid region (liver, spleen, bone marrow).
- Hodgkin.
- Nodular sclerosing (46%—most common).
- Mixed cellularity (31%).
- Lymphocyte predominance (16%).
- Lymphocyte depletion (7%).
- Non-Hodgkin (10% of all pediatric tumors).
- Lymphoblastic.
- Burkitt's (39%).
- Large cell or histiocytic.

SIGNS AND SYMPTOMS

- Fever, night sweats.
- Weight loss, loss of appetite.
- Cough, dysphagia, dyspnea.
- Lymphadenopathy—lower cervical, supraclavicular.
- Hepatosplenomegaly.

DIAGNOSIS

- CBC, erythrocyte sedimentation rate (ESR).
- Serum electrolytes, uric acid, LDH.
- Chest x-ray.
- Computed tomography (CT) of chest, abdomen, and pelvis.
- Lymph node or bone marrow biopsy.

STAGING

- Stage I: One lymph node involved.
- Stage II: Two lymph nodes on same side of diaphragm.
- Stage III: Lymph node involvement on both sides of diaphragm.
- Stage IV: Bone marrow or liver involvement.

TREATMENT

- Radiation for stage I or II disease.
- Chemotherapy for stage III or IV.

Reed-Sternberg cells are characteristic of Hodgkin lymphoma.

Suspicious lymph nodes are:
- Painless, firm, and rubbery
- In the posterior triangle

Endocrine Disease

A 10-year-old girl has 2-hour postprandial blood glucose of 300 mg/dL and a large amount of glucose and trace ketones in her urine. She has lost 1 kg of weight. *Think: Type 1 diabetes,* and start treatment with insulin.

Typical history: Polyuria, polydipsia, polyphagia, and weight loss over a period of time. The initial symptoms due to hyperglycemia may be nonspecific. Exogenous insulin is required to correct the metabolic derangement due to insulin deficiency. Children with type 2 diabetes mellitus are usually overweight and may show signs of insulin resistance such as acanthosis nigricans. Family history of type 2 diabetes in first- and second-degree relative may also be present.

See Table 16-1.

DEFINITION

Syndrome characterized by disturbance of metabolism of carbohydrate, protein, and fat, resulting in hyperglycemia and glucosuria from deficiency in insulin secretion or its action.

EPIDEMIOLOGY

- Diabetes is one of the most common endocrine disorders of the pediatric age group.

Think of testing urine glucose with the onset of enuresis in a previously toilet-trained child.

TABLE 16-1.   Diabetes

TYPE I (INSULIN DEPENDENT)	TYPE II (NON–INSULIN DEPENDENT)
Absolute insulin deficiency (require insulin for survival)	Insulin is ↑, normal, or ↓ (insulin is not required for survival)
Immune mediated	Insulin resistance
Juvenile onset	Usually adult onset but incidence is rising in children
Shorter duration of symptoms with history of weight loss at diagnosis	Mild symptoms, 85% overweight at diagnosis
Ketosis common	Ketosis infrequent but occurs under stressful conditions
DKA is a complication of uncontrolled diabetes	Hyperglycemic hyperosmolar state is a rare complication
HLA-DR3 and -DR4 (chromosome 6)	Not HLA associated
5% have diabetic relative	74–100% have a diabetic relative

DKA, diabetic ketoacidosis; HLA, human leukocyte antigen.

- Classification:
  - **Type 1 diabetes:** Caused by absolute insulin deficiency. It has abrupt onset with classic symptoms of polyuria, polydipsia, polyphagia, and weight loss. Most children have positive urine ketones at onset. Incidence is roughly 1 in 400 children. It is prevalent in Caucasians of northern European decent and caused by autoimmune destruction of pancreatic islet cell. Over 80% of children are positive for immune marker of beta cell destruction (examples: islet cell antibodies, anti-glutamic acid decarboxylase antibodies, and insulin autoantibody).
  - **Type 2 diabetes:** A heterogeneous disorder mainly caused by insulin resistance with relative insulin deficiency. It is insidious in onset and diagnosis is usually delayed because of lack of symptoms early in the course of disease. It is prevalent in certain minorities such as Hispanic-American, Native American, and African-American. Its incidence is increasing in children with increasing obesity. Most of them have acanthosis nigricans (hyperpigmentation with thickening of skin into velvety irregular folds in flexural or opposed areas), which is a cutaneous manifestation of insulin resistance.

PATHOPHYSIOLOGY

Revolves around insulin deficiency or insulin resistance leading to:

- ↓ glucose utilization.
- ↑ hepatic glucose production.

SIGNS AND SYMPTOMS

- Triad of polyuria, polydipsia, and polyphagia (more abrupt in type 1 diabetes).
- Weight loss and enuresis are common symptoms in type 1 diabetes.
- Vomiting, dehydration, and abdominal pain are hallmark of acute complication → diabetic ketoacidosis.

DIAGNOSIS

- Fasting blood glucose ≥ 126 mg/dL (7 mmol/L).
- Random blood glucose ≥ 200 mg/dL along with symptoms of diabetes.
- Two-hour plasma glucose > 200 during a 75-g oral glucose tolerance test.
- To diagnose type 2 diabetes early in children, the American Diabetes Association recommends testing children every 2 yr if they are overweight and have two or more risk factors such as:
  - Obesity (body mass index > 85th percentile for age)
  - Family history of type 2 diabetes (first- and second-degree relatives).
  - Race (Native American, African-American, Hispanic, and Asian).
  - Signs and symptoms associated with insulin resistance (acanthosis nigricans, dyslipidemia, hypertension [HTN], and polycystic ovarian syndrome).

TREATMENT

- Patient education and counseling.
- Diet.
- Exercise.
- Insulin (0.5–1 U/kg).
- Oral hypoglycemics in type 2 diabetes (such as metformin, sulfonylurea, thiazolidinediones).

A 3½-year-old boy is found unconscious. He has a flushed face, pulse of 160/min, respiratory rate of 30/min with shallow breaths, blood pressure 40/20 mmHg, and an unusual odor on his breath. He has a generalized tonic-clonic seizure. His mucous membranes are dry. His parents report a weight loss of 5 lb in the past month and noted that he was asking for juice. *Think: DKA, and check serum glucose.*

Polyuria, polydipsia, and weight loss are common symptoms in diabetes mellitus. Weight loss is due to hyperglycemia and glucosuria → lipolysis. Shallow breathing is a respiratory compensation for metabolic acidosis secondary to ketoacid accumulation. Severe dehydration is due to glucosuria → osmotic diuresis and volume depletion. Seizure may occur due to cerbrovascular event, which is a known complication of diabetic ketoacidosis.

DEFINITION

- Hyperglycemia > 200 mg/dL.
- Acidosis pH < 7.30.
- Bicarbonate < 15 mmol/L.
- Ketonemia > 3 mmol/L.

ETIOLOGY/PATHOPHYSIOLOGY

- Relative or absolute insulin deficiency → accelerated hepatic and renal glucose production and impaired glucose utilization, release of free fatty acids into circulation (from lipolysis) and ↑ fatty acid oxidation to ketone bodies.
- Precipitating factors—stress, infection, trauma.

Insulin-dependent diabetes mellitus in children is associated with islet cell antibodies and ↑ prevalence of human leukocyte antigen (HLA)-DR3 and -DR4 or both.

SIGNS AND SYMPTOMS

Polyuria, polydipsia, dehydration, fatigue, headache, nausea, vomiting, abdominal pain, tachycardia, tachypnea.

OTHER LABORATORY FINDINGS

- ↑ anion gap (>12–16 mEq).
- ↑ hemoglobin (Hgb) and hematocrit (Hct) (hemoconcentration).
- ↑ white blood cell (WBC) count.
- ↓ serum sodium (Na) (pseudohyponatremia from hyperglycemia and/or hypertriglyceridemia).
- Normal or ↑ potassium (K) (from shift of K from intracellular to extracellular compartment due to acidosis).
- Urinalysis reveals glucose and ketones (acetoacetate/acetone).

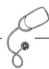

Dehydration in DKA is primarily intracellular and is often underestimated.

TREATMENT

- Careful fluid and electrolyte replacement to avoid cerebral edema. Rehydration fluid should not exceed 4000 mL/m²/day.
- Bolus should be 10–20 cc/kg/hr normal saline. Repeat bolus if needed. Subsequent replacement fluid can be 0.45% or 0.9% saline with potassium.
- Potassium should be given as half KCl and half KPO₄.
- Insulin regular (0.1 U/kg/hr).
- Glucose (add glucose when blood glucose is < 250–300 mg/dL).

Serum Na ↓ 1.6 mEq/L for every 100 mg/dL rise in glucose.

371

COMPLICATIONS

- Hypoglycemia.
- Hypokalemia.
- Cerebral edema: Cause of death in patients with DKA (get a head CT for headache/mental status changes indicative of acute intracranial pressure elevation). Treatment includes immediate reduction in intravenous fluid rate, hyperventilation, and mannitol 0.5–2 g/kg q4–6h as needed.

Total body potassium may be considerably depleted even when serum K^+ is normal or ↑.

HYPERINSULINISM

A 2-hour-old newborn has plasma glucose of 20 mg/dL. Physical examination shows a large plethoric newborn with macrocephaly. Birth weight is > 90th percentile. *Think: Hyperinsulinism.*

Hyperinsulinism is a common cause of hypoglycemia in early infancy. These infants may have macrosomia. Hypoglycemia may develop on the first day of life, and there may be rapid development after a few hours of feeding. The diagnostic criterion is the presence of signs and symptoms of hypoglycemia with low plasma glucose level and an inappropriately elevated insulin level. Macrosomia is due to hyperinsulinemia, as insulin is an important growth factor in intrauterine life. Transient hyperinsulinism may usually occur due to maternal diabetes. Persistent hyperinsulinism is due to genetic mutation (autosomal recessive) in the sulfonylurea receptor–inwardly rectifying K channel.

EPIDEMIOLOGY

Hyperinsulinemia is the most common cause of severe hypoglycemia in early infancy. Sixty percent develop hypoglycemia during the first month of life, 30% in the first year.

Transient Hyperinsulinemia

- Excessive insulin secretion in infants from transient dysfunction in islet cell function.
- Risk factors include:
  - Small-for-gestational-age (SGA) or premature infants.
  - Fetal hypoxia/asphyxia.
  - Infant of diabetic mother (born to mother with poorly controlled diabetes (type 1, type 2, or gestational).
  - Erythroblastosis fetalis.
- Other causes include surreptitious insulin administration.

Permanent Hyperinsulinemia

- Most common variety is an autosomal recessive defect caused by mutation in the genes coding component of K_{ATP} channel involved in glucose-regulated insulin release.
- Autosomal-dominant forms of hyperinsulinism are usually milder and caused by activating mutation in glucokinase (GCK) gene and glutamate dehydrogenase gene (GLUD1).

- Sporadic form of hyperinsulinism can result in either focal or diffuse hyperplasia of β-cell. Focal adenomatous hyperplasia is caused by loss of heterozygosity of 11p15 from somatic loss of maternal allele.

TREATMENT

- Frequent feeding (feed q3–4h).
- IV glucose if necessary.
- In severe, prolonged cases, diazoxide, somatostatin, and/or pancreatectomy.

HYPOGLYCEMIA

A 14-year-old boy with an 8-year history of diabetes mellitus has had frequent admissions for DKA in the past 18 months. His school performance has been deteriorating. Recently, he has had frequent episodes of hypoglycemia. He is Tanner stage 2 in pubertal development, is growing at a normal rate, and has mild hepatomegaly. *Think: Poorly controlled diabetes mellitus due to noncompliance.*

Adolescence is a difficult age for management of any chronic disease such as diabetes. Not adhering to the treatment regimen is common in teenagers. Often, blood sugar levels are high because of missing the dose of insulin. In addition, inappropriate administration of insulin doses may result in secondary hypoglycemia. Recurrent hospitalization is the hallmark of noncompliance. Hepatomegaly is most likely due poorly controlled diabetes mellitus (Mauriac syndrome).

ETIOLOGY

- Hyperinsulinism.
- Hormone deficiencies (glucocorticoid, growth hormone).
- Glycogen storage disease.
- Defect in gluconeogenesis.
- Fatty acid oxidation defects.
- Organic acidemias.
- Ketotic hypoglycemia.
- Malnutrition, prematurity, SGA.
- Liver failure.
- Congenital heart diseases.
- Tumors.
- Poisons/drugs (salicylates, alcohol).
- Systemic disease—sepsis, burns, cardiogenic shock.

TREATMENT

- Acute symptomatic hypoglycemia: 0.3 g/kg glucose (3 mL/kg $D_{10}W$) IV over 10 min to restore plasma glucose concentration to normal, followed by 10% dextrose at 6–8 mg/kg/min.
- In patients with hyperinsulinemia, subcutaneous glucagon 0.03 mg/kg can reverse the hypoglycemia.

DEFINITION

- ↑ storage of iron in the form of hemosiderin in parenchymal cells.
- Liver, heart, gonad, skin, and joints.

ETIOLOGY

- Hereditary
- Neonatal
- Transfusion induced

SIGNS AND SYMPTOMS

- Cirrhosis
- Bronzing of skin
- Diabetes mellitus

LABORATORY FINDINGS

- ↑ serum ferritin
- ↑ transferrin saturation

TREATMENT

Chelation with desferoxamine, phlebotomy.

DEFINITION

↑ secretion of thyroid hormone.

Juvenile Graves Disease

Juvenile Graves disease causes 95% of thyrotoxicosis in children.

- Occurs more frequently in females (male-to-female ratio 3:1–5:1).
- Triad of:
  - Hyperthyroidism with diffuse goiter (almost always present; goiter is usually symmetrical, smooth, soft, and nontender).
  - Ophthalmopathy (present in over one-half of the patients).
  - Dermopathy: Pretibial myxedema is present in 1–2% of adults; it rarely occurs in children.

ETIOLOGY

- Autoimmune disorder with antibodies against thyroid-stimulating hormone (TSH) receptor—thyrotropin-binding inhibitory immunoglobulin (TBII).
- TBII can either stimulate or inhibit thyroid cell function.
- Thyroid-stimulating immunoglobulin (TSI): Present in Graves disease.
- TSH receptor–blocking antibodies: Cause hypothyroidism.
- Clinical presentation is determined by the net effect of interaction between stimulating and blocking antibodies.

SIGNS AND SYMPTOMS

- Gradual onset (6–12 months).
- Emotional disturbance, change in academic performance.
- Insomnia.
- Palpitations.
- Fatigue, muscle weakness, ↑ sweating.
- ↑ appetite with ↓ or no weight gain.
- Goiter.
- Heat intolerance.
- Fine tremors.
- Exophthalmos.
- Menstrual irregularities.
- **Thyroid storm:** Characterized by:
  - Fever (usually > 101.3°F [38.5°C]).
  - Severe tachycardia out of proportion to fever, leading to high-output cardiac failure.
  - Central nervous system (CNS) manifestations (confusion, obtundation, coma, and convulsions).

LABORATORY FINDINGS

- Elevated total and free thyroxine (T_4) and total and free triiodothyronine (T_3) levels.
- ↓ TSH.
- Elevated TBII (receptor assay).
- Elevated TSI (bioassay).

TREATMENT OF HYPERTHYROIDISM

- Pediatric endocrine consultation.
- Propylthiouracil (PTU) 5–10 mg/kg/day q8h PO or methimazole 0.5–1 mg/kg/day q8h. Side effects occur in 20–30% and include agranulocytosis, hepatotoxicity, urticaria, arthralgia, and very rarely vasculitis.
- Propranolol 1–2 mg/kg/day PO in divided doses q6–8h (0.01–0.15 mg/kg/dose IV).
- Treatment with ^{131}I (radioactive iodine) for juvenile Graves disease is increasing.
- Surgical—thyroidectomy.
- For thyroid storm, besides PTU and propranolol also give iodides (SSKI) 5 drops PO q8h and hydrocortisone. Both PTU and hydrocortisone inhibit the peripheral conversion of T_4 to T_3.

HYPOTHYROIDISM

DEFINITION

- ↓ production of thyroid hormone either from primary defect at the level of thyroid or secondary to hypothalamic pituitary disorder.
- In serum, 99.8% of T_4 and 99.7% of T_3 are bound to thyroxine-binding protein. Only 0.02% of T_4 and 0.3 % of T_3 are present as free fractions, which are biologically active (see Table 16-2).

TABLE 16-2. Thyroid Functions in Different Thyroid Conditions

	T₄	T₃	FT₄	FT₃	TSH	rT₃	T₃U
Primary hypothyroidism	L	L	L	L	H	L	L
Secondary hypothyroidism	L	L	L	L	N or L	L	L
Subclinical hypothyroidism	N	N	N	N	Slightly H	N	N
Subclinical hyperthyroidism	N	N	N	N	L	N	N
Euthyroid sick syndrome	L	L	L or N	L	N	H	L
TBG deficiency	L	L	N	N	N	N	H
TBG excess – TSH normal	H	H	N	N	H	N	L
Hypothyroxinemia of prematurity	L	L	L	L	N	L	L

H = high, L = low, N = normal.

FT₃, free triiodothyronine fraction; FT₄, free thyroxine fraction; rT₃, reverse T₃; T₃, triiodothyronine; T₃U, T₃ resin uptake; T₄, thyroxine; TBG, thyroxine-binding globulin.

Classic findings of congenital hypothyroidism are rare in the early neonatal period due to placental transfer of some maternal thyroid hormone.

Early diagnosis of congenital hypothyroidism is crucial to prevent or minimize cognitive impairment.

Congenital Hypothyroidism

Incidence is same worldwide (1 in 4000).

ETIOLOGY

- Sporadic: Thyroid dysgenesis (absent thyroid, hypoplastic thyroid, ectopic thyroid).
- Iodine deficiency remains a major cause worldwide.
- Prenatal exposure to radioiodine or antithyroid medications.
- Rarely hereditary: Thyroid dyshormonogenesis (defect in synthesis of thyroid hormone) and generalized thyroid hormone resistance.

SIGNS AND SYMPTOMS

- Most cases are asymptomatic at birth.
- Postmaturity, macrosomia.
- Wide fontanelle.
- Prolonged jaundice.
- Macroglossia.
- Hoarse cry.
- Abdominal distention, constipation.
- Umbilical hernia.
- Hypotonia.
- Goiter (in some dyshormonogenesis).
- If left untreated:
  - Slowed development, late teeth, late milestones, short stature.
  - Eventual mental retardation.

Newborn screening:

- **Primary T$_4$–sequential TSH:**
  - Used by most North American programs.
  - Initial filter paper blood spot: T$_4$ with TSH measurement in specimens with low T$_4$ values.
  - Uses a percentile as the cutoff, with 10th percentile being the usual standard.
- **Primary TSH–sequential T$_4$:**
  - Used in all European countries (except the Netherlands), Japan, Australia, and parts of North America.
  - Initial TSH measurement, supplemented by T$_4$ in cases of high TSH.
  - Cutoff point for recall is TSH 20–50 μU/mL with low T$_4$ (< 5 μg/dL) or TSH > 50 μIU/mL.

TREATMENT

- Both early and high-dose treatment appear necessary.
- L-thyroxine 10–15 μg/kg/day.

Acquired Hypothyroidism

A 10-year-old girl has a 3-year history of growth failure. A moderate-sized goiter is palpated. T$_4$ is 3.1 μg/dL, and TSH 322 μU/mL. *Think: Acquired hypothyroidism.*

Congenital hypothyroidism is generally diagnosed in neonatal life because of newborn screening. Hypothyroidism that begins in childhood is usually Hashimoto disease. Initial signs and symptoms of hypothyroidism may be subtle. Growth retardation is usually not severe. However, if it remains unrecognized and untreated, linear growth is severely retarded and sexual maturation is also delayed. Goiter is the hallmark of classic Hashimoto disease. The results of the thyroid function test depend on stage of disease. TSH is elevated. Antithyroglobulin and anti–thyroid peroxidase (anti-TPO antibody) may be present. Iodine deficiency is one of the most common causes of acquired hypothyroidism worldwide.

- Prevalence in children is 0.15% with a female-to-male ratio of 3:1.
- Lymphocytic thyroiditis (Hashimoto) is the most common cause. It is an autoimmune disorder characterized by lymphocytic infiltration of thyroid and presence of:
  - Antithyroglobuin antibodies
  - Anti-TPO antibodies
- Other causes include thyroid surgery and irradiation, medications (iodine, lithium, amiodarone, etc.), pituitary or hypothalamic dysfunction (secondary or tertiary acquired hypothyroidism).

Look for hypothyroidism in Down syndrome, Turner syndrome, and Klinefelter syndrome.

SIGNS AND SYMPTOMS

- Goiter.
- Growth deceleration.
- Delayed skeletal maturation.
- Fatigue, lethargy.
- Constipation.
- Cold intolerance.
- Bradycardia.
- Dry skin.
- Weight gain.
- Delayed deep tendon reflexes.

TREATMENT

L-thyroxine 2–4 µg/kg/day.

THYROID NEOPLASM

EPIDEMIOLOGY

- Rare in children.
- Most common pediatric endocrine tumor (differentiated thyroid cancer).
- Family history (in medullary thyroid cancer).
- Prior irradiation (in papillary thyroid cancer).

TYPES

- Thyroid adenoma (approximately 1% are toxic adenoma and cause hyperthyroidism).
- Thyroid carcinoma: Arise from:
  - Follicular epithelium:
    - Papillary carcinoma (most common; focal calcification [ie, psammoma in 40–50%]).
    - Follicular carcinoma (higher prevalence in areas with iodine deficiency).
    - Insular carcinoma (poorly differentiated).
  - C cells: Medullary carcinoma (produce calcitonin). Associated with type 2 multiple endocrine neoplasia (MEN).

Cervical lymphadenopathy: Rapid and painless enlargement of a thyroid growth may suggest neoplasia.

SIGNS AND SYMPTOMS

Solitary or multiple thyroid nodules (risk of malignancy in solitary nodules in children is 30–50%).

DIAGNOSIS

Incidence of malignancy of a thyroid neoplasm is higher in children than in adults.

- Thyroid profile (thyroid functions are usually normal).
- Calcitonin (for medullary cancer).
- Thyroid ultrasound.
- Fine-needle aspiration.
- Definite diagnosis by surgical excision.

- Papillary and follicular cancer:
  - Near total or total thyroidectomy (complications include bleeding, hypoparathyroidism, damage to recurrent laryngeal nerve) with modified neck dissection, if needed.
  - Postoperative ^{131}I ablation if the risk for recurrence is high.
  - Replacement thyroxine (higher doses in patients with ↑ risk of recurrence).
- Medullary thyroid cancer:
  - Total thyroidectomy.
  - Prophylactic thyroidectomy if positive for MEN mutation, before age 5 yr in MEN 2A and before age 6 months in MEN 2B.

HYPERPARATHYROIDISM

 A 10-year-old girl has severe abdominal pain and gross hematuria. She passes a calculus in her urine. She had received no medication and has no family history of renal stones. *Think: Primary hyperparathyroidism.*

Symptoms of primary hyperparathyroidism include painful bones, renal stones, abdominal groans, and psychic moans. It is a common cause of hypercalcemia. Hypercalcemia in the presence of elevated serum parathyroid hormone level confirm the diagnosis of primary hyperparathyroidism. Other biochemical findings include hypercalciuria and hypophosphatemia.

DEFINITION

Hypercalcemia accompanied by increased or inappropriately normal parathyroid hormone (PTH) level.

EPIDEMIOLOGY

Uncommon in children.

ETIOLOGY

- Primary (defect of parathyroid gland):
  - Parathyroid adenoma.
  - Generalized hyperplasia of all glands (MEN 1 and MEN 2A).
  - Parathyroid carcinoma.
- Secondary (response to hypocalcemia):
  - Chronic renal failure (CRF).
  - Renal tubular acidosis.
  - Vitamin D–deficiency rickets.
  - Treatment (with phosphorus) for hypophosphatemic rickets.
  - Liver failure.
- Tertiary hypoparathyroidism: Adenomatous change in parathyroid in the setting of CRF.

SIGNS AND SYMPTOMS

- Clinical manifestation of hypercalcemia.
- Muscle weakness, anorexia, nausea, vomiting, constipation, polydipsia, polyuria, dehydration, failure to thrive, coma, seizures, fever, renal stones.

DIAGNOSIS

- ↑ serum Ca.
- ↓ serum phosphorus.
- ↑ urinary calcium.
- ↑ PTH.
- Shortened QTc interval.
- Subperiosteal absorption (with prolonged hyperparathyroidism).
- ^{99m}Tc-sestamibi scanning for parathyroid adenoma.

TREATMENT

- Hypercalcemia:
  - Hydration (IV NS at 2–3 times maintenance).
  - Furosemide 1 mg/kg q6h (↑ Na and Ca excretion).
  - Prednisone (↓ intestinal absorption of Ca).
  - Calcitonin 4 U/kg SQ q12h.
  - Pamidronate 0.5 mg/kg infusion.
  - Calcimimetics suppress PTH secretion in affected gland.
- Primary hyperparathyroidism:
  - Resection of isolated adenoma.
  - For generalized hyperplasia resection of 3½ glands.
  - Vitamin D and calcium for postop hypocalcemia, which can be severe and prolonged due to hungry bone syndrome in cases of severe hyperparathyroidism.
- Secondary hyperparathyroidism: Treatment of the underlying cause.

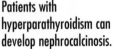

Patients with hyperparathyroidism can develop nephrocalcinosis.

HYPOPARATHYROIDISM

DEFINITION

Decreased PTH.

ETIOLOGY

- Autoimmune.
- Familial: Autosomal dominant, autosomal recessive, and X-linked recessive.
- DiGeorge/velocardiofacial syndrome (deletion of chromosome 22q.11.2).
- Acute illness (PTH secretion is impaired in critical illness).
- Severe hypomagnesemia (usually < 1 mg/dL).

SIGNS AND SYMPTOMS

- Most common presentation is numbness, tingling, paresthesia, muscle cramps.
- In severe cases, seizure, tetany, and mental status changes.
- In older asymptomatic patients, hyperreflexia, Chvostek's (facial twitching), and Trousseau's (carpopedal spasm) signs can be elicited.

Hypoparathyroidism can be seen with polyglandular autoimmune endocrinopathy: Thyroiditis, diabetes, adrenal insufficiency, mucocutaneous candidiasis.

DIAGNOSIS

- ↓ serum total Ca and ionized Ca.
- ↑ serum P.
- Markedly ↓ PTH.
- Prolonged QTc interval.
- Total Ca ↓ by 0.8 mg/dL for each 1 g/dL ↓ in albumin below 4 g/dL.
- ↑ or ↓ in pH by 0.1 units ↓ and ↑ ionized Ca by 0.03 mmol/L, respectively.

DIFFERENTIAL DIAGNOSIS

Pseudohypoparathyroidism (PTH unresponsiveness). Markedly ↑ PTH.

TREATMENT

- Correct hypocalcemia:
  - Intravenous (IV) 10% calcium gluconate 2 cc/kg gradually over 10 min for acute symptomatic hypocalcemia.
  - To maintain normocalcemia: Continuous IV infusion (20–80 mg Ca/kg/24 hr).
  - Transition to PO calcium as soon as possible (25–100 mg Ca/kg/day).
- Correct hypomagnesemia.
- Vitamin D (calcitriol).

Pay attention to heart rate with treatment for hypoparathyroidism: Bradycardia is an indication to stop calcium infusion.

CONGENITAL ADRENAL HYPERPLASIA (CAH)

DEFINITION

- Genetic defect of adrenal corticosteroid and/or mineralocorticoid synthesis.
- ↓ in cortisol secretion results in a ↓ in negative feedback at the level of hypothalamus and pituitary gland.
- ↑ ACTH secretion results in markedly elevated production of the precursors before the block.

EPIDEMIOLOGY

- Most common cause of ambiguous genitalia.
- Incidence of classical 21-hydroxylase CAH is 1 in 15,000 live births.

A newborn with ambiguous genitalia is a medical and social emergency.

ETIOLOGY

- 21-hydroxylase deficiency (90% of all CAH):
  - Three-quarters of cases are salt wasters.
  - Ambiguous genitalia in the females; normal genitalia in males.
  - Milder form (nonclassical variant) has normal genitalia in females and presents late with premature pubarche.
- 11β-hydroxylase deficiency: HTN with low K frequently present because of excessive deoxycorticosterone (DOC).
- 3β-hydroxysteroid dehydrogenase:
  - Ambiguous genitalia in both sexes.
  - Salt wasting is present.
- 17-hydroxylase/17,20-lyase deficiency:
  - Normal genitalia in females; undervirilized genitalia in males.
  - HTN with low K frequently present.

- Congenital lipoid adrenal hyperplasia:
  - Normal genitalia in females; undervirilized genitalia in males.
  - Salt wasting is present.
  - All adrenal hormones and their precursors are low.

SIGNS AND SYMPTOMS

- Clinical features result from both the hormonal deficiencies (cortisol and aldosterone) and excessive production of precursors (17-hydroxy-progesterone, androstenedione, DOC).
- Female pseudohermaphroditsm: Ambiguous genitalia in female with normal 46,XX chromosome (21-hydroxylase, 11β-hydroxylase, 3β-hydroxysteroid dehydrogenase deficiency).
- Male pseudohermaphroditism: Ambiguous genitalia in male with 46,XY chromosome (3β-hydroxysteroid dehydrogenase, 17-hydroxylase/17,20-lyase deficiency, and congenital lipoid adrenal hyperplasia).
- Hypoglycemia (from cortisol deficiency).
- Salt wasting (21-hydroxylase, 3β-hydroxysteroid dehydrogenase, and congenital lipoid adrenal hyperplasia).
- HTN with hypokalemia (11β-hydroxylase and 17 hydroxylase/17,20-lyase deficiency).
- Vomiting, dehydration, and shock at 2–4 weeks of age.

Combination of hyperkalemia and hyponatremia clue to diagnosis of classical CAH of salt-wasting variety.

DIAGNOSIS

- Newborn screening (elevated 17-hydroxyprogesterone level for 21-hydroxylase).
- Karyotype.
- Hyponatremia, hyperkalemia, hypochloremia, hypoglycemia.
- Markedly ↑ 17-hydroxyprogesterone for gestational age and weight (for 21-hydroxylase).
- Low baseline cortisol and low cortisol 60 min after 1–24 ACTH (Cortrosyn) stimulation.
- Elevated plasma renin activity (PRA).
- Genetic testing (DNA analysis for genetic mutations in the affected gene).
- Prenatal diagnosis (in pregnancy with ↑ risk).

Most urgent tests for congenital adrenal hyperplasia:
1. **Serum glucose**
2. **Serum electrolytes**
Other tests: cortisol, testosterone, 17-OH progesterone.

TREATMENT

- Fluid and electrolyte replacement.
- Normal saline (NS) 20 mL/kg bolus, then maintenance plus ongoing fluid losses with D5NS.
- Management of hypoglycemia.
- Hydrocortisone 25 mg IV bolus, then 50–100 mg/m²/24 hr (preferably as IV infusion) for acute adrenal crisis. Once crisis is improved, switch to PO 10–15 mg/m²/24 hr).
- Fludrocortisone 0.1–0.2 mg/day.
- Salt replacement (8–10 mEq/kg/day in the first few months of life, as Na content of formula and breast milk is quite low).
- Prenatal treatment: Treat mother with a pregnancy at risk for 21-hydroxylase deficiency, with dexamethasone.

In CAH, blood should be drawn for steroid profile before the administration of hydrocortisone.

DEFINITION

Characteristic pattern of obesity with or without HTN due to excessive gluco-corticoid production/exposure.

ETIOLOGY

- Iatrogenic from exogenous corticosteroid (most common cause of hypercortisolism).
- Cushing disease: Bilateral adrenal hyperplasia due excessive secretion of ACTH, usually by pituitary corticotroph adenoma. It is the most common cause of endogenous hypercortisolism in children.
- Cushing syndrome: Excess cortisol secretion by unilateral adrenocortical tumors (adenoma, carcinoma) or bilateral adrenal hyperplasia (primary pigmented micronodular adrenal hyperplasia).
- Ectopic ACTH syndrome: Malignant nonendocrine tumor produces an excessive amount of ACTH. Extremely rare in children.

Cushing disease is a state of hypercortisolism secondary to adrenocorticotropic hormone (ACTH)-producing pituitary adenoma.

SIGNS AND SYMPTOMS

Truncal obesity, rounded moon facies, buffalo hump, purple striae, easy bruising, muscle weakness, osteopenia, statural growth retardation, acne, hirsutism, hyperpigmentation, HTN, hyperglycemia, depression, cognitive impairment.

DIAGNOSIS

- Elevated 24-hour urine test for free cortisol (UFC) and 17-hydroxycorticosteroid (17-OHS).
  - Mean rate of UFC in normal children is < 70 mg/m²/day.
  - Mean rate of 17-OHS is < 7 mg/g of creatinine per day.
- 8:00 A.M. ACTH and cortisol: Elevated ACTH level (> 29 pg/mL with elevated UFC) suggests Cushing disease or ectopic ACTH production.
- Midnight plasma cortisol and ACTH (midnight cortisol > 4.4 μg/dL is highly suggestive of Cushing but does not differentiate between Cushing syndrome vs. Cushing disease).
- Low-dose dexamethasone suppression test:
  - Overnight dose 0.03 mg/kg (max 1 mg) at 11 P.M. X1 dose *or*
  - 0.03 mg/kg/day (max 0.5 q6h) for 2 days.
  - Normal if suppression results in plasma cortisol of < 5 μg/dL.
  - Nonsuppression with elevated UFC suggests the diagnosis of Cushing but does not differentiate between Cushing syndrome vs. Cushing disease.
- High-dose dexamethasone suppression test:
  - Overnight dose of 0.12 mg/kg/day (max 8 mg) *or*
  - 0.12 mg/kg/day (max 2 mg q6h) for 2 days.
  - Suppression (cortisol < 5 μg/dL) suggests Cushing disease, while non-suppression suggests Cushing syndrome.
  - 24 UFC paradoxically rises in primary pigmented nodular adrenal disease after high-dose dexamethasone suppression test.
- Ovine corticotropin-releasing hormone (CRH) stimulation test/bilateral petrosal sinus sampling: ↑ in ACTH after IV CRH suggests Cushing disease.

Growth retardation may be the early manifestation of Cushing syndrome. Virilization may indicate adrenal carcinoma.

- Polycythemia, lymphopenia, and eosinopenia can be associated findings.
- Abdominal computed tomography (CT) (adrenal tumors).
- Pituitary magnetic resonance imaging (MRI) (pituitary adenoma).

DIFFERENTIAL DIAGNOSIS

- Exogenous obesity (pseudo-Cushing state).
- Normal growth rate.
- Cortisol level suppressed by dexamethasone.

TREATMENT

- Pediatric endocrine, surgical, and neurosurgical consultation.
- Adrenalectomy (unilateral or bilateral for adrenal tumors or bilateral nodular hyperplasia, respectively).
- Chemotherapy with mitotane for adrenal cancer with metastasis (after surgery).
- Transsphenoidal resection of pituitary adenoma.
- Fractionated radiotherapy for recurrent pituitary adenoma.

ADRENAL INSUFFICIENCY

DEFINITION

- Adrenal cortex fails to produce enough glucocorticoid to mount response to stress.
- May be primary adrenal disorder or secondary to ACTH deficiency/resistance.
- Mineralocorticoid deficiency is present in primary adrenal disorder but is not part of secondary adrenal insufficiency, as aldosterone secretion depends on renin/angiotensin system.

ETIOLOGY

Primary Adrenal Insufficiency (Low Cortisol/Elevated ACTH)
- **Congenital:**
  - CAH.
  - Congenital adrenal hypoplasia (X-linked).
  - ACTH resistance.
  - Adrenal leukodystrophy (X-linked-recessive disorder of metabolism of very long chain fatty acids).
- **Acquired (Addison disease):**
  - Autoimmune destruction (80%).
  - Tuberculosis (TB).
  - Bilateral adrenal hemorrhages (meningococcal septicemia).
  - AIDS (opportunistic infections).
  - Antiphospholipid antibody syndrome.

Secondary Adrenal Insufficiency (Low Cortisol/Low ACTH)

- **Congenital:**
  - Congenital hypopituitarism
  - Septo-optic dysplasia
- **Acquired:**
  - Iatrogenic: Adrenal insufficiency from abrupt discontinuation of glucocorticoids after prolonged use.
  - Pituitary or hypothalamic tumors.

SIGNS AND SYMPTOMS

- Weakness, fatigue, anorexia, nausea, vomiting, weight loss.
- Postural hypotension (more marked in primary adrenal insufficiency).
- Hyperpigmentation of skin and mucosal surfaces (in primary adrenal insufficiency due to elevated ACTH/melanocyte-stimulating hormone [MSH]).
- Salt craving (in primary adrenal insufficiency).
- Adrenal crisis (fever, vomiting, dehydration, and shock precipitated by infection, trauma, or surgery in susceptible patient).

DIAGNOSIS

- Hyponatremia, hyperkalemia, acidosis, hypoglycemia.
- A.M. plasma cortisol and ACTH level:
  - A.M. plasma cortisol < 3 μg/dL is indicative of adrenal insufficiency while value > 19 μg/dL makes it unlikely.
  - Basal plasma ACTH level invariably exceeds 100 pg/mL in primary adrenal insufficiency, while normal ACTH level does not rule out secondary adrenal insufficiency.
- Antiadrenal antibodies (in autoimmune destruction of adrenal glands).
- ACTH stimulation test:
  - 1-24 ACTH (Cortrosyn) given IV or IM and cortisol level measured at baseline and 30–60 min after the injection.
  - For primary and severe/prolonged adrenal insufficiency use 250 μg Cortrosyn.
  - For secondary adrenal insufficiency that is mild or recent onset use 1 μg.
  - Normal response is plasma cortisol concentration of 18–20 μg/dL at 30-60 min post Cortrosyn.
- CT scan of adrenal glands (in primary adrenal insufficiency).
- MRI of the pituitary gland and hypothalamus (in secondary adrenal insufficiency).

TREATMENT

- Hydrocortisone (10–15 mg/m²/24 hr divided in 2–3 doses). Double or triple the oral dose of glucocorticoids for febrile illness or injury.
- Fludrocortisone (0.05–0.2 mg PO daily).
- In acute adrenal insufficiency (adrenal crisis):
  - Volume replacement.
  - Hydrocortisone 50–100 mg IV, then 50–100 mg/m²/24 hr or methylprednisolone 7.5 mg/m²/24 hr.
  - Switched to oral therapy in 2–3 days.

Tumors arising in the adrenal medulla produce both epinephrine and norepinephrine. Extra-adrenal tumors produce only norepinephrine.

Siblings of a patient with a pheochromocytoma should be periodically evaluated because of ↑ familial incidence.

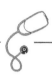

The most useful screening test for pheochromocytoma is blood pressure. Hypertensive paroxysms are an important diagnostic clue.

Increased urinary norepinephrine indicates an extra-adrenal site of a pheochromocytoma, whereas increased epinephrine indicates an adrenal lesion.

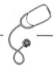

After successful surgery of a pheochromocytoma, catecholamine excretion returns to normal in about 1 week.

DEFINITION

- Catecholamine-producing tumor of chromaffin tissue of adrenal medulla and sympathetic ganglia (paraganglioma).
- Adrenal medulla (80–85%).
- Extra-adrenal (15–20%), also called paragangliomas.
- Usually benign, well encapsulated (< 10% malignant).
- In children: Frequently familial, bilateral, and multifocal.
- Recurrent tumor may appear years after initial diagnosis.

ETIOLOGY

- May occur in isolation (sporadic).
- Also seen in the MEN 2 (bilateral), von Hippel–Lindau, neurofibromatosis type 1, and familial carotid body tumor syndromes.

SIGNS AND SYMPTOMS

- Nonspecific symptoms.
- Headache, palpitations, ↑ sweating, anxiety.
- Nausea, vomiting, weight loss, tremor, fatigue, chest or abdominal pain, and flushing.
- Sustained HTN (in children).
- Hyperglycemia.
- Epinephrine-producing tumor may present with postural hypotension.

DIAGNOSIS

- Plasma free metanephrines (metanephrine and normetanephrine): Unequivocally elevated, 4–5 times the upper limit of the reference range.
- ↑ urinary catecholamines or metabolites (24-hour urinary excretion of fractionated metanephrines), vanillylmandelic acid (VMA).
- Serum chromogranin A.
- Abdominal ultrasound (US).
- Abdominal CT and MRI.
- ^{123}I MIBG (metaiodobenzylguanidine) scan.
- FDG PET (Flourodeoxyglucose positron emission tomography) scan.
- Octreoscan.

DIFFERENTIAL DIAGNOSIS

- Ganglioneuroma
- Neuroblastoma
- Ganglioneuroblastoma

TREATMENT

- Surgical excision.
- Preoperative α_1 and α_2 adrenoreceptor blockade (phenoxybenzamine) and β adrenoreceptor blockade (propranolol, atenolol) are required to prevent hypertensive crisis and arrhythmias, respectively.
- Yearly follow-up evaluation for assessment of recurrence for at least 5 years (indefinitely in children with familial pheochromocytoma).

Gigantism/Acromegaly

- ↑ GH.
- If occurs before epiphyses close, → gigantism.
- If after epiphyses close, → acromegaly.

ETIOLOGY

Most commonly caused by growth hormone (GH)-secreting adenoma.

CLINICAL FEATURES

- Accelerated rate of linear growth.
- Coarsening of facial features and mandibular prominence.
- Enlargement of hands and feet.

DIAGNOSIS

- Elevated insulin-like growth factor 1 (IGF-1) and IGF-binding protein 3 (IGFBP-3).
- GH may be normal or elevated. GH not suppressed by glucose.
- MRI of the pituitary.

TREATMENT

- Transsphenoidal resection of adenoma.
- Somatostatin and dopamine agonist for incomplete resection.

ETIOLOGY

- Prolactin-secreting adenoma: Microadenoma (< 1 cm) or macroadenoma (> 1 cm).
- Tumor that disrupt pituitary stalk preventing inhibitory control.
- Drugs (phenothiazines, estrogen, cocaine).
- Hypothyroidism.
- Liver or renal failure.
- Macroprolactinemia (variant molecule).
- Physical stress.

CLINICAL FEATURES

- Galactorrhea
- Menstrual irregularities/amenorrhea
- Decreased libido

DIAGNOSIS

- Prolactin level (> 20 ng/mL).
- MRI (hypothalamic-pituitary region).

TREATMENT

- Treatment of the cause.
- Dopamine agonists (bromocriptine, cabergoline) are the first line of treatment.
- Transsphenoidal surgery if medical treatment is unsuccessful.

Prolactin secretion chronically inhibited by dopamine in pituitary—prolactinomas responds to dopamine agonists such as bromocriptine.

> An infant has hypoglycemia and a micropenis. *Think: Hypopituitarism.*
> Hypopituitarism—growth hormone deficiency + deficiencies of other pituitary hormones. Severe hypoglycemia may be an initial presentation. Most infants present in the first few days of life with severe hypoglycemia. In males, microphallus is important diagnostic information. It is due to LH deficiency as LH stimulates testosterone production from testes during the last trimester of pregnancy causing lengthening of penis. Prolonged jaundice may be present which is due to associated central (hypothalamic or pituitary) hypothyroidism. Children who remain unrecognized may present later with failure to thrive and poor weight gain.

DEFINITION

Deficiency of more than one pituitary hormone.

PHYSIOLOGY

- ACTH → adrenal glucocorticoids.
- TSH → thyroid hormone.
- Luteinizing hormone (LH) and follicle-stimulating hormone (FSH) → gonadal function.
- Prolactin → lactation
- GH → growth.
- Antidiuretic hormone (ADH) → diabetes insipidus.

ETIOLOGY

- **Congenital:**
  - Inherited (mutation in the gene encoding pituitary transcription factor Pit-1).
  - Sporadic developmental defects: Midline anomalies (septo-optic dysplasia, cleft palate), holoprosencephaly.
- **Acquired:**
  - Tumors and their treatment (craniopharyngioma).
  - Head trauma.
  - CNS irradiation.
  - Histiocytosis X.
  - Autoimmune hypophysitis.
  - Hemochromatosis.
  - Disseminated tuberculosis or sarcoidosis.

SIGNS AND SYMPTOMS

- Depends on missing hormone and or etiological cause.
- GH deficiency (poor linear growth, hypoglycemia).
- In neonates (hypoglycemia and micropenis).
- LH and FSH (pubertal delay).
- ADH (polyuria, polydipsia).
- Visual and neurologic complaints.

Cortisol and GH are insulin counterregulatory hormones.

TREATMENT

Replacement directed toward the hormonal deficiency.

HIGH-YIELD FACTS

ENDOCRINE DISEASE

DEFINITION

Height below the 5th percentile for age and gender: (> 2 standard deviations below the mean).

Normal
- Chronological age (CA) = Bone age (BA) = Height age (HA)
- Normal growth velocity depends on age and pubertal stage:
  - First year: 25 cm/yr
  - 1–2 years: 12 cm/yr
  - 2–3 years: 10 cm/yr
  - 3–4 years: 7 cm/yr
  - 4–5 years: 6 cm/yr
  - After 5 years: 5 cm/yr
  - During puberty (girls Tanner II–III): 10 cm/yr
  - During puberty (boys Tanner IV): 12 cm/yr

Genetic Potential
- For males: Add 5 inches to mother's height and average it with father's height.
- For females: Subtract 5 inches from father's height and average it with mother's height.

Familial (Genetic Short Stature)
- Common cause of short stature.
- Growth rate ↓ between 6 and 18 months.
- Height within family norm (usually at least one parent has short stature).
- Normal rate of growth (follow steady channel after 2–3 yr).
- Normal bone age.
- Puberty at average age.

The most common causes of short stature are normal variants including familial short stature and constitutional delay.

Constitutional
- Most common cause of short stature.
- Normal variant of growth.
- Normal at birth, then growth decelerate during first 2 yr of life.
- Both length and weight gain decelerate until age 2–3 yr.
- Resume growth rate by 2–3 yr paralleling a lower percentile curve.
- Delayed puberty (second growth deceleration at age 12–14 yr).
- Delayed bone age (bone age = height age).

Children with constitutional delay are the so-called "late bloomers."

Nutritional
- Inflammatory bowel disease.
- Celiac disease.
- HIV infection.
- Other conditions causing malnutrition.

Psychosocial Deprivation
- Children with psychosocial deprivation clinically resemble children with GH deficiency with retardation of bone age and similar findings on GH stimulation testing; however, testing and growth revert to normal when the child is removed from the deprived environment.

Small for Gestational Age
- Birth weight and length < 10th percentile for gestational age.

Intrauterine Growth Retardation
- Pathologically growth restricted infants.

Growth Hormone Deficiency (GHD)

- Pathologic cause of short stature.
- Hypoglycemia and micropenis (especially if associated with hypopituitarism).
- Height below genetic potential.
- ↓ growth velocity (< 25th percentile for age).
- Downward crossing of percentiles on growth chart after age 2–3 yr.
- ↓ muscle mass, ↑ fat mass.
- Pubertal delay.
- Causes—idiopathic, hereditary, hypothalamic/pituitary malformation, hypothalamic/pituitary tumor, head trauma, CNS surgery, CNS radiation, meningitis/encephalitis, autoimmune hypophysitis, histiocytosis X, sarcoidosis, and hemochromatosis.

DIAGNOSIS

- Delayed bone age.
- Low IGF-1, low IGFBP-3, inadequate response to GH stimulation.

TREATMENT

Biosynthetic human GH.

Children with poor growth due to nutritional definiencies are generally short and have low birth weight, whereas children with endocrinologic causes for poor (linear) growth are usually disproportionately heavy.

Growth Hormone Insensitivity (Laron Syndrome)

- Features similar to GHD.
- GH receptor defect.
- Elevated GH level.
- Low IGF-1, IGF-2, and IGFBP-3.
- Absent or low growth hormone binding protein (GHBP).

TREATMENT

Biosynthetic IGF-1.

Hypothyroidism

- Pathologic cause of short stature.
- ↓ growth velocity.
- Delayed bone age.

DIAGNOSIS

Elevated TSH, decreased T_4.

TREATMENT

Synthroid (T_4).

Thyroid hormone is the most important hormone for linear growth in the first 2 years of life.

Cushing Syndrome

- Pathologic cause of short stature.
- ↑ cortisol inhibits growth.
- Abnormal weight gain.
- Truncal obesity, rounded moon facies, buffalo hump, purple striae.

ETIOLOGY

Endogenous or exogenous steroids.

DIAGNOSIS

Elevated 24-hr urine test for free cortisol is the best screening test.

TREATMENT

Treat the cause.

Chromosomal Disorders

- Turner syndrome
- Down syndrome
- Silver-Russell syndrome
- Prader-Willi syndrome

TALL STATURE

DEFINITION

Height more than 2 standard deviations above the mean for age and gender.

Familial
- Most common.

Hormonal
- GH excess.
- Early puberty: ↑ sex steroids (tall as child, short as adult from early epiphyseal closure).
- CAH: ↑ adrenal androgens (tall as child, short as adult from early epiphyseal closure).
- Hyperinsulinism/obesity.
- Hypogonadotrophic hypogonadism (Kallmann syndrome).

Syndromes
- Marfan syndrome.
- Homocystinuria.
- Klinefelter syndrome.
- Sotos syndrome (not truly endocrine, associated mental retardation)—cerebral gigantism: In utero and postnatal overgrowth.
- Beckwith-Wiedmann syndrome: Macrosomia with in utero and postnatal somatic overgrowth, macroglosia, hemihypertrophy and abdominal wall defect. Hypoglycemia due to hyperinsulinemia. ↑ incidence of tumors.

Beckwith-Weidemann syndrome: Large babies due to overproduction of IGF-2.

DIABETES INSIPIDUS (DI)

DEFINITION

Inability of kidneys to concentrate urine.

ETIOLOGY

- Central (↓ ADH):
  - Congenital hypothalamic/pituitary defects (septo-optic dysplasia, holoprosencephaly).
  - Idiopathic, accidental or surgical trauma, infections (meningitis).
  - Neoplasms (suprasellar tumors).
  - Infiltrative and autoimmune diseases (histiocytosis X).
  - Drugs (ethanol, phenytoin).
- Nephrogenic (renal unresponsiveness to ADH):
  - X-linked recessive (vasopressin type 2 receptor mutation): Males—early infancy.
  - Autosomal recessive (mutation in the renal water channel—aquaporin-2).
  - Idiopathic.
  - Renal diseases.
  - Hypercalcemia.
  - Hypokalemia.
  - Drugs (lithium, demeclocycline).

SIGNS AND SYMPTOMS

- Central:
  - Polyuria (> 1.5 L/m^2/day).
  - Polydipsia (excessive thirst).
  - Enuresis.
  - Hypernatremic dehydration.
- Nephrogenic:
  - Polyuria, failure to thrive (FTT), hyperpyrexia, vomiting.
  - Hypernatremic dehydration.

DIAGNOSIS

- ↑ serum osmolality (normal: < 290 mOsm/kg).
- ↑ serum Na (normal: < 145 mmol/L).
- ↓ urine osmolality.
- Water deprivation test: Withhold fluids for 8–10 hr (may need to be done in hospital). Serum osmolality > 300 mOsm/kg with urine osmolality < 600 mOsm/kg establishes the diagnosis. Once diagnosis is established, give pitressin 1 U/m^2 SQ.
  - Urine volume falls and osmolality doubles—central DI.
  - Less than twofold rise in urine osmolality—nephrogenic DI.
- Plasma vasopressin (low in central DI and high in nephrogenic DI).
- MRI: Posterior pituitary bright spot is diminished or absent in both forms of DI.

TREATMENT

- Central:
  - Fluids (3–4 L/m^2/day without vasopressin, 1 L/m^2/day with vasopressin).
  - Vasopressin (desmopressin [DDAVP]) 0.025-0.2 mg bid orally, 2.5–30 µg intranasally divided qd-bid, or 0.08 µg/kg subcutaneously divided q 12).
- Nephrogenic:
  - Fluids.
  - Thiazide diuretic (promotes Na excretion in the distal tubule and alters inner medullary osmolality → ↑ proximal tubular reabsorption of Na and ↑ free water reabsorption from the collecting duct).

In diabetes insipidus, there is high urine output despite significant dehydration.

- Indomethacin 2 mg/kg/day further enhances proximal tubular sodium and water reabsorption.

DEFINITION

Hyponatremia with ↑ ADH.

ETIOLOGY

- Encephalitis/meningitis.
- Brain tumor.
- Head trauma.
- Psychiatric diseases.
- Postictal period.
- Positive pressure ventilation.
- Rocky Mountain spotted fever.
- Pneumonia.
- AIDS.
- Drugs (carbamazepine, chlorpropamide, vincristine, tricyclic antidepressant).

In SIADH, there is an absence of edema and dehydration.

SIGNS AND SYMPTOMS

- Asymptomatic until Na < 120.
- Headache, nausea, vomiting, irritability, seizure.
- ↓ urine output.

DIAGNOSIS

- Hyponatremia (Na < 135 mmol/L).
- ↓ serum osmolality (< 275 mOsm/kg).
- ↑ urine osmolality (>100 mOsm/kg).
- ↑ urine Na (usually > 80 mEq/L).
- Low serum uric acid level.
- Normal renal, adrenal, and thyroid function.

Urine osmolality < 100 mOsm/kg excludes diagnosis of SIADH.

TREATMENT

- **Symptomatic with hyponatremia:** Hypertonic (3%) saline 6 mL/kg bolus ↑ Na by 5 mmol/L. Repeat bolus until patient stops seizing.
- **Asymptomatic:**
  - Fluid restriction (1000 mL/m^2/day).
  - Demeclocycline if resistant (rarely used).
  - Selective V2 receptor antagonist (tolvaptan).
  - Oral urea (0.1–2.0 g/kg/day divided q6h) at low doses reduces natriuresis and at higher doses causes osmotic diuresis.

DEFINITION

Renal loss of Na during intracranial disease.

TABLE 16-3. Comparison Between SIADH and CSW

	SIADH	CSW
Body weight	↑	↓
Plasma volume	↑	↓
Serum Na	↓	↓
Serum osmolality	↓	↓
Urine osmolality	Higher than plasma	Isotonic with plasma
Urine flow rate	↓	↑
Plasma renin	↓	↓
Plasma aldosterone	↑	↓
Plasma ADH	↑	↓
Plasma ANP	↑	↑
Serum uric acid	↓	Normal

ADH, antidiuretic hormone; ANP, atrial natriuretic peptide; CSW, cerebral salt wasting; SIADH, syndrome of inappropriate secretion of antidiuretic hormone.

ETIOLOGY

High atrial natriuretic peptide (ANP) → natriuresis and diuresis.

SIGNS AND SYMPTOMS

- Acute, intermittent excessive fluid and salt loss.
- ↑ urine output.
- Onset within first week of CNS insult.
- Duration variable usually lasts 2–4 weeks.
- Dehydration (↓ extracellular fluid).

DIAGNOSIS

- Hyponatremia (Na < 130 mmol/L).
- Urine osmolality isotonic with plasma.
- ↑ urine Na (usually > 150 mEq/L).
- See Table 16-3 for comparison between SIADH and CSW.

TREATMENT

- Water and salt replacement (0.9 or 3% NS).
- Urea.

- Pubertal events are classified by Tanner staging. Puberty progresses usually with an average duration of 3–4 yr, spending roughly about one year in each stage.
- See Table 16-4 and Figure 16-1.

Normal Female Progression

Thelarche → height growth spurt → pubic hair → menarche (12.5–13 yr). (In 20 % of girls, pubarche may precede thelarche).

Normal Male Progression

Testicular enlargement → pubic hair → penile enlargement → height growth spurt (14–15 yr) → axillary hair.

> The ↑ in height velocity in boys occurs at a later chronologic age than in girls (Tanner IV in boys, Tanner II–III in girls).

Precocious Puberty

A 6½-year-old girl develops enlarged breasts. Six months later she begins to develop pubic and axillary hair. Her menses began at age 9. *Think: Idiopathic precocious puberty.*

Puberty in girls is now recognized to be occurring at earlier age. The exact cause of the precocious puberty in most cases remains unknown. Evaluation should include serum FSH, LH, estradiol, and bone age. Brain MRI should be obtained to rule out possible underlying intracranial cause.

TABLE 16-4. Tanner Stages

STAGE	BREAST DEVELOPMENT (FEMALE)	GENITAL DEVELOPMENT (MALE)	PUBIC HAIR (FEMALE AND MALE)
I	Preadolescent	Preadolescent	Preadolescent
II	Breast bud (11 yr)	Enlargement of scrotum and testes, darkening of scrotum and texture change (12 yr)	Sparse, long, slightly pigmented downy hair (female 12, male 13.5)
III	Continued enlargement, no contour separation (12 yr)	Enlargement of penis (13 yr)	Darker, coarser, and more curled (female 12.5, male 14)
IV	Secondary mound, projection of areola and papilla (13 yr)	Increase in penis breadth and development of glans (14 yr)	Hair resembles adult, distributed less than adult and not to medial thighs (female 13, male 14.5)
V	Mature stage (15 yr)	Mature stage (15 yr)	Mature stage (female 14.5, male 15)

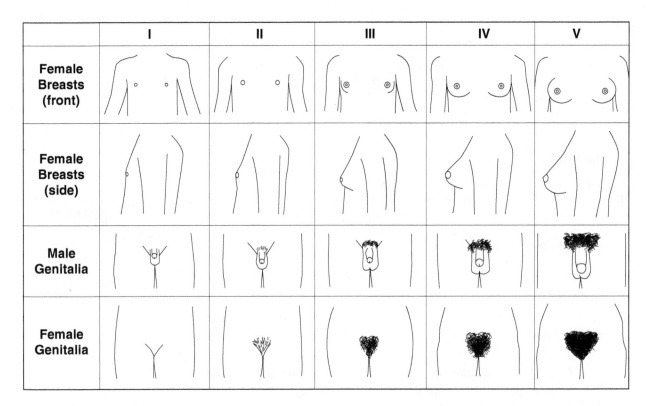

FIGURE 16-1. Tanner stages

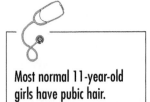

Most normal 11-year-old girls have pubic hair.

DEFINITION

- Onset of secondary sexual characteristics.
- Girls (< 8 yr for white girls, < 7 for African-American and Hispanics).
- Boys (< 9 yr).
- Premature breast development (thelarche).
- Premature pubic hair development (pubarche/adrenarche).

ETIOLOGY

Central or True Precocious Puberty
- Premature activation of the hypothalamic-pituitary-gonadal axis.
- Gonadotropin dependent: Pubertal (high) FSH and LH and sex steroids (testosterone or estradiol).
- Usually idiopathic in girls, while secondary to organic lesion in boys.
- CNS abnormalities:
  - Hypothalamic hamartoma.
  - Head injury.
  - Hydrocephalus.
  - Radiation.
  - Surgical trauma.
  - Tumors (astryocytoma, glioma, pinealoma, LH-secreting adenoma).

Peripheral or Pseudo Precocious Puberty
- Gonadotropin independent: Prepubertal (low) FSH and LH, pubertal (high) sex steroids.
- **Male:**
  - Testotoxicosis: Familial male limited precocious puberty (bilateral testicular enlargement).

- Tumors.
  - Testicular Leydig cell tumor (unilateral testicular enlargement).
  - Choriocarcinoma, dysgerminoma, hepatoblastoma (human chorionic gonadotropin [HCG] producing).
  - Adrenal tumors (testosterone secreting).
- CAH.
- McCune-Albright syndrome.
- Exogenous sex steroid.
- **Female:**
  - McCune-Albright syndrome: Ovarian cysts secreting estrogen.
  - Tumors:
    - Ovarian tumors (granulosa cell tumor, gonadoblastoma).
    - Choriocarcinoma, dysgerminoma, hepatoblastoma (HCG producing).
  - Adrenal tumors (estrogen secreting).
  - Exogenous sex steroids.

Precocious puberty in girls is usually idiopathic, while in boys it usually has an organic cause.

SIGNS AND SYMPTOMS

- Growth acceleration.
- Significantly advanced bone age.
- Sexual development is progressive (in some children, particularly girls, such changes may be very slowly progressive—a variant of normal development).

DIAGNOSIS

- FSH, LH.
- Estradiol, testosterone.
- Dehydroepiandrosterone sulfate (DHEAS), 17-hydroxyprogesterone, androstenedione.
- α-fetoprotein (AFP), HCG.
- Prepubertal levels (low) of gonadotropins and pubertal (high) level of estrogen or testosterone suggest gonadotropin-independent process.
- Gonadotrpins may be pubertal or prepubertal at baseline while testosterone or estrogen is usually pubertal in gonadotrpin-dependent precocious puberty.
- No ↑ in gonadotropins after gonadotropin-releasing hormone (GnRH) in gonadotrpin-independent precocious puberty.
- Pubertal LH-dominant response (LH > 5 mIU/mL and LH-to-FSH ratio > 1) after GnRH in true, central, gonadotropin-dependent precocious puberty.
- Pelvic ultrasound to evaluate ovarian and uterine size and rule out any pathology (ovarian cyst, tumor).
- MRI of the head to rule out CNS abnormality in central precocious puberty.
- CT abdomen and pelvis if tumor is the likely cause of peripheral precocious puberty.

TREATMENT

- Treatment of underlying cause (in both central and peripheral puberty).
- GnRH analogues (in central precocious puberty).
- Androgen antagonist (flutamide) and aromatase inhibitor (blocks conversion of androgen to estrogen) in peripheral precocious puberty.

Premature Thelarche

DEFINITION

- Isolated breast development.
- Most commonly noted during the first 2 yr of life.
- May occur after 2 yr due to temporary increase in FSH. Breast development is usually limited and often regresses.

SIGNS AND SYMPTOMS

- Normal growth rate and bone age.
- Prepubertal level of gonadotropins and estrogen.

TREATMENT

Nonprogressive and self-limiting.

Premature Adrenarche

DEFINITION

Early appearance of sexual hair (premature pubarche) without other signs of sexual development.

- < 8 yr in girls (< 7 yr in African-American and Hispanic).
- < 9 yr in boys.
- Adult body odor is other associated feature.

ETIOLOGY

- Early onset of increased adrenal androgen production (premature adrenarche).
- In girls it is a risk factor for later development of polycystic ovarian syndrome (PCOS).
- Nonclassical CAH may present similarly and can lead to early puberty.

DIAGNOSIS

- Adrenal androgen (DHEAS): Normal for pubertal stage but elevated for chronologic age.
- If androgens are significantly elevated, CAH and adrenal tumor need to be excluded.

TREATMENT

Self-limiting.

Delayed Puberty

DEFINITION

Absence of pubertal development by 14 yr in girls and 15 yr in boys.

EPIDEMIOLOGY

More common in boys.

ETIOLOGY

- **Female:**
  - Constitutional.
  - Primary ovarian failure (idiopathic, autoimmune, chemotherapy, radiation, galactosemia, fragile X syndrome, mutation in gonodotropin receptor).
  - Turner syndrome.
  - Hypogonadotropic hypogonadism (Kallmann syndrome).
  - 17-hydroxylase deficiency CAH.
  - Hypopituitarism (congenital or acquired).
  - Dysfunction of hypothalamic-pituitary-gonadal axis secondary to systemic illness, undernutrition, or strenuous physical activity.
  - Prader-Willi syndrome.
- **Male:**
  - Constitutional.
  - Primary testicular failure (vanishing testis syndrome, bilateral cryptorchidism/torsion, infection, chemotherapy, radiation, surgical trauma, hemochromatosis, fragile X syndrome, mutation in gonodotropin receptor).
  - Klinefelter syndrome.
  - Hypogonadotropic hypogonadism (Kallmann syndrome).
  - Dysfunction of hypothalamic-pituitary-gonadal axis secondary to systemic illness or undernutrition.
  - Hypopituitarism (congenital or acquired).
  - Prader-Willi syndrome.

DIAGNOSIS

- FSH, LH, estradiol, testosterone.
  - Elevated gonadotropin levels (FSH, LH) suggest primary gonadal failure—hypergonadotrophic hypogonadism.
  - Low gonadotropin levels suggest hypogonadotrophic hypogonadism or constitutional delay. No test definitely differentiates constitutional delay from gonadotropin deficiency until age is well into adolescence.
- Chromosome analysis (for primary gonadal failure).
- MRI of the head (in hypogonadotrophic hypogonadism or hypopituitarism).

TREATMENT

- Treatment of the cause.
- Females: Estrogen initially; later, cyclic estrogen progesterone.
- Males: Testosterone.

Kallmann syndrome:
Usually sporadic; 5%
X-linked hypogonadotropic hypogonadism affecting males and rarely females, associated with anosmia, cleft lip/palate, and other midline defects.

MENSTRUATION

- The mean age for menarche in American is 12.8 yr +/– 1.2 yr.
- Menarche occurs about 2–3 yr after the initiation of puberty. Two-thirds of females reach menarche at Tanner stage IV puberty.
- Fifty to sixty percent of cycles in the first 2 yr after menarche in most girls are anovulatory.
- The length of a cycle is between 21 and 45 days (average is 28 days).
- The length of flow is 2–7 days (average is 3–5 days).
- Blood loss is on average 40 mL (range, 25–70 mL).

Turner syndrome is the most common cause of primary amenorrhea.

Amenorrhea

PRIMARY AMENORRHEA

Lack of spontaneous uterine bleeding regardless of secondary sexual characteristics by age 16 yr.

ETIOLOGY

- **Primary ovarian failure** (elevated FSH and LH).
- Chromosomal:
  - Turner syndrome.
  - Triple X syndrome.
  - Pure gonadal dysgenesis (46,XX or 46,XY).
  - Fragile X.
- Classical galactosemia.
- Autoimmune oophoritis.
- Radiation.
- Chemotherapy.
- Gonadal trauma.
- 17-hydroxylase deficiency (CAH).
- Congenital lipid hyperplasia.
- FSH/LH receptor mutation.
- Idiopathic.
- **Hypogonadotropic hypogonadism** (low FSH and LH): Isolated or with hypopituitarism.
- Prader-Willi syndrome.
- Anorexia nervosa.
- Strenuous exercise.
- **Structural anomalies:**
  - Imperforate hymen.
  - Agenesis of Müllerian structure (Mayer-Rokitansky-Hauser syndrome).
- Other:
  - Complete androgen insensitivity (testicular feminization syndrome).
  - True hermaphroditism.

SECONDARY AMENORRHEA

A 16-year-old female had the onset of breast development at the age of 12 years and menses at age 14. She has not had menses for 2 months. She is active in sports. Physical examination is normal. *Think: Rule out pregnancy, then consider the sports contribution to her secondary amenorrhea.*

Pregnancy is the most common cause of amenorrhea and should be excluded in any female patient of reproductive age. After pregnancy, thyroid disease and hyperprolactinemia should be considered as potential diagnoses. Amenorrhea can also occur due to exercise and participation in athletic activity. Female athlete triad (disordered eating, amenorrhea, and osteoporosis) is a well-recognized entity. Athletic amenorrhea is due to hypothalamic-pituitary axis suppression, but it is a diagnosis of exclusion. Other causes must be excluded, and evaluation should include pregnancy test, prolactin, FSH, LH, TSH, T_4 DHEAs, 17 Hydroxprogesterone and testosterone levels.

Absence of menstruation for 6 months or a length of time equal to three cycles after menstrual cycles have already been established.

ETIOLOGY

- Pregnancy.
- Turner syndrome (mosaicism).
- Hyperandrogenic states (PCOS, CAH).
- Hyperprolactinemia.
- Hypothalamic amenorrhea.
- Causes of primary amenorrhea.

DIFFERENTIAL DIAGNOSIS

- **Normal/low FSH:**
  - Consider hypothalamic amenorrhea related to stress, weight loss, an eating disorder, competitive athletics, phenothiazine use, or substance abuse.
  - Also consider chronic disease, CNS tumor (ie, prolactinoma), pituitary infiltration or infarction as in postpartum hemorrhage or sickle cell disease, and Asherman syndrome (following endometrial curettage).
- **High FSH:** Consider gonadal dysgenesis as in mosaic Turner syndrome or autoimmune oophoritis.

The most common causes of secondary amenorrhea include pregnancy, stress, and PCOS.

Dysmenorrhea

DEFINITION

Painful menstruation.

PRIMARY OR ESSENTIAL DYSMENORRHEA

Dysmenorrhea in the absence of any specific, pelvic pathologic condition. Associated with ovulatory cycles.

ETIOLOGY

- Progesterone produced during ovulatory cycle ↑ the synthesis of the prostaglandins.
- Excessive amounts of prostaglandins F_2 and E_2, which cause uterine contractions, tissue hypoxia and ischemia, and ↑ sensitization of pain receptors.

TREATMENT

Recommend prostaglandin inhibitors for dysmenorrhea at the onset of flow or pain.

Dysmenorrhea is the most common gynecologic complaint.

SECONDARY DYSMENORRHEA

ETIOLOGY

- Underlying structural abnormality of the vagina, cervix, or uterus (endometrial polyps, fibroids).
- Congenital anomalies.
- Pelvic adhesions.
- Endometriosis.
- Foreign body such as an intrauterine device.

- Endometritis: Infection, especially secondary to sexually transmitted diseases (STDs).
- Complications of pregnancy such as ectopic pregnancy.

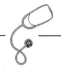

Mittelschmerz

- Mid-menstrual cycle pain due to ovulation
- Not pathologic
- Treat symptomatically

TESTICULAR FEMINIZATION

DEFINITION

- Androgen insensitivity syndrome (complete and partial form).
- X-linked.
- In complete insensitivity, XY male appears as unambiguous female with a short, blind-ending vaginal pouch and no uterus. Androgen receptor is either absent or unable to bind androgen.
- In partial insensitivity, XY cases have either ambiguous or female genitalia with no uterus. Considerable virilization occurs at puberty, but gynecomastia also develops. Androgen receptor binding is low or normal.

SIGNS AND SYMPTOMS

- Primary amenorrhea.
- Normal breast development.
- Pubic hair absent or sparse.
- Presence of testes in inguinal hernia.

DIAGNOSIS

- Testosterone level is elevated.
- LH is normal or elevated.
- Sex hormone binding globulin (SHBG) test: IM testosterone (2 mg/kg) unable to suppress SHBG to < 80% of the basal value suggests androgen insensitivity.
- HCG stimulation (3000 mg/m^2/day) every other day for 2 days shows normal testosterone response (double from baseline at 48 hr, then double again 2 days after the second injection) helps differentiate partial androgen sensitivity from causes of ambiguous genitalia due to testosterone synthesis defect.
- Androgen receptor binding studies in cultured genital skin fibroblast.
- DNA analysis for mutation in AR gene.

TRUE HERMAPHRODITISM

DEFINITION

- Gonads comprised of both ovarian and testicular elements (ovotestis).
- Most are 46,XX.
- Can be familial.

ETIOLOGY

Abnormal gonadal differentiation.

- Ambiguous genitalia—significant masculinization (raised as male).
- Risk of malignant transformation of gonadal tissue is much lower (2%) than XY gonadal dysgenesis.

PSEUDOHERMAPHRODITISM

Female

DEFINITION

Normal gonads and uterus (both gonads are ovaries) with virilization of external genitalia in a patient with a 46,XX karyotype.

ETIOLOGY

- CAH (21-hydroxylase deficiency, 11 β-hydroxylase deficiency, 3 β-hydroxysteroid dehydrogenase deficiency).
- Placental aromatase deficiency (conversion of androgens to estrogens is blocked). Estriol level is undetectable. Maternal virilization during pregnancy.
- Luteoma of pregnancy: Maternal virilization during pregnancy.

SIGNS AND SYMPTOMS

Virilization of external genitalia (clitoral hypertrophy, labioscrotal fusion).

Male

DEFINITION

Normal testes (both gonads are testes) with undervirilization or completely female appearing external genitalia in a patient with 46,XY karyotype.

ETIOLOGY

- Androgen insensitivity.
- CAH: 3β-hydroxysteroid dehydrogenase deficiency, 17-hydroxylase deficiency, and congenital lipoid adrenal hyperplasia.
- Enzyme defects in testosterone synthesis (17-ketoreductase deficiency).
- 5α-reductase deficiency: Conversion of testosterone to dihydrotestosterone is blocked.

SIGNS AND SYMPTOMS

Undervirilization of external genitalia (small phallus, hypospadias, undescended testes) or completely female appearing genitalia.

METABOLIC BONE DISEASE

- **Osteopenia:** Deficiency in bone mass relative to age, sex, and race norms.
- **Osteoporosis:** Loss of bone mineral and matrix due to disproportionately low osteoblastic activity.

- **Osteomalacia:** Defective mineralization in bone.
- **Rickets:** Defective mineralization of cartilage in the growth plate.

Classification of Rickets

CALCIOPENIC

ETIOLOGY

- Nutritional:
  - Vitamin D deficiency
  - Calcium deficiency
- Genetic:
  - Vitamin D–dependent rickets type 1 (1α-hydroxylase deficiency causing defect in the conversion of 25(OH) vitamin D to 1,25(OH)$_2$ vitamin D).
  - Vitamin D–dependent rickets type 2 (mutation in the gene coding the vitamin D receptor causing hereditary vitamin D resistance).
- Drugs:
  - Corticosteroids
  - Anticonvulsants
- Prematurity.

PHOSPHOPENIC

- Genetic:
  - X-linked hypophostemic rickets (mutation in the *PHEX* gene).
  - Autosomal-dominant hereditary hypophosphatemic ricket (mutation in the gene for fibroblast growth factor 23).
  - Autosomal-recessive hereditary hyperphosphatemic rickets with hypercalciuria (mutation in the gene for renal sodium phosphate cotransporter NaP(i)-IIc).
- Tumor-induced hypophostemia (tumor mostly of mesenchymal origin).
- Dietary:
  - Intestinal malabsorption.
  - Breast-fed premature infants.
- Fanconi syndrome (renal loss of glucose, phosphate, amino acids, and bicarbonate).

CLINICAL FEATURES

- Genu varum (bow-legged deformity) during early childhood.
- Genu valgum (knocked-knee deformity) in older children.
- Enlargement of wrists and knees.
- Rachitic rosary (bulging of costochondral junctions).
- Harrison grooves (groove extending laterally from xiphoid process, corresponds to the diaphragmatic attachment).
- Frontal bossing.
- Craniotabes (generalized softening of calvaria).
- Craniosynostosis.
- Bone pain.
- Proximal muscle weakness.

RADIOLOGICAL FEATURES

- Widening of epiphyseal plates.
- Cupping.
- Deformities in shaft of long bones.

- Serum calcium, phosphorous, alkaline phosphatase level:
  - Alkaline phosphatase is elevated in most cases of rickets. Elevation is marked in calcium and vitamin D deficiency and mild in hypophosphatemic rickets.
  - Serum calcium and phosphorus tend to be low or low normal in all form of calciopenic rickets.
  - Low serum phosphate with normal calcium level suggests the diagnosis of hypophosphatemic rickets.
- 25(OH) vitamin D and 1,25(OH)$_2$ vitamin D level:
  - Low 25(OH) vitamin D is seen in all forms of vitamin D deficiency.
  - Normal 25(OH) vitamin D level with low 1,25(OH)$_2$ vitamin D level point to 1α-hydroxylase deficiency.
  - 1,25(OH)$_2$ vitamin D level is elevated in hereditary vitamin D resistance.
  - 1,25(OH)$_2$ vitamin D level is inappropriately normal in the setting of hypophosphatemia in X-linked and autosomal-dominant hypophosphatemic rickets.
- PTH level:
  - Moderate to severe hyperparathyroidism is characteristic of calciopenic rickets.
  - In hypophosphatemic rickets, PTH level may be normal or modestly elevated.
- Tubular reabsorption of phosphorous (TRP).

$$[1-\{(Urine\ P \times Serum\ creatinine)\ /$$
$$(Serum\ P \times Urine\ creatinine)\}] \times 100$$

- Normal TRP value 85–95% for children.
- A nomogram is used to determine the renal tubular threshold maximum for phosphate as expressed per glomerular filtration rate (TMP/GFR).
- Low TMP/GFR in the setting of low serum phosphate confirms inappropriate renal loses, characteristic of hypophosphatemic rickets.

TREATMENT

- **Nutritional rickets:**
  - 5000–15,000 IU of vitamin D PO for 4 weeks.
  - 600,000 IU in a single dose PO/IM for noncompliance (stoss therapy).
  - Ensure adequate calcium intake (350–1500 mg elemental calcium per day for 6 months).
- **1α-hydroxylase deficiency rickets:**
  - 1,25(OH)$_2$ vitamin D (calcitriol) 0.5–3 μg/day.
  - Adequate dietary calcium intake.
- **Hereditary vitamin D resistance:**
  - High doses of 1,25(OH)$_2$ vitamin D.
  - IV calcium in patients who do not respond to vitamin D.
- **Hypophosphatemic rickets:**
  - Phosphate (250–1000 mg elemental phosphorus in 2–3 divided doses).
  - 1,25(OH)$_2$ vitamin D is important for successful outcome. It enhances Ca and P absorption and dampens phosphate stimulated PTH secretion.

DEFINITION

- Symptom of brain dysfunction (not an etiologic diagnosis).
- A paroxysmal electrical discharge of neurons in the brain resulting in an alteration of function or behavior.
- The most common neurologic disorder in children:
  - 4–10% of children
  - 1% of all ED visits
- Highest incidence: < 3 yr.

ETIOLOGY

Multiple etiologies have been identified for seizures. Provoked causes include:

- Fever.
- Metabolic:
  - Hypoglycemia
  - Hyponatremia
  - Hypocalcemia
  - Inborn errors of metabolism
- Medications and illegal drugs.
- Trauma (intracranial hemorrhage).
- Infections (encephalitis, meningitis, abscess).
- Vascular events (strokes).
- Hypoxic ischemia encephalopathy.

Types of Seizures

See Table 17-1.

PARTIAL (FOCAL) SEIZURES

Begin in one brain region.

1. Simple partial seizures:
   - Average duration is 10–20 sec.
   - Restricted at onset to one focal cortical region.

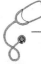

The diagnosis of clinical epilepsy requires two or more unprovoked seizures.

- Recurrence risk after a first unprovoked episode is 45% (27–52%).
- The risk of epilepsy is > 70% after two unprovoked episodes.

In most children with seizures, an underlying cause cannot be determined and a diagnosis of idiopathic epilepsy is given.

Partial seizures: Onset in one brain region. Generalized seizures: Onset simultaneously in both cerebral hemispheres.

Aura: Abnormal perception or hallucination that precede seizures.

HIGH-YIELD FACTS

NEUROLOGIC DISEASE

TABLE 17-1. Types of Seizures

Absence	Sudden brief discontinuation of activity and unresponsiveness
Tonic-Clonic	Bilateral symmetrical tonic contraction, then bilateral clonic contractions
Tonic	Sustained muscle contraction for seconds to minutes
Clonic	Repetitive, rhythmic myoclonus at 2–3 Hz
Myoclonic	Sudden, brief (< 100 ms) involuntary contraction of muscles or group of muscles
Atonic	Sudden, brief, 1–2 sec ↓ in tone without preceding myoclonic or tonic event

In seizure, as opposed to migraine, the aura is part of the seizure.

Both simple and complex partial seizures may become generalized.

The first step in evaluating any seizure disorder is determining the type of seizure.

Motor activity is the most common symptom of simple partial seizures.

- Consciousness is not altered.
- Tend to involve the face, neck, and extremities.
- Patients may complain of preictal aura, which is characteristic for the brain region involved in the seizure (ie, visual aura, auditory aura, etc.).
- Seizures can also be somatosensory/visual or auditory.

2. Complex partial seizures:
   - Average duration is 1–2 min.
   - Hallmark feature is *alteration* or loss of consciousness.
   - Automatisms are seen in 50–75% of cases (psychic, sensory, or motor phenomena carried out while unconscious and not recalled postictally).
   - May begin as a simple partial seizure and progress until consciousness is affected.

GENERALIZED SEIZURES

Begins simultaneously in both cerebral hemispheres. Consciousness is impaired from seizure onset.

1. Typical absence seizures (formerly "petit mal"):
   - Generalized seizure.
   - Characterized by sudden cessation of motor activity or speech.
   - Brief stares (usually < 10 sec), rarely longer than 30 sec.
   - More common in girls. Male-to-female ratio: 2:1.
   - Onset 2–6 yr.
   - Frequency: Dozens/day.
   - There is no aura.
   - There is no postictal state.
   - Childhood absence epilepsy is associated with characteristic 3-Hz spike-and-wave pattern (Figure 17-1) on EEG.

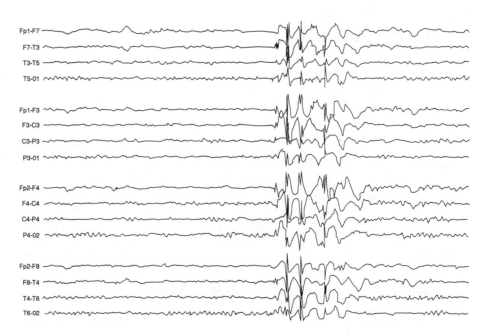

FIGURE 17-1. Absence seizure EEG.

Characteristic 3-Hz spike and wave pattern.

2. Generalized tonic-clonic (GTC, formerly "grand mal") seizures:
   - Extremely common and may follow a partial seizure with focal onset.
   - Patients suddenly lose consciousness, their eyes roll back, and their entire musculature undergoes tonic contractions, rarely arresting breathing.
   - Gradually, the hyperextension gives way to a series of rapid clonic jerks.
   - Finally, a period of flaccid relaxation occurs, during which sphincter control is often lost (incontinence).
   - Prodromal symptoms (not aura) often precede the attack by several hours and include mood change, apprehension, insomnia, or loss of appetite. (Unclear if these are warning signs or part of the cause).

ABSENCE VERSUS COMPLEX PARTIAL SEIZURES

While examining an 8-year-old girl in your office, the child suddenly develops a blank stare and flickering eyelids. Twenty seconds later she returns to normal and acts as if nothing out of the ordinary has occurred. *Think: Absence seizure.*

You are reviewing the history before seeing a patient. She is a 7-year-old bright girl with no significant past medical history. The schoolteacher noted that she sometimes does not respond when her name is called. Also, she stares in space with a blank look momentarily. *Think: Absence seizures.*

Absence seizures are the second most common type of generalized seizure in children. Common age of presentation is between 4 and 12 yr. Since these seizures develop in childhood, schoolteachers are often the first to notice. There is no aura and no postictal symptoms. It may be accompanied by brief eye blinking or myoclonic movement. Electroencephalogram (EEG) shows spike-and-wave activity at 3/sec. These seizures are not associated with progressive neurologic disease.

Pediatric Seizure Disorders

SIMPLE FEBRILE SEIZURE

- The most common seizure disorder during childhood. Occur in 2–5% of children 6 months to 6 years of age.
- Present as a brief tonic-clonic seizure associated with a fever.
- Risk of recurrence is 30% after first episode and 50% after second episode.
- Highest recurrence before 1 year of age (50%).
- There are no long-term sequelae, and children will outgrow by age 6.
- Risk of epilepsy (1–2% as opposed to 0.5–1% in the general population) not statistically significant.
- ↑ risk of epilepsy (up to 13%) in the presence of:
  - Abnormal neurologic examination.
  - Complex febrile seizure.
  - Family history of epilepsy.
- An autosomal-dominant inheritance pattern with incomplete penetrance is demonstrated in some families (19p and 8q13–21).

Benign neonatal familial convulsions ("fifth day fits") are a brief self-limited autosomal-dominant condition with generalized seizures beginning in the first week of life and subsiding within 6 weeks. There is a normal interictal EEG. There is a 10–15% chance of future epilepsy, but otherwise carries an excellent prognosis. Always elicit a family history in neonatal seizures usually revealed after interviewing grandparents.

Immature neonatal brain is more excitable than older children.

If you are present during a tonic–clonic seizure:

- Keep track of the duration.
- Place the patient between prone and lateral decubitus to allow the tongue and secretions to fall forward.
- Hyperextend the neck and jaw to enhance breathing.
- Loosen any tight clothing or jewelry around the neck.
- **Do not try to force open the mouth or teeth!**

NEONATAL SEIZURE

- The most common neurologic manifestation of impaired brain function.
- **Occurs in 1.8–3.5 of every 1000 newborns.**
- Higher incidence in low-birth-weight infants.
- Metabolic, toxic, hypoxic, ischemic, and infectious diseases are commonly present during the neonatal period, placing the child at an ↑ risk for seizures.
- Myelination is not complete at birth; thus, GTC seizures are very uncommon in the first month of life.
- May manifest as tonic, myoclonic, clonic, or subtle (prolonged nonnutritive sucking, nystagmus, color change, autonomic instability).
- EEG may show burst suppression (alternating high and very low voltages), low-voltage invariance, diffuse or focal background slowing, and focal or multifocal spikes.
- Neonatal seizures are typically treated acutely with phenobarbital (drug of choice), fosphenytoin, or benzodiazepines.
- Phenytoin not a first-line agent due to depressive effect on the myocardium and variable metabolism in newborns.
- Prophylaxis usually with phenobarbital, but also topiramate or levetiracetam.

INFANTILE SPASM

- Onset: 4–8 months.
- Clusters of brief symmetric flexor/extensor contractions of the neck, trunk, and extremities up to 100/day.
- Symptomatic type is most commonly seen with central nervous system (CNS) malformations, brain injury, tuberous sclerosis, or inborn errors of metabolism, and typically has a poor outcome.
- Cryptogenic type has a better prognosis and children typically have an uneventful birth history and reach developmental milestones before the onset of the seizures.
- Treated with adrenocorticotropic hormone (ACTH) in the United States.
- Vigabatrin (equally as effective as ACTH therapy).
- EEG has characteristic hypsarrhythmia pattern: Large amplitude chaotic multifocal spikes and slowing (see Figure 17-2).

Epilepsy

DEFINITION

- A history of two or more unprovoked seizures.
- After a nebulous period (on the order of 5–10 yr) of seizure freedom without the aid of antiepileptic medications or devices, the epilepsy can be considered to have resolved, particularly if the patient fits an epilepsy syndrome that is known typically to resolve.

EPIDEMIOLOGY

Epilepsy occurs in 0.5–1% of the population and begins in childhood in 60% of the cases.

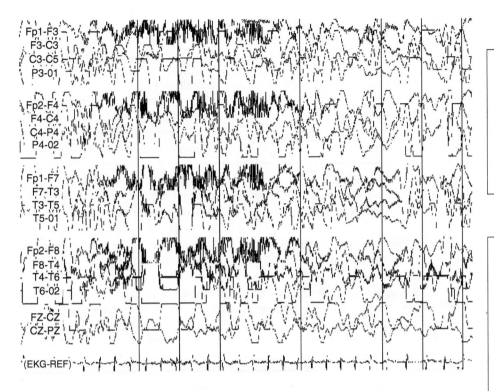

FIGURE 17-2. EEG demonstrating hypsarrhythmia pattern.

Often seen in tuberous sclerosis, for example.

SIGNS AND SYMPTOMS

- Vary depending on the seizure pattern. See above discussion of types of seizures.
- A seizure is defined electrographically as a hypersynchronous, hyperrhythmic, high-amplitude signal that evolves in both frequency and space.
- An aura is a stereotyped symptom set that immediately precedes the onset of a clinical seizure and does not affect consciousness.
- Physiologically, the aura is the true beginning of the seizure, and as such its character can be quite useful for localizing seizure onset.
- A seizure prodrome is a set of symptoms, much less stereotyped than an aura, that precedes a seizure by hours to days. Symptoms such as headache, mood changes, and nausea are reported by over 50% of patients in some series.

TREATMENT

- Therapy is directed at preventing the attacks.
- See Table 17-2 for current pharmacologic treatments for epilepsy.

Common Epilepsy Syndromes

See Table 17-3 for localizing/lateralizing seizure semiologies.

A febrile seizure lasting > 15 min suggests an organic cause such as meningitis or toxin exposure. Always get cerebrospinal fluid (CSF) if suspicion of infection.

If the seizure is brief with fever and immediate complete recovery consistent with febrile seizure, then only good examination and laboratory evaluation to find the cause of fever. CT/ EEG is not indicated.

Etiologies of neonatal seizure:
- Hypoxic-ischemic encephalopathy (35–42%)
- Intracranial hemorrhage/infarction (15–20%)
- CNS infection (12–17%)
- Metabolic and inborn errors of metabolism (8–25%)
- CNS malformation (5%)

Unprovoked seizure: Unrelated to current acute CNS insult such as infection, ↑ intracranial pressure (ICP), trauma, toxin, etc.

TABLE 17-2. Epilepsy Drugs and Their Use in Different Seizure Types

DRUG (U.S. BRAND NAME)	SEIZURE TYPE	SIDE EFFECTS
Carbamazepine (Tegretol, Carbatrol)	Focal-onset	Aplastic anemia
Ethosuxamide (Zarontin)	Absence, some generalized	Drowsiness
Phenytoin (Dilantin)	Generalized or focal	Stevens-Johnson, gingival hyperplasia
Phenobarbital	Focal, generalized	Hyperactivity
Valproate (Depakote, Depacon)	Generalized, focal-onset	Hepatic failure, low platelets, pancreatitis
Topiramate (Topamax)	Partial, generalized	Renal stones, weight loss
Levetiracetam (Keppra)	Partial, generalized, Lennox-Gastaut	Behavior change
Lamotrigine (Lamictal)	Focal, generalized	Stevens-Johnson syndrome
Zonisamide (Zonigran)	Focal, generalized	Don't use if sulfa allergic
Felbamate (Felbatol)	Focal, generalized	Hepatic failure, aplastic anemia

LOCALIZATION-RELATED EPILEPSY

- Seizures secondary to a focal CNS lesion, not necessarily visible on imaging, best candidates for epilepsy surgery.
- Common examples include masses (particularly cortical tubers of tuberous sclerosis [TS]), cortical dysplasia, postencephalitic gliosis, and arteriovenous malformations (AVMs).

BENIGN ROLANDIC EPILEPSY

A 5-year-old boy was noted to have facial twitching and facial drooling noted at a day care center during a nap followed by generalized shaking of the body lasting 1–2 min. The mother also reported noticing facial twitching during sleep. In the ED, he is awake and his neurological examination is normal. You order an EEG, which shows centrotemporal spikes. *Think: Benign rolandic epilepsy.*

Benign rolandic epilepsy is partial epilepsy of childhood. The usual age of presentation is 3–13 years. Typical presentation: seizure occurs during sleep (nighttime) with facial involvement. EEG shows central temporal spikes. Seizures typically resolve spontaneously by early adulthood.

- Most common partial epilepsy.
- Onset 3–13 years.
- Particularly nocturnal (early morning hours before awakening).
- EEG: Central temporal spikes (Figure 17-3).
- Excellent prognosis; most resolve by age 16 yr.
- **Treatment:** Carbamazepine, phenytoin, and valproic acid.

TABLE 17-3. Localizing/Lateralizing Seizure Semiologies

CLINICAL EVENT	LATERALIZATION	LOCALIZATION
Ipsilateral indicates phenomenon is directed toward the seizing hemisphere.		
Head turn		
Early nonforced	Ipsilateral	Temporal
Forced		
Early forced		Frontal (less likely to generalize)
Late forced	Contralateral	Temporal (more likely to generalize)
Ocular version	Contralateral	Occipital
Focal clonus	Contralateral	Frontal = temporal
Dystonic limb	Contralateral	Temporal > frontal
Unilateral tonic limb	Contralateral	
M2e fencing	Contralateral	Frontal > temporal
Figure 4	Contralateral	
Ictal paresis	Contralateral	
Todd's (postictal) paresis	Contralateral	
Unilateral blinking	Ipsilateral	
Unilateral automatism	Ipsilateral	
Postictal nose rubbing	Ipsilateral (to hand used)	Temporal > frontal
Postictal cough		Temporal
Bipedal automatism		Frontal > temporal
Hypermotoric state		Supplementary motor area
Ictal spitting	Right	Temporal
Automatism with preserved responsiveness	Right	Temporal
Gelastic		Hypothalamic, mesial temporal
Ictal vomiting/retching	Right	Temporal
Ictal urinary urgency	Nondominant	Temporal
Loud vocalization		Frontal > temporal
Ictal speech arrest		Temporal
Postictal aphasia	Dominant	

Epilepsy History

- Age, sex, handedness
- Seizure semiology (what the seizures look like, details about right/left). If more than one type, the pattern of progression (if any)
- Seizure duration/history of status epilepticus
- Postictal lethargy or focal neurologic deficits
- Current frequency/ tendency to cluster
- Age at onset
- Date of last seizure
- Longest seizure-free interval
- Known precipitants (don't forget to ask if the seizures typically arise out of sleep)
- History of head trauma, difficult birth, intrauterine infection, hypoxic/ischemic insults, meningoencephalitis, or other CNS disease
- Developmental history (delay strongly correlated with poorer prognosis)
- Family history of epilepsy, febrile seizures
- Psychiatric history
- Current AEDs
- AED history (maximum doses, efficacy, reason for stopping)
- Previous EEG, MRI findings

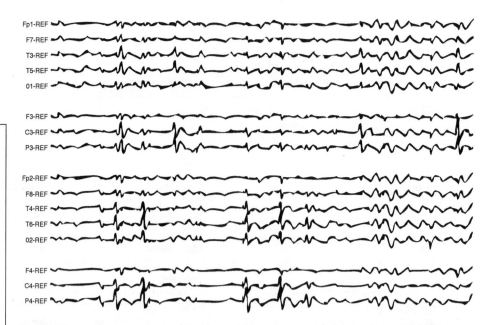

FIGURE 17-3. EEG demonstrating central temporal spikes characteristic of benign Rolandic epilepsy.

WEST SYNDROME

- Two percent of childhood epilepsies, but 25% of epilepsy with onset in the first year of life.
- Onset is at age 4–8 months.
- Triad: Infantile spasms, mental retardation (MR), and hypsarrhythmia.
- Boys are more commonly affected but not significantly; generally poor prognosis.
- Differential includes TS (largest group), CNS malformation, intrauterine infection, inborn metabolic disorders, and idiopathic. Idiopathic group fares the best.
- **Treatment** in the United States is restricted to ACTH.

JUVENILE MYOCLONIC EPILEPSY (JME)

- Onset: 12–16 yr.
- Characteristic history: Usually early morning on awakening, while hair combing and tooth brushing.
- Seizures: Myoclonus, absence, GTC.
- EEG: 4- to 6-Hz irregular spike-and-wave pattern (Figure 17-4 and Table 17-4).
- Treatment: Valproate, lamotrigine.
- Prognosis: Good Rx response but lifelong.
- High rate of recurrence if antiepileptic drug (AED) discontinued.

CHILDHOOD ABSENCE EPILEPSY (CAE; PYKNOLEPSY)

- See absence seizures above. GTC seizures often develop in adolescence; spontaneous resolution is the rule, however.
- Juvenile absence epilepsy (JAE): Similar to CAE except beginning in adolescence and have more GTC seizures, sexes affected equally, EEG spike and wave often faster than 3 Hz.

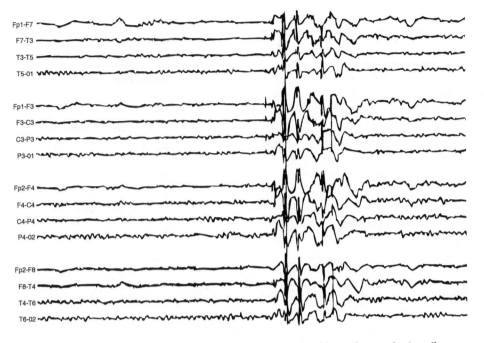

FIGURE 17-4. **EEG demonstrating characteristic pattern of juvenile myoclonic epilepsy.**

LENNOX-GASTAUT SYNDROME (LGS)

- A generalized epilepsy syndrome.
- Multiple seizure types (tonic, atonic, absence, and myoclonic seizures).
- EEG: 1.5- to 2.5-Hz spike-and-wave pattern.
- Cognitive impairment.
- Infantile spasms may evolve to LGS (30%).
- Seizures are frequent and resistant to treatment with AEDs.

LANDAU-KLEFFNER SYNDROME (LKS; ACQUIRED EPILEPTIC APHASIA)

- Language regression.
- Aphasia (primarily receptive or expressive).
- Seizures of several types (focal or GTC, atypical absence, partial complex).
- EEG: High-amplitude spike-and-wave discharges. Obtain EEG during sleep (more apparent during non–rapid eye movement sleep).
- **Differential diagnosis:** Autism.
- **Treatment:** Valproic acid.

Loss of language skills in a previously normal child with seizure disorder. *Think: LKS.*

PROGRESSIVE MYOCLONIC EPILEPSIES

- This group of diseases includes Unverricht-Lundborg disease, myoclonic epilepsy with ragged-red fibers (MERRF), Lafora disease, neuronal ceroid lipofuscinosis, and sialidosis/mucolipidosis, and Ramsay Hunt syndrome.
- Begin in late childhood to adolescence, and entail progressive neurologic deterioration with myoclonic seizures, dementia, and ataxia. Death within 10 yr of onset is common, but survival to old age occurs.

Evaluate patients following their first seizure (for mass, lesion, etc.) prior to diagnosing and treating epilepsy.

TABLE 17-4.   **Characteristic EEG Patterns in Various Seizure Conditions**

SEIZURE CONDITION	EEG	DRUG OF CHOICE
Simple febrile seizure Brief GTC with complete rapid recovery	Not required	Reassurance
Complex partial seizure > 15 min, focal, recurrent	Not required *Get MRI if focal prolonged*	Rectal valium (Diastat®) if recurrent
Infantile spasms (IS) See above	Hypsarrythmia	ACTH
West syndrome Hypsarrythmia, IS, mental retardation	Hypsarrythmia	ACTH
Benign myoclonus of epilepsy Clinically similar to IS but resolves in 3 months, rare after 2 yr	Normal	–
Benign myoclonic epilepsy 4 months–2 yr, brief myoclonic activity or neck and legs flexion with arms extension	3-Hz spike/polyspike and wave	Valproate Levetiracetam is safer in young
Benign rolandic epilepsy See above	Central-temporal spikes	–
Juvenile myoclonic epilepsy See above	4- to 6-Hz generalized polyspike/wave with photo-paroxysmal response	Valproate Lamotrigine
Childhood absence epilepsy See above	3-Hz spike and wave (first second may be 4 Hz, then ↓ to 2.5 by end)	Ethosuximide Carbamazepine contraindicated
Juvenile absence epilepsy See above	3- to 3.5-Hz spike and wave	Valproate
Lennox-Gastaut syndrome See above	1.5- to 2.5-Hz spike and wave	Valproate Clonazepam Vigabatrin
Landau-Kleffner syndrome See above	Generalized spike and wave, 1.5- to 3-Hz range	Benzodiazepines Valproate
Mesial temporal sclerosis See above	5–7 Hz, rhythmic, sharp theta activity	Phenytoin, phenobarbital, carbamazepine, and valproate

MESIAL TEMPORAL SCLEROSIS/TEMPORAL LOBE EPILEPSY

■ Gliotic scarring and atrophy of the hippocampal formation, creating a seizure focus. Abnormality is often apparent on high-resolution magnetic resonance imaging (MRI).

- Rhythmic, 5–7 Hz, sharp theta activity.
- Phenytoin, phenobarbital, carbamazepine, and valproate are equally effective. Curative resection is often possible if refractory to treatment.

DEFINITION

A neurodegenerative disorder of unknown cause.

EPIDEMIOLOGY

- X-linked recessive with *MECP2* gene mutation occurs almost exclusively in females. Rett syndrome does exist in males with 47,XXY and *MEP2* gene mutation. However, males with 46,XY and *MECP2* gene mutation do not survive.
- Prevalence: 1 in 15,000 to 1 in 22,000.

ETIOLOGY

- Most cases result from defect in *MECP2*. Gene testing available.
- *CDKL5* gene mutations can also cause Rett syndrome.

SIGNS AND SYMPTOMS

- Normal development until 12–18 months (can appear as early as 5 months)
- The first signs are deceleration of head growth, lack of interest in environment, and hypotonia, followed by a regression of language and motor milestones.
- Ataxia, hand-wringing, reduced brain weight, and episodes of hyperventilation are typical.
- Autistic behavior.

The hallmark of Rett syndrome is repetitive hand-wringing and loss of purposeful and spontaneous hand movements.

PROGNOSIS

- After the initial period of regression, the disease appears to plateau.
- Death occurs during adolescence or the third decade of life (cardiac arrhythmias).

Dermato-oculo-neural syndrome.

EPIDEMIOLOGY

Occurs sporadically in 1 in 50,000.

ETIOLOGY

- Abnormal development of the meningeal vasculature, resulting in hemispheric vascular steal phenomenon and resultant hemiatrophy.
- Facial capillary hemangioma usually accompanies in V1 distribution.

If you see "port-wine stain," *think:* Sturge-Weber syndrome.

SIGNS AND SYMPTOMS

- Cutaneous facial nevus flammeus (distribution of the trigeminal nerve) → port-wine stain.
- Ipsilateral diffuse cavernous hemangioma of the choroid → glaucoma.
- Ipsilateral meningeal hemangiomatosis (seizures and mental retardation).
- The lesions in the eye, skin, and brain are always present at birth.
- Contrast-enhanced MRI to look for meningeal angioma.
- Seizures are usually refractory, and hemispherectomy improves the prognosis.
- It is very unlikely to have meningeal involvement without port-wine stain, but most children with a facial port-wine nevus do not have an intracranial angioma.

STATUS EPILEPTICUS (SE)

DEFINITION

Any seizure or recurrent seizures without return to baseline lasting 20 min.

ETIOLOGY

- Febrile seizures, idiopathic status epilepticus, and symptomatic SE.
- Febrile SE accounts for 5% of febrile seizures and one-third of all episodes of SE.

PATHOPHYSIOLOGY

Prolonged neural firing may result in neuronal cell death, called excitotoxicity.

TREATMENT

- Initial treatment includes assessment of the respiratory and cardiovascular systems (ABCs).
- Obtain rapid bedside glucose level.

PROTOCOL

1. Airway, breathing, circulation (ABCs); give O_2.
2. Vitals, particularly blood pressure (BP).
3. Intravenous (IV) access.
4. Obtain rapid bedside glucose level.
5. Labs: Basic metabolic panel, ammonia (NH_3), aspartate transaminase (AST), alanine transaminase (ALT), AED levels, toxicology screen, blood cultures, complete blood count (CBC). Obtain blood cultures if febrile (consider lumbar puncture).
6. If seizing for > 5 min: Lorazepam 0.1 mg/kg IV (benzodiazepines #1).
7. If lorazepam fails, fosphenytoin 20 mg/kg IV (doses of fosphenytoin are in "phenytoin equivalents" by convention).
8. If fosphenytoin fails, give a second dose of 5 mg/kg IV.

In children under age 3, febrile seizures are the most likely etiology of status epilepticus.

Neonatal status that is refractory to the usual measures may respond to pyridoxine. This is seen in pyridoxine dependency (due to diminished glutamate decarboxylase activity, a rare autosomal-recessive condition) or pyridoxine deficiency in children born to mothers on isoniazid.

9. If second fosphenytoin fails, either:
   - Load with phenobarbital 20 mg/kg IV *or*
   - Load with midazolam 0.1 mg/kg IV and start drip at 2 µg/kg/min and titrate to effect.
10. Consider EEG and computed tomography (CT) head in case of new-onset SE in otherwise stable child.

Obstructive Sleep Apnea (OSA)

- Occurs in 2–5 % of children, most often between ages 2 and 6.
- Characterized by chronic partial airway obstruction with intermittent episodes of complete obstruction during sleep, resulting in disturbed sleep.
- Snoring is the most common symptom, occurring in most of them (12% of general pediatric population has snoring without OSA).
- **Symptoms:** Fatigue/hyperactivity, headache, daytime somnolence.
- **Signs:** Narrow airway, tonsillar hypertrophy, often obese.
- **Diagnosis:** History and physical examination, polysomnography (> 1 apnea/hypopnea per hour).

Obstructive sleep apnea due to adenotonsillar hyperplasia is an indication for tonsillectomy and adenoidectomy.

Night Terrors

DEFINITION

- Transient, sudden-onset episodes of terror in which the child cannot be consoled and is unaware of the surroundings, usually lasting for 5–15 min.
- There is total amnesia following the episodes.

Since obstructive sleep apnea causes hypoxia, it may be associated with polycythemia vera, growth failure, and serious cardiorespiratory pathophysiology.

EPIDEMIOLOGY

Occur in 1–3% of the population, primarily in boys between ages 5 and 7.

PATHOPHYSIOLOGY

- Fifty percent complete recovery by age 8.
- Fifty percent are also sleepwalkers.
- Often, incontinence and diaphoresis.
- Occurs in stage 4 (deep) sleep.

DIAGNOSIS

PSG (polysomnography).

TREATMENT

Reassurance; usually self-limited and resolve by age 6.

Night terrors, sleepwalking, and nightmares are associated with disturbed sleep, but have no known neurologic disorder.

Sleep deprivation causes attention deficit, hyperactivity, and behavior disturbances in children — often mistaken for attention deficit/hyperactivity disorder (ADHD).

Somnambulance (Sleepwalking)

- Occurs during slow-wave sleep.
- Occurs during first third of the night.
- Onset: 8–12 yr.
- Awakened only with difficulty and may be confused when awakened.
- Fifty percent also have night terrors.

Night Terrors
- NREM sleep
- No memory of the event; goes back to sleep
- 2 hours after falling sleep (between midnight and 2 AM)
- Disappears by age 6

- 50% also are sleepwalkers

Nightmares
- REM sleep
- Remembers dream and afraid to sleep
- Close to morning (last one-third of sleep time)
- Peak 3–6 yr; may continue in adolescence but less frequent
- No sleepwalking

Insomnia

- Affects 10–20% of adolescents.
- Depression is a common cause and should be ruled out.

COMA

- Consciousness refers to the state of awareness of self and environment.
- Pediatric evaluation of consciousness is dependent on both age and developmental level.

DEFINITION

Pathologic cause of loss of normal consciousness.

PATHOPHYSIOLOGY

- Consciousness is the result of communication between the cerebral cortex and the ascending reticular-activating system.
- Coma can be caused by:
  - One medial cerebral hemisphere with ispilateral, striatum, thalamus, and tegmentum of midbrain and rostral pons.
  - Bilateral medial hemispheres, striatum, thalami, tegmentum of rostral pontomesencephalic tegmentum impairs consciousness.
  - Lesions of the medullary reticular-activating system or its ascending projections. Ventral pontine lesions can → the locked-in syndrome, which is not coma.

ETIOLOGY

- Structural causes include trauma, vascular conditions, and mass lesions involving directly or mass effects.
- Metabolic and toxic causes include hypoxic-ischemic injury, toxins, infectious causes, and seizures.

Herniation syndromes that may result in coma:
- Ipsilateral oculomotor dysfunction. *Think: Uncal herniation.*
- Cheyne-Stokes respirations. *Think: Transtentorial (central) herniation.*

EVALUATION

- Administer glucose via IV line so that the brain has an adequate energy supply.
- Treat underlying cause (toxin antidote, reduce ICP, antibiotics, etc.).

PROGNOSIS

- Overall, children tend to do better than adults.
- Several measurement scales have been published attempting to predict outcome. The most widely accepted is the Glasgow Coma Scale (see Table 17-5).

TABLE 17-5. Glasgow Coma Scale (GCS)

EYE OPENING (TOTAL POINTS: 4)

Spontaneous	4
To Voice	3
To Pain	2
None	1

VERBAL RESPONSE (TOTAL POINTS: 5)

INFANTS AND YOUNG CHILDREN		OLDER CHILDREN	
Appropriate words; smiles, fixes, and follows	5	Oriented	5
Consolable crying	4	Confused	4
Persistently irritable	3	Inappropriate	3
Restless, agitated	2	Incomprehensible	2
None	1	None	1

MOTOR RESPONSE (TOTAL POINTS: 6)

Obeys	6
Localizes pain	5
Withdraws	4
Flexion	3
Extension	2
None	1

Note minimum score is 3, not 0.

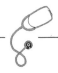
Prognosis depends on the etiology of the insult and the rapid initiation of treatment!

■ Another scale that you should know exists is the Pediatric Cerebral Performance Category Scale, which, unlike the Glasgow, was specifically designed for pediatric patients.

CNS INFECTION

Meningitis

DEFINITION

■ Diffuse inflammation of the meninges, particularly arachnoids and pia mater.
■ **Bacteria:**
  ■ < 3 months: Group B streptococci and gram-negative organisms, *Escherichia coli*, *Listeria*.
  ■ > 3 months: *Streptococcus pneumoniae*, *Haemophilus influenzae* type b, and *Neisseria meningitidis* (two life-threatening clinical syndromes: meningococcemia and meningococcal meningitis).
■ **Virus:** The term *aseptic meningitis* is used to describe the syndrome of meningism and CSF leukocytosis usually caused by viruses or bacteria.

SIGNS AND SYMPTOMS

If immunocompromised, these signs and symptoms will be not prominent.

■ Fever, headache, and nuchal rigidity (most important features).
■ Photophobia or myalgia may be present.
■ Meningism (Brudzinski and Kernig signs) (see Figures 17-5 and 17-6).
■ Altered consciousness, petechial rash, seizures, cranial nerve, or other abnormal neurological findings.

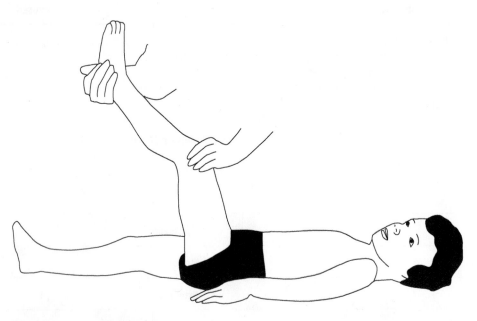

FIGURE 17-5. **Kernig sign.**

Flex patient's leg at both hip and knee, and then straighten knee. Pain on extension is a positive sign.

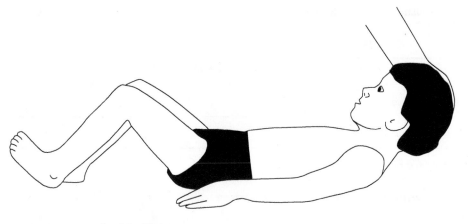

FIGURE 17-6. **Brudzinski sign.**

Involuntary flexion of the hips and knees with passive flexion of the neck while supine.

DIAGNOSIS

Analysis of the CSF is not always predictive of viral or bacterial infection since there is considerable overlap in the respective CSF findings, especially at the onset of the disease (Table 17-6).

Take some time to familiarize yourself with Tables 17-6 and 17-7: *You will be asked this!*

BACTERIAL MENINGITIS

- See Table 17-7 for common meningitis-causing bacteria.
- Associated with high rate of complications and chronic morbidity.

TABLE 17-6. **Cerebrospinal Fluid (CSF) Findings in Meningitis**

	NORMAL LEVELS	BACTERIAL	VIRAL	FUNGAL	TB
Appearance		Turbid	Clear	Clear	Fibrinous
Cells	Mononuclear	Polymorphs	Mononuclear	Mononuclear	Mononuclear
Leukocytes (mm³)	< 5	100–1000	50–1000	> 100	100–500
Protein (mg/dL)	20–45	100–500	50–200	25–500	1–5 g/dL
Glucose (mg/dL)	> 50 or 75% serum glucose	↓ < 40 or 66% serum	Generally normal	< 50; continues to decline if untreated	Less than half of the serum
Lab cultures		▪ Gram stain of CSF	▪ Hard to detect ▪ PCR of CSF may show HSV or enteroviruses	▪ Budding yeast may be seen ▪ Cryptococcal antigen may be positive in serum and CSF	Ziehl Neelsen AFB stain PCR

CSF, cerebrospinal fluid; PCR, polymerase chain reaction; HSV, herpes simplex virus.

TABLE 17-7. Common Causes of Pediatric Bacterial Meningitis

AGE	BACTERIA	TREATMENT
Neonates (< 1 month)	Group B streptococcus	Ampicillin and a third-generation cephalosporin
	Gram-negative enteric bacilli	
	Listeria monocytogenes	
	Escherichia coli	
Infants (1–24 months) and children <10 yr)	*Streptococcus pneumoniae*	Third-generation cephalosporin
	Neisseria meningitidis	Vancomycin should be added until susceptibility is known
	Haemophilus influenzae type B	
Children ages 10–19 yr	*Streptococcus pneumoniae*	Third-generation cephalosporin
	Neisseria meningitidis	Vancomycin should be added until susceptibility is known

Chronic meningitis:
Bacterial: TB, Lyme, syphilis
Viral: *Cryptococcus*, histoplasmosis, coccidioidomycosis, and *Nocardia*
Noninfectious: Cardiovascular disease

- Pathogenesis: 95% blood-borne. Organism enters the CSF, multiplies, and stimulates an inflammatory response. Direct toxin from organism, hypotension, or vasculitis → thrombotic event; vasogenic/cytotoxic edema causes ↑ ICP and ↓ blood flow, which all may contribute to further damage.

VIRAL MENINGITIS

- Enterovirus (85%): Echovirus, coxsackievirus, and nonparalytic poliovirus.
- Other classic causes are herpes simplex virus type 1 (HSV-1), Epstein-Barr virus (EBV), mumps, influenza, arboviruses, and adenoviruses.
- Clinical presentation is similar but symptoms are less severe than that of bacterial meningitis.
- Children are not toxic looking.
- Children show typical viral-type infectious signs (fever, malaise, myalgia, nausea, and rash) as well as meningeal signs.
- Typically is a self-limited process with complete recovery, and treatment is supportive.

FUNGAL MENINGITIS

Treat all acute cases of meningitis as if they are bacterial until cultures return.

- Although relatively uncommon, the classic organism is *Cryptococcus*.
- Encountered primarily in the immunocompromised patient (with transplants, AIDS, or on chemotherapy).
- May be rapidly fatal (as quickly as 2 weeks) or evolve over months to years.
- Tends to cause direct lymphatic obstruction, → hydrocephalus.

TREATMENT

- Third-generation cephalosporin (cefotaxime/ceftriaxone).
- Add ampicillin for *Listeria* in neonates. Neonates can be treated with ampicillin + gentamicin or ampicillin + cefotaxime.
- Add vancomycin, considering the increasing resistance of pneumococci to cephalosporins and carbapenems until the sensitivities are known.
- If viral etiology is suspected or CSF is not clearly differentiating between bacterial and viral etiologies, consider adding acyclovir until viral polymerase chain reaction (PCR) comes back negative.
- Steroid use is controversial.

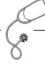

Nuchal rigidity. *Think:* Meningitis.

ENCEPHALITIS

DEFINITION

- A disease process in the brain primarily affecting the brain parenchyma.
- Because patients often have symptoms of both meningitis and encephalitis, the term *meningoencephalitis* is often applied.

Congenital syphilis may manifest around age 2 with Hutchinson's triad:
- Interstitial keratitis
- Peg-shaped incisors
- Deafness (cranial nerve [CN] VIII)

ETIOLOGY

Chronic Bacterial Meningoencephalitis

1. *Mycobacterium tuberculosis, M bovis,* and *M avium-intracellulare.*
   - Nonspecific features develop over days to weeks. Patients have generalized complaints of headache, malaise, and weight loss initially.
   - This is followed by confusion, focal neurological signs, cranial nerve palsies, and seizures or, in advanced cases, hemiparesis, hemiplegia, or coma.
   - Serious complications include arachnoid fibrosis, → hydrocephalus, and arterial occlusion, → infarcts.
   - *M avium-intracellulare* is common in AIDS patients.

Argyll Robertson pupil is discrepancy in pupil size seen in neurosyphilis.

2. Neurosyphilis (tabes dorsalis).
   - Causative organism is *Treponema pallidum.*
   - May present with aseptic meningitis only.
   - Tertiary syphilis (late-stage syphilis) manifests with neurologic, cardiovascular, and granulomatous lesions.
   - Congenital syphilis presents with a maculopapular rash, lymphadenopathy, and mucopurulent rhinitis.
   - Routine prenatal screening for syphilis is now mandatory in most states to prevent congenital syphilis.

Pupil reacts poorly to light but accommodation is normal.

Viral Meningoencephalitis

1. **Herpes simplex virus:**
   - HSV-1: Most cases after the neonatal period.
   - HSV-2: Usually blood-borne and results in diffuse meningoencephalitis and other organ involvement. It is the congenitally acquired form, transmitted to 50% of babies born to a mother with active vaginal lesions.

2. **Herpes zoster virus:**
   - Can occur after primary infection or as a result of reactivation later in life.
   - Usually with a rash, but outcome is poor in those without a rash.
   - In immunocompetnt hosts, after 2–6 months of primary infection, the dormant virus in the ganglia becomes activated in and causes large-vessel vasculitis → infarcts.

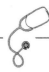

The transmission rate of syphilis from infected mother to infant is nearly 100%. Treat infant with IV penicillin G.

Acyclovir is the treatment of choice for herpetic meningitis.

- In immunocompromised hosts, the dormant virus causes small-vessel vasculitis and results in hemorrhagic infarcts of gray and white matter.
- EEG will show diffuse slowing and periodic lateralizing epileptiform discharges (PLEDs).

3. **Rabies:**
   - Causes severe encephalitis, coma, and death due to respiratory failure.
   - Transmitted via bite from an infected animal, usually associated with dogs, bats, skunks, raccoons, or squirrels.
   - The virus travels up the peripheral nerves from the bite site and enters the brain.
   - Nonspecific symptoms (fever, malaise) and paresthesia around the bite site are pathognomonic. This is followed by more specific neurologic symptoms of hydrophobia, aerophobia, agitation, **hypersalivation,** and seizures. This proceeds to coma and death.
   - Hydrophobia is a classic, late finding but is not consistently present.

TRANSVERSE MYELITIS

DEFINITION

- An acute focal infectious or immune-mediated illness causing swelling and demyelination of the spinal cord. This most commonly affects the thoracic spinal cord (80%) followed by cervical cord.
- It is a neurological emergency and requires prompt diagnosis and treatment to prevent permanent damage.

SIGNS AND SYMPTOMS

- Fever, lethargy, malaise, muscle pains.
- Begins acutely and progresses within 1–2 days.
- Back pain at the level of the involved cord and paresthesias of the legs are common.
- Anterior horn involvement may cause lower motor neuron dysfunction.
- Bladder and bowel dysfunction is present.

DIAGNOSIS

- MRI: Enhanced T2 signals.
- CSF: Pleocytosis.
- Electromyogram (EMG): Anterior horn cell dysfunction in involved segments.

TREATMENT

IV steroids, intravenous immune globulin (IVIG), may require surgical intervention.

PROGNOSIS

Most make good recovery; however, it is slow.

Numerous viruses as well as the rabies vaccination and smallpox vaccination have been linked to transverse myelitis.

A 1-week-old child born to an immunocompromised mother presents with difficulty feeding, trismus, and other rigid muscles. *Think: tetanus.*

Tetanus is a toxin-mediated disease characterized by severe skeletal muscle spasms. It is a serious infection in neonatal life. Initial symptoms can be nonspecific. Inability to suck and difficulty in swallowing are important clinical features followed by stiffness and seizures. Neonatal tetanus can be prevented by immunizing mothers before or during pregnancy and providing sterile care throughout the delivery.

DEFINITION

- An acute illness with painful muscle spasms and hypertonia caused by the neurotoxin produced by *Clostridium tetani*.
- These symptoms usually starts in the jaw and facial muscles and progressively involve other muscle groups.

SIGNS AND SYMPTOMS

- Trismus (masseter muscle spasm) is the characteristic sign and is present in 75% of cases.
- **Risus sardonicus,** a grin caused by facial spasm, is also classic.
- Dysphagia due to pharyngeal spasm develops over a few days; laryngospasm may result in asphyxia.
- The muscles are involved in a descending order and once the paralysis involves the trunk and thigh, the patient may exhibit an arched posture in which only the head and heels touch the ground.
- Late stages manifest with recurrent seizures consisting of sudden severe tonic contractions of the muscles with fist clenching, flexion, and adduction of the upper limb and extension of the lower limb.
- The development of seizures is associated with poor prognosis.
- Autonomic dysfunction may be seen as ↑ sweating, heart rate, blood pressure, and temperature.
- Can also present with localized spasms at the site of infection or with abdominal pain mimicking acute abdomen.
- Incubation period varies from 2 to 14 days (average 7 days).

DIAGNOSIS

- Diagnosis is clinical, with the presence of trismus, dysphagia, ↑ rigidity, and muscle spasms.
- Laboratory studies are usually normal, but a moderate leukocytosis may be present.
- CSF is normal.
- Gram stain is positive in only one-third of cases.

TREATMENT

- Admit to ICU for prophylactic intubation.
- Rapid administration of human tetanus immune globulin.
- IV penicillin G, metronidazole, or doxycycline.

- Surgical excision and debridement of the wound.
- Muscle relaxants such as diazepam, phenobarbital should be used to promote relaxation and seizure control. Neuromuscular blocking agents like vecuronium are also used.

Tetanic contractions can be triggered by minor stimuli, such as a flashing light. Patients should be sedated, intubated, and put in a dark room in severe cases.

PROGNOSIS

- Mortality rate: 5–35%.
- Neonatal tetanus mortality ranges from 10% to 75%, depending on quality of care received.

Tetanus is an entirely preventable disease via immunization.

ENCEPHALOPATHIES

DEFINITION

A syndrome of generalized dysfunction of the brain.

TYPES

Two main groups:

1. Progressive encephalopathies with onset before age 2 years.
   - If other systems are involved in addition to nervous system then it is lysosomal, peroxisomal, or mitochondrial disorders.
   - If peripheral nervous system and muscles involved in addition to central nervous system is likely lysosomal or mitochondrial.
   - Gray matter or white matter disease.
2. Encephalopathies that begin during childhood after age 2 years.
   - Lysosomal disorders: Gaucher type 3, late onset Krabbe disease, juvenile Tay-Sachs disease, Niemann-Pick disease type C.
   - Infectious disease: AIDS, congenital syphilis, subacute sclerosing panencephalitis.
   - Grey matter disorders: Ceroid lipofuscinosis, Huntington disease, mitochondrial disorders (late-onset poliodystrophy, myoclonic epilepsy, and ragged-red fibers), xeroderma pigmentosa.

Mitochondrial Encephalopathy

A group of disorders that can be caused by mutations in either nuclear or mitochondrial DNA, resulting in a variety of symptoms:

1. **Mitochondrial encephalopathy, lactic acidosis, and strokelike episodes (MELAS):**
   - The most common of mitochondrial encephalopathies.
   - Onset between ages 2 and 10 yr; initial development normal, but short stature is present.
   - The most initial feature is GTC seizure (often associated with hemiparesis and cortical blindness), recurrent headache, and vomiting.
   - The neurologic abnormalities are transient initially, but later become progressive and → coma and death.
   - MRI shows multiple strokes not in vascular distribution pattern. ↑ lactic acid in blood and CSF. Muscle biopsy is diagnostic (ragged-red fibers).
2. **Myoclonic epilepsy with ragged-red fibers (MERRF):**
   - Onset may be in childhood or adult life.
   - Four cardinal features are myoclonus, myoclonic epilepsy, ataxia, and ragged-red fibers on muscle biopsy.

- The initial feature is progressive insidious decline in school performance. GTC seizures or myoclonus is usually the first symptom to seek medical attention. Later, they develop progressive epilepsy, cerebellar ataxia, and dysarthria. Clinical myopathy may not be present.
  - Diagnosis is by gene testing and muscle biopsy.

3. **Reye syndrome:**
- A disorder of mitochondrial dysfunction associated with viral infection and aspirin ingestion.
- Sporadic syndrome can occur with varicella-zoster or influenza B infection.
- Recurrent Reye-like syndrome is seen in children with inborn errors of metabolism, medium-chain acyl Co-A dehydrogenase (MCAD) deficiency, urea cycle disorders, pyruvate metabolism disorders.
- **Diagnosis:** Liver biopsy is diagnostic. ↓ blood glucose, ↑ ammonia and liver enzymes without jaundice.

MELAS and MERRF are caused by point mutations in transfer RNA (tRNA) in mitochondrial DNA.
MELAS = leucine
MERRF = lycine
MERRF is often confused with Friedreich ataxia.

Hepatic Encephalopathy

- Acute hepatic failure caused by viral hepatitis, drugs, toxins, or Reye syndrome results in altered consciousness (due to cerebral edema and accumulation of toxins, ammonia).
- In children, most commonly related to fulminant viral hepatitis (50–75%).
- Early symptoms are malaise, lethargy, jaundice, dark urine, and abnormal liver function tests (LFTs). The encephalopathy can be acute or chronic.
- Other features include, sleep disturbance, change in affect, drowsiness, asterixis (flapping tremor). Decerebrate posturing may occur in the terminal stages.
- Hepatic encephalopathy is reversible with treatment, and most therapies are aimed at controlling the cerebral, renal, and cardiovascular functions until the liver regenerates or liver transplantation can be done. These are achieved by lowering:
  - Ammonia level (↓ dietary protein, stop gastrointestinal [GI] bleed, treat constipation).
  - Cerebral edema with fluid restriction and the use of hyperosmolar agents (mannitol).
- Patients who recover typically have no long-term sequelae.

In general, salicylates should be avoided in children to prevent Reye syndrome.

HIV/AIDS Encephalopathy

- There is a 40–90% incidence of CNS involvement in perinatally infected children.
- Ninety percent of infected infants are symptomatic by 18 months of age.
- Develops 2–5 months after infection.
- Commonly presents with progressive encephalopathy and hepatosplenomegaly, → failure to meet developmental milestones, impaired brain growth, and symmetrical motor dysfunction.
- Imaging techniques reveal cerebral atrophy in 85% of children and ventricular enlargement.
- Basal ganglia calcifications may be present.
- Opportunistic infections such as toxoplasmosis typically occur later in adolescence.

Old lead paint is the number one cause of lead toxicity.

- PCR analysis of HIV DNA or RNA is used to detect HIV infection in infants < 18 months.
- **Diagnosis:** Via immunoglobulin G (IgG) antibody to HIV for patients > 18 months and a confirmatory test HIV DNA PCR.
- **Treatment:** Highly active antiretroviral therapy (HAART).
- All pregnant mothers are tested for HIV infection and are treated to ↓ the transmission.

PANDAS (pediatric autoimmune neuropsychiatric disorder) has been suggested for the syndrome of behavioral problems, obsessive-compulsive behavior, and tics with an antecedent group A β-hemolytic streptococcal infection.

Lead Encephalopathy

- There is no direct correlation to the level of lead and clinical manifestations. Lead interferes with porphyrin metabolism in red blood cells (RBCs).
- **Acute:** Vomiting, abdominal pain, seizures, impaired consciousness, and respiratory arrest are common.
- **Chronic:** Gradual confusion, behavior changes, sleep problems, seizures, ataxia. Peripheral neuropathy, while common in adults, is rarely seen in children unless they also have sickle cell anemia.
- Pica is common in these children (eg, eating paint chips).
- Diagnosis is made primarily through history and also via blood lead testing. Microcytic hypochromic anemia, basophilic stippling, and azotemia also present.
- Treatment: Removing the source of lead, and chelation therapy.

Sydenham's Chorea

Posited to fall in a disease spectrum including Syndenham chorea, in which there is an autoimmune attack of the basal ganglia triggered by a group A strep infection.

- Rapid, brief, unsustained, nonstereotypical movements of the body.
- Autoimmune mediated.
- Twice as common in females.
- Onset: Age 3–17 yr.
- Postinfectious chorea appearing 4–8 weeks after a group A streptococcal pharyngitis.
- Resolves after 8–9 months; 50% have persistent chorea.
- **Diagnosis:** Recent throat infection (anti-streptolysin O, DNase B), ↑ T2 signals in basal ganglia.
- **Treatment:**
  - Valproate: First choice.
  - Dopamine-blocking agents: Second choice.
  - Also treat primary infection.

Adrenoleukodystrophy

- A progressive disease, characterized by demyelination of the CNS and peripheral nerves and adrenal insufficiency.
- X-linked recessive, peroxisomal disorder, defect in the ability to catabolize long-chain fatty acids (LCFAs).
- It presents between 4 and 10 yr with behavioral and cognitive decline with visual loss, followed by motor symptoms.
- **Diagnosis:** White matter abnormality on MRI, ↑ serum very-long-chain fatty acids (VLCFA), labs for adrenal insufficiency.
- **Treatment:** Bone marrow transplantation if only radiological changes are present and no appearance of the neurological symptoms.

Methylphenidate may unmask Tourette syndrome but does not cause it.

Tourette Syndrome

- A lifelong condition affecting 1 in 2000 that presents before age 15.
- Diagnostic criteria: Multiple motor and vocal tics for > 1 year with tic-free period not more than 3 consecutive months.
- Often associated with other conditions like obsessive-compulsive disorder (OCD), attention deficit/hyperactivity disorder (ADHD).
- Symptoms are enhanced by stress and anxiety.
- Treatment with medications should be avoided.
- Treat when tics interfere with child's developmental learning or cause undue social stress. Also treat comorbid conditions.

CEREBRAL PALSY (CP)

DEFINITION

- A **nonprogressive** disorder of movement and posture resulting from damage to the developing brain prior to or surrounding birth. If progressive, consider another diagnosis.
- Most cases occur in the absence of identifiable causes.

ETIOLOGY

- Prematurity with intraventricular hemorrhage.
- Birth or other asphyxia.
- Intrauterine growth retardation (IUGR), placental insufficiency.
- Infection: Prenatal/postnatal.
- Twin pregnancy.
- Chromosomal and genetic disorders.
- Head trauma.

CP is a static disorder, meaning that it does not result in the loss of previously acquired milestones.

SIGNS AND SYMPTOMS

- Prenatal and perinatal history.
- Delayed motor, language, or social skills.
- Not losing skills previously acquired.
- Feeding difficulties.
- Late-onset dystonia (age 7–10).

EXAMINATION

- Hypertonia.
- Hyperreflexia.
- Posture and movement: May be spastic, ataxic, choreoathetoid, and dystonic.
- Abnormal primitive reflexes.
- Abnormal gait.
- Impaired growth of affected extremity.

When there are no risk factors, family history of neurologic disease, presents late infancy or early childhood, ataxic CP, or atypical features, then consider other diagnosis.

ASSOCIATED PROBLEMS

- Seizure disorder
- Mental retardation
- Developmental disorders

CLASSIFICATION

- Hemiplegic cerebral palsy: Upper limb involvement > lower limb; many walk before 2 years.
- Diplegic cerebral palsy.
- Quadriplegic cerebral palsy: Majority does not walk.
- Dystonic/athetoid cerebral palsy.
- Ataxic cerebral palsy.
- Monoplegic cerebral palsy: Usually lower limb and appears late.

TREATMENT

- Multidisciplinary approach with goals of maximizing function and minimizing impairment.
- Team includes general pediatrician, physiotherapist, occupational therapist, language therapist, neurologist, and social and educational support services.
- Orthopedic interventions are sometimes helpful.

MENTAL RETARDATION (MR)

DEFINITION

- Below average intellectual functioning in association with deficits in adaptive behavior prior to 18 years of age.
- Intelligence quotient (IQ) or developmental quotient (DQ) < 70 or < 2 standard deviations (SDs).

EPIDEMIOLOGY

- Affects 1–3% of the population.
- Approximately 75% are mild cases.
- Males are affected more than females.

SIGNS AND SYMPTOMS

- Significant delay in reaching developmental milestones.
- Delayed speech and language skills in toddlers with less severe MR.
- The child will continue to learn new skills depending on severity of MR.

DIAGNOSIS

Classification is based on IQ:

- Mild: IQ 55–70, 85% of cases.
- Moderate: IQ 40–55, 10% of cases.
- Severe: IQ 25–40, 3–5% of cases.
- Profound: IQ < 25, 1–2% of cases.

LEARNING DISABILITY (LD)

- Significant discrepancy between a person's intellectual ability and academic achievement.
- Often learn best in unconventional ways.

Extensor plantar response (presence of Babinski sign) can be present up to 1 year of age, but should be present symmetrically.

DQ is often used as a rough estimator of IQ in infants and younger children. It is simply the mental age (estimated from historical milestones and exam) divided by the chronologic age, × 100.

The IQ is scaled such that the mean is 100 and the standard deviation (SD) is 15. So MR is simply defined as an IQ two SDs below the mean.

Earlier classification:
- Moron: IQ 51–75
- Imbecile: IQ 26–50
- Idiot: IQ ≤ 25
This is no longer considered politically correct.

- Often restricted to a particular realm such as reading or mathematics with correspondingly discrepant scores on standardized measures of intelligence or academic achievement.
- Significant improvement with appropriate interventions.

ATAXIAS

Inability to coordinate muscle activities to regulate posture and also strength and direction of extremity movements (see Table 17-8).

> **Titubations** are a disturbance of body equilibrium in standing or walking, resulting in an uncertain gait and trembling, especially resulting from diseases of the cerebellum.

Types

ACUTE CEREBELLAR ATAXIA

- A diagnosis of exclusion occurring in children 2–7 years old.
- Often follows viral infection by 2–3 weeks; thought to be autoimmune response and has been seen with live inactivated vaccines like varicella vaccine.
- Sudden onset of severe truncal ataxia; often, the child cannot stand or sit.
- Severity is maximum at the onset with clear sensorium.
- Horizontal nystagmus in 50%.
- **Diagnosis:** Diagnosis of exclusion; exclude other serious causes first.
- **Treatment:** Self-limited disease.
- **Prognosis:** Complete recovery typically occurs within 2 months (1–5 months).

TABLE 17-8. Ataxias

TYPE	COMMON FEATURES	EXAMPLES
Sensory	Gait: Wide based and high stepping Falls in dark or eyes closed (Romberg +) Difficulty of fine finger movements	Posterior column involvements like B_{12} deficiency
Cerebellar	Gait: Wide based and crunchy so cannot perform Romberg test. Intention tremors, nystagmus, dysmetria, titubations, hypotonia	Spinocerebellar ataxia Pontocerebellar hypoplasia Vermian agenesis or dysgenesis Cerebellar degeneration in trisomies, etc.
Mixed	Both sensory and cerebellar components	Friedreich ataxia Vincristine side affect

FREIDREICH'S ATAXIA

- Autosomal-recessive mutation (usually a triplet expansion) in Frataxin gene on chromosome 9.
- Degeneration of the dorsal columns and rootlets, spinocerebellar tracts, and, to a lesser extent, the pyramidal tracts and cerebellar hemispheres.
- Onset before age 10 (2–16 yr).
- Slow progression of ataxia involving the lower limbs > upper limbs associated with dysarthria, ↓ tendon reflexes, positive Babinki sign, high-arch foot with loss of dorsal column sensations.
- Romberg test is positive.
- Associated abnormalities include skeletal abnormalities (scoliosis), cardiomyopathy, and optic atrophy.
- Elevated α-fetoprotein (AFP).
- Clinical features establish the diagnosis, which is confirmed with genetic testing. There is no curative treatment available but symptomatic treatment to improve quality of life.

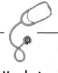

Myoclonic epilepsy with ragged-red fibers (MERRF) is often confused with Friedreich ataxia.

ATAXIA-TELANGIECTASIA

- Autosomal-recessive disorder of nervous and immune system due to gene mutation at chromosome 11.
- The most common degenerative ataxia.
- A slowly progressive ataxia beginning during first year of life resulting in inability to walk by adolescence.
- Oculomotor apraxia is a present in 90% of the patients.
- Telangiectasia becomes evident after 2 yr or in the teenage years and is most prominent on the bulbar conjunctiva (first), bridge of nose, and exposed surfaces of the extremities. Sun exposure exacerbates the telangiectasia.
- Sinopulmonary infection is another important feature. ↓ or absent IgA, IgE, and especially IgG$_2$ subclass. IgM may be ↑.
- ↑ AFP and peripheral acanthocytes.
- Have a 50- to 100-fold greater chance of brain tumors and lymphoid tumors, so avoid radiation exposure by limiting imaging studies.

PERIPHERAL NEUROPATHIES

- Injuries to the peripheral nerves may be either:
  - Demyelinating (injury to Schwann cells).
  - Degenerating (injury to the nerve or axon).
- Peripheral neuropathy is the most common cause of progressive distal weakness.
- Most common are hereditary causes and slow progression.
- The most common acquired cause is Guillain-Barré syndrome (GBS) with rapid progression.

Types

Guillain-Barré Syndrome

> A 6-year-old boy with no significant past medical history presents to the ED with difficulty walking for past few days and is now unable to walk. He also has some weakness in his upper extremities but he does not have any respiratory distress. There is no clear history of any recent illness, vaccination, or sick contacts. He had upper respiratory infection symptoms a few weeks ago. On examination, he is weaker more in the lower extremities than upper, and deep tendon reflexes are absent at knee and ankle. *Think: Guillain-Barré syndrome (GBS).*
>
> GBS is an ascending paralysis. History of prior upper respiratory tract or viral infection or recent vaccination may be present. Initial symptoms are pain, numbness, paresthesia, or weakness in the lower extremities, which rapidly progresses to bilateral and relatively symmetric weakness. ↓ or absent deep-tendon reflexes are often present. Lumbar puncture typically shows ↑ protein with normal CSF and white cell count (cyto-albuminologic dissociation).

- A postinfection demyelinating neuropathy affecting predominantly the motor neurons.
- It is due to immune cross-reactivity to a secondary illness within 4 weeks. Most commonly seen after upper respiratory infection (URI), *Campylobacter jejuni, Mycoplasma pneumoniae,* cytomegalovirus (CMV), Epstein-Barr virus (EBV), varicella, influenza, hepatitis A and B infection.
- Weakness begins in the legs and progresses symmetrically upward to the trunk, arms, then bulbar and ocular muscles.
- Tendon reflexes are absent.
- Respiratory muscles in 50%, autonomic dysfunction, pain, paresthesias can be present.
- ↑ proteins in CSF with no ↑ in lymphocytes.
- Nerve conduction will be slow with conduction blocks, and enhancement of nerve roots can be seen on MRI.
- Treatment includes close monitoring for respiratory weakness and IVIG or plasmapheresis in more severe cases.

Botulism

- Botulinum toxin is disseminated through the blood and, due to the rich vascular network in the bulbar region, symmetric flaccid paralysis of the cranial nerves is the typical manifestation.
- Infant botulism: The first sign is usually absence of defecation. The head control is lost and the weakness descends.
- Most dreaded complication is respiratory paralysis, and approximately 50% of patients are intubated.
- Prognosis is good in noncomplicated cases.
- Antibiotics and blocking antibodies have not been shown to affect the course of the disease.
- Electromyogram (EMG) with high frequency (20–50 Hz) reverses the presynaptic blockade and produces an incremental response.

It is not possible to have botulism without having multiple cranial nerve palsies.

Infantile botulism is associated with ingestion of honey (honey contains botulism spores).

MYASTHENIA GRAVIS

- ↓ in postsynaptic acetylcholine receptors due to autoimmune degradation, resulting in rapid fatigability of muscles.
- Ptosis and extraocular eye weakness are the earliest and most diagnostic symptoms.
- Onset usually after age 8, as early as 6 months. Prepubertal male bias, postpubertal female bias.
- Diagnosis is made by EMG with repetitive stimulation, edrophonium (Tensilon) test, a quick test (acetylcholinesterase inhibitor). Acetylcholine receptor-binding or -blocking antibodies are detected in the seropositive forms and are an indication for thymectomy. May be associated with autoimmune thyroid disease and seizures.
- Cholinesterase drugs are the mainstay of treatment, with oral steroids used as needed for immune suppression (initially may exacerbate the disease).
- Prognosis varies, with some children undergoing spontaneous remission, while in others the disease persists into adulthood.

Children with myasthenic syndromes cannot tolerate neuromuscular blocking drugs, such as succinylcholine, and various other drugs. Most offenders are in the antibiotic, cardiovascular, and psychotropic categories.

TRANSITORY NEONATAL MYASTHENIA

- Passive transfer of antibodies from myasthenic mothers (10–15% incidence).
- Self-limited disease consisting of generalized weakness and hypotonia for 1 week to 2 months. Symptoms develop a few hours after birth. If develop after 3 days, then are unlikely.
- Poor suck and respiratory problems are addressed with supportive care. Neostigmine or exchange transfusion can be used in more severe cases.

FAMILIAL INFANTILE MYASTHENIA

- Rare disorder.
- Collection of autosomal-recessive seronegative disorders of the neuromuscular junction. Most defects are postsynaptic, but presynaptic forms are described.
- Onset can be neonatal. Diagnosis by EMG with repetitive stimulation, response to edrophonium, specialized testing for identification of the specific defect.
- Long-term treatment with neostigmine or pyridostigmine useful in some forms (acetylcholinesterase inhibitors). Thymectomy and immunosuppression are of no benefit.

Remember, rapid correction of hyponatremia can result in cerebellar pontine myelinosis.

ELECTROLYTE IMBALANCES

See Table 17-9 for common electrolyte imbalances affecting the nervous system.

HEADACHES

Migraine

The most common type of headache in the pediatric population with female predominance.

TABLE 17-9. Electrolyte Disturbances and the Nervous System

DISTURBANCE	MANIFESTATION	COMMON CAUSES
Hyponatremia	▪ Rapid onset: Brain swelling, lethargy, coma, and seizures ▪ Slow onset: Usually asymptomatic	▪ Typically impaired renal water excretion in the presence of normal water intake
Hypernatremia	▪ Intracranial bleeding is common in children (dehydrated brain shrinks and can tear bridging veins)	▪ Most common cause is dehydration or inadequate intake of water ▪ Rare
Hypokalemia	▪ Neuromuscular: Weakness, paralysis, rhabdomyolysis ▪ Gastrointestinal: Constipation, ileus ▪ Nephrogenic diabetes insipidus ▪ ECG changes: Prominent U waves, T-wave flattening ▪ Arrhythmias	▪ Uptake into cells ▪ Renal loss ▪ Severe diarrhea, laxative abuse ▪ Magnesium depletion is an important and often overlooked cause

Hyperkalemia	▪ Severe cases are a medical emergency!
	▪ Neuromuscular: Weakness, ascending paralysis, respiratory failure
	▪ Progressive ECG changes with increasing potassium:
	  ▪ Peaked T waves
	  ▪ Flattened P waves
	  ▪ Long PR interval
	  ▪ Idioventricular rhythm
	  ▪ Wide QRS and deep S waves
	  ▪ Sine-wave pattern and ventricular fibrillation
		▪ Shift out of cells
		▪ Aldosterone deficiency/unresponsiveness
		▪ Renal failure

DEFINITION

A recurrent headache with symptom-free intervals and associated with the following:

- Abdominal pain.
- Nausea and/or vomiting.
- Throbbing headache.
- Often bilateral (vs. unilateral in adults).
- Associated aura.
- Relieved by sleep.
- Family history of migraines.

CLASSIFICATION

Migraines may be classified into the following subgroups:

- The diagnosis of migraine in children is based on clinical symptoms, and usually we do not follow the International Headache Society criteria in young children.
- Diagnosis of migraine is clinical and no neuroimaging is necessary unless it is persistently occipital or with abnormal neurologic examination.

COMMON MIGRAINE

- The most prevalent type of migraine in children.
- Intense nausea and vomiting are classic.

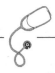

- Aura is absent.
- Family history is present in 80%, most often on the maternal side.

CLASSIC MIGRAINE

- An aura precedes the headache by 5–20 min and nearly always disappears before the headache begins.
- The auras most often manifest as paresthesias and visual disturbances such as flashing lights, black dots, zig-zag lines.

COMPLICATED MIGRAINE

Transient neurologic signs develop during a headache and persist after the resolution of the headache for a few hours to days.

TREATMENT

- Avoid the possible triggers: Often, migraines occur in response to specific triggers, such as psychological stress, strenuous exercise, sleep deprivation, cheese, chocolate, processed meat, or moving vehicles, and minimizing these factors may have great therapeutic effect.
- Consider nonpharmacologic treatment with biofeedback techniques in chronic stress headache.
- For acute attacks:
  - Dark, quiet environment and sleep.
  - Adequate fluid intake.
  - Pharmacologic therapy: Acetaminophen and nonsteroidal anti-inflammatory drugs (NSAIDs) are first line.
  - Second-line drugs include triptans, caffeine, and ergot alkaloids (status migrinosus).
  - Antiemetics are helpful at the start of headache.
  - Treatment should be instituted as early as possible in an attack.

PROPHYLAXIS

- Antiepileptic drugs, such as topiramate, valproate, levetiracetam.
- Tricyclic antidepresssants such as amitriptyline.
- β blockers such as propranolol.

Cluster Headache

- Brief, severe, unilateral stabbing headaches that occur multiple times daily over a period of several weeks and tend to be seasonal.
- Onset after 10 yr of age.
- Male predominance.
- Conjunctival injection, tearing, rhinorrhea.
- Prophylaxis with lithium or calcium channel blocker.
- Acute treatment with 100% oxygen or sumatriptan and dihydroergotamine (DHE).

Tension Headache

Tension or stress headaches are rare in children prior to puberty and are often difficult to differentiate from migraines.

- Most often occur with a stressful situation, such as an exam.
- Described as "hurting" but not "throbbing."
- It presents like a band around the head. It is present most of the times of the day.
- Unlike migraines and ↑ intracranial pressure, tension headaches are not associated with nausea and vomiting,
- However, it is sometimes difficult to differentiate them from migraine.

DIAGNOSIS

- Diagnosis of exclusion.
- EEG or CT is not necessary.
- A poor self-image, fear of failure, and low self-esteem are common factors.

TREATMENT

Steps should be taken to minimize anxiety and stress:

- Mild analgesics often are ample.
- Other options include counseling and biofeedback.
- Sedatives or antidepressants are rarely necessary.

Increased Intracranial Pressure (ICP)

Headache due to tension of the blood vessels or dura may be the first symptom of an ↑ in intracranial pressure.

SYMPTOMS

- It usually presents as headache, nausea, vomiting, diplopia, personality changes.
- It can present as bulging fontanelle, impaired upward gaze in infants.
- The presentation depends also on rate at which the ICP increases. If it increases slowly, then the intracranial structures have time to accommodate for the change.
- Coughing or Valsalva maneuver tends to make the pain worse by increasing ICP further.

ETIOLOGY

Common causes include posterior fossa brain tumors (and other brain tumors), obstructive hydrocephalus, hemorrhage, meningitis, venous sinus thrombosis, pseudotumor cerebri, abscesses, and chronic lead poisoning.

DIAGNOSIS

- Thorough history and physical exam are vital.
- Papilledema (if ↑ pressure is present for some time) and nuchal rigidity are helpful signs.
- Obtain CBC, erythrocyte sedimentation rate (ESR), and CT/MRI to narrow the differential.
- If CT/MRI is negative, consider lumbar puncture (LP).

Headaches can occur in children secondary to refractive errors. It is therefore imperative to perform a visual acuity determination.

Normal ICP
Newborns: 6 mmHg
Children: 6–13 mmHg
Adolescents/adults: 0–15 mmHg

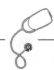

Any time you see papilledema, think ↑ ICP.

A classic textbook finding due to compression of the brain stem is **Cushing triad:**
1. ↓ respiratory rate
2. ↓ heart rate
3. ↑ BP (actually seen in 20–30%)

MRI is the best test for a posterior fossa tumor.

Never perform an LP if papilledema is present.

Must obtain CT before LP if suspicion of ↑ ICP.

Subarachnoid hemorrhage can present as subacute or repeated headaches.

CT reveals hemorrhage in two-thirds of patients. LP reveals ↓ RBCs in tube 4 and xanthochromia.

Relatively more children have aneurysms in the vertebrobasilar circulation (23%) compared to adults (12%).

TREATMENT

- Varies with particular diagnosis, and should be directed at the underlying etiology.
- Techniques to lower ICP acutely are as follows:
  1. Intubation and subsequent hyperventilation results in cerebral vasoconstriction, effective for about 30 min.
  2. Elevating the head 30 degrees facilitates venous return.
  3. Hyperosmolar agents such as mannitol (osmotic diuretic), avoid hypovolemia.
  4. Extraventricular drain provides temporary relief and can provide continuous monitoring of ICP.
  5. Surgical decompression if persistently remains ↑.

ANEURYSMS

- The pathogenesis of the aneurysms is multifactorial and controversial; however, it is believed that focal congenital weakness of the internal elastic lamina and muscular layers in the cerebral arteries → to aneurysmal formation.
- Most common in internal carotid artery followed by middle cerebral artery, anterior communicating artery, and basilar artery.
- Saccular aneurysms are the most common type and often at bifurcation of the internal carotid artery.
- Early warning signs are headaches or localized cranial nerve compression.
- Most common presentation is subarachnoid hemorrhage (SAH).
- More likely to rupture in patients < 2 years of age or > 10 years.
- More common in males 2:1.
- Familial occurrence is common.

ETIOLOGY

- Most often are related to a congenital diseases:
  - Ehlers-Danlos syndrome.
  - Marfan syndrome, tuberous sclerosis.
  - AVMs.
  - Coarctation of the aorta.
  - Polycystic kidney disease (likely develop secondary to hypertension in this condition); called **berry aneuryms.**
- Acquired aneurysms are most often related to bacterial endocarditis:
  - Embolization of bacteria results in mycotic aneurysms in the cerebral vasculature.
  - Twenty-five percent present with bleeding, such as a subarachnoid or intraparenchymal hemorrhage.

DIAGNOSIS

- Angiography is the gold standard for aneurysms in both children and adults.
- Magnetic resonance angiography (MRA) may also be used and is becoming more reliable.

TREATMENT

- Surgical clipping or endovascular coiling is the treatment of choice.
- Risk for rebleeding.

- True AVMs consist of an abnormal communication of arteries and veins without intervening capillaries that arises during development in prenatal period or just after birth.
- It grows in size with time and varies in size from several millimeters to several centimeters.
- The larger ones create a significant atrioventricular (AV) shunt (steal phenomenon) and considerable damage if they rupture.
- Supratentorial (90%).

PRESENTATION

- Small unruptured malformations present with headache or seizures.
- Larger malformations may present with progressive neurologic deficit.
- Hemorrhage is most often presentation (subarachnoid or intraparenchymal).

DIAGNOSIS

- Angiography is the test of choice and is required to direct the future therapy. MRA is also available.
- MRI or CT with contrast can demonstrate an AVM but provide less information than angiography.
- Photon knife is the treatment.

Common AVM Variants

VEIN OF GALEN MALFORMATIONS

- Normal vein of Galen does not develop from its primitive vein, which persists and communicates with superior saggital sinus.
- Typically present during infancy with high-output congestive heart failure (CHF), failure to thrive, or enlarging head size.
- Mortality is 50%.
- Treatment is difficult embolization is preferred over surgery.
- A cranial bruit is often present with vein of Galen malformations.

CAVERNOUS HEMANGIOMAS

- Low-flow AVM with tendency to leak (cause seizure) but usually do not result in massive intracerebral hemorrhage.
- Retinal cavernous hemangiomas may be also present.
- Surgical resection is indicated if symptomatic.

VENOUS ANGIOMAS

- Rarely symptomatic (seizures are the most common presenting sign).
- Surgery is not indicated unless complications arise.

TREATMENT

- Treatment consists of surgical resection or embolization.
- Focused gamma knife radiation has some benefit in smaller lesions.

Gamma knife radiation typically takes up to 2 yr to see resolution of the AVM, during which time the patient is at risk for hemorrhage; thus, surgery is the treatment of choice.

- Transient ischemic attacks (TIAs): Neurologic deficits that resolves in < 24 hr.
- Stroke: Neurological deficits persists beyond 24 hr.

EPIDEMIOLOGY

- 2.6–13 cases per 100,000 per yr.
- Hemorrhagic stroke 1.5–5 per 100,000 children per yr.
- Ischemic stroke 1.2 and 8 per 100,000 children per yr.

SIGNS AND SYMPTOMS

- Sudden onset of neurologic deficit or seizures in neonates.
- Headache, neck pain, and visual symptoms.

ETIOLOGY

- Pediatric causes of stroke differ from those in the adult population.
- Types of stroke include:
  - Ischemic: Thrombosis (both arterial and venous) or embolic (arterial).
  - Hemorrhage.
- A variety of conditions or risk factors exist for stroke, including:
  - AVMs.
  - Antiphospholipid antibodies/lupus anticoagulant.
  - Congenital coagulopathies such as factor V Leiden and deficiencies of protein C, S, and antithrombin III.
  - Hemoglobinopathies, sickle cell disease (SCD).
  - Sickle cell anemia at risk for ischemic stroke (sickling RBCs may → thrombosis or endothelial injury).
  - Cardiac conditions: Arrhythmias, myxoma, paradoxical emboli through a patent foramen ovale, and septic emboli from bacterial endocarditis.
  - Blunt trauma to the head and neck → arterial dissection.
  - Vasculitis, such as Kawasaki, hemolytic-uremic syndrome, systemic lupus erythematosus (SLE), meningitis.
  - Mitochondrial diseases.
  - Extracorporeal membrane oxygenation (ECMO) is a risk for both intracranial hemorrhage and embolic ischemic stroke.

Cardiac abnormalities are the most common cause of thromboembolic stroke in children.

Clinically Relevant Types of Stroke

ARTERIAL THROMBOSIS/EMBOLISM

History and physical exam are critical to search for the etiology.

- Intracerebral arterial dissection after trivial trauma to head and neck due to a tear in the intima.
- The cerebral area supplied by the vessel distal to lesion undergoes infarction and produces symptoms (loss of functions)
- Cerebral symptoms such as a progressive hemiplegia, lethargy, or aphasia result from the shedding of small emboli into the carotid circulation.
- Seizures are the most common presenting symptom in neonates.
- Cardiac source usually.

VENOUS THROMBOSIS

- May be subdivided into septic and nonseptic causes.
- Septic causes include bacterial meningitis, otitis media, and mastoiditis.
- Aseptic causes are numerous and include severe dehydration, hypercoagulable states, congenital heart disease, and hemoglobinopathies (SCD).
- Neonates present with diffuse neurologic signs and seizures.
- In children, focal neurologic signs are more common.

CLOSED HEAD TRAUMA

See Table 17-10 for a comparison of subdural and epidural hematomas.

Subdural Hematoma (SDH)

EPIDEMIOLOGY

- The most frequent focal brain injury in sports and the most common form of sports-related intracranial hemorrhage. Seen most often in infants, with a peak at 6 months.

ETIOLOGY

- Occurs when a bridging vein is torn between the dura and the brain.
- In neonates due to a tear in tentorium near its junction with the falx.
- Trauma is usually the cause. Skull fracture is not seen commonly.
- An SDH should be ruled out if changes in conscious level are present after head injury.
- Typically frontoparietal location. It can be acute, subacute, or chronic.

SIGNS AND SYMPTOMS

- These depend on age of the child and also severity of the SDH.
- Neonates: Seizures, a bulging fontanelle, and ↓ activity.
- Retinal and preretinal hemorrhages common in children, especially in abused children.
- ↑ ICP (irritability, lethargy, vomiting, papilledema, headache).

DIAGNOSIS

Gold standard is CT scan.

Epidural Hematoma

EPIDEMIOLOGY

Seen most often in children > 2 years of age.

ETIOLOGY

- Most commonly results from a fracture in the temporal bone, lacerating the middle meningeal artery.
- Can be acute (arterial bleed) or chronic (venous bleed).
- Skull fracture is seen commonly.
- Nearly always unilateral; however, bilateral case has been described.

A typical workup for a stroke syndrome will include head CT or MRI scan, followed by an angiogram (if the CT/MRI is nondiagnostic), and a cardiac echo to exclude cardiac causes.

Low-molecular-weight heparin has been shown to be safe, effective, and well tolerated in children.

The extent of brain damage directly attributable to impact is the most important prognostic factor.

Subdural hematomas appear crescent shaped (concave) on CT and will not cross the midline, but will cross ipsilateral suture lines.

SIGNS AND SYMPTOMS

- Classic progression involves an initial loss of consciousness, followed by a lucid interval, and then abrupt deterioration and death (not as helpful in younger children).
- Hemorrhage and acute brain swelling cause ↑ ICP that can result in herniation with ispilateral ptosis, dilated pupil, and ispilateral hemiparesis due to contralateral compression of crus cerebri.
- Retinal and preretinal hemorrhages are not common.
- ↑ ICP is seen (irritability, lethargy, vomiting, papilledema, headache).

Lucid interval. *Think: Epidural hematoma.*

DIAGNOSIS

Gold standard is CT scan.

TREATMENT

Epidural hematomas may progress rapidly, and immediate neurosurgical treatment is indicated.

Epidural hematomas appear lens shaped (convex) on CT and will not cross the midline or other cranial sutures.

Coup/Contrecoup Injuries

Cerebral contusion injury mainly occurs when the head is subjected to a sudden acceleration or deceleration.

COUP INJURIES

- Located directly at the point of impact.
- More common in acceleration injuries such as being hit with a baseball bat.
- Multiple microhemorrhages as blood leaks into the brain tissue.

Old contusions develop an orange color secondary to hemosiderin deposition and are referred to as *plaques jaunes* by pathologists.

TABLE 17-10. Features of Acute Epidural and Subdural Hematomas

Clinically it is not easy to differentiate the two, so head imaging helps differentiate between the two.	

SUBDURAL HEMATOMA	EPIDURAL HEMATOMA
Follows inner layer of dura	Follows outer layer of dura (periosteum)
"Rounds the bend" to follow to follow falx or tentorium	Crosses falx or tentorium
Not affected by sutures of skull	Limited by sutures of skull (typically)
Tendency for crescentic shapes	Tendency for lentiform shapes
More mass effect than expected for their size	
Typical source of SDH: cortical vein	Typical source of EDH: skull fracture with arterial or sinus laceration

CONTRECOUP INJURIES

- Located opposite (180 degrees) from the point of impact.
- More common in deceleration injuries, such as striking one's head on the pavement after a fall.

Contrecoup injuries tend to be more severe than coup injuries.

Diffuse Axonal Injury

EPIDEMIOLOGY

- Tissues with differing elastic properties shear against each other, tearing axons.
- Caused by rapid deceleration/rotation of head.
- Locations:
    - Cerebral hemispheres near gray-white junction.
    - Basal ganglia.
    - Corpus callosum, especially splenium.
    - Dorsal brain stem.
- High morbitity and mortality—common cause of posttraumatic vegetative state.
- Initial CT often normal despite poor GCS.
- Lesions often nonhemorrhagic and seen only on MRI.
- Survivors often have substantial long-term cognitive and behavioral morbidity.

Diffuse axonal injury is best visualized on a T2-weighted MRI.

HYDROCEPHALUS

Head circumference > 2 SD above the mean is macrocephaly, and if due to ↑ CSF in the CSF spaces, it is called hydrocephalus.

PHYSIOLOGY

- CSF is made by the choroid plexus in the walls of the lateral, third, and fourth ventricles.
- CSF flows in the following direction: lateral ventricles → foramen of Monro → third ventricle → cerebral aqueduct → fourth ventricle → foramina of Magendie and Luschka → subarachnoid space of spinal cord and brain → arachnoid villi.
- CSF is absorbed primarily by the arachnoid villi through tight junctions.

Choroid plexus papilloma is the only rare cause of hydrocephalus from ↑ CSF production.

ETIOLOGY

- **Obstructive (noncommunicating) hydrocephalus:**
    - Most commonly due to stenosis or narrowing of the aqueduct of Sylvius.
    - An obstruction in the fourth ventricle is a common cause in children, including posterior fossa brain tumors, Arnold-Chiari malformations (type II), and Dandy-Walker syndrome.
    - Also seen in brain abscess, hematoma, infectious, vein of Galen malformation.
- **Nonobstructive (communicating) hydrocephalus:**
    - Most commonly follows a subarachnoid hemorrhage or meningitis.
    - Blood in the subarachnoid spaces may obliterate the cisterns or arachnoid villi and obstruct CSF flow.

- Venous sinus thrombosis, meningeal malignancy, and intrauterine infections are other causes.
- **Ex vacuo:** Hydrocephalus resulting from ↓ brain parenchyma.

CLINICAL MANIFESTATIONS

- Infants:
  - Accelerated rate of enlargement of the head is most prominent sign.
  - Bulging anterior fontanelle (fontanelles can provide some pressure relief in infants, delaying symptoms of ↑ ICP). Widening of cranial sutures, sun-setting sign, and Parinaud syndrome.
  - Upper motor neuron signs such as brisk reflexes are common findings due to stretching of the descending cortical spinal tract.
  - ↑ ICP signs (lethargy, vomiting, headache, etc.) may be present, especially acutely ↑ ICP.
  - Ocular bobbing.
- Children and adolescents:
  - Signs are more subtle because the cranial sutures are partially closed.
  - ↑ ICP signs may be present. Visual fields particularly peripheral fields are involved gradually. Papilledema can be present.
  - A gradual change in school performance may be the first clue to a slowly obstructing lesion.

DIAGNOSIS

- A detailed history and physical exam is key to discovering the underlying etiology.
- Ultrasound and head CT/MRI are the most important studies to identify the cause of hydrocephalus.
- Familial cases of aqueductal stenosis have been reported and have an X-linked pattern of inheritance.
- Neurofibromatosis and meningitis have also been linked to aqueductal stenosis.

TREATMENT

- Medical management with acetazolamide (may ↓ CSF production) and furosemide may provide temporary relief.
- Placement of an extraventricular drain (EVD) or ventriculoperitoneal shunt (VPS), if the etiology is permanent, may be required.

NEOPLASMS

Pediatric Brain Tumors

EPIDEMIOLOGY

- Most common solid tumors of the childhood.
- Third most common pediatric tumors (#1 leukemia, #2 lymphoma).
- Supratentorial tumors are as common as infratentorial tumors.
- Glial cell tumors are the most common tumors in childhood and consist of astrocytomas, ependymomas, olidodendrioglioma, and primitive neuroectodermal tumor (PNET).
- Medulloblastoma is a common PNET only in childhood.

CLINICAL MANIFESTATIONS

- Generally present with either signs and symptoms of ↑ ICP (infants) or with focal neurologic signs (adolescents).
- Alterations in personality are often the first symptoms of a brain tumor.
- Nystagmus is the classic finding in posterior fossa tumors.
- Clinical signs depending on location of the tumor (loss/alteration in the functions of the brain area).
- Tumors in the posterior fossa tend to result in hydrocephalus secondary to CSF flow obstruction.

CEREBELLAR ASTROCYTOMA

- The most common posterior fossa tumor of childhood.
- It is a slow-growing poilocytic astrocytoma and more benign than the adult-onset astrocytomas.
- Histologically shows fibrillary astrocytes with dense cytoplasmic inclusions called Rosenthal fibers.
- Associated with neurofibromatosis type 2 (NF2).
- Good prognosis; 5-year survival > 90% after gross total resection which is achieved in 70% of the cases.
- Treatment is surgical resection.

> Rosenthal fibers are also seen in Alexander disease, a progressive leukodystrophy with mental retardation, spasticity, and megalencephaly.

MEDULLOBLASTOMA (PNET)

- The second most common posterior fossa tumor and the most prevalent brain tumor in children under the age of 7 yr. More common in males.
- Rapidly growing malignant tumor, arises from the undifferentiated neural cells in the region of cerebellar vermis.
- Tends to invade the fourth ventricle and spread along CSF pathways and involves the spine, so consider imaging the spine.
- Histologic analysis shows deeply staining nuclei with scant cytoplasm arranged in pseudorosettes.
- Presents with intracranial hypertension and ataxia, symptoms evolving in few weeks; papilledema is absent.
- MRI: Brightly enhancing mass with cystic lesion.
- **Treatment:** Surgical resection followed by irradiation.
- **Prognosis:** Dependent on size and dissemination of the tumor, 5-year survival rate is > 80%.

CRANIOPHARYNGIOMA

- One of the most common supratentorial brain tumors of childhood which arises from cells in the Rathke's pouch.
- It is locally aggressive and recurs.
- Short stature or other endocrine-associated problems are common initial signs.
- Typically slow growing and benign.
- The tumor may be confined to the sella turcica or extend through the diaphragma sellae and compress the optic nerve or, rarely, obstruct CSF flow.
- Due to location, surgical resection is often subtotal.

DIAGNOSIS

- Ninety percent of craniopharyngiomas show calcification on CT scan; MRI provides better images of surrounding structures.
- Baseline endocrine studies and visual fields should be done prior to surgery.

NEUROBLASTOMA (NB)

EPIDEMIOLOGY

- A common tumor of neural crest origin, representing the most common neoplasm in infants and 8% of all childhood malignancies.
- Malignant tumor that arises from the neural crest cells.
- Ninety percent are diagnosed before age 5, with a peak at 2 yr.

PATHOGENESIS

- NB is a small, round blue cell tumor with varying degrees of neuronal differentiation.

CLINICAL PRESENTATION

- The tumor may arise at any site of sympathetic nervous tissue.
- The adrenals, retroperitoneal sympathetic ganglia, and abdomen are the most common sites.
- Thirty percent arise in the cervical or thoracic region and may present with Horner syndrome.
- Opsoclonus-myoclonus: "Dancing eyes, dancing feet"—the telltale symptom of this disease (secondary to paraneoplastic antibodies).

DIAGNOSIS

- Typically, a mass is seen on CT or MRI.
- Ninety-five percent of cases have elevated tumor markers, most often homovanillic acid (HVA) and vanillylmandelic acid (VMA) in the urine.
- Metaiodobenzylguanidine (MIBG) radioisotope scan for detecting small primaries and metastases.
- Stage 4: Infantile form, self-limited with good prognosis.
- Unfavorable prognosis is associated with ↑ neuron-specific enolase and amplification of N-Myc gene.
- Treatment is surgical resection followed by radio + chemotherapy.

von Hippel–Lindau Disease

DEFINITION

A neurocutaneous syndrome (usually no cutaneous involment) affecting many organs, including the cerebellum, spinal cord, medulla, retina, kidneys, pancreas, and epididymis.

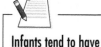

Infants tend to have localized NB in the cervical or thoracic region, whereas older children tend to have disseminated abdominal disease.

The major neurologic manifestations are:

- **Cerebellar/spinal hemagioblastomas:** Present in early adult life with signs of ↑ ICP.
- **Retinal angiomata:** Small masses of thin-walled capillaries in the peripheral retina.
- Multiple congenital cysts of the pancreas and polycythemia are also associated with it.
- Early detection and resection is the best management.
- Photocoagulation for retinal detachment.

Renal carcinoma is the most common cause of death associated with von Hippel–Lindau disease.

Neurofibromatosis (NF)

EPIDEMIOLOGY

Both types display autosomal recessive inheritance patterns.

- **Type 1:** The most prevalent type (~90%) with an incidence of 1 in 4000 (chromosome 17).
- **Type 2:** Accounts for 10% of all cases of NF, with an incidence of 1 in 40,000 (chromosome 22).

CLINICAL MANIFESTATIONS

Type 1
- Diagnosis is made by the presence of two or more of the following:
  - Six or more café-au-lait macules (must be > 5 mm prepuberty, > 15 mm postpuberty).
  - Axillary or inguinal freckling (Crowe sign).
  - Two or more iris Lisch nodules (melanocytic hamartomas).
  - Two or more cutaneous neurofibromas.
  - A characteristic osseous lesion (sphenoid dysplasia, thinning of long-bone cortex).
  - Optic glioma.
  - A first-degree relative with confirmed NF-1.
- Learning disabilities, abnormal speech development, and seizures are common.
- Patients are at a higher risk for other tumors of the CNS such as meningiomas and astrocytomas (optic nerve gliomas in 20%) (but not as significantly as in NF-2).
- Risk of malignant transformation to neurofibrosarcoma is < 5%.

Type 2
- Diagnosis is made when one of the following is present:
  - Bilateral CN VIII masses (most of the cases).
  - A parent or sibling with the disease and either a neurofibroma, meningioma, glioma, or schwannoma.
- Café-au-lait spots and skin neurofibromas are not common findings.
- Patients are at significantly higher risk for CNS tumors than in NF-1 and typically have multiple tumors.

About 50% of NF-1 results from new mutations. Parents should be carefully screened before counseling on the risk to future children.

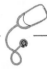

NF-1: Café-au-lait spots, childhood onset.
NF-2: Bilateral acoustic neuromas, teenage onset, multiple CNS tumors.

Café-au-lait is French for "coffee with milk," which is the color of these lesions.

Prenatal diagnosis and genetic confirmation of diagnosis is available in familial cases of both NF-1 and NF-2, but not new mutations.

In general, the younger that a child presents with signs and symptoms, the greater the likelihood of mental retardation.

Tuberous sclerosis is the most common cause of infantile spasms, an ominous seizure pattern in infants.

Hamartoma: A tumor-like overgrowth of tissue normally found in the area surrounding it.

TREATMENT

- Treatment is mainly aimed at preventing future complications and early detection of malignancies. Resection of the schwanomas can be done to preserve hearing.

Tuberous Sclerosis

EPIDEMIOLOGY

- Inherited as an autosomal-dominant trait, with a frequency of 1:6,000.
- Two-third are new mutations.

PATHOLOGY

- Characteristic brain lesions consist of tubers, which are located in the convolutions of the cerebrum, where they undergo calcification and project into the ventricles.
- There are two recognized genes: TSC1 on chromosome 9, encoding a protein called hamartin; and TSC2 on chromosome 16, encoding a protein called tuberin.
- Tubers may obstruct the foramen of Monro, → hydrocephalus.

CLINICAL MANIFESTATIONS

- Hypopigmented macules (Ash leaf skin lesions) are seen in 90% and are best viewed under a Wood's lamp (violet/ultraviolet light source).
- CT scan shows calcified hamartomas (tubers) in the periventricular region.
- Seizures and infantile spasms (IS) are common. Seizures usually present as IS before age 1 and are difficult to control. Children develop autistic features and have developmental disabilities and learning difficulties.
- Adenoma sebaceum—small, raised papules resembling acne that develop on the face between 4 and 6 years of age, actually are small hamartomas.
- A Shagreen patch (rough, raised lesion with an orange-peel consistency in the lumbar region) is also a classic finding; typically does not develop until adolescence.
- Fifty percent of children also have rhabdomyomas of the heart, which may → CHF or arrhythmias. They can be found on prenatal ultrasonography but usually regress after birth.
- Hamartomas of the kidneys and the lungs are also frequently present.

DIAGNOSIS

- A high index of suspicion is needed, but all children presenting with infantile spasms should be carefully assessed for skin and retinal lesions.
- CT or MRI will confirm the diagnosis.
- Genetic testing is available for mutations in TSC1 and TSC2.

Agenesis of the Corpus Callosum

- Associated with numerous syndromes and several inborn errors of metabolism, including patients with lissencephaly, Dandy-Walker syndrome, Arnold-Chiari type 2 malformations, and Aicardi syndrome.
- Imaging techniques reveal that the lateral ventricles are shifted laterally.
- Normal intelligence is not unusual, and often only mild clinical signs are seen.
- The severity of the disease varies greatly, from only mild deficits to marked retardation and severe epilepsy.

Syringomyelia

 A teenage girl has a headache and a cape-like distribution of pain and temperature sensory loss that developed after a minor motor vehicle accident. *Think: Cervical syringomyelia with undiagnosed Chiari I.*

The Chiari type I malformation is characterized by herniation of the cerebellar tonsils through the foramen magnum and may → the development of syringomyelia. Common presentations include headache, neck pain, vertigo, sensory changes, and ataxia. Typical scenario is occipital pain precipitated by cough or Valsalva maneuver. MRI is the modality of choice.

- A slowly progressive paracentral cavity formation within the brain or spinal cord, most often in the cervical or lumbar regions.
- Thought to arise from incomplete closure of the neural tube during the fourth week of gestation.
- MRI is the test of choice for diagnosis.
- Often develops post-traumatically in the setting of an undiagnosed Chiari I malformation or tethered cord.
- Symptoms include bilateral impaired pain and temperature sensation due to decussation of these fibers near the central canal. Also weakness of the hand muscles and progressive symptoms as the cavity enlarges. It contains a yellow fluid.
- Called *syringobulbia* when present in brain stem.

Dandy-Walker Malformation

- Results from a developmental failure of the roof of the fourth ventricle to form, resulting in a cystic expansion into the posterior fossa.
- Ninety percent of patients have hydrocephalus.
- Agenesis of the cerebellar vermis and corpus callosum is also common.
- Infants present with a rapid ↑ in head size.
- Management is via shunting of the cystic cavity to prevent hydrocephalus.

Arnold-Chiari Malformations

- Four variations exist (see Figure 17-7), with type 2 being the most common, in which the cerebellum and medulla are shifted caudally, resulting in crowding of the upper spinal column.
- Type 2 is also associated with meningomyelocele in > 95% of cases.
- Syringomyelia is associated in 70% of type 1, and 20–50% overall.
- Management includes close observation with serial MRIs and surgery as required.

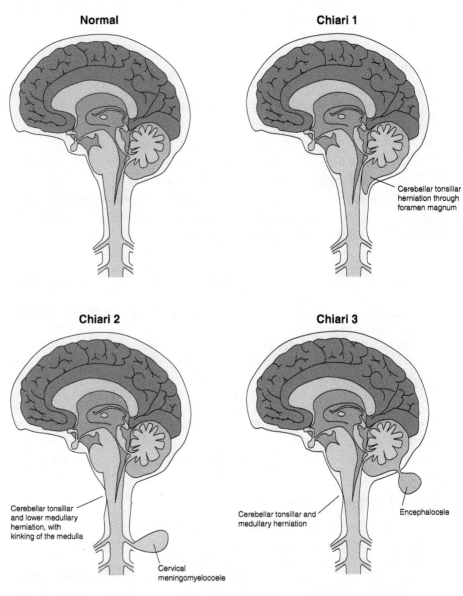

Normal

Chiari 1

Cerebellar tonsillar herniation through foramen magnum

Chiari 2

Cerebellar tonsillar and lower medullary herniation, with kinking of the medulla

Cervical meningomyelocoele

Chiari 3

Cerebellar tonsillar and medullary herniation

Encephalocele

FIGURE 17-7.   The Chiari malformations.

Schematic representations of the Chiari malformations. Commonly associated hydrocephalus and syringomyelia not depicted.

Special Organs—Eye, Ear, Nose

Amblyopia has been called "lazy eye."

Strabismus is the most common cause of amblyopia.

Amblyopia is usually asymptomatic and can be detected only by screening examination.

Younger children are more susceptible to the development of amblyopia.

For the best results, amblyopia should be treated by age 4.

Amblyopia can be reversed more rapidly in younger children.

A deviated eye is described as being turned "eso" (inward), "exo" (outward), "hypo" (downward), or "hyper" (upward).

Amblyopia

DEFINITION

A ↓ in visual acuity in one or both eyes caused by blurred retinal images, which → failure of the visual cortex to develop properly.

ETIOLOGY

- Strabismus.
- Refractive errors.
- Opacity in the visual path (eg, cataract, ptosis, eyelid hemangioma).

DIAGNOSIS

Diagnosis is made by visual acuity testing.

TREATMENT

- Removal of the pathology such as a cataract.
- Prescription glasses to correct refractive errors.
- Patching the good eye until the ambylopic eye has improved its vision.

Strabismus   *check for retinoblestoma*

DEFINITION

- Deviation or misalignment of the eye (see Figure 18-1).
- "To squint or to look obliquely."
- Strabismus can lead to vision loss (amblyopia).

DIAGNOSIS   *poor eye muscle control*

- **Corneal light reflex:** The child looks directly into a light source and the doctor observes where the reflex lies in both eyes; if the light is off center in one pupil or asymmetric, then strabismus exists.
- **Alternative cover test:** The child stares at an object in the distance and the doctor covers one of the child's eyes; if there is movement of the uncovered eye once the other eye is covered, then strabismus exists.

TREATMENT

- Prescription glasses may help if the strabismus is secondary to refraction.
- Eye muscle surgery may be necessary.

eso - in
exo - out

Optic Neuritis

DEFINITION

- Inflammation of the optic nerve.
- Retrobulbar optic neuritis: Without ophthalmoscopically visible signs of disc inflammation.
- Papillitis or intraocular optic neuritis: Ophthalmoscopically visible evidence of inflammation of the **nerve head.**
- Neuroretinitis: Inflammation of both the **retina and papilla.**

SPECIAL ORGANS—EYE, EAR, NOSE

HIGH-YIELD FACTS

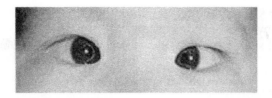

FIGURE 18-1. Child with strabismus.

ETIOLOGY

- Idiopathic.
- Recent immunization or viral infection (measles, chickenpox, influenza).
- Extension from an infection involving the teeth, sinuses, or meninges.
- Side effect of treatment with vincristine or chloramphenicol.
- Secondary to a toxin such as lead.

SIGNS AND SYMPTOMS

- Loss of vision.
- Pain with extraocular motion.
- Pain to palpation of the globe.
- Afferent papillary defect.
- Bilateral in children (unilateral in adults).

COMPLICATIONS

- Color deficits.
- Motion perception deficits.
- Brightness sense deficits.

TREATMENT

A trial of intravenous (IV) steroids may ↓ the length of time for symptoms but has no effect on the outcome.

In children, optic neuritis is rarely associated with multiple sclerosis.

Conjunctivitis

DEFINITION

Inflammation of the conjunctiva.

TYPES

Allergic
- Immunoglobulin E (IgE)-mediated reaction caused by triggers such as pollen or dust.
- **Signs and symptoms:** Include watery, itchy, red eyes with edema to the conjunctiva and lids.
- Pruritus and chemosis are common.
- **Treatment:** Includes removal of the trigger, cold compresses, and antihistamines.

Viral
- Adenovirus and coxsackievirus are typical causes.
- Adenovirus: Pharyngoconjunctival fever—triad: pharyngitis, fever, and conjunctivitis.

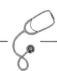
Adenovirus is the most common viral cause of conjunctivitis.

- Epidemic keratoconjunctivitis: Fulminant vision threatening condition with the involvement of cornea.
- **Signs and symptoms:** Include watery, red eyes with preauricular lymph nodes.
- **Treatment:** Includes supportive treatment with constant hand washing to prevent transmission.

Bacterial

- Three organisms: Nontypeable *Haemophilus influenzae*, *Streptococcus pneumoniae*, and *Staphylococcus aureus*.
- Highly contagious, outbreaks can occur.
- **Signs and symptoms:** Include a mucopurulent discharge, red eyes, and edema of the conjunctiva.
- **Treatment:** Topical antibiotics (drops or ointment).

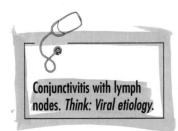

Conjunctivitis with lymph nodes. Think: Viral etiology.

[handwritten: Hflu Strep pNa staph a.]

[handwritten: Bactrim + polymixin]

Episcleritis/Scleritis

DEFINITION

Inflammation of the episclera or sclera.

ETIOLOGY

High association with autoimmune diseases.

[handwritten: unilateral/confined to one area of eye.]

SIGNS AND SYMPTOMS

- Eye pain.
- Photophobia.
- Erythema.
- ↓ visual acuity.
- Perforation is associated only with scleritis.

Episcleritis/scleritis is usually unilateral.

TREATMENT

- Topical steroids.
- Nonsteroidal anti-inflammatory drugs (NSAIDs).
- Immunosuppressive drugs in case of failure of steroids.
- Surgery for thinning or perforated sclera

Blepharitis

DEFINITION

Inflammation of the eyelid margins.

ETIOLOGY

- *Staphylococcus aureus.*
- *Staphylococcus epidermidis.*
- Seborrheic.
- A combination of the above.

SIGNS AND SYMPTOMS

- Burning.
- Itching.
- Erythema.
- Scaling.
- Ulceration of the lid margin.

TREATMENT

- Daily eyelid cleansing to remove scales.
- Topical antibiotics.

Dacryostenosis

> 🧍 A 4-month-old child presents with an exudative eye discharge and a painful, red lacrimal sac. *Think: Dacrocystitis.*
>
> Dacrocystitis is the most common infection of the lacrimal system. It is often a complication of dacryocystocele. Excessive tearing, purulent eye discharge, and fever are the common symptoms. *S aureus* and streptococci are the common organisms. Most patients require admission for intravenous antibiotics. An incision and drainage may be needed in the presence of a lacrimal sac abscess.

DEFINITION

A congenital nasolacrimal duct obstruction.

EPIDEMIOLOGY

Occurs in 5% of infants; appears a few weeks after birth.

ETIOLOGY

Failure of the epithelial cells of tear duct to come apart.

SIGNS AND SYMPTOMS

- Chronic tearing.
- Erythema occurs secondary to rubbing the tears.

COMPLICATIONS

Dacrocystitis—inflammation of the nasolacrimal sac; this must be treated with topical or systemic antibiotic and warm compresses.

TREATMENT

- Digital massage of the lacrimal sac.
- Eyelid cleansing.
- Probing if still present after 1 year of age to rupture the membrane.

> Dacryostenosis is the most common disorder of the lacrimal system.

> Most dacryostenosis will resolve by 8 months of age.

Chalazion

DEFINITION

Inflammation of a meibomian (tarsal) gland leading to the formation of a granuloma.

SIGNS AND SYMPTOMS

- Firm nodule on the eyelid.
- Nontender.

TREATMENT

- Warm compresses.
- Excision if necessary.
- Most subside spontaneously over months.

Hordeolum

TYPES

- **External hordeolum,** or stye, is an infection of the glands of Zeis or Moll.
- **Internal hordeolum** is infection of the meibomian gland.

ETIOLOGY

S aureus.

erythromycin

SIGNS AND SYMPTOMS

- Localized swelling
- Tenderness
- Erythema

TREATMENT

- Warm compresses.
- Topical antibiotics (eg, erythromycin).
- Incision and drainage if there is no spontaneous rupture.

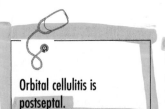

Orbital cellulitis is postseptal.

Orbital Cellulitis

MCC ethmoid sinusitis

DEFINITION

Inflammation of the orbital tissues behind the septum.

ETIOLOGY

- Extension of a local infection including paranasal sinusitis, facial cellulitis, or dental abscess.
- Trauma.
- The most common organisms are *H influenza*, *S aureus*, and *S pneumoniae*.
- Most common site: Medial orbital wall.
- ↑ incidence secondary to ↑ in methicillin-resistant *S aureus* (MRSA).
- Orbital cellulitis is caused most commonly by ethmoid sinusitis.

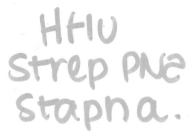

Periorbital cellulitis is much more common than orbital cellulitis.

SIGNS AND SYMPTOMS

- Proptosis, ophthalmoplegia, and ↓ vision differentiate it from preseptal cellulitis.
- Painful extraocular motion.
- Proptosis.
- ↓ vision.
- Erythema.
- Edema.

Hflu
strep PNe
stapha.

painful EOM

COMPLICATIONS

- Loss of vision.
- Meningitis.
- Central nervous system (CNS) abscess.

TREATMENT

- Orbital computed tomography (CT) scan.
- Ophthalmology consultation.
- Intravenous antibiotics, possible surgical drainage.

Periorbital Cellulitis

DEFINITION

Inflammation of the eyelids and periorbital tissue anterior to the septum.

ETIOLOGY

- Extension of local infections including upper respiratory infection (URI), sinusitis, facial cellulitis, or eyelid infection.
- Trauma: Skin trauma is the most likely etiology.

SIGNS AND SYMPTOMS

- Erythema.
- Edema.
- No pain with extraocular movements.

COMPLICATIONS

Development of an orbital cellulitis.

TREATMENT

- Oral or IV antibiotics (eg, ceftriaxone).
- The most common cause of leukocoria is a cataract.

Corneal Ulcer

ETIOLOGY

- Trauma (sand, contact lens, etc.) with secondary infection. Often preceded by a traumatic corneal abrasion.
- Bacterial: *Pseudomonas aeruginosa, Neisseria gonorrhoeae.*
- Fungal: Especially in contact lens users.

SIGNS AND SYMPTOMS

- Corneal haze
- Painful
- Photophobia
- Tearing

COMPLICATIONS

- Perforation
- Scarring
- Blindness

Periorbital cellulitis is preseptal.

The most common organisms causing both preorbital and orbital cellulitis—

SHIP

S *aureus*
H *influenzae*
S *Pneumoniae*

DIAGNOSIS

- Slit-lamp exam: Fluorescein staining reveals an epithelial defect.
- Scraping of the cornea to identify infectious etiology.

TREATMENT

- Local antibiotics.
- In some cases, systemic treatment may be required.

Retinoblastoma gene: Mutation in the long arm of chromosome 13.

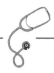

Must evaluate for the presence of retinoblastoma in a child presenting with strabismus.

Retinoblastoma is the most common primary malignant intraocular tumor in children.

Family members of a patient with retinoblastoma should be checked because it may be hereditary.

Retinoblastoma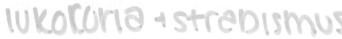

lukocoria + strebismus

- The most common primary ocular malignancy in children.
- Average age: 18 months (90% < 5 years).

SIGNS AND SYMPTOMS

- Leukocoria: White pupillary reflex is the most common presentation.
- Strabismus is the second most common presentation.
- Orbital inflammation.
- Hyphema: Blood layering anterior to the iris.
- May be bilateral (40%).

DIAGNOSIS

- Direct visualization during eye exam.
- Computed tomography (CT) or ultrasound (US) can help confirm and evaluate spread.

TREATMENT

- Chemotherapy.
- Laser photocoagulation.
- Cryotherapy.
- Enucleation for unresponsive tumors.
- Referral for genetic counseling in parents with a family history of retinoblastoma.

EAR

Otitis Media

DEFINITION

Inflammation of the middle ear.

EPIDEMIOLOGY

- The incidence of otitis media is higher in:
  - Boys.
  - Children in day care.
  - Children exposed to secondhand smoke.
  - Non-breast-fed infants.
  - Immunocompromised children.
  - Children with craniofacial defects like cleft palate.
  - Children with a strong family history for otitis media.

- The incidence of infection is higher in children because of their eustachian tube anatomy:
  - Horizontal
  - Short in length
  - ↓ tone

ETIOLOGY

- *S pneumoniae*
- *H influenzae*
- *Moraxella catarrhalis*

Media
- HFlu
- strep pNa
- Mox

COMPLICATIONS

- Hearing loss. *MC*
- Perforation.
- Mastoiditis.
- Cholesteatoma: Saclike epithelial structures.
- Facial nerve paralysis: The facial nerve may not be completely covered with bone in the middle ear; therefore, infection can spread to the nerve.
- Labyrinthitis.
- Abscess formation.
- Tympanosclerosis: Scarring of the tympanic membrane.
- Meningitis. *MC*

Acute Otitis Media

Eustachian tube dysfunction is the most important factor.

SIGNS AND SYMPTOMS

- Ear tugging
- Ear pain
- Fever
- Malaise
- Irritability
- Hearing loss
- Nausea and vomiting

amoxicillin

DIAGNOSIS

- Diagnosis is made with a pneumatic otoscope—the tympanic membrane will have ↓ mobility and will appear hyperemic and bulging with loss of landmarks.
- Tympanocentesis should be used as an adjunct in patients who are < 8 weeks old, are immunocompromised, have a complication, or were treated with multiple courses of antibiotics without improvement; the fluid is sent for culture and sensitivity.

TREATMENT

- Typically, the first-line antibiotic is amoxicillin. High dose can be used for cases most likely to be resistant.
- Antipyretics: Ibuprofen and/or acetaminophen.
- Topical anesthetic eardrops (eg, benzocaine).
- For healthy children > 2 yr old with milder case, watchful waiting for 24–48 hr is an option.
- Pneumococcal vaccine has reduced the incidence of acute otitis media.

The most common overall complication of otitis media is hearing loss.

The most common intracranial complication of otitis media is meningitis.

Remember that younger children who are unable to communicate may have only nonspecific signs like nausea and vomiting with an acute illness such as acute otitis media.

A red eardrum in a crying child is normal; the most specific sign of acute otitis media is ↓ mobility of the tympanic membrane.

Recurrent Acute Otitis Media

DEFINITION

Three to four episodes of acute otitis media in 6 months or six episodes in a year.

TREATMENT

- Prophylactic antibiotics.
- Myringotomy and ventilating tubes should be considered.

Otitis Media with Effusion

SIGNS AND SYMPTOMS

- Hearing loss
- Dizziness
- No fever
- No ear pain

DIAGNOSIS

Pneumatic otoscope shows a retracted eardrum with loss of landmarks and air-fluid levels or bubbles.

TREATMENT

- If asymptomatic, a child is observed for 3 months to see if effusion resolves.
- If symptomatic after 3 months of observation, treatment includes antibiotics and possibly myringotomy and insertion of tympanostomy tubes.

Otitis Externa

A 4-year-old boy presents with what looks like herpetic vesicles in the ear canal and tympanic membrane. *Think: Ramsay Hunt syndrome* (facial paralysis + herpes zoster oticus). CN VIII involved = sensorineural hearing loss or vertigo.

It is due to herpetic involvement of the facial (geniculate), vestibulocochlear, or trigeminal ganglia which results in pain and vesicular eruptions about the auricle and external ear canal.

DEFINITION

- Inflammation of the external auditory canal.
- Occurs when trauma introduces bacteria into an area that is excessively wet or dry.

Otitis externa is known as "swimmer's ear."

ETIOLOGY

- Bacterial: *P aeruginosa, S aureus, Proteus mirabilis, Klebsiella pneumoniae.*
- Viral: Herpes.
- Fungal: *Candida.*

SIGNS AND SYMPTOMS

- Ear pain with movement of the pinna.
- Pruritus of the ear canal.
- Edema of the ear canal.
- Otorrhea: Usually white in color.
- Palpable lymph nodes: Peri- and preauricular.
- Normal tympanic membrane.

COMPLICATIONS

- Malignant otitis externa leads to hearing loss, vertigo, and facial nerve paralysis.
- Temporary hearing loss secondary to swelling.
- Necrotizing otitis externa:
  - *Pseudomonas* osteomyelitis in the temporal bone.
  - Risk factor: Diabetes, immunocompromised (*Aspergillus fumigatus*).

CORTISPORIN

DIAGNOSIS

Diagnosis is made by otoscopic examination.

TREATMENT

Topical antibiotics and steroids to reduce edema (eg, Cortisporin suspension [hydrocortisone-polymyxin-neomycin-bacitracin]).

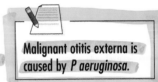

Malignant otitis externa is caused by *P aeruginosa*.

Mastoiditis

DEFINITION

- Inflammation of the mastoid air cells in the temporal bone.
- Most common pathogen: *S pneumoniae.*

ACUTE MASTOIDITIS

- Mostly seen in children after/with an acute otitis media.
- If resolution does not occur, may → acute mastoiditis with periosteitis, acute mastoid osteitis, or chronic mastoiditis.
- Fever.
- Pain behind the ear.
- Erythema and tenderness over the mastoid area.

ACUTE MASTOIDITIS WITH PERIOSTEITIS

- Includes the involvement of the periosteum.
- **Treatment:** Includes myringotomy with ventilation tube placement and IV antibiotics.

ACUTE MASTOID OSTEITIS

- Occurs when there is destruction of the mastoid cells and empyema is present.
- The child will have a tender, swollen, red mastoid process with the ear displaced down and out.
- **Treatment:** Includes IV antibiotics, and mastoidectomy may be necessary.

CHRONIC MASTOIDITIS

Involves treatment with antibiotics and possibly a mastoidectomy if osteitis is present.

COMPLICATIONS

- Hearing loss.
- Facial nerve palsy.
- Subperiosteal abscess.
- Cranial osteomyelitis.
- Labyrinthitis.
- Intracranial spread (meningitis, epidural or cerebellar abscess, subdural empyema).
- Dural sinus thrombosis.

Tinnitus

DEFINITION

- Ringing heard in the ear.
- Commonly found in children who have middle ear disease or hearing loss.

Vertigo

DEFINITION

Dizziness with the feeling that one's body is in motion.

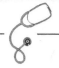

Benign positional vertigo (BPV) will present with ataxia and horizontal nystagmus.

SIGNS AND SYMPTOMS

- Difficulty walking straight or stumbling.
- Spinning sensation.

ETIOLOGY

May occur secondary to the following conditions:

- Otitis media
- Labyrinthitis
- Trauma
- Cholesteatoma
- BPV
- Ménière disease
- CNS disease

Ménière triad includes vertigo, tinnitus, and hearing loss.

TREATMENT

Address the underlying cause.

Ototoxic Drugs

See Table 18-1.

TABLE 18-1. Ototoxic Drugs

Diuretics	**Furosemide**
	Ethacrynic acid
Antibiotics	**Aminoglycosides**
	Minocycline
	Quinolones
Chemotherapeutics	Cisplatin
	Vinblastine
Antimalarials	Quinine
	Chloroquine
	Mefloquine
Antiarrhythmics	Quinidine
Salicylates	Aspirin

NOSE

Sinusitis

DEFINITION

Inflammation of the membranes covering the sinuses.

SINUS DEVELOPMENT

- Ethmoid sinus at birth.
- Maxillary sinus at birth.
- Sphenoid sinus 5 yr.
- Frontal sinus 7 yr.

ETIOLOGY

- A child may be at ↑ risk for sinusitis if there is an obstruction or cilia impairment.
- *S pneumoniae.*
- *H influenzae.*
- *M catarrhalis.*
- Rhinovirus is the most common viral pathogen.
- Bacterial sinusitis is usually preceded by a viral upper respiratory infection.

PREDISPOSITIONS

- Occlusion of the sinus ostium.
- Cystic fibrosis.
- Allergy/asthma.
- Cyanotic congenital heart disease.
- Dental infections.

At birth, only the maxillary and ethmoid sinuses are present.

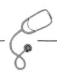

The most common location for epistaxis in children is from the anterior nasal septum because Kiesselbach's plexus is located there.

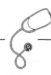

Blood in vomit may be present if a child has swallowed blood from an epistaxis; always ask about epistaxis if a patient presents with hematemesis.

Allergic rhinitis is the most common atopic disease.

SIGNS AND SYMPTOMS

- Headache.
- Sinus tenderness to palpation.
- Persistent nasal discharge (purulent) > 10 days' duration.
- Halitosis.
- Cough secondary to postnasal drip.

COMPLICATIONS

- Cellulitis.
- Abscess formation.
- Osteomyelitis.
- Meningitis may occur through spread of the ethmoid, sphenoid, or frontal sinuses.

DIAGNOSIS

- Diagnosis is made clinically.
- If a test is required, a CT scan is preferred over plain films, which are not as sensitive.

TREATMENT

- Antibiotics (eg, amoxicllin) for 14–21 days.
- If no improvement, a macrolide or amoxicillin-clavulanate may be used.
- Decongestants.
- Nasal saline drops/mist.

Epistaxis

DEFINITION

- Nosebleed.
- Common age: 2–10 yr.
- Unusual during infancy. Must consider coagulopathy or nasal organic causes (eg, choanal atresia).

ETIOLOGY

- The most common location for a nosebleed in children is the anterior septum.
- The most common cause is trauma secondary to a fingernail.
- Other causes may include foreign bodies, inflammation, or dry air.
- If a child has recurrent, severe epistaxis, other, more serious causes should be looked into such as thrombocytopenia, clotting deficiencies, and angiofibromas.

SIGNS AND SYMPTOMS

Bleeding may occur from one or both nostrils.

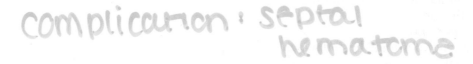

sinusitis

amoxacillin → augmentin

complication: septal hematome

TREATMENT

- Compression for 10 min with head tilted forward.
- Cold compresses to the nose.
- Topical vasoconstrictors may allow visualization of the bleeding site.
- Cauterization using silver nitrite.
- Packing the nose.

Allergic Rhinitis

DEFINITION

An IgE-mediated response to an allergen causing an inflammation of the nasal mucous membranes.

SIGNS AND SYMPTOMS

- Generally don't develop until 2–3 yr of age.
- Sneezing.
- Watery nasal discharge.
- Red, watery eyes.
- Itchy ears, eyes, nose, and throat.
- Nasal obstruction secondary to edema.

DIAGNOSIS

Characteristic findings on physical exam, including:

- Boggy, bluish mucous membranes of the nose.
- Dark circles under the lower eyelids ("allergic shiners").
- Allergic salute.
- Rabbit nose.
- A smear of nasal secretions will show a high number of eosinophils.

TREATMENT

- Avoid triggers
- Antihistamines
- Decongestants
- Cromolyn nasal solution
- Topical steroids

Choanal Atresia

DEFINITION

- A separation of the nose and pharynx by a membrane or bone (90%); may be unilateral or bilateral.
- The most common congenital anomaly of the nose.

The "allergic salute," seen in allergic rhinitis — horizontal crease on the nose that occurs from constant rubbing.

Children with allergic rhinitis may exhibit rabbit-like nose wrinkling because of pruritus.

Allergic rhinitis in children may be a precursor for the development of asthma.

Fifty percent of children with choanal atresia have other associated congenital anomalies —

CHARGE syndrome
Coloboma
Heart disease
Atresia choanae
Retarded growth
Genital anomalies
Ear involvement

SIGNS AND SYMPTOMS

- Each child's presentation will differ depending on his or her ability to mouth breathe.
- Respiratory distress that improves as the child cries because the mouth is open.
- Cyanosis, especially when the child is feeding or sucking. Crying relieves the cyanosis.

DIAGNOSIS

- Inability to pass a catheter through one or both nostrils.
- CT will show the extent of the atresia.

TREATMENT

- Prompt placement of an oral airway, maintaining the mouth in an open position or intubation.
- The ultimate treatment is surgical correction.
- Maintaining an open airway by an orogastric tube or large nipple.
- Tracheostomy or intubation may be required depending on the severity.

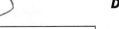

Restenosis of corrected choanal atresia is common.

Musculoskeletal Disease

- The growth plate in the newborn is generally not constituted as an effective structure until 12–24 months.
- The metaphysis is the most metabolically active area.

PEDIATRIC SKELETON

- The anatomy, biomechanics, and physiology of the child's skeleton are very different when compared to adults, → differences in fracture pattern, diagnostic problems, and treatment regimens.
- Bone is more porous and elastic.
- The most obvious anatomic differences in the pediatric bones are the presence of growth plates and the thick periosteum.
- The physis (growth plate) is the weakest site in a child's bone.
- A thick periosteal sleeve makes fractures more stable.
- Remodeling capabilities and rapid healing.

OSTEOMYELITIS

A previously ambulatory 18-month-old girl refuses to walk. She has marked tenderness over the distal left femur. The child has a temperature of 101.6°F (38.7°C), erythrocyte sedimentation rate (ESR) of 72 mm/hr, and white blood cell count (WBC) of 18.5. Radiographs reveal no bony abnormalities. *Think: Osteomyelitis.*

The initial signs and symptoms are often nonspecific. Refusal to walk, limping, or reluctance to move the affected extremity is common presentation. Fever is usually present. Focal tenderness over a long bone may be an important clue for diagnosis. The WBC count is usually ↑ and ESR is elevated. Initial plain radiograph may be normal or show only soft tissue swelling. Radionuclide bone scans usually are positive within 48–72 hr of onset of illness. Bone aspiration may reveal an etiologic agent.

DEFINITION

- Inflammation of the bone caused by infection.
- Can be acute (< 2 weeks) or chronic.

EPIDEMIOLOGY

- Preschool-age children (50%).
- Male preponderance.
- More common in African-American children.

ETIOLOGY

- Most often bacterial.
- See Table 19-1 for causes of osteomyelitis by age group.
- Overall, *Staphylococcus aureus* is the most common bug.

Children with sickle cell disease are prone to *Salmonella* osteomyelitis (but remember, the most common cause even in these children is *Staphylococcus aureus*).

In addition to *S aureus*, young infants may develop osteomyelitis caused by *Streptococcus agalactiae* or enteric gram-negative bacteria.

Consider *Kingella kingae* in children who attend day care. (Remember, *K kingae* is a fastidious organism found in normal respiratory flora.)

Cultures for *K kingae* may need to be incubated longer than usual laboratory protocol.

Puncture wounds to the foot may result in osteomyelitis caused by mixed flora, including *Pseudomonas.*

HIGH-YIELD FACTS

MUSCULOSKELETAL DISEASE

TABLE 19-1. Causes of Osteomyelitis by Age

AGE GROUP	ORGANISMS
Infants < 1 yr, especially under age 3 months	*Staphylococcus aureus* *Streptococcus agalactiae* *Escherichia coli*
< 5 yr	*S aureus* *Streptococcus pyogenes* *Streptococcus pneumoniae* *Kingella kingae*
> 5 yr	*S aureus* *S pyogenes*
Adolescent	*Neisseria gonorrhoeae*

The most common site for osteomyelitis is the rapidly growing end (metaphysis) of long bones.

Nearly 50% of hematogenous osteomyelitis occurs in the tibia or femur.

Consider osteomyelitis in any child with ↓ use of a limb and fever.

Every attempt should be made to establish a microbiologic diagnosis.

PATHOPHYSIOLOGY

- Primarily hematogenous.
- Spread from contiguous infected structures.
- Direct inoculation.

SIGNS AND SYMPTOMS

- Infants and young children:
  - Fever, irritability, and lethargy.
  - Refusal to walk or bear weight.
- Older children:
  - May localize pain
  - Limping
- Physical examination:
  - Painful local swelling
  - Point tenderness
  - Local warmth
  - Erythema

DIAGNOSIS

- Leukocytosis.
- Elevated ESR: Sensitive marker for osteomyelitis, mean ~70 mm/hr. Peaks 3–5 days.
- Elevated C-reactive protein (CRP): peaks at 48 hr.
- CRP typically returns to normal 7–10 days after appropriate therapy but the ESR may remain elevated for 3 or 4 weeks, even with appropriate therapy.
- Growth on blood culture.
- Radiographic findings (see Figure 19-1):
  - Lucent areas in bone represent cortical destruction.
  - Periosteal elevation. Periosteal and lytic changes in the bone may not be seen until substantial bone destruction has occurred.
  - Plain films may be normal for 7–10 days in up to two-thirds of children.

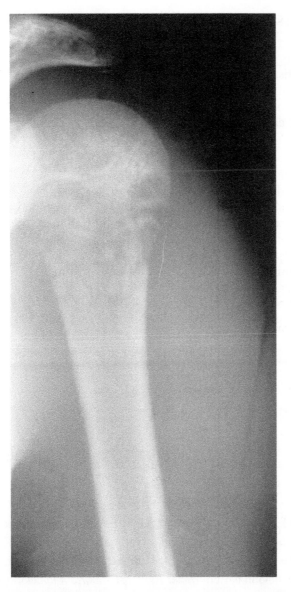

FIGURE 19-1. **Acute hematogenous osteomyelitis of the proximal humerus.**

Mottling and patchy radiolucencies are present in the metaphyseal region. (Reproduced, with permission, from Wilson FC, Lin PP. *General Orthopedics.* New York: McGraw-Hill, 1997.)

- Radionuclide scintigraphy (bone scan):
  - Common isotopes used include technetium, gallium, and indium.
  - Can detect osteomyelitis within 24–48 hr of onset with ~90% sensitivity.
  - *Caution:* Radionuclide scans may be positive in other illnesses that result in ↑ osteoblastic activity, including malignancy, trauma, cellulitis, postsurgery, and arthritis.
- Magnetic resonance imaging (MRI):
  - Provides anatomic detail not seen with bone scan.
  - Useful for visualizing soft tissue abscess associated with osteomyelitis, bone marrow edema, and bone destruction.
  - Contrast enhancement with gadolinium.

The ESR and CRP can be followed to assess response of osteomyelitis to therapy. They should ↓ if treatment is working.

Osteomyelitis without radiographic change should not be treated with antibiotics until an osseous specimen is obtained.

DIFFERENTIAL DIAGNOSIS

- Septic arthritis (can coexist).
- Fracture.
- Cellulitis.
- Transient synovitis.
- Acute leukemia or neuroblastoma.
- Slipped capital femoral epiphysis (SCFE).

TREATMENT

- Admit all children with osteomyelitis.
- Orthopedic consultation.
- Parenteral antibiotics pending cultures (obtain blood, bone, and joint aspirate cultures before antibiotic administration).
- Infants and children: Penicillinase-resistant penicillin (oxacillin) and cephalosporin (cefotaxime).
- Older children (> 5 yr): nafcillin or vancomycin.
- Consider surgical drainage if:
  - Pus is obtained from aspirate.
  - No response to 24–48 hr of antibiotics.

COMPLICATIONS

- Pathologic fractures.
- Chronic osteomyelitis.
- Leg length discrepancy.

SEPTIC ARTHRITIS

Most common cause of polyarticular septic arthritis is *Neisseria gonorrhoeae.*

A 14-year-old boy presents to the emergency department (ED) because of right knee pain for the past 2 days. Three days prior to the onset of the pain, he hit his knee on a pool table. Vitals: Temperature 100.6°F (38.1°C), pulse rate 100, respirations 24. On physical exam, the knee is slightly swollen and tender and is held in flexion. *Think: The most important initial diagnostic procedure is aspiration of the knee for smear and culture.*

Although more common in children, it can occurs in all ages. Trauma can be the precipitant of infection. *Staphylococcus aureus* is the most common cause of septic arthritis. Physical examination may show local erythema, warmth, and swelling. The key to the diagnosis is the detection of bacteria in the synovial fluid either by Gram stain or by a culture; therefore, synovial fluid aspiration should be performed.

A 5-year-old boy who has a definite history of penicillin allergy develops osteomyelitis. Smear of the aspirate shows gram-positive cocci in clusters. *Think: Treat child with vancomycin.*

Vancomycin is directed against gram-positive organisms and can be given to patients who can not receive penicillins and cephalosporins.

DEFINITION

A microbial invasion of joint space.

ETIOLOGY

- Neonates:
  - *S aureus* (most common cause of septic arthritis in all ages).
  - *S agalactiae.*
  - Gram-negative enteric bacilli (*K kingae* has replaced *Haemophilus influenzae* type b [Hib] as the most common gram-negative arthritis in the child 2 months to 5 years old).
- Older children (very similar to osteomyelitis):
  - *S aureus: Remember*—infection with community-acquired methicillin-resistant *S aureus* (CA-MRSA) is becoming more common.
  - *S pyogenes.*
  - *S pneumoniae.*
  - Gonococcus.

Adolescent intravenous (IV) drug abusers are at risk for gram-negative septic arthritis.

EPIDEMIOLOGY

Relatively common in infancy and childhood; can occur in all ages.

Candida albicans must also be considered in neonates and premature infants with septic arthritis.

PATHOPHYSIOLOGY

Organisms may invade the joint by:

- Direct inoculation.
- Contiguous spread.
- Bacteremia (most common route).

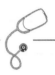

Septic arthritis is an orthopedic emergency.

SIGNS AND SYMPTOMS

- Pain.
- Joint stiffness.
- Erythema.
- Edema.
- Limp and unable to bear weight.

Two-thirds of cases of septic arthritis occur in weight-bearing (hip or knee) joints and involve a single joint (monoarticular).

LABORATORY

- Complete blood count (CBC)—a normal WBC does not rule out diagnosis.
- Elevated ESR.
- Blood culture.
- Joint aspiration.

The knee is the most frequently infected pediatric joint, but the hip is known to have the most severe consequences.

MANAGEMENT

- Admit all children with septic arthritis.
- Orthopedic consultation (it is an orthopedic emergency)
- Joint aspiration.
- Parenteral antibiotics immediately after joint aspiration.

COMPLICATIONS

Potential for severe complications:

- Spread—results in osteomyelitis.
- Avascular necrosis.
- Angular deformities.
- Leg length discrepancy.

Fever is not necessary for diagnosis of septic arthritis.

An 18-month-old infant develops a temperature of 105°F (40.6°C) and refuses to bear weight on her right leg. Physical exam reveals a swollen and warm right knee that the infant will not allow to be flexed or extended. The infant was diagnosed with varicella 3 weeks prior to the onset of this illness. *Think: The most appropriate diagnostic test would be a synovial fluid analysis.*

This patient has a high suspicion for septic arthritis. Joint aspiration is the gold standard for diagnosing septic arthritis and should be performed whenever septic arthritis is suspected. Septic arthritis (due to group A β-hemolytic streptococcus) can occur after a viral infection such as varicella. Children with septic arthritis usually have a history of high fever and restriction of movements.

DEFINITION

- ▓ A reactive arthritis.
- ▓ The most common cause of hip pain in childhood.
- ▓ Predominates in children 5–10 years old.

ETIOLOGY

- ▓ Cause remains uncertain.
- ▓ Often follows an upper respiratory infection (URI).

SIGNS AND SYMPTOMS

- ▓ Unilateral hip or groin pain is the most common complaint.
- ▓ Painful limp.
- ▓ Usually afebrile and nontoxic appearance.

DIAGNOSIS

- ▓ Diagnosis of exclusion. Transient synovitis must be distinguished from septic arthritis. The two disorders present on a continuum and may overlap. Where doubt exists, ultrasound-guided or fluoroscopically guided diagnostic aspiration should be performed.
- ▓ Radiographs are usually normal.
- ▓ Plain films do not diagnose or exclude a hip effusion.
- ▓ The appearance of a septic arthritis of the hip may be identical.

MANAGEMENT

- ▓ First, rule out septic arthritis.
- ▓ Supportive therapy.
- ▓ Nonsteroidal anti-inflammatory drugs (NSAIDs).
- ▓ Complete recovery occurs within a few weeks.

Most common mimic of septic arthritis is transient synovitis. Examining the joint aspirate can differentiate.

A 16-year-old boy complains of right knee pain. On examination, there is significant tenderness and swelling over the tibial tuberosity. He is otherwise healthy. *Think: Osgood–Schlatter disease;* treat with activity restriction.

Osgood-Schlatter disease is a chronic overuse injury and a common cause of knee pain. It occurs due to forceful contraction of the extensor mechanism in sports such as jumping. It is a clinical diagnosis. Tenderness over the proximal tibial tuberosity at the site of patellar insertion is often present. However, plain radiographs are helpful to rule out other causes of knee pain.

DEFINITION

- An inflammatory disorder of the proximal tibial physis where the patellar tendon inserts on the tibia.
- Benign, self-limited extra-articular disease.

ETIOLOGY

- Traction apophysitis/repetitive trauma.
- Chronic microtrauma to the tibial tuberosity secondary to overuse of the quadriceps muscle.

RISK FACTORS

- Boys between ages 11 and 18 yr.
- Rapid skeletal growth.
- Involvement in repetitive jumping sports.

SIGNS AND SYMPTOMS

- Knee pain (tibial tuberosity pain).
- Reproduced by extending the knee against resistance.
- Knee joint examination is normal.
- Tibial tuberosity swelling.
- Absence of effusion or condylar tenderness.

DIAGNOSIS

- Diagnosis is primarily clinical.
- X-ray of the knee may show evidence of fragmentation of the tibial tubercle (see Figure 19-2). Compare with opposite side.

TREATMENT

- Relative rest.
- Restriction of activities as tolerated (patients can still engage in activities even with pain; they will eventually grow out of it).
- Knee immobilizer only for severe cases.
- Complete resolution through physeal closure.

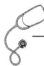
Pain is most pronounced over the tibial tubercle in Osgood-Schlatter disease.

Typical history: Nonspecific aching knee pain exacerbated by exercise.

Osgood-Schlatter disease is a common cause of knee pain in the adolescent.

Septic arthritis may coexist with osteomyelitis at sites where the metaphysis lies *within* the joint capsule:
- Proximal femur–hip joint
- Proximal humerus–shoulder joint
- Distal lateral tibia–ankle joint
- Proximal radius–elbow joint

The major consequence of bacterial invasion of a joint is permanent damage to joint cartilage.

HIGH-YIELD FACTS

MUSCULOSKELETAL DISEASE

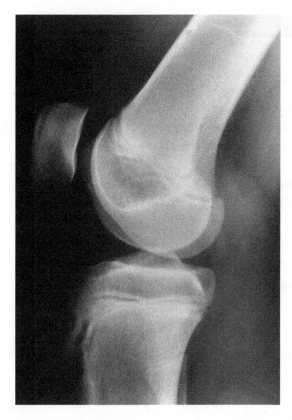

FIGURE 19-2.   Osgood-Schlatter disease.

Note the elevation and irregularity of the tibal tubercle. (Reproduced, with permission, from Wilson FC, Lin PP. *General Orthopedics*. New York: McGraw-Hill, 1997.)

LEGG-CALVÉ-PERTHES DISEASE

A 6-year-old boy presents with hip and knee pain. He has been limping. On examination, he is unable to abduct or internally rotate his hip. *Think: Legg-Calvé-Perthes disease.*

Legg-Calvé-Perthes disease is osteonecrosis of the capital femoral epiphysis of the femoral head. It is due to vascular changes within the proximal femur. Limping is the most common symptom. Pain may be poorly localized in the groin or referred to the thigh or knee joint. It is therefore important to recognize that thigh or knee pain in the child may be due to hip pathology. Plain x-rays of the hip are helpful in making the diagnosis. It occurs at an earlier age than slipped capital femoral epiphysis (SCFE).

DEFINITION

Avascular necrosis of femoral head (occurs when blood supply to the proximal femoral epiphysis is disrupted).

ETIOLOGY

- Idiopathic.
- Some precipitants include sickle cell disease, steroids, trauma, and infection.

Toxic synovitis is the most common cause of limping and acute hip pain in children aged 3–10 yr.

EPIDEMIOLOGY

- Male-to-female ratio: 4:1.
- Highest incidence is during periods of rapid growth of the epiphyses (ages 4–8 yr). *younger child*

SIGNS AND SYMPTOMS

- Insidious onset. Symptoms generally begin with minor trauma.
- Limp with or without pain.
- Pain (activity related and relieved by rest).
- Limited hip motion, particularly abduction and medial rotation. *cannot abduct or internally rotate*
- ↓ range of motion.
- Knee pain is common.

> Classic presentation of Legg-Calvé-Perthes disease is a "painless limp."

RADIOLOGY

- Anteroposterior (AP) and frog-leg lateral position. X-ray findings correlate with the progression and extent of necrosis (see Figure 19-3).
- Early: Effusion of the joint, widening of the joint space and periarticular swelling.
- Few weeks: ↓ bone density around the joint, collapse of the femoral head (affected side appears smaller than the unaffected femoral head).
- Late: New bone replaces necrotic bone.

MANAGEMENT

- Pediatric orthopedic consultation.
- Protect joint.
- Abduction orthoses to "contain" the femoral head on the acetabulum.
- Rest and NSAIDs.
- Surgery for 6- to 10-year-olds with large areas of necrosis.

COMPLICATIONS

Limb length discrepancy.

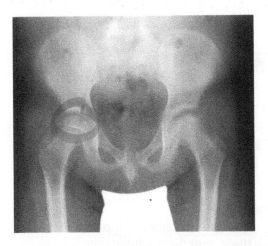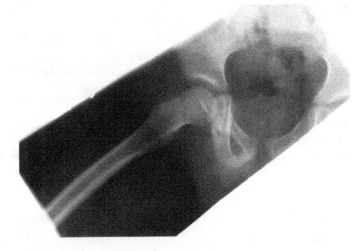

FIGURE 19-3. Radiograph of pelvis demonstrating changes of Legg-Calvé-Perthes disease.

Note the sclerotic, flattened, and fragmented right femoral head.

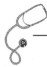

An obese 14-year-old boy has pain in the left anterior thigh for 2 months. On physical exam, there is limited passive flexion and internal rotation of his hip. *Think: The most likely diagnosis is SCFE.*

SCFE is the most common hip disorder of adolescence and occurs at the time of the pubertal growth spurt. Referred pain (groin, thigh, or knee pain) is a common presentation. AP and frog-leg lateral views of the pelvis should be obtained.

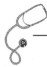

Knee pain in a child warrants a complete hip examination.

SCFE is the second most commonly missed time-sensitive pediatric orthopedic problem (fracture is most common).

Remember, slips can occur in children of normal weight.

MRI can reveal avascular necrosis, whereas conventional radiographs may appear normal.

SCFE is the most common orthopedic hip disorder occurring in adolescence.

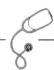

In the presence of suspicion for SCFE, both hips should be imaged.

DEFINITION

- Type of Salter I fracture of the proximal femoral growth plate.
- Disruption of the proximal femoral epiphysis through the physeal plate.
- Epiphysis is usually displaced medially and posteriorly.

ETIOLOGY

- Most cases are idiopathic.
- Weak growth plate (physis is weak prior to closure).
- Local trauma. *Older child (male)*

TYPES

- Acute (< 3 weeks).
- Chronic (> 3 weeks).

RISK FACTORS

- Obesity.
- Hypothyroidism.
- Hypogonadism.
- Growth hormone (GH) administration.
- Renal osteodystrophy.
- Radiation therapy. *cannot abduct or internally rotate*

SIGNS AND SYMPTOMS

- Pain can be located anywhere between the groin and medial knee.
- Limping.
- Internal rotation, flexion, and abduction are lost.
- Painful limp.
- Leg tends to roll into external rotation.

DIAGNOSIS

- AP and frog-leg lateral of both hips (Figure 19-4).
  - Ice cream scoop (epiphysis) falling off its cone.
  - The frog-leg lateral film demonstrates subtle displacement more clearly.
- Earliest sign is widening of epiphysis.
- Always examine and obtain x-ray of the contralateral hip.
- A diagnosis of a preslip can be made with bone scintigraphy.

COMPLICATIONS

- Avascular necrosis of capital femoral epiphysis.
- Chondrolysis.

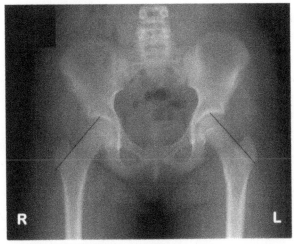

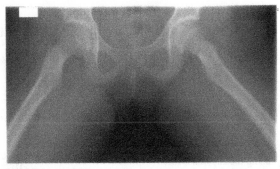

FROG LEG VIEW

R L

ANTERO-POSTERIOR (AP) VIEW

FIGURE 19-4. Hip radiographs in a 13-year-old girl with mildly slipped capital femoral epiphysis (SCFE) on the right.

Note on the AP view that a line drawn along the superior border of the femoral neck (Klein line) shows less femoral head superior to the line on the right than it does in the normal hip on the left.

- Nonunion.
- Premature closure of the epiphyseal plate.

TREATMENT

- Orthopedic consultation.
- Removal of weight bearing from the affected limb (crutches or wheelchair in overweight patients).
- Internal fixation using central percutaneous pin fixation with one or more cannulated screws is the treatment of choice (Figure 19-5).

surgery

Fifteen percent of children who have SCFE have mostly knee or distal thigh pain.

Bilateral SCFE is common.

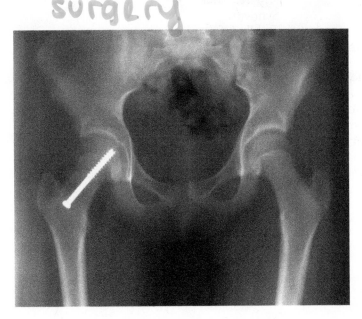

FIGURE 19-5. SCFE after screw fixation (same patient as Figure 19-4).

DEFINITION

Inflammation of the tendon and tendon sheath.

ETIOLOGY

- Trauma
- Overuse

TYPES

- de Quervain tenosynovitis of the wrist (ie, abductor pollicis longus and extensor pollicis brevis tendons).
- Volar flexor tenosynovitis (ie, trigger finger).

MANAGEMENT

- Rest.
- NSAIDs.
- Thumb spica wrist splint.

Klein line: On the AP view of the hip, a line drawn along the superior border of the femoral neck should pass through a portion of the femoral head. If not, consider SCFE.

THE LIMPING CHILD

- Thorough history and physical.
- Assess gait with patient barefoot based on age.
- Plain-film radiographs typically initial study.
- Consider lab work based on differential diagnosis (ie, CBC, ESR).

DIFFERENTIAL DIAGNOSIS

Age Range	Differential Diagnosis
0–4	Hip dysplasia
	Synovitis
	Toddler's fracture
4–10 years old	Juvenile rheumatoid arthritis
	Legg-Calvé-Perthes
10–18 years old	SCFE
	Osgood-Schlatter
	Gonococcal arthritis
	Fracture
All ages	Sprain
	Contusion
	Osteomyelitis
	Septic arthritis
	Neoplasm

DEFINITION

Chronic disease characterized by inflammation of the joints.

ETIOLOGY

Unknown.

CLASSIFICATION

- **Polyarticular (35%):**
  - Five or more joints.
  - Symmetric distribution.
  - Both large and small joints.
- **Pauciarticular (50%):**
  - Fewer than five joints.
  - Asymmetric distribution.
  - Often large weight-bearing joints.
  - Iridocyclitis (50%).
- **Systemic (20%):**
  - Fever, rash, arthritis, and visceral involvement.
  - Also known as Still disease.

MC - <5 (pauc)

DIAGNOSTIC CRITERIA

- Age of onset under 16 yr.
- Arthritis in one or more joints.
- Duration ≥ 6 weeks.
- Exclusion of other causes.
- See Table 19-2 for diagnosis based on joint fluid analysis.

SIGNS AND SYMPTOMS

- Polyarticular:
  - Symmetric, chronic pain and swelling of joints.
  - Systemic features are less prominent.
  - Long-term arthritis; symptoms wax and wane.
- Pauciarticular:
  - Asymmetric chronic arthritis of a few large joints.
  - Systemic features are uncommon.

Seek help from your radiology and orthopedic colleagues if clinical suspicion for SCFE is high but the films are negative.

The most common cause of chest pain in children is idiopathic.

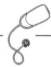

Rheumatoid factor (RF) tends to be negative in early childhood in JRA. RF is positive in about 15% of patients, usually when onset of polyarticular disease occurs after the age of 8 yr.

HIGH-YIELD FACTS

MUSCULOSKELETAL DISEASE

TABLE 19-2. Joint Fluid Analysis

DISORDER	CELLS/mL	GLUCOSE
Trauma	RBC > WBC < 2000 WBC	Normal
Reactive arthritis	2000–10,000 mononuclear WBC	Normal
Juvenile rheumatoid arthritis	5000–60,000 WBC, mostly neutrophils	Low to normal
Septic arthritis	> 60,000 WBC > 90% neutrophils	Low to normal

(Reproduced, with permission, from Hay WW, et al. *Current Pediatric Diagnosis and Treatment*, 14th ed. New York: McGraw-Hill, 2002.)

- **Systemic:**
    - Salmon-pink macular rash.
    - Systemic symptoms: Arthritis, hepatosplenomegaly, leukocytosis, and polyserositis.
    - Episodic, remission of systemic features within 1 yr.

TREATMENT

The goal of treatment is to restore function, relieve pain, and maintain joint motion.

- NSAIDs.
- Range-of-motion and muscle-strengthening exercises.
- Methotrexate, anti–tumor necrosis factor (TNF) antibodies, or antipyrimidine medication for patients who do not respond to NSAIDs.

A normal ESR does not exclude the diagnosis of JRA.

REITER SYNDROME

DEFINITION

Triad of asymmetric arthritis, urethritis, and uveitis.

ETIOLOGY

Thought to be a reactive arthritis after infection with gram-negative (*Salmonella, Shigella, Yersinia, Campylobacter, Chlamydia, Mycoplasma,* and *Ureaplasma*) in persons with human lymphocyte antigen (HLA)-B27.

DIAGNOSIS

- Bone density is preserved.
- Proliferative bone formation is present.

The presence of HLA-B27 is a major determinant of disease severity in Reiter syndrome and a predictor of recurrence.

CHILDHOOD FRACTURES (NOT RELATED TO ABUSE)

Torus Fracture (Figure 19-6)

- Latin *torus* = buckle.
- Buckle fracture: A buckle in the concave cortex of malleable bone under compression.
- Impaction injury in children in which the bone cortex is buckled but not disrupted.
- Stable fracture.

Routine ophthalmologic screening should be performed every 3–6 months for 4 yr for all children with arthritis to look for iridocyclitis.

Greenstick Fracture (Figure 19-7)

- **Definition:** A break in the convex cortex under tension caused by the bending of malleable bone.
- Angulation beyond the limits of plastic deformation.
- Incomplete fracture in which cortex is disrupted on only one side.
- Represents bone failure on the tension side and a plastic or bend deformity on the compression side.

Reiter syndrome: Can't pee, can't see, can't climb a tree.

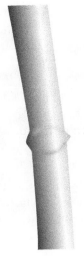

TORUS

FIGURE 19-6. Torus fracture.

Toddler Fracture (Figure 19-8)

- Nondisplaced spiral fracture of the tibia.
- Symptoms include pain, refusal to walk, and minor swelling.
- There is often no history of trauma, or a history of a twisting motion of the leg with a planted foot.
- **Differential diagnosis:** Should include nonaccidental trauma.
- **Treatment:** Immobilization for a few weeks to protect the limb and to relieve pain.

Salter-Harris Fracture Classification

See Figure 19-9.

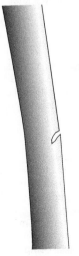

GREENSTICK

FIGURE 19-7. Greenstick fracture.

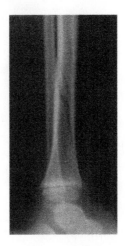

FIGURE 19-8. Toddler fracture.

(Reproduced, with permission, from Schwartz DT, Reisdorff BJ. *Emergency Radiology.* New York: McGraw-Hill, 2000: 602.)

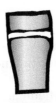

Salter-Harris Type I:
- Fracture throught the physis (growth plate only)
- Often seen in children < 5 years
- Only visible radiographically if the physis is widened, distorted or the epiphysis is distorted *twisting*

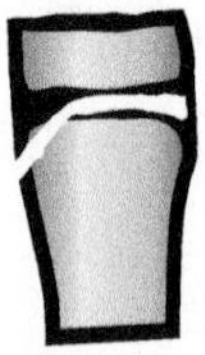

Salter-Haris Type II:
- Through the metaphysis and the physis
- Most common sites are distal radius & tibia

 M

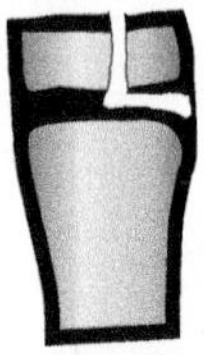

Salter-Harris Type III:
- Through the epiphysis and physis
- Most common sites are knee ankle

 E

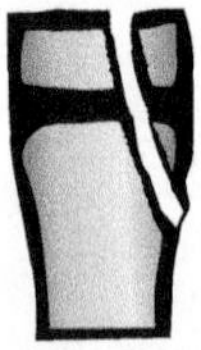

Salter-Harris Type IV:
- Through the epiphysis, physis, and metaphysis
- Most common site is lateral condyle of humerus ME
- Can produce joint defomity and chronic disability

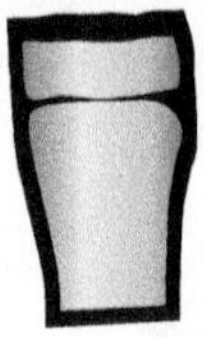

Salter-Harris Type V:
- Crush injury of the physis *crush*
- May appear as a narrowing of the growth plate lucency
- Often not radiographically visible
- May lead to premature fusion
- The proximal tibia is the most common site for growth disturbance
- Mechanism is axial compression

FIGURE 19-9. Salter-Harris fracture classification.

DEFINITION

- **Sprain:** Injury to ligament.
- **Strain:** Injury to muscle-tendon unit.

Ankle Sprain

- **Inversion:** Injury to lateral ligament (85%).
  - Anterior talofibular injures first.
  - Posterior talofibular—severe pain.
- **Eversion:** Injury to medial ligament (15%).
  - Deltoid ligament injury most common.
  - More severe than inversion.

Sprain is a diagnosis of exclusion in children.

SIGNS AND SYMPTOMS

- Grade I: Pain/tenderness without loss of motion.
- Grade II: Pain/tenderness, ecchymosis with some loss of range of motion.
- Grade III: Ligament is completely disrupted; pain/tenderness, swelling and ecchymosis, joint instability, and complete loss of range of motion.

MANAGEMENT

- The goal of treatment is to ↓ local edema and residual stiffness.
- RICE therapy—rest, ice, compression, elevation.
- Protection includes joint immobilization at a right angle, elastic (Ace) bandage wrap, and Jones's dressing for more severe injuries. Splinting the affected joint protects against injury and relieves swelling and pain.
- Crutches and crutch gait training.
- NSAIDs as needed for analgesia.
- Early use of joint and appropriate rehabilitation is key to healing process.

NurseMaids Elbow

A 2-year-old boy complains of left arm pain. He holds his arm in a flexed, pronated position and refuses to supinate his forearm during examination. His mother remembers pulling him by the arm yesterday. *Think: Subluxation of the radial head (nursemaid's elbow).*

Subluxation of the radial head is a common traumatic elbow injury in children. Average age is between 2 and 4 yr. It is due to a sudden longitudinal pull on the forearm while the child's arm is in pronation. Child keeps his arm in passive pronation, with slight flexion at the elbow. Radiographs are not required if the history suggestive of this injury.

DEFINITION

Subluxation of the radial head.

presents-
fixed +
pronated
↓
tx supination

ETIOLOGY

- Slippage of the head of the radius under the annular ligament.
- Most common cause is axial traction.
- Sudden longitudinal pull on the forearm while the child's arm is in pronation.
- Stretching of the annular ligament allows fibers to slip between the capitellum and the head of the radius.

EPIDEMIOLOGY

- Common age: 1–4 yr.
- More frequent under 2 yr.
- Left arm predominance.
- Rare after the age of 6 yr (annular ligament becomes thick and strong by age 5 yr).

SIGNS AND SYMPTOMS

- Child suddenly refuses to use an arm.
- Elbow fully pronated/inability of the child to supinate the arm.

DIAGNOSIS

- Diagnosis is made primarily by history.
- Imaging studies are unnecessary.

MANAGEMENT

- Elbow is placed in full supination and slowly moved to full flexion.
- Alternatively, overpronation of the forearm is also effective.
- A click at the level of the radial head signifies reduction (see Figure 19-10).
- Relief of pain is remarkable.

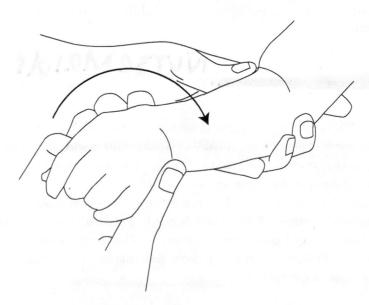

FIGURE 19-10. **Reduction of nursemaid's elbow.**

A patient has had dull, aching pain for several months that has suddenly become more severe. *Think: Osteosarcoma.*

Osteosarcoma is a common cancer in adolescence. Symptoms may be present for a significant period of time before it is diagnosed. Pain, particularly with activity, is a common symptom. Distal femur and proximal tibia are commonly involved bones. On examination, palpable mass may be present. Since osteosarcoma is not radiosensitive, surgery may be needed.

DEFINITION

Malignant tumor arising from osteoblasts.

EPIDEMIOLOGY

- The most frequent sites of origin are the metaphyseal regions.
- Most osteosarcomas develop in patients 10–20 years of age.
- Osteosarcomas most frequently occur during periods of maximal growth.

SIGNS AND SYMPTOMS

- Bone pain.
- Typically long bones (distal femur and proximal tibia) and flat bones (pelvis 10%).

Osteosarcoma is the sixth most common malignancy in children and the third most common in adolescents.

Osteosarcoma is the most common primary malignant neoplasm of bone (60%).

HIGH-YIELD FACTS

MUSCULOSKELETAL DISEASE

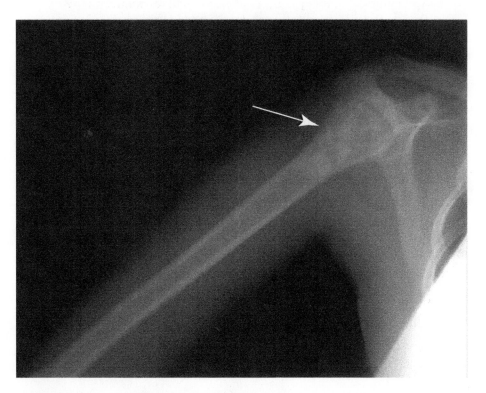

FIGURE 19-11.   Osteosarcoma of proximal humerus.

Note disorganized appearance of bony cortex (arrow).

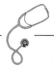

RADIOLOGY

Radiographs show mixed sclerotic and lytic lesion arising in the metaphyseal region, often described as a *sunburst pattern* (Figure 19-11).

MANAGEMENT

- Bone tumors generally are sensitive to radiation and chemotherapy.
- Amputation and limb salvage are effective in achieving local control.

PROGNOSIS

- Seventy-five percent survival in nonmetastatic disease.
- Death is usually due to pulmonary metastasis.
- Widely metastatic disease carries poor prognosis.

EWING SARCOMA

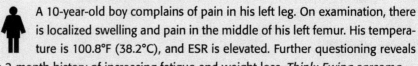

A 10-year-old boy complains of pain in his left leg. On examination, there is localized swelling and pain in the middle of his left femur. His temperature is 100.8°F (38.2°C), and ESR is elevated. Further questioning reveals a 2-month history of increasing fatigue and weight loss. *Think: Ewing sarcoma.*

Ewing sarcoma is a common malignant bone tumor in young patients. Most patients present with either pain or a mass. Most common site for metastases is lung. Periosteal reaction and new bone formation with an onion-skin appearance are suggestive of Ewing sarcoma. Most tumors are considered radiosensitive.

DEFINITION

Malignant tumor of bone arising in medullary tissue.

EPIDEMIOLOGY

- Most common bone lesion in first decade.
- Second to osteosarcoma in second decade.
- However, still rare—only 200 new cases/yr.
- Very strong Caucasian and male predilection, hereditary.

SIGNS AND SYMPTOMS

- Bone pain.
- Systemic signs: Fever, weight loss, fatigue.

RADIOLOGY

- Calcified periosteal elevation, termed *onion skin*.
- Radiolucent lytic bone lesions in the diaphyseal region.
- Evaluation of patients with Ewing's sarcoma should include a CT to define the extent of metastatic disease.

TREATMENT

- Radiotherapy.
- Chemotherapy.
- Surgical resection.
- Autologous bone marrow transplant for high-risk patients.

PROGNOSIS

- Patients with a small localized tumor have a 50–70% long-term disease-free survival rate.
- Patients with metastatic disease have a poor prognosis.

Metastasis is present in 25% of patients with Ewing's sarcoma at diagnosis. The most common sites of metastasis are the lungs, bone (spine), and bone marrow.

BENIGN BONE TUMORS

Osteoid Osteoma

DEFINITION

Reactive lesion of bone.

SIGNS AND SYMPTOMS

- Pain (evening or at night), relieved with aspirin.
- Point tenderness.
- Predominantly found in boys.

RADIOLOGY

Osteosclerosis surrounds small radiolucent nidus.

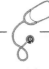

Osteoid osteomas are most common in the femur and tibia.

MANAGEMENT

- Salicylates relieve pain.
- Surgical incision of the nidus is curative.

PROGNOSIS

Prognosis is excellent. There have been no known cases of malignant transformation, although the lesion has been known to reoccur.

Enchondroma

DEFINITION

Cartilaginous lesions.

SIGNS AND SYMPTOMS

- Tubular bones of hands and feet.
- Pathologic fractures.
- Swollen bone.
- Ollier disease (if multiple lesions are present).

RADIOLOGY

- Radiolucent diaphyseal or metaphyseal lesion.
- Often described as "fingernail streaks in bones."

Enchondromas have a predilection for the phalanges.

Mafurci syndrome is multiple enchondromas and aniomas of the soft tissue.

MANAGEMENT

Surgical curettage and bone grafting.

PROGNOSIS

Prognosis is excellent. Malignant transformation may occur, but is very rare in childhood.

Osteochondroma (Exostosis)

DEFINITION

- Most common bone tumor in children.
- Disturbance in enchondral growth.
- Benign cartilage-capped protrusion of osseous tissue arising from the surface of bone.

SIGNS AND SYMPTOMS

- Painless, hard, nontender mass.
- Distal metaphysis of femur, proximal humerus, and proximal tibia.
- Grows with child until skeletal maturity

RADIOLOGY

Pedunculated or sessile mass in the metaphyseal region of long bones.

MANAGEMENT

Excision if symptomatic.

PROGNOSIS

Prognosis is excellent. Malignant transformation is very rare.

Baker cysts are the most common mass in the popliteal fossa.

Baker Cysts

DEFINITION

- Herniation of the synovium in the knee joint into the popliteal region.
- A Baker cyst is lined by a true synovium, as it is an extension of the knee joint.

SIGNS AND SYMPTOMS

- Popliteal mass
- Commonly transilluminates

DIAGNOSIS

Aspiration of mucinous fluid from popliteal fossa.

It is important to exclude deep vein thrombosis (DVT) in patients with a popliteal cyst and leg swelling.

MANAGEMENT

- Baker cysts are benign.
- Nearly always disappears with time in children.
- Avoid surgery (only for significant pain).

While doing a physical exam on a 3-month-old female infant, the physician notices that her left knee is lower when her hips are flexed. The infant was born to a P1G1 mother via a breech vaginal delivery. *Think: DDH.*

It is called Galeazzi sign, which is an apparent shortening of the femur on the side of the dislocated hip and is noted by placing both hips in 90 degrees of flexion and comparing the height of the knees. Screening examination should include the Ortolani test and the provocative maneuver of Barlow. Risk factors include female gender, breech presentation, and positive family history for DDH. Ultrasound can be obtained in infants younger than 6 months. It is a treatable condition with successful treatment if intervention starts early. Pavlik harness is the treatment of choice in the first 6 months of life.

[handwritten: ortolani- abduct tx]
[handwritten: barlow - adduct dx]

DEFINITION

Abnormal growth and development of the hip resulting in an abnormal relationship between the proximal femur and the acetabulum.

EPIDEMIOLOGY

- One in 1000 live births.
- Tenfold ↑ risk in sibling of child with DDH.
- Female > male. Breech female is at highest risk.

*[handwritten: *Breech delivery]*

PATHOPHYSIOLOGY

- At birth there is a lack of development of both acetabulum and femur.
- Progressive with growth.
- Reversible if corrected in first few days or weeks.

SIGNS AND SYMPTOMS

- Newborn:
  - Ortolani: Reduction maneuver. *[handwritten: abd]*
  - Barlow: Provocative test → potential for dislocation of a nondisplaced hip. *[handwritten: add]*
  - Asymmetric skin folds (40%).
- 3–6 months:
  - Limited abduction.
  - Allis's or Galeazzi's sign: Knee is lower on affected side when hips are flexed.
- 12 months (unilateral dislocation): Trendelenburg sign—painless limp and lurch to the affected side with ambulation. When the child stands on the affected leg, there is a dip of the pelvis on the opposite side, due to a weakness of the gluteus medius muscle.
- 12 months (bilateral dislocation):
  - Waddling gait.
  - Lumbar lordosis due to flexion contractures.

Associated anomalies with DDH:

- Torticollis
- Clubfeet
- Metatarsus adductus

[handwritten: <6mo]

Ortolani test: Slowly abduct flexed hip. The femoral head will shift into the acetabulum producing a clunk.

[handwritten: <6mo]

Barlow test: Dislocate the hip by flexing and adducting the hip with axial pressure.

Forced abduction of the hips in DDH is contraindicated because of risk of avascular necrosis.

Signs of instability are more reliable than x-ray in DDH.

In DDH, after 3–6 months, muscle contractures develop, and the Barlow and Ortolani tests become negative.

Triple diapers have no place in the treatment of DDH.

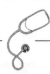

Double or triple diapers are not adequate to obtain a proper position and are no longer indicated treatment of DDH.

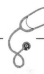

X-ray is not helpful in the newborn. After 6–8 weeks, x-rays begin to show signs of dislocation (lateral displacement of the femoral head).

OI is the most common osteoporosis syndrome in children.

Type I collagen fibers are found in bones, organ capsules, fascia, cornea, sclera, tendons, meninges, and the dermis.

IMAGING

- < 6 months: Ultrasound (acetabulum and proximal femur are predominantly cartilaginous).
- > 6 months: Radiographs (proximal femoral epiphysis ossifies by 4–6 months).

TREATMENT

- **Newborn to 6 months:** Pavlik harness (flexion and abduction of the hip).
- **6 months to 3 years:** Skin traction for 3 weeks to relax soft tissues around the hip prior to closed or open reduction. After 6 months of age, the failure rate for the Pavlik harness is > 50%.
- **> 3 yr:** Operations to correct deformities of the acetabulum and femur.

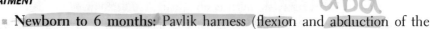

OSTEOGENESIS IMPERFECTA (OI)

 A 2-year-old child is brought in with a right radial fracture after lightly bumping his arm. An x-ray shows multiple healing fractures. On examination, the child has blue sclera, thin skin, and hypoplastic teeth. *Think: OI.*

OI is also called brittle bone disease. Triad: fragile bones, blue sclerae, and early deafness. The teeth frequently have dentinogenesis imperfecta. The enamel is normal, but the dentin is dysplastic. Radiographic appearance may vary according to the type of disease and its severity and include osteopenia and fractures. In infancy, these features may result in evaluation for nonaccidental injury.

DEFINITION

- Rare, inherited disorder of connective tissue, characterized by multiple and recurrent fractures.
- OI is an autosomal-dominant disorder that occurs in all racial and ethnic groups.

ETIOLOGY

- Molecular genetics have identified more than 150 mutations in the genes that encode for type 1 collagen.
- There are four types of OI: Types I and IV are mild and present with an ↑ risk of fractures. Type II is lethal in the newborn period, and type III is a severe form causing significant bony deformity secondary to multiple fractures.
- Ten percent of OI patients have the severe neonatal form of the disease.

SIGNS AND SYMPTOMS

- Bone fragility.
- Easy bruising.
- Repeated fracture after mild trauma.
- Deafness.
- Blue sclera.
- Hyperextensibility of ligaments.
- Normal intelligence.

DIAGNOSIS

Radiographic findings:

- Osteopenia.
- Wormian bones.
- Thin cortices.
- Bowing.
- Normal callus formation.
- Collagen synthesis analysis.

TREATMENT

- Bisphosphonates.
- Surgical correction of long-bone deformities.
- Trauma prevention.

PROGNOSIS

Prognosis is poor, and most patients are confined to wheelchairs by adulthood.

GENETIC COUNSELING

- Genetic counseling should be offered.
- Risk of an affected individual passing the gene to his or her offspring is 50%.

KLIPPEL-FEIL SYNDROME

DEFINITION

Congenital fusion of a variable number of cervical vertebrae.

ETIOLOGY

Failure of normal segmentation in the cervical spine.

Children with Klippel-Feil syndrome are at risk for:
- Atlantoaxial instability
- Neurologic impairment

SIGNS AND SYMPTOMS

- Classic clinical triad:
  - Short neck.
  - Low hairline.
  - Limitation of neck motion.
- Associated with:
  - Renal anomalies.
  - Scoliosis.
  - Spina bifida.
  - Deafness.

DIAGNOSIS

Children with Klippel-Feil syndrome should have the following tests performed:

- Renal ultrasound.
- Hearing test.
- Lateral flexion-extension radiographs of cervical spine.

TREATMENT

- Annual evaluation.
- Avoid violent activities.
- Close evaluation of immediate family members.

TORTICOLLIS

DEFINITION

Twisted or wry neck.

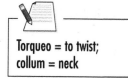

Torqueo = to twist; collum = neck

ETIOLOGY

- **Congenital:** Injury to the sternocleidomastoid muscle during delivery.
- **Acquired:** Rotatory subluxation of the upper cervical spine.

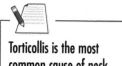

Torticollis is the most common cause of neck muscle strain.

MANAGEMENT

- **Congenital:** Physical therapy for stretching.
- **Acquired:**
  - Warm soaks.
  - Analgesics.
  - Mild anti-inflammatory agents.
  - Soft cervical collar.
  - Passive stretching.

MUSCULAR DYSTROPHIES

Duchenne Muscular Dystrophy (DMD)

A 3-year-old boy must use his hands to push himself up when rising from a seated position. *Think: Gower's maneuver.*

The Gower test indicates proximal muscle weakness, which is described as a ↓ in the ability to rise from the floor without assistance of the upper extremities. DMD is a sex-linked recessive inherited trait that occurs in males. Since children with DMD usually reach early motor milestones at appropriate times, diagnosis may be delayed. However, the diagnosis becomes evident between 3 and 6 years of age. Creatine kinase (CK) should be obtained, which is elevated (50–100 times normal). DNA analysis confirms the diagnosis.

DEFINITION

Degenerative disease of muscles. DMD is characterized by early childhood onset, typically within the first 5 yr.

INHERITANCE

- X-linked recessive.
- One in 3600 males.

Signs and Symptoms

- Clumsiness.
- Easy fatigability.
- Symmetric involvement.
- Axial and proximal before distal.
- Pelvic girdle, with shoulder girdle usually later.
- Rapid progression.
- Loss of ambulation by 8–12 yr.
- Pseudohypertrophy of calves.
- Cardiomegaly—varied severity.

Diagnosis

- Serum CK is markedly elevated.
- Muscle biopsy is pathognomonic—degeneration and variation in fiber size and proliferation of connective tissue. No dystrophin present.

Management

- Encourage ambulation.
- Prevent contractures with passive stretching.

Becker Muscular Dystrophy (BMD)

Definition

Milder form of muscular dystrophy.

Inheritance

X-linked recessive.

Signs and Symptoms

- Late childhood onset, typically between 5 and 15 yr.
- Slow progression.
- Proximal muscle weakness.
- Prominence of calf muscles.
- Inability to walk occurs after 16 yr.

Diagnosis

Muscle biopsy shows degeneration of muscle fibers. Dystrophin is reduced or abnormal.

Myotonic Muscular Dystrophy (MMD)

Inheritance

Autosomal dominant.

Signs and Symptoms

- Congenital MMD affects infants and is more severe than the adult form.
- Adult-onset MMD has a variable onset, typically in the teens to adulthood.
- Muscle weakness of voluntary muscles in the face, distal limbs, and diaphragm.
- Involuntary clenching of hands and jaw, ptosis, and respiratory difficulty.

DMD is the most common muscular dystrophy.

DMD is associated with:
- Mental retardation
- Cardiomyopathy

Death in patients with DMD occurs through cardiac or respiratory failure.

Limb Girdle Muscular Dystrophy

DEFINITION

Two types:

- Pelvifemoral (Leyden-Möbius).
- Scapulohumeral (Erb's juvenile).

INHERITANCE

Autosomal recessive, with high sporadic incidence.

SIGNS AND SYMPTOMS

- Variable age of onset; childhood to early adult (present in second or third decade).
- Pelvic girdle usually involved first and to greater extent.
- Shoulder girdle often asymmetric.

DIAGNOSIS

Muscle biopsy shows dystrophic muscle changes. Dystrophin is normal.

MANAGEMENT

- Promote ambulation.
- Physiotherapy.
- Mildly progressive, life expectancy mid to late adulthood.

Facioscapulohumeral Muscular Dystrophy

INHERITANCE

Autosomal dominant.

SIGNS AND SYMPTOMS

- Variable.
- Slow progression.
- Diminished facial movements: inability to close eyes, smile, or whistle.
- Weakness of the shoulder girdle: Difficulty raising arms over head.
- Normal life span.

DERMATOMYOSITIS/POLYMYOSITIS

In adults, dermatomyositis and polymyositis are associated with malignancy and rheumatic disease. Myositis is not associated with cancer in children.

DEFINITION

- **Polymyositis** primarily affects skeletal muscle.
- **Dermatomyositis:** Skin eruption + myopathy.

EPIDEMIOLOGY

- Female > male.
- Age 5–14 yr.

SIGNS AND SYMPTOMS

- Symmetric proximal muscle weakness.
- Violaceous rash—symmetric, erythematous rash on extensor surfaces, upper eyelids, and knuckles. Rash around eyes called *heliotrope rash*.
- Worrisome triad (not common):
  - Dysphagia
  - Dysphonia
  - Dyspnea

DIAGNOSIS

- ESR, serum CK, and aldolase reflect the activity of the disease.
- Electromyography (EMG) is used to distinguish myopathic from neuropathic causes of muscle weakness.

TREATMENT

- Prednisone.
- Intravenous immune globulin (IVIG), cyclosporine, or methotrexate in refractory cases.

PROGNOSIS

Most children will recover in 1–3 yr.

Dermatomyositis affects proximal muscles more than distal muscles, and weakness usually starts in the legs. An inability to climb stairs may be the first warning sign.

CONNECTIVE TISSUE DISEASES

Marfan Syndrome

DEFINITION

Genetic defect of genes coding for the connective tissue protein fibrillin.

INHERITANCE

Autosomal dominant.

SIGNS AND SYMPTOMS

- **Musculoskeletal:**
  - Tall stature.
  - Long, thin digits (arachnodactyly).
  - Hyperextensible joints.
  - High arched palate.
- **Cardiac:** Dilation of the aorta.
- **Ocular:** Ectopia lentis—lens dislocation (which progresses over time).

The most worrisome complications of Marfan syndrome are aortic dilation, aortic regurgitation, and aortic aneurysms.

Ehlers-Danlos Syndrome (EDS)

DEFINITION

Group of genetically heterogenous connective tissue disorders.

ETIOLOGY

- Quantitative deficiency of collagen causing poor cross-linking of collagen.
- Autosomal dominant.

Type IV EDS is associated with a weakened uterus, blood vessels, or intestines. It is important to identify patients with EDS type IV because of the grave consequences of the disease. Women with EDS type IV should be counseled to avoid pregnancy.

SIGNS AND SYMPTOMS

- Children with EDS are normal at birth.
- Skin hyperelasticity.
- Fragility of the skin and blood vessels.
- Joint hypermobility.
- Propensity for tissue rupture.

MANAGEMENT

- Symptomatic.
- Preventive.
- Prolonged wound fixation.
- Genetic counseling.

Scoliosis

DEFINITION

More than 10-degree curvature of spine in the lateral plane due to the rotation of the involved vertebrae (see Figure 19-12).

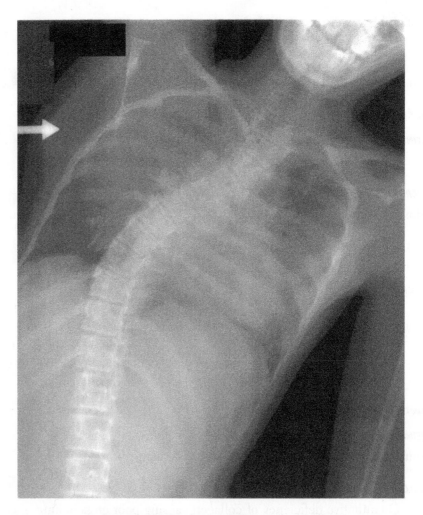

FIGURE 19-12. Radiograph of spine demonstrating marked scoliosis.

ETIOLOGY

- Eighty percent of cases are idiopathic.
- Scoliosis is associated with:
  - Neurofibromatosis.
  - Marfan syndrome.
  - Cerebral palsy.
  - Muscular dystrophy.
  - Poliomyelitis.
  - Myelodysplasia.
  - Congenital vertebral anomalies (hemivertebrae, unilateral vertebral bridge).

EPIDEMIOLOGY

- Four to five times more common in girls.
- Age of onset: 9–10 yr for girls, 11–12 yr for boys.

SIGNS AND SYMPTOMS

- Usually asymptomatic.
- Severe curvature may → impairment of pulmonary function.

DIAGNOSIS

- X-ray of entire spine in both the AP and lateral planes.
- To examine children, have the patient bend forward 90 degrees with the hands joined in the midline. An abnormal finding consists of asymmetry of the height of the ribs or paravertebral muscles on one side.

MANAGEMENT

Treatment depends on the curve magnitude, skeletal maturity, and risk of progression:

- Curve < 20 degrees: Physical therapy and back exercises aimed at strengthening back muscles.
- Curve 20–40 degrees in a skeletally immature child: Orthopedic back brace. A back brace does not ↓ the curve, but prevents further curve progression.
- Curve > 40 degrees: Spinal fusion to correct deformity.

PROGNOSIS

- Curve > 60 degrees: Associated with poor pulmonary function. Large thoracic curves are associated with a shortened life span.
- Curve < 40 degrees: Usually do not progress. Small curves are well tolerated.
- Risk of progression higher in younger childhood.

Thirty percent of family members of patients with scoliosis are also affected. Siblings of affected children should be carefully examined.

Screening for scoliosis should begin at age 6–7 yr.

Kyphosis

DEFINITION

Posterior curvature of the spine.

ETIOLOGY

Scheuermann thoracic kyphosis is a structural deformity of the thoracic spine.

SIGNS AND SYMPTOMS

- Pain
- Progressive deformity
- Neurologic compromise
- Cardiovascular complaints
- Cosmetic issues

RADIOLOGY

- Diagnosis is confirmed on lateral radiographs.
- X-ray shows anterior wedging of at least 5 degrees of three or more adjacent thoracic vertebral bodies.

Spondylolysis

DEFINITION

Fracture of the pars interarticularis due to repetitive stress to this area.

ETIOLOGY

Spondylosis occurs as a result of new bone formation in areas where the annular ligament is stressed.

TYPES

- **Congenital:** Cervical.
- **Acquired:** Lumbar, most often at L5 (85% of cases).

SIGNS AND SYMPTOMS

- Cervical pain.
- Low back pain, worse during the adolescent growth spurt and with spine extension.
- Radicular symptoms are not common.

DIAGNOSIS

Oblique x-ray view of the spine will show the characteristic "Scottie dog sign."

TREATMENT

- NSAIDs.
- Strength and stretching exercises.
- Lumbosacral back brace.

Spondylolisthesis

DEFINITION

Anterior or posterior displacement of one vertebral body on the next due to bilateral pars interarticularis injury.

SIGNS AND SYMPTOMS

- A palpable "step-off" at the lumbosacral area.
- Limited lumbar flexibility.

DIAGNOSIS

Lateral x-ray views show displacement of one vertebral body from another.

Spondylolysis is the most common cause of low back pain in adolescent athletes. This injury is most commonly seen in gymnasts, dancers, and football players.

Grade 1: < 25% displacement
Grade 2: 25–50%
Grade 3: 50–75%
Grade 4: 75–100%
Grade 5: Complete displacement

MANAGEMENT

Treatment depends on grade of lesion:

- < 30% displacement: No restrictions on sports activities, but requires routine follow-up.
- > 50% displacement: In situ posterior spinal fusion or bracing.

COMPLICATIONS

- Deformity
- Disability

Diskitis

DEFINITION

- Pyogenic infection of the intervertebral disk space.
- An uncommon primary infection of the nucleus pulposus, with secondary involvement of the cartilaginous end plate and vertebral body.

ETIOLOGY

- Most present prior to 10 years of age.
- Spontaneous.

SIGNS AND SYMPTOMS

- Moderate to severe pain.
- Pain is localized to the level of involvement and exacerbated by movement.
- Radicular symptoms.

LABS

- MRI is the radiographic study of choice.
- Elevated ESR.

MANAGEMENT

- Intravenous antibiotics.
- Surgery is often not necessary.

RENAL OSTEODYSTROPHY

DEFINITION

Bone diseases resulting from defective mineralization due to renal failure.

SIGNS AND SYMPTOMS

- Growth retardation
- Muscle weakness
- Bone pain
- Skeletal deformities
- Slipped epiphyses

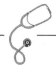

Children at highest risk for diskitis:

- Immunocompromised
- Systemic infections
- Postsurgery

The lumbar spine is the most common site of involvement for diskitis.

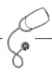

S aureus is the most common organism causing diskitis.

Plain radiographs are usually not helpful for early diagnosis of diskitis.

HIGH-YIELD FACTS

MUSCULOSKELETAL DISEASE

In children, renal osteodystrophy resembles rickets.

DIAGNOSIS

- Normal to ↓ serum calcium.
- Normal to ↑ phosphorus.
- ↑ alkaline phosphatase.
- Normal parathyroid hormone (PTH) levels.
- Radiographs of the hands, wrists, and knees show subperiosteal resorption of bone with widening of the metaphyses.

TREATMENT

- Low-phosphate formula.
- Enhance fecal phosphate excretion with oral calcium carbonate, an antacid that also binds phosphate in the intestinal tract.
- The goals of treatment include normalization of the serum calcium and phosphorus levels and maintenance of the intact PTH level in the range of 200–400 pg/mL.

OSTEOCHONDRITIS DISSECANS

DEFINITION

Avascular necrosis of bone adjacent to articular cartilage.

SIGNS AND SYMPTOMS

- Vague pain (typically in the knee or ankle).
- With joint flexed, may be able to palpate defect below articular cartilage.
- May present as a loose body in the joint.
- Most common in the lateral portion of medial femoral condyle.

DIAGNOSIS

- X-rays show characteristic appearance of subcondylar osteonecrosis.
- MRI may be useful to confirm diagnosis.

TREATMENT

- Children < 11 years—typically observed with serial radiographs to assess healing.
- Adolescents—excision of loose fragments if small. Replacement with fixation if large. Sometimes area can be drilled to promote revascularization and healing.

PROGNOSIS

Typically good with appropriate intervention.

Dermatologic Disease

Primary Skin Lesions

- **Macule:** Flat, nonpalpable, skin discoloration.
- **Plaque:** Elevated, > 2 cm diameter.
- **Wheal:** Elevated, round or flat-topped area of dermal edema, disappears within hours.
- **Vesicle:** Circumscribed, elevated, fluid-filled, < 0.5 cm diameter.
- **Bullae:** Circumscribed, elevated, fluid-filled, > 0.5 cm diameter.
- **Pustule:** Circumscribed, elevated, pus-filled.
- **Papule:** Elevated, palpable, solid, < 0.5 cm diameter.
- **Nodule:** Elevated, palpable, solid, > 0.5 cm.
- **Petechiae:** Red-purple, nonblanching macule, < 0.5 cm diameter, usually pinpoint.
- **Purpura:** Red-purple, nonblanching macule, > 0.5 cm diameter.
- **Telangiectasia:** Blanchable, dilated blood vessels.

Secondary Skin Lesions

- **Scale:** Accumulation of dead, exfoliating epidermal cells.
- **Crust (scab):** Dried serum, blood, or purulent exudate on skin surface.
- **Erosion:** Superficial loss of epidermis, leaving a denuded, moist surface; heals without scar.
- **Ulcer:** Loss of epidermis extending into dermis; heals with scar.
- **Scar:** Replacement of normal skin with fibrous tissue as a result of healing.
- **Excoriation:** Linear erosion produced by scratching.
- **Atrophy:** Thinning of skin.
- **Lichenification:** Thickening of epidermis with accentuation of normal skin markings.

- **Diascopy:** Glass slide pressed firmly against red lesion—blanchable (capillary dilatation) or nonblanchable (extravasation of blood).
- **Gram stain:** Identifies some bacterial infections. Identifies infectious agent and finds antimicrobial susceptibilities.
- **KOH prep:** Identifies fungi and yeast under microscope.
- **Tzanck prep:** Identifies vesicular viral eruptions under microscope.
- **Scabies prep:** Skin scraping to identify mites, eggs, or feces under microscope.
- **Wood's lamp:** Tinea capitis will fluoresce green/yellow on hair shaft.
- **Patch testing:** Detects type IV hypersensitivity reactions (allergic contact dermatitis).

Psoriasis (Figure 20-1)

DEFINITION

- Chronic, noninfectious, hyperproliferative inflammatory disorder.
- Polygenic, chronic, relapsing, T cell–mediated inflammatory skin disease.

ETIOLOGY

- Unknown, but with genetic predisposition.
- Triggering factors: Trauma, infection, and medications.

PATHOPHYSIOLOGY

↑ epidermal cell proliferation due to a shortened epithelial cell cycle.

EPIDEMIOLOGY

- Rare under 10 years of age.
- Worse in winter.

SIGNS AND SYMPTOMS

- **Classic:** Thick, silvery-scaled, sharply defined, pink plaques occurring on the scalp, elbows, and knee.
- Thick, adherent, well-demarcated, salmon-pink plaques with adherent silver-white scale.
- On extensor surfaces of extremities, trunk, and scalp.
- Nails commonly involved—pitting, "oil spots," onycholysis, subungual hyperkeratosis.
- May be associated with arthritis (psoriatic arthritis).
- Higher streptococcal and staphylococcal skin carriage rates.

DIAGNOSIS

- Clinical diagnosis.
- Potassium hydroxide (KOH) test to differentiate from fungal infection.

TREATMENT

- Topical coal tar, anthralin, corticosteroids, synthetic vitamin D analogue.
- If extensive or resistant—ultraviolet B (UVB) phototherapy, PUVA (psoralen and ultraviolet A [UVA]), retinoids, methotrexate, cyclosporine.

Salmon-pink plaques with silvery scale. *Think: Psoriasis.*

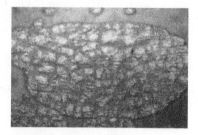

FIGURE 20-1. **Silvery scale plaque of psoriasis.**

(Reproduced, with permission, from Fauci KS, Kasper DL, Braunwald E, et al. *Harrison's Principles of Internal Medicine*, 17th ed. New York: McGraw-Hill, 2008: 311.)

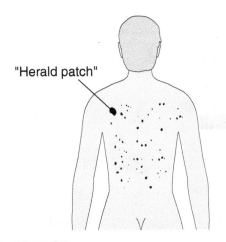

"Herald patch"

FIGURE 20-2. Pityriasis rosea.

Note "Christmas tree" distribution of macules. Note "herald patch" that precedes other lesions.

Pityriasis Rosea (Figure 20-2)

DEFINITION

Common, self-limited eruption of single herald patch followed by a generalized secondary eruption.

ETIOLOGY

Suspected infectious agent.

EPIDEMIOLOGY

Affects children and young adults.

SIGNS AND SYMPTOMS

- Herald plaque—2- to 10-cm solitary, oval, erythematous, with collarette of scale.
- After few days to a few weeks, followed in 80% by generalized eruption of multiple smaller, pink, oval, scaly patches over trunk and upper extremities in "Christmas tree" distribution.
- Can occur in an inverse form (extremities affected and trunk spared).
- Pruritus.

DIAGNOSIS

- Clinical.
- Rapid plasma reagin (RPR) to differentiate from syphilis if suspected, KOH to differentiate from fungal infection.

TREATMENT

- Self-limited, resolves in 6–12 weeks.
- Symptomatic: The goal is to control pruritus (baths, calamine, topical corticosteroids, oral antihistamines).

Herald patch followed by a rash in a Christmas tree distribution (oriented parallel to the ribs). *Think: Pityriasis rosea.*

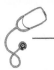

Absence of herald patch does not exclude the diagnosis of pityriasis rosea.

Must consider secondary syphilis in a sexually active adolescent if the rash involves palms and soles.

The herald patch may be mistaken for tinea corporis.

HIGH-YIELD FACTS

DERMATOLOGIC DISEASE

Eczema: Broad term used to describe several inflammatory skin reactions; used synonymously with dermatitis.

Atopic Dermatitis (AD)

DEFINITION

Hypersensitivity inflammatory reaction.

ETIOLOGY

Type 1 (IgE) immediate hypersensitivity response.

PATHOPHYSIOLOGY

Sensitized mast cells release vasoactive mediators.

EPIDEMIOLOGY

- Up to 17% of all children in the United States.
- Affects all ages, but onset usually in first 6 months of life.
- Two-thirds outgrow by age 10.
- Familial tendency and ↑ risk for other atopic disorders (allergic rhinoconjunctivitis, asthma, and food allergy).
- AD may be the initial manifestation of the "atopic march."

SIGNS AND SYMPTOMS

- Pruritic.
- Lesions vary with patient's age.
- Infantile—red, exudative, **crusty**, and **oozing** lesions primarily affecting face (especially cheeks) and extensor surfaces.
- Nose and **paranasal** areas often spared.
- Diaper area is also spared.
- Juvenile/adult: Dry, lichenified, pruritic plaques distributed over flexural areas (antecubital, popliteal, neck).
- Susceptible to secondary bacterial (*S aureus*) and viral (herpes simplex virus) infections.

DIAGNOSIS

Clinical; supported by personal or family history of atopy.

TREATMENT

- Sensitive skin cares (nonperfumed lotions, soaps detergents).
- Avoid scratching.
- Lubricate dry skin.
- Avoid wool, fragrances, and harsh cleansers.
- Oral antihistamines.
- Oral antibiotics *only* if clinical signs of secondary infection.
- Topical corticosteroids are the mainstay of therapy.
- Avoid oral corticosteroids: Patients become steroid dependent or rebound when discontinued.

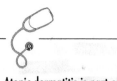

Atopic dermatitis is part of the atopic triad: allergic rhinitis, asthma, and eczema.

You can think of atopic dermatitis as "the itch that rashes."

Don't culture skin in atopic dermatitis—90% of atopic patients are carriers of *Staphylococcus aureus*.

Contact Dermatitis

DEFINITION

Inflammatory skin reaction resulting from contact with an external agent.

ETIOLOGY

Irritant or allergic types.

SIGNS AND SYMPTOMS

- Sharply demarcated, erythematous vesicles and plaques at site of contact with agent.
- Chronic lesions may be lichenified.

DIAGNOSIS

- Clinical: Consider location, relationship to external factors, particular configurations.
- History alone can identify the sensitizing agent in only 10–20%.
  - Nickel.
  - Plant associated (poison ivy).
- KOH to differentiate from fungal infection.

TREATMENT

- Remove offending agent.
- Topical lubrication.
- Wet dressings soaked in Burow's solution (aluminum acetate).
- Topical corticosteroids.

Rhus dermatitis is an allergic dermatitis caused by contact with poison ivy or oak.

Seborrheic Dermatitis

DEFINITION

Chronic and recurrent skin disease occurring at sites with sebaceous gland activity, characterized by erythema and scaling.

ETIOLOGY

Unknown; however, *Malassezia furfur* has been implicated.

PATHOPHYSIOLOGY

Unknown.

EPIDEMIOLOGY

- Affects children and adults.
- Occurs more often in winter months.

SIGNS AND SYMPTOMS

- Children age 0–3 months: "Cradle cap"—greasy scales covering scalp, forehead, cheeks, neck, chin, shoulders ("shawl distribution").
- Adults: Flaking, greasy scales on erythematous background over scalp (dandruff), ears, eyelids (blepharitis), nasolabial fold, and central chest.

DIAGNOSIS

- Clinical.
- KOH to differentiate from fungal infection.

TREATMENT

- Symptomatic: Antiseborrheic shampoo (selenium sulfide), topical corticosteroids (brief course) in the presence of inflamed lesions.
- Topical immunomodulatory agents (tacrolimus, pimecrolimus) > 2 yr.
- Consider **Langerhans cell histiocytosis X** and HIV in the presence of chronic seborrhea.

BULLOUS DISEASES

Pemphigus Vulgaris

DEFINITION

Potentially fatal, chronic, autoimmune, blistering disease of the skin and mucous membranes.

ETIOLOGY

Autoimmune.

PATHOPHYSIOLOGY

Circulating antibodies adhere to cell surface glycoproteins that hold epidermal cells together, causing intraepidermal blisters.

EPIDEMIOLOGY

Very rare in children, but may occur. Often follows a viral infection.

SIGNS AND SYMPTOMS

- Initial development of oral blisters that rupture easily (see Figure 20-3).
- Months later, flaccid bullae emerge and rupture, leaving eroded, denuded, and crusted surfaces.
- Localizes to mouth, or generalized on scalp, face, axillae, chest, and groin, sparing palms and soles.

DIFFERENTIAL DIAGNOSIS

Bullous pemphigoid:

- Rare in children.
- Blisters in crops (flexural aspects of the extremities, in the axillae, and on the groin).
- Large, tense bullae (smaller, flaccid bullae in pemphigus vulgaris).
- Oral lesions less frequent.
- Biopsy: Subepidermal bulla and a dermal inflammatory infiltrate, predominantly of eosinophil.

DIAGNOSIS

- Clinical.
- Confirm by biopsy showing acantholysis (separation of keratinocytes).

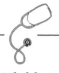

Nikolsky's sign: Direct pressure applied to surface of bulla causes it to extend laterally.

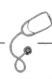

Painful oral ulcers may be the only presentation of pemphigus for the first few weeks.

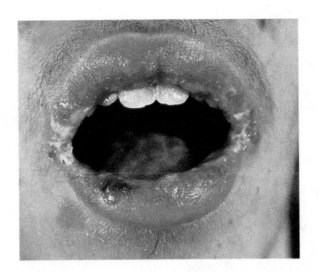

FIGURE 20-3. **Pemphigus.**

(Reproduced, with permission, from Weinberg S, Prose NS, Kristal L. *Color Atlas of Pediatric Dermatology.* New York: McGraw-Hill, 2008: 180.)

- Intercellular immunoglobulin G (IgG) deposits on direct immunofluorescence.
- Circulating antibodies levels that correlate with disease activity.

TREATMENT

- Often fatal if not treated.
- Systemic corticosteroids, immunosuppressive agents.

Best site for biopsy: Fresh small blisters show acantholytic epidermal cells (cell-cell dyshesion).

Erythema Multiforme (Figure 20-4)

DEFINITION

General name used to describe an immune complex–mediated hypersensitivity reaction to different causative agents.

ETIOLOGY

- Drugs (eg, penicillin, sulfonamides, barbiturates, nonsteroidal anti-inflammatory drugs [NSAIDs], thiazides, phenytoin, vaccinations).
- Viruses (herpes simplex, hepatitis A and B).
- Bacteria (*Streptococcus*).
- Fungi, mycoplasma, malignancy, radiotherapy, pregnancy.
- Idiopathic in 20–50%.
- Morphologically, two types: *Iris type* (target lesions) and *vesiculo-bullous type.*
- Clinically, three groups:
  - Erythema multiforme "minor": "Target lesions."
  - Erythema multiforme "major": Rash + mucosal involvement + constitutional symptoms.
  - Maximal variant erythema multiforme (Stevens-Johnson syndrome): Erythema major + systemic complications.

Herpes simplex viruses account for most cases of recurrent erythema multiforme that are not idiopathic.

Mycoplasma pneumoniae can cause a similar presentation.

Minor - ©

Major - Mucosal involvement + constitutional sx

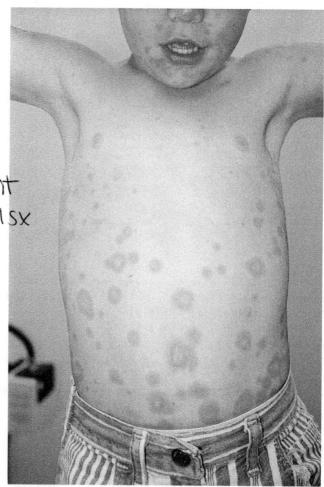

FIGURE 20-4. Erythema multiforme.

Note the many different-sized lesions. (Reproduced, with permission, from Stead LG, Stead SM, Kaufman MS. *First Aid for the Emergency Medicine Clerkship*, 2nd ed. New York: McGraw-Hill, 2006: 356.)

PATHOPHYSIOLOGY

Unknown, likely hypersensitivity reaction.

EPIDEMIOLOGY

Older children and adults.

SIGNS AND SYMPTOMS

Pruritus or pain.

Stevens-Johnson Syndrome (Erythema Multiforme Major)

DEFINITION

Severe variant of erythema multiforme with systemic illness.

ETIOLOGY

Often viruses (herpes) or drugs (see above).

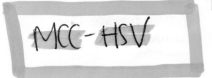

MCC - HSV

SIGNS AND SYMPTOMS

- Systemic illness (fever, malaise).
- Severe mucous membrane involvement (oral, vaginal, conjunctival).
- Extensive target-like lesions and mucosal erosions covering < 10% of body surface area.
- Ocular involvement (purulent uveitis/conjunctivitis) may result in scarring or corneal ulcers.
- May evolve to toxic epidermal necrolysis.

TREATMENT

- Discontinue offending agent (if identified).
- Symptomatic and supportive.
- Observe closely for strictures developing upon mucous membrane healing.
- Mouthwashes, topical anesthetics, pain control.

Toxic Epidermal Necrolysis (TEN)

DEFINITION

↑ severe variant/progression of erythema multiforme with widespread involvement:

- Widespread blister formation and morbilliform or confluent erythema with skin tenderness.
- Absence of target lesions.
- Sudden onset and generalization within 24–48 hr.
- Full-thickness epidermal necrosis and a minimal to absent dermal infiltrate.

ETIOLOGY

Hypersensitivity, triggered by many of above list.

PATHOPHYSIOLOGY

Damage to basal cell layer of epidermis.

SIGNS AND SYMPTOMS

- Widespread, full-thickness necrosis of skin, covering > 30% body surface area.
- Abrupt onset of fever and influenza-like symptoms.
- Pruritus, pain, tenderness, and burning.
- Complications: Secondary skin infections, fluid and electrolyte abnormalities, prerenal azotemia.
- Thirty percent mortality rate.

DIAGNOSIS

Clinical; confirm by biopsy.

TREATMENT

- Removal and/or treatment of causative agent.
- Hospitalization for severe disease.
- Fluid and electrolyte replacement.
- Systemic corticosteroids.
- Antibiotics (for secondary bacterial infection).

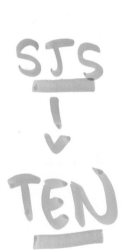

< 10% SJS
> 30% TEN

SJS
↓
TEN

Impetigo (Figure 20-5)

A 3-year-old girl had an upper respiratory infection for the past week. Two days ago, her parents noted a rash immediately under her nose. On examination, she is afebrile with multiple round and oval areas of erythema with golden-colored crusts. *Think: Impetigo.*

Impetigo is a highly contagious superficial skin infection that is limited to the epidermis. It is transmitted by direct contact. The nonbullous form is more common, which begins as a single papule that quickly becomes a vesicle. When this vesicle ruptures and the contents dry, characteristic honey or golden-colored crusts develops.

DEFINITION

- Contagious, superficial, bacterial infection transmitted by direct contact.
- Nonbullous impetigo (70%).
- Bullous impetigo (most commonly affects neonates).

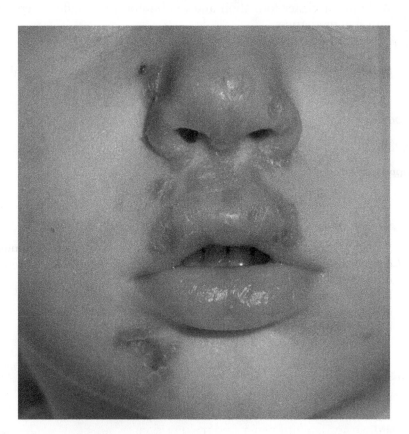

FIGURE 20-5.   Impetigo.

Note characteristic honey-colored crusted lesion, typically seen at corners of mouth and over face. (Reproduced, with permission, from Wolff K, Johnson RA, Suurmond D. *Fitzpatrick's Color Atlas & Synopsis of Clinical Dermatology*, 6th ed. New York: McGraw-Hill, 2009: 599.)

ETIOLOGY

- *Staphylococcus aureus* (bullous lesions).
- Group A β-hemolytic *Streptococcus pyogenes* (GAS) (nonbullous lesions).

[handwritten: gm ⊕ < clusters sa / chains sp]

PATHOPHYSIOLOGY

Only epidermis is affected.

EPIDEMIOLOGY

- Common in children.
- Warm and humid climates.
- Crowded conditions.

SIGNS AND SYMPTOMS

- Mild burning or pruritus.
- Initial lesion is a transient erythematous papule or thin-roofed vesicle that ruptures easily and forms a honey-colored crust.
- Lesions can progress for weeks if untreated.

"Honey-colored crust" is classic for impetigo.

DIAGNOSIS

Clinical; can confirm with Gram stain and culture showing gram-positive cocci in clusters (*S aureus*) or chains (GAS).

TREATMENT

- Remove crusts by soaking in warm water.
- Antibacterial washes (benzoyl peroxide).
- Topical antibiotic if disease is limited (Bactroban).
- Oral antibiotics (cephalexin or macrolide) if more severe.

Cellulitis

DEFINITION

Acute, deep infection of dermis and subcutaneous tissue.

ETIOLOGY

- *S aureus* (rapidly changing epidemiology now places community-acquired methicillin-resistant *S aureus* [CA-MRSA] as one of the common organisms).
- Group A β-hemolytic *S pyogenes*.
- *Haemophilus influenzae* (children).

PATHOPHYSIOLOGY

- Precipitating factors include injury, abrasions, burns, surgical wounds, mucosal infections, bites, underlying dermatosis, and preexisting lymphatic stress.
- Risk factors include cancer, chemotherapy, immunodeficiency, diabetes, cirrhosis, neutropenia, and malnutrition.

EPIDEMIOLOGY

Any age.

SIGNS AND SYMPTOMS

- Erythematous, edematous, shiny area of warm and tender skin with poorly demarcated, nonelevated borders.
- Fever, chills, and malaise can develop rapidly.

DIAGNOSIS

- Clinical; confirmed by Gram stain demonstrating gram-positive cocci in clusters or chains.
- Culture of lesion or blood will be positive only 25% of the time.

TREATMENT

- First-generation cephalosporin or oxacillin.
- Vancomycin if allergic or if MRSA is involved.
- Cefotaxime or ceftriaxone for *H influenzae*.

Erysipelas

DEFINITION

- Variant of cellulitis.
- Others include erysipeloid (hands from handling infected food) and necrotizing fasciitis (medical emergency).
- Clear line of demarcation between involved and uninvolved tissue.
- Raised lesions above the surrounding normal skin.

ETIOLOGY

GAS.

EPIDEMIOLOGY

↑ incidence in young children and adults.

SIGNS AND SYMPTOMS

- Local pain and tenderness.
- Acute onset of fever, malaise, and shivering may precede lesion.
- Well-demarcated, indurated, and elevated advancing border; less edematous (versus cellulitis).
- High morbidity if untreated.

DIAGNOSIS

Clinical; Gram stain reveals gram-positive cocci in chains.

TREATMENT

Oral antibiotics (penicillin, cephalosporin, macrolide, vancomycin).

TOXIN-MEDIATED DISEASES

Staphylococcal Scalded Skin Syndrome

DEFINITION

Toxin-mediated blistering disease.

ETIOLOGY

- *S aureus.*
- Epidermolytic toxins that separate the epidermal cells → blisters.

PATHOPHYSIOLOGY

- Pathogen colonizes nose or conjunctivae without causing clinical signs of infection, but produces exfoliatin and epidermolytic toxins that spread hematogenously to skin, resulting in blistering and sloughing of the epidermis.
- Begins with localized infection, usually around the umbilicus, perioral region conjunctivae, or perineum.
- Toxin is produced at the primary site of infection and then spreads hematogenously to distant sites.

EPIDEMIOLOGY

Newborns and infants (< 2 years old).

SIGNS AND SYMPTOMS

- Skin is initially red and tender with flaccid bullae.
- Epidermis sloughs off and appears wrinkled, usually beginning in the face, neck, axillae, and groin.
- Becomes widespread within 24–48 hours, resembling scalding.
- Direct pressure applied to surface of bulla causes it to extend laterally (Nikolsky's sign).
- Self-limited in 5–7 days, though death can occur in neonates with extensive disease.

> Culture of epidermolytic skin in staphylococcal scalded skin syndrome will not demonstrate the pathogen.

DIAGNOSIS

Clinical; confirmed by culture of colonized site (nose, eyes, throat) revealing gram-positive cocci.

TREATMENT

- Hospitalize newborns with extensive skin sloughing.
- Warm baths for debridement of necrotic epidermis.
- Systemic antibiotics (oxacillin, dicloxacillin).
- Pain control.
- Intravenous (IV) fluids in severe cases.

Scarlet Fever

DEFINITION

Toxin-mediated disease characterized by sore throat, high fever, and mucous membrane erythema.

ETIOLOGY

GAS.

PATHOPHYSIOLOGY

Toxin mediated.

EPIDEMIOLOGY

- Children.
- Untreated streptococcal infection of pharynx, tonsils, or wound.

SIGNS AND SYMPTOMS

- Finely punctate pink-scarlet exanthem first appears on upper trunk 12–48 hr after onset of fever.
- As exanthem spreads to extremities, it becomes confluent and feels like rough sandpaper-like texture.
- Fades in 4–5 days, followed by desquamation.
- Circumoral pallor.
- Linear petechiae evident in body folds (Pastia's sign).
- Pharynx is beefy red and tongue is initially white, but within 4–5 days the white coating sloughs off and tongue becomes bright red.

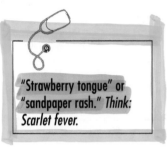

"Strawberry tongue" or "sandpaper rash." *Think: Scarlet fever.*

DIAGNOSIS

- Clinical; confirmed by culture from throat or wound.
- Rapid direct antigen tests detect GAS antigens.
- Gram stain reveals gram-positive cocci in chains.

ᴸ Strep

TREATMENT

- Acetaminophen for fever and pain.
- Antibiotics (penicillin, macrolide, or cephalosporin).
- Follow-up recommended if history of rheumatic fever present.

CUTANEOUS VIRAL INFECTIONS

Verrucae (Warts)

DEFINITION

Viral infection of skin and mucous membranes spread by direct contact.

ETIOLOGY

Human papillomavirus (HPV).

EPIDEMIOLOGY

↑ incidence in atopic and immunocompromised patients.

SIGNS AND SYMPTOMS

- Tender if irritated.
- Types:
  - Verrucae vulgaris: Hands, fingers, knees; skin-colored papule.
  - Verrucae plantaris: Rough; over pressure points on plantar aspect of foot.
  - Verrucae planar: Flat; on face and dorsum of hands and fingers.
  - Condyloma acuminata: Anogenital warts.

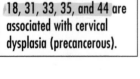

HPV subtypes 6, 11, 16, 18, 31, 33, 35, and 44 are associated with cervical dysplasia (precancerous).

DIAGNOSIS

Clinical—absence of normal skin lines and presence of black dots.

522

TREATMENT

Cryotherapy, topical keratolytic agents (eg, salicylic acid), destructive agents (podophyllin), curettage and desiccation, topical imiquod.

Herpes Gingivostomatitis (Fever Blisters, Cold Sores)

DEFINITION

Highly contagious viral eruption characterized by painful vesicles, commonly occurring around the mouth (type 1) and genitals (type 2).

ETIOLOGY

Herpes simplex virus (HSV) types 1 and 2.

PATHOPHYSIOLOGY

- Transmitted by direct contact with skin and mucous membranes.
- After primary infection, virus remains latent in a neural ganglion.
- Reactivation of latent virus results in recurrent disease commonly occurring in the same area.
- Recurrences become less frequent over time.

EPIDEMIOLOGY

- Primary infection affects children and young adults.
- ↑ incidence of infection in immunocompromised patients.

SIGNS AND SYMPTOMS

- Grouped vesicles on an erythematous base, occurring primarily on lips, mouths, genitals, and eyes, but can occur at any site.
- Erosions and crusted lesions form after a couple of days.
- Fever, malaise, headache, and adenopathy may occur with primary infection.
- Prodrome of burning, tingling, or itching occurs with recurrent infection.
- Complications include ocular disease, secondary infection, and dissemination (especially in immunocompromised patients).

Herpetic whitlow (herpes-infected finger) — can occur in children with herpes gingivostomatitis secondary to sucking of fingers.

DIAGNOSIS

- Clinical.
- Confirmed by Tzanck preparation, revealing multinucleated giant cells.
- Viral culture of vesicle fluid.

TREATMENT

- Oral acyclovir, valacyclovir, or famciclovir ↓ viral shedding time and accelerate healing time. Consider if herpetic whitlow or at risk for severe disease.
- Suppressive therapy with acyclovir for more than six recurrences per year.

Do not try to excise herpetic whitlow — opening the lesion will only serve to spill more virus onto surrounding skin and spread the infection.

Molluscum Contagiosum (Figure 20-6)

DEFINITION

Self-limited, contagious, viral infection transmitted by direct contact.

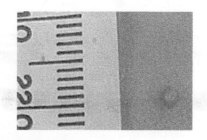

FIGURE 20-6. **Molluscum contagiosum.**

(Courtesy of Danial Stuhlberg, MD, Utah Family Practice Residency, Provo, UT.)

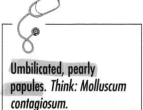

Umbilicated, pearly papules. *Think: Molluscum contagiosum.*

ETIOLOGY

Molluscum contagiosum virus (poxvirus).

EPIDEMIOLOGY

- Affects children and sexually active adults.
- ↑ incidence in atopic and immunocompromised patients.

SIGNS AND SYMPTOMS

- Single or multiple, 2- to 5-mm, firm, umbilicated, skin-colored or pearly-white papules.
- Commonly found on face, eyelids, axillae, and anogenital region.
- Multiple lesions on face suggest human immunodeficiency virus (HIV) infection.

DIAGNOSIS

Clinical.

TREATMENT

Curettage, cryosurgery, electrodesiccation, laser surgery, or tincture of time.

CUTANEOUS FUNGAL INFECTIONS

Tinea (Dermatophytoses)

Tinea corporis lesions are annular with peripheral scale and central clearing.

DEFINITION

- Group of noninvasive fungi that can infect keratinized tissue of epidermis, nails, and hair.
- Clinical presentation depends on anatomic site of infection and is named accordingly.

ETIOLOGY

Trichophyton, Microsporum, Epidermophyton.

EPIDEMIOLOGY

Exacerbated by warm, humid climates.

Signs and Symptoms

- Tinea pedis ("athlete's foot").
- Tinea cruris ("jock itch"): Groin.
- Tinea corporis ("ringworm"): Body (see Figure 20-7).
- Tinea manuum: Hand.
- Tinea facialis: Face.
- Tinea capitis: Scalp.
- Tinea barbae: Beard/mustache area.
- Onychomycosis: Nails.
- Tinea versicolor: Superficial, asymptomatic.

Diagnosis

- Clinical presentation and history.
- KOH preparation reveals multiple, septated hyphae.
- Wood's lamp reveals bright green fluorescence of hair shaft in tinea capitis.
- Fungal culture of affected area may demonstrate dermatophyte.

Treatment

- **Prevention:** Wearing well-ventilated shoes and clothing.
- Topical antifungal agents (imidazoles and terbinafine).
- Systemic antifungal agents if unresponsive to topical or if involvement of nails or hair (griseofulvin, systemic azoles, terbinafine).
- Mild-potency topical corticosteroids if inflammation and pruritus are severe.

Tinea versicolor has hyphae and yeast forms in a "spaghetti-and-meatball" distribution on KOH preparation.

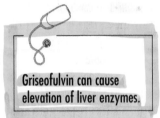

Griseofulvin can cause elevation of liver enzymes.

Candidal Skin Infections (Candida)

Definition

Superficial infection occurring in moist cutaneous sites.

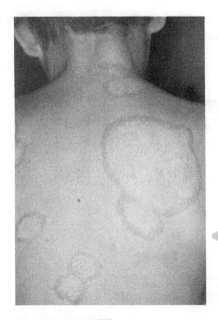

annular lesions + central clearing. Tinea coporis

FIGURE 20-7. **Tinea corporis (ringworm).**

HIGH-YIELD FACTS

DERMATOLOGIC DISEASE

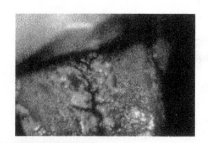

FIGURE 20-8. Oral candidiasis (thrush).

(Reproduced, with permission, from Yong-Kwang T, Seow C. What syndrome is this? *Pediatric Dermatology* 2001;18(4): 353.)

> Thrush is a candidal infection of mucosal surfaces, presenting as creamy white, easily removable papules on an erythematous mucosal surface (see Figure 20-8).

> Diaper rash is often superinfected with *Candida*, which manifests as erythematous satellite lesions.

ETIOLOGY

Candida albicans.

PATHOPHYSIOLOGY

Predisposing factors: Diabetes mellitus, obesity, immunosuppression, chronic debilitation, recent use of antibiotics.

SIGNS AND SYMPTOMS

- Pruritus and soreness.
- Confluent, bright red papules and pustules forming a sharply demarcated eroded patch with pustular lesions at the periphery (satellite lesions).
- Distributed over intertriginous regions, including axillae; groin; web spaces; genital, anal, and inframammary areas.
- Oral form is thrush: Thick white plaque on tongue or inside of cheeks that can't be scraped off (Figure 20-8).

DIAGNOSIS

Clinical; confirmed by KOH preparation revealing pseudohyphae and budding spores and cultures of lesion.

TREATMENT

- Keep intertriginous areas dry.
- Topical antifungals (azoles).
- Topical corticosteroids for symptomatic relief.

INFESTATIONS

Lice (Pediculosis)

DEFINITION

1. Pediculosis corporis—body.
2. Pediculosis capitis—scalp hair.
3. Pediculosis pubis—pubic hair.

ETIOLOGY

1. *Pediculus humanus corporis.*
2. *Pediculus humanus capitis.*
3. *Pthirus pubis.*

PATHOPHYSIOLOGY

Lice are obligate parasites, feeding on human blood.

EPIDEMIOLOGY

1. Poor hygiene.
2. Head-to-head contact, sharing hair items.
3. Sexual contact.

SIGNS AND SYMPTOMS

- Pruritus.
- Pyoderma may develop from scratching.
- Corporis—primary lesion is an intensely pruritic, small, red macule or papule with central hemorrhagic punctum on shoulders, trunk, or buttocks; secondary lesions include excoriations, wheals, and eczematous, secondarily infected plaques.

DIAGNOSIS

Nits detectable on hair/fibers.

TREATMENT

- Hot water laundering.
- Boil or dispose of implements.
- Comb hair.
- Permethrin rinse—once, then again at 1 week (alternatives—pyrethrin, lindane).

Cutaneous Larva Migrans (Figure 20-9)

DEFINITION

Eruption caused by several larval nematodes not usually parasitic to humans.

ETIOLOGY

Most often *Ancylostoma braziliense* (hookworm of dogs and cats).

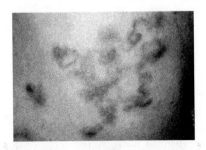

FIGURE 20-9. Cutaneous larva migrans.

(Reproduced, with permission, from Berger MS. A serpiginous eruption on the buttocks. *American Family Physician* 2000;62: 2493.)

PATHOPHYSIOLOGY

Parasite eggs are deposited in feces of animals, then hatch. Larvae penetrate human skin, then migrate along epidermal-dermal junction.

EPIDEMIOLOGY

Warm, moist areas.

SIGNS AND SYMPTOMS

- Raised, erythematous, serpiginous tracks, occasionally forming bullae.
- Single or multiple.
- Usually on an extremity or the buttocks, but can occur anywhere on the body.

DIAGNOSIS

Clinical.

TREATMENT

- Self-limited in weeks to months.
- Thiabendazole if symptoms warrant treatment.

Scabies

A 4-year-old boy has been treated with hydrocortisone cream for eczema on and off for the last 3 years. Over the past 2 months, parents have noted a pruritic, papular rash that improves when hydrocortisone cream is used but returns when hydrocortisone is discontinued. On examination, he is afebrile with diffusely distributed papules on the trunk and extremities, concentrated in the intertriginous areas. Burrows are noted as well. *Think: Scabies.*

Scabies. It is a highly contagious disease caused by the mite *Sarcoptes scabiei* and spreads in households with intimate personal contact or sharing of inanimate object. Schoolchildren are especially at higher risk. Typical presentation is generalized, intense nocturnal itching, and classic sites are hairless areas with a thin stratum corneum (interdigital web spaces of fingers and toes, popliteal fossae, flexor surfaces of the wrists, and gluteal region). Presence of skin burrows is the most supportive finding. Definitive diagnosis is established by finding the scabies mites. The most effective topical treatment is 5% permethrin. One application is usually effective but a second treatment 1 week after the first application may be required.

ETIOLOGY

Female mite *Sarcoptes scabiei hominis.*

PATHOPHYSIOLOGY

- Pregnant female mite exudes keratolytic substance and burrows into the stratum corneum, depositing eggs and feces daily.
- Eggs hatch; larvae molt into nymphs, mature in 2–3 weeks, and repeat the cycle.

2 - 3 weeks

- Physical contact with infected individual.
- Rarely transmitted by fomites, as isolated mites dies within 2–3 days.

SIGNS AND SYMPTOMS

- Pruritus at initial infestation.
- First sign: 1- to 2-mm red papules, some of which are excoriated, crusted, or scaling.
- Threadlike burrows.
- Multiple types of lesions.

DIAGNOSIS

Scraping for microscopic identification of mites, ova, and feces.

TREATMENT

- Permethrin, neck down, scalp only if involved; leave on 8–12 hr; may be repeated after 1 week.
- Infants are particularly susceptible to the neurotoxicity of lindane; therefore avoid.
- Alternatives include permethrin or sulfur ointment.

lindane - neurotoxic

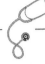

Threadlike burrows are classic for scabies, but may not be seen in infants.

Transmission of scabies mites is unlikely 24 hr after treatment.

GROWTHS

Hemangioma

DEFINITION

Benign vascular proliferation that is usually present at birth or appears soon afterward (eg, capillary hemangioma, port-wine stain, cavernous hemangioma) (Figure 20-10).

ETIOLOGY/PATHOPHYSIOLOGY

Abnormal angiogenesis, perhaps incited by cytokines, such as basic fibroblast growth factor (bFGF) and vascular endothelial growth factor (VEGF).

EPIDEMIOLOGY

Approximately 0.5% of infants.

SIGNS AND SYMPTOMS

- Capillary ("strawberry") hemangioma: Red or purple papules or nodules that develop soon after birth and spontaneously involute by fifth year (see Figure 20-11).
- If multiple hemangiomas, may also have visceral hemangiomas (hemangomatosis).

TREATMENT

- Most resolve without treatment.
- Involvement of bone, soft tissue, or organ parenchyma may warrant excision of the hemangioma.

HIGH-YIELD FACTS

DERMATOLOGIC DISEASE

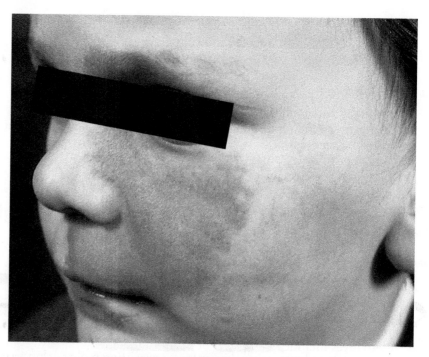

FIGURE 20-10. Port-wine stain seen in Sturge-Weber syndrome.

(Reproduced, with permission, from Wolff K, Johnson RA, Suurmond D. *Fitzpatrick's Color Atlas & Synopsis of Clinical Dermatology*, 5th ed. New York: McGraw-Hill, 2005: 187.)

Melanocytic Nevus (Mole) (Figure 20-12)

DEFINITION

Benign proliferation of melanocytes, which are classified according to location of clustering: dermal-epidermal junction (junctional), dermis (dermal), or both (compound).

EPIDEMIOLOGY

Nevi usually arise in childhood, peak during adolescence, and spontaneously regress during adulthood.

TREATMENT

- Serial observation for early recognition of premalignancy.
- Early excision of suspicious lesions.

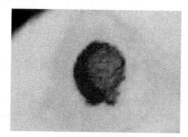

FIGURE 20-11. Capillary hemangioma.

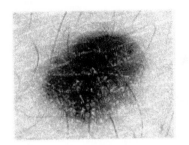

FIGURE 20-12. **Melanocytic nevus.**

(Reproduced, with permission, from Wang SQ, Katz B, Rabinovitz H, Kopf AW, Oliviero M. Lessons on dermoscopy. *Dermatologic Surgery* 2000;26[4]: 397.)

Malignant Melanoma

DEFINITION

Malignant proliferation of melanocytes.

ETIOLOGY

May arise from normal-appearing skin or from preexisting mole or skin lesion.

PATHOPHYSIOLOGY

- Horizontal growth phase: Lateral extension within the epidermis and dermis.
- Vertical phase: Penetrates into dermis, greatly increasing risk of metastasis.

EPIDEMIOLOGY

- ↑ incidence in fair-skinned people and with sun exposure.
- Adolescents.

SIGNS AND SYMPTOMS

Characteristics of a mole suspicious for melanoma:

- Asymmetric.
- Border (irregular).
- Color (variegated and mottled).
- Diameter (> 0.6 cm).
- Elevated.
- Enlarging.

DIAGNOSIS

Prognosis based on thickness of the primary tumor.

TREATMENT

- Surgical excision with margins at least 1 cm beyond borders, depending on depth of lesion.
- Close follow-up.

Characteristics of mole
suspicious for melanoma:
- Asymmetric
- Borders irregular
- Color uneven
- Diameter > 0.6 cm
- Elevated
- Enlarging

Xeroderma Pigmentosum

DEFINITION

Genetic defect in DNA repair mechanisms, predisposing to certain skin cancers.

ETIOLOGY

Autosomal recessive.

PATHOPHYSIOLOGY

Failure to repair ultraviolet-damaged DNA.

SIGNS AND SYMPTOMS

Predisposes patients to basal and squamous cell skin cancers.

OTHER SKIN CONDITIONS

Henoch-Schönlein Purpura (Figure 20-13)

DEFINITION

Classic example of vasculitis in children.

Iga

ETIOLOGY/PATHOPHYSIOLOGY

- Immunoglobulin A (IgA) mediated.
- Occurs most commonly following streptococcal or viral infection.

EPIDEMIOLOGY

Pediatric age group.

post strep/viral
→ PALPABLE

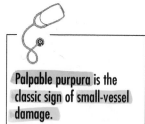

Palpable purpura is the classic sign of small-vessel damage.

SIGNS AND SYMPTOMS

- Palpable purpura
- Arthritis
- Abdominal pain

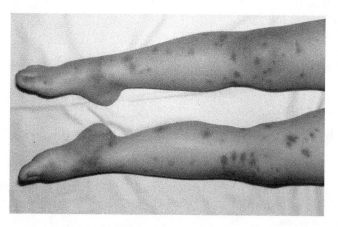

FIGURE 20-13. Henoch-Schönlein purpura.

(Reproduced, with permission, from Knoop KJ, Stack LB, and Storrow AB et al. *Atlas of Emergency Medicine*, 3rd ed. New York: McGraw-Hill, 2010: 429. Photo contributor: Lawrence B. Stack, MD.)

DIAGNOSIS

Clinical; may biopsy.

TREATMENT

- Usually benign, self-limited.
- If severe, consider systemic steroids.
- Monitor for renal dysfunction.

Intestinal wall purpura can serve as a lead point for intussussception.

Acne Vulgaris

DEFINITION

- Disorder of pilosebaceous glands.
- Develops in areas with the greatest concentration of sebaceous glands.

ETIOLOGY/PATHOPHYSIOLOGY

- Results from a combination of hormonal (androgens), bacterial (*Propionibacterium acnes*), and genetic factors.
- Initial pathology is microscopic microcomedo.

EPIDEMIOLOGY

Adolescents.

open - black
closed - white

SIGNS AND SYMPTOMS

- Comedone: Plug of sebaceous and dead skin material stuck in the opening of a hair follicle; open follicle (blackhead) or almost closed (whitehead).
- Pustules, papules.
- Painful nodules and cysts if severe.
- Seborrhea of face and scalp (greasy skin).
- Depressed or hypertrophic scars may develop with healing.

DIAGNOSIS

Clinical; confirmed by presence of comedones.

TREATMENT

- Benzoyl peroxide wash.
- Topical antibiotics (clindamycin or erythromycin).
- Intralesional corticosteroid injections (triamcinolone acetonide).
- Topical retinoid: ↑ cell turnover and prevent follicle occlusion.
- Oral isotretinoin (Accutane) for severe, recalcitrant, nodular acne.
- Dermabrasion for treatment of scars.

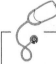
Accutane is teratogenic and **must** be prescribed with oral contraceptives; it also has many side effects.

trimacnelone SQ

Diaper Rash

DEFINITION

Rash occurring in the diaper area.

ETIOLOGY

- Irritant contact dermatitis: Prolonged dampness, interaction of urine (ammonia) and feces with the skin, reactions to medications/creams, type of diaper.

- Candidal or bacterial secondary infection can occur.
- Atopic dermatitis.
- May be any other dermatologic condition in diaper distribution.

PATHOPHYSIOLOGY

Overhydration, friction, maceration, allergy, etc.

EPIDEMIOLOGY

Most children who wear diapers, to some degree.

SIGNS AND SYMPTOMS

- Red, scaly, fissured, eroded skin.
- Patchy or confluent.
- If secondarily infected: Impetiginous or candidal.
- Check for oral candidiasis if present in diaper area.

TREATMENT

- Keep infant dry, change diapers often.
- Avoid harsh detergents, wipes with alcohol, and plastic pants.
- Ointments can reduce friction and protect skin from irritation.
- Avoid powders, as they can injure infants' lungs if inhaled accidentally.
- Nystatin or other antifungal cream for yeast infection.

Recurrent Minor Aphthous Ulcers/Stomatitis (Canker Sores)

DEFINITION

Chronic inflammatory disease causing recurrent oral ulcers of varying frequency.

ETIOLOGY

Local cell-mediated immunity, elevated inflammatory mediators, abnormal cell communication/epithelial integrity.

PATHOPHYSIOLOGY

Triggers may include toothpaste/mouthwash with sodium lauryl sulfate, mechanical trauma, stress, nutritional deficiencies, food sensitivities/allergies, hormones, infection, genetics, medical conditions, and medications.

EPIDEMIOLOGY

Twenty percent of the general population.

SIGNS AND SYMPTOMS

- Round/ovoid ulcer with grayish membrane and edges surrounded by reddish halo.
- Occur on nonkeratinized skin: Inside of the lips and cheeks, floor of the mouth, under the tongue, soft palate, and tonsillar areas.
- High recurrence rate.
- Painful.
- Usually heal uneventfully in 4–14 days.

DIAGNOSIS

Clinical; rule out herpes stomatitis.

TREATMENT

- Avoid individual triggering factors.
- Symptomatic: Oral numbing or coating medications.
- Antibacterial/cleansing rinses.
- Home remedies: Milk of Magnesia, warm salt water, alum rinses.
- Prescription anti-inflammatory or antibacterial collagenase inhibitors.

Vitiligo

DEFINITION

Pigmentary defect.

ETIOLOGY/PATHOPHYSIOLOGY

- Unknown, possibly autoimmune.
- Trauma may be associated with initiation of the lesions.

EPIDEMIOLOGY

Half of cases present before 20 years of age.

SIGNS AND SYMPTOMS

- Depigmented macules.
- Predilection for hyperpigmented areas.

DIAGNOSIS

Clinical, though melanocyte absence can be confirmed by electron microscopy of biopsy specimen.

TREATMENT

- Many months of psoralen and ultraviolet therapy can partially or completely repigment areas.
- Potent topical steroids are used on areas such as lips not amenable to phototherapy.

Urticaria-Angioedema

A 12-year-old boy with a history of multiple food allergies ate a candy bar given to him by a friend at school. He complained of throat discomfort and a rash. On examination, he is afebrile. He is wheezing. Multiple discrete erythematous papules are noted on trunk and extremities. *Think: Urticaria.*

Urticaria with or without angioedema is frequently seen in pediatric practice. Angioedema is due to an urticarial process that involves deeper layers of the skin. Acute urticaria is more common in children. History is often able to identify an inciting factor, especially if the hives occur shortly after ingestion of a food or drug. Common foods that cause urticaria are milk, eggs, peanuts, and shellfish. The mast cell is the mediator in the development of urticaria. These lesions are typically pruritic and erythematous, often showing central clearing. Systemic symptoms develop if it is associated with anaphylaxis.

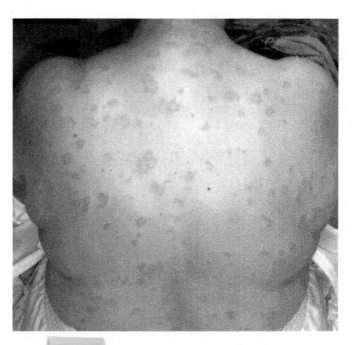

FIGURE 20-14. Urticaria.

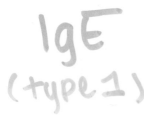

DEFINITION

Allergic response → edema of the tissues.

ETIOLOGY/PATHOPHYSIOLOGY

Type 1 hypersensitivity reaction of immunoglobulin E (IgE) with mast cells causes the release of histamine, → vasodilation, ↑ vascular permeability, and axonal response.

EPIDEMIOLOGY

Can occur in response to a large number of entities—ingestion, contact, infectious agents, environmental factors, or genetic conditions.

SIGNS AND SYMPTOMS

- **Urticaria:** Well circumscribed, but can be coalescent, erythematous, raised lesions (wheals or welts) (see Figure 20-14).
- **Angioedema:** Involves the deeper layers of skin, submucosa, and subcutaneous tissues.

TREATMENT

- Usually self-limited.
- Antihistamines to relieve pruritus.
- Watch for signs of airway compromise (especially with angioedema).
- Epinephrine for severe cases.

FIGURE 12-3. Streptococcal pharyngitis.

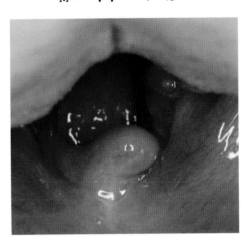

Note white exudates on top of erythematous swollen tonsils. (Reproduced, with permission, from Knoop KJ, Stack LB, and Storrow AB, et al. *Atlas of Emergency Medicine*, 3rd ed. New York: McGraw-Hill, 2010: 115.)

FIGURE 20-1. Silvery scale plaque of psoriasis.

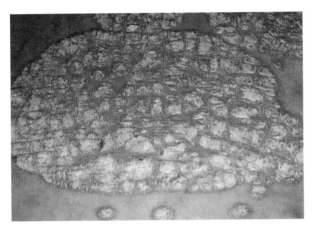

(Reproduced, with permission, from Fauci KS, Kasper DL, Braunwald E, et al. *Harrison's Principles of Internal Medicine*, 17th ed. New York: McGraw-Hill, 2008: 311.)

FIGURE 10-1. Meningococcemia.

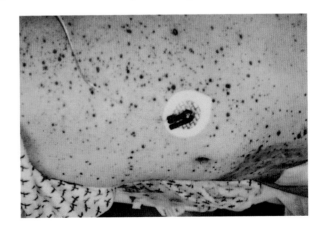

(Reproduced, with permission, from Knoop KJ, Stack LB, and Storrow AB, et al. *Atlas of Emergency Medicine*, 3rd ed. New York: McGraw-Hill, 2010: 423. Photo contributor: Richard Strait, MD.)

FIGURE 10-2. Koplik spots (rubeola).

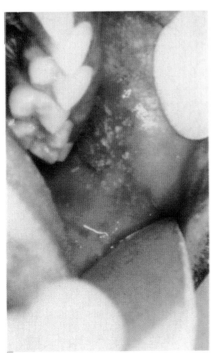

(Reproduced, with permission, from Knoop KJ, Stack LB, and Storrow AB. *Atlas of Emergency Medicine*, 1st ed. New York: McGraw-Hill, 1997: 174.)

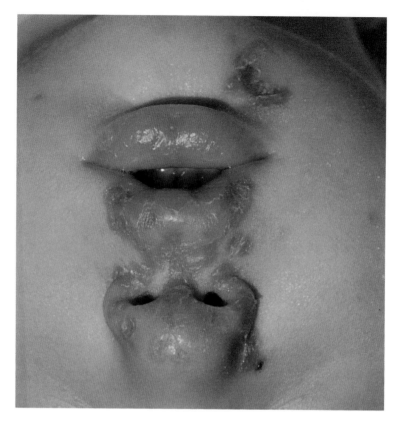

FIGURE 20-5. Impetigo.

Note characteristic honey-colored crusted lesion, typically seen at corners of mouth and over face. (Reproduced, with permission, from Wolff K, Johnson RA, Suurmond D. Fitzpatrick's Color Atlas & Synopsis of Clinical Dermatology, 6th ed. New York: McGraw-Hill, 2009:599.)

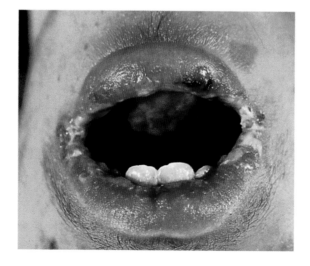

FIGURE 20-3. Pemphigus.

(Reproduced, with permission, from Weinberg S, Prose NS, and Kristal L. Color Atlas of Pediatric Dermatology. New York: McGraw-Hill, 2008: 180.)

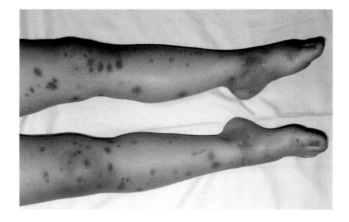

FIGURE 20-13. Henoch-Schönlein purpura.

(Reproduced, with permission, from Knoop KJ, Stack LB, and Storrow AB et al. *Atlas of Emergency Medicine*, 3rd ed. New York: McGraw-Hill, 2010: 429. Photo contributor: Lawrence B. Stack, MD.)

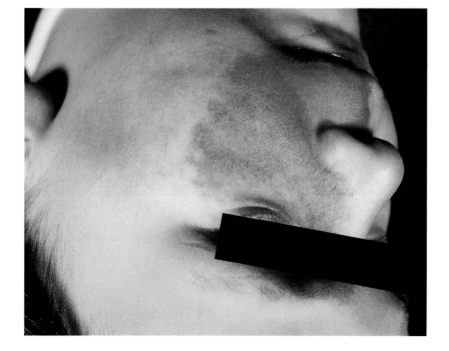

FIGURE 20-10. Port-wine stain seen in Sturge–Weber disease.

(Reproduced, with permission, from Wolff K, Johnson RA, Suurmond D. *Fitzpatrick's Color Atlas & Synopsis of Clinical Dermatology*, 5th ed. New York: McGraw-Hill, 2005: 187.)

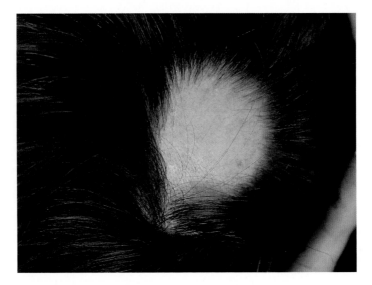

FIGURE 20-15. Alopecia areata of scalp: solitary lesion.
A sharply outlined portion of the scalp with complete alopecia without scaling, erythema, atrophy, or scarring. Empty follicles can still be seen on the involved scalp. The short, broken-off hair shafts (so-called exclamation point hair) appear as very short stubs emerging from the bald scalp. (Reproduced, with permission, from Wolff K, Johnson RA, Suurmond D. *Fitzpatrick's Color Atlas & Synopsis of Clinical Dermatology*, 5th ed. New York: McGraw-Hill, 2005: 956.)

See Table 20-1.

Hair Loss

MOST COMMON ETIOLOGIES

- Tinea capitis (see p. 524).
- Trichotillomania.
- Alopecia areata.

Trichotillomania (Hair Pulling)

DEFINITION

- Traumatic hair pulling resulting in breaking of hair shafts at different lengths.
- Can also involve eyebrows or eyelashes.

ETIOLOGY

- Habitual.
- Sign of psychiatric disorder.
- Reaction to stress.

SIGNS AND SYMPTOMS

- Patchy hair loss of scalp (often on side of dominant hand).
- Loss of eyebrows, eyelashes.
- Close examination of hair demonstrates hair shafts broken at different lengths.

TABLE 20-1. Neonatal Dermatologic Conditions

CONDITION	ETIOLOGY	APPEARANCE	RESOLUTION
Sebaceous hyperplasia	Maternal hormones	Shiny, yellow papules	A few weeks
Acne neonatorum	Maternal hormones	Similar to minor acne vulgaris	Peaks at 2 months
Milia	Retention of dead skin and oily material in hair follicles	White papules on face	Within first month
Erythema toxicum	Unknown, possible hypersensitivity	Blotchy red spots with overlying white or yellow papules or pustules	A few days
Mongolian spots	Melanocytes arrested in migration from neural crest to epidermis	Congenital, blue-gray macules, especially in nonwhite infants	First few years of life, though some never disappear

Note: All of these conditions are diagnosed clinically, are self-limited, and rarely require treatment.

HIGH-YIELD FACTS

DERMATOLOGIC DISEASE

TREATMENT

- Behavioral modification.
- Consider psychiatry/psychology referral.

Alopecia Areata (Figure 20-15)

DEFINITION

Total hair loss in localized area.

ETIOLOGY

Immunologic mediated loss of hair. Infiltration of lymphocytes may be relapsing/remitting in some children.

SIGNS AND SYMPTOMS

- Loss of every hair within area.
- Exclamation point hairs.

TREATMENT

- High rates of spontaneous resolution/regrowth within 12 months.
- In some cases, steroids (systemic, topical, or local injection).
- Minoxidil or other immune modulation.

Dermatologic Manifestations of Some Infectious Diseases

See Table 20-2.

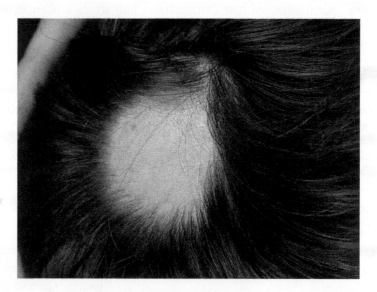

FIGURE 20-15. Alopecia areata of scalp: solitary lesion.

A sharply outlined portion of the scalp with complete alopecia without scaling, erythema, atrophy, or scarring. Empty follicles can still be seen on the involved scalp. The short, broken-off hair shafts (so-called exclamation point hair) appear as very short stubs emerging from the bald scalp. (Reproduced, with permission, from Wolff K, Johnson RA, Suurmond D. *Fitzpatrick's Color Atlas & Synopsis of Clinical Dermatology*, 5th ed. New York: McGraw-Hill, 2005: 956.)

TABLE 20-2. Dermatologic Manifestations of Some Infectious Diseases

Rubella (German measles)	■ Pink macules and papules, initially on face and spread inferiorly within 24 hr *Face*
Measles (rubeola; a paramyxovirus)	■ Erythematous macules and papules initially along hairline, spreading inferiorly within 2–3 days, fade within 4–6 days with subsequent desquamation *Hairline* ■ Koplik's spots: Bluish-white papules on erythematous base appear on day 1–2 of fever, over buccal mucosa, adjacent to second molars
Hand, foot, and mouth disease (coxsackie A virus)	■ Vesicles rapidly open to painful ulcers, soft palate is common location ■ Gray blisters on hands and feet on background erythema
Rocky Mountain spotted fever (*Rickettsia rickettsii*)	■ 2- to 6-mm blanchable macules that first appear peripherally on wrists, forearms, ankles, palms, and soles ■ Spreads to trunk, proximal extremities, and face within 6–18 hr ■ Evolve to deep red papules and petechiae over 1–3 days Within 2–4 days, exanthem is no longer blanchable
Erythema infectiosum (fifth disease; parvovirus B19)	■ "Slapped cheeks"—red papules coalesce on face *Reticulate* ■ Reticulate rash on buttocks and upper arms that spreads ■ Palms and soles may be involved ■ Mucous membranes may have red spots
Meningococcemia (*Neisseria meningitidis*)	■ Discrete, pink macules, papules, and petechiae over trunk, extremities, and palate
Gonococcemia (*Neisseria gonorrhoeae*)	■ Erythematous macules over arms and legs evolve into hemorrhagic, painful pustules within 2–3 days
Syphilis (*Treponema pallidum*)	■ Primary: Painless "button-like" chancre with indurated borders ■ Secondary: Multiple, discrete, firm, "ham-colored" papules scattered symmetrically over trunk, palm, soles, and genitals; condyloma lata—soft, flat-topped, pink papules in anogenital region ■ Tertiary: Some untreated develop brown, firm plaques on body
Lyme disease (*Borrelia burgdorferi*)	■ Erythema chronicum migrans—expanding, erythematous, annular plaque with central clearing
Kawasaki disease (etiology unknown)	■ Erythematous macules and plaques appear in a stocking-and-glove distribution 1–3 days after onset of fever ■ Spreads to involve trunk and extremities within 2 days, lasts an average of 12 days

See Table 20-3.

TABLE 20-3. **Dermatologic Manifestations of Systemic Disease**

Tuberous sclerosis	**Ash leaf:** Hypopigmented lesions anywhere on body
	Shagreen patches: Raised patches on lower back with orange-peel texture
	Adenoma sebaceum: Red, vascular nodules on face that may resemble aggravated acne
	Periungual fibromas
Neurofibromatosis	**Café-au-lait spots:** Flat, sharply demarcated, ovoid, light brown macules, with the long axis oriented along a cutaneous nerve track
Sturge-Weber syndrome	**Port-wine stain:** Hemangioma variant; appears as a sharply marginated, red or purple macule, commonly distributed unilaterally on the face; present at birth and never disappears; lesion grows proportionately to the size of the individual and may develop papular and nodular areas (see Figure 20-13)
Bacterial endocarditis	**Osler's nodes:** Tender, violaceous subcutaneous nodules on palms and soles
	Janeway lesions: Multiple, hemorrhagic, nontender macules on fingers and toes
	Subungual splinter hemorrhages
	Multiple, nonblanching red macules (petechiae) on upper chest and mucous membranes
Obesity, endocrinopathy, malignancy (GI)	**Acanthosis nigricans:** Velvety, hyperpigmented plaques; occur in axillae and groin
Peutz-Jeghers syndrome	**Lentigines:** Hyperpigmented macules on nose, mouth, oral cavity, hands, and feet

- Consult multiple sources:
  - Child: Young children usually report information in concrete terms but give accurate details about their emotional states.
  - Parents.
  - Teachers.
  - Child welfare/justice.
- Methods of gathering information:
  - Play, stories, drawing.
  - Kaufman Assessment Battery for Children (K-ABC): Intelligence test for ages 2½ to 12.
  - Wechsler Intelligence Scale for Children–Revised (WISC-R): Intelligence quotient (IQ) for ages 6–16.
  - Peabody Individual Achievement Test (PIAT): Tests academic achievement.

MENTAL RETARDATION (MR)

See Neurologic Disease chapter.

LEARNING DISORDERS

See Neurologic Disease chapter.

BEHAVIORAL DISORDERS

DEFINITION

Behavioral disorders include oppositional defiant disorder and conduct disorder.

Oppositional Defiant Disorder (ODD)

 A 9-year-old boy's mother has been called to school because her son is defiant toward the teacher and does not comply with her requests to follow the rules. His parents reports similar scenarios at home, and he often becomes argumentative with them. *Think: Oppositional defiant disorder.*

ODD is a common mental health condition in children. It is more common in boys. A certain degree of oppositional behavior may be normal in childhood. However, normal defiance should not impair significant social relationship or academic performance. Children with this condition have substantially impaired relationships with parents, teachers, and peers. They might not show oppositional behavior in the pediatrician office. The diagnosis is therefore based on reports from the parents or teachers. Attention deficit/hyperactivity disorder (ADHD) and other mood disorders may coexist.

DIAGNOSIS

- *Diagnostic and Statistical Manual of Mental Disorders*, 4th ed. (DSM-IV) definition: Recurrent pattern of negativistic, defiant, disobedient, and hostile behavior for 6 months.
- Consistent pattern of disobedience toward parent or teacher
- Four or more of the following criteria are usually present:
  - Loses temper.
  - Argues with adults.
  - Refuses to follow rules.
  - Deliberately annoys others.
  - Does not take responsibility for mistakes or behavior.
  - Sensitive, touchy, easily annoyed.
  - Angry, resentful.
  - Spiteful, vindictive.
  - Behavior causes impairment in social and academic functioning.
- Rule out other causes of clinical presentation.

PATHOPHYSIOLOGY

Low self-esteem, low frustration tolerance, precocious use of substances.

EPIDEMIOLOGY

- Prevalence: 2–16%.
- May be a precursor of a conduct disorder.
- ↑ incidence of substance abuse, mood disorders, disorder (ADHD).

TREATMENT

- Behavioral therapy, problem-solving skills.
- Early intervention is more effective than waiting for a child to grow out of it.
- Parental management training.

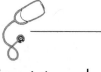

Temper tantrums and breath holding are manipulative behaviors.

ODD can be a developmental antecedent to conduct disorder. The former does not involve violation of the basic rights of others.

Conduct Disorder

 A 9-year-old boy's mother has been called to school because her son has been hitting other children and stealing pens. She reports that he often pokes their family cat with sharp objects. *Think: Conduct disorder.*

This disorder involves a variety of problematic behaviors, including oppositional and defiant behaviors and antisocial activities such as lying, stealing, running away, and physical violence. It is a pattern of behavior that violates the basic rights of others. The basic problem is a chronic conflict with parents, teachers, and peers. It is two to three times more common in boys. Conduct disorder is difficult to treat, and these behaviors are more likely to persist into adulthood.

DIAGNOSIS

- Chronic conflict with parents, teachers, or peers.
- A repetitive and persistent pattern of behavior that involves violation of the basic rights of others or of social norms and rules, with at least three of the following in 1 year:
  - Aggression toward people and animals.
  - Destruction of property.

- Deceitfulness or theft.
- Serious violation of rules.
- The change in behavior causes significant impairment in social, academic, or occupational functioning.
- A closely linked behavior is juvenile delinquency, which is a tendency to break the law or engage in illicit behavior.

ETIOLOGY

- Lack of empathy is an important risk factor.
- Involves genetic and psychosocial factors.

EPIDEMIOLOGY

- Prevalence: 6–16% in boys, 2–9% in girls.
- Up to 40% risk of developing antisocial personality disorder in adulthood.
- ↑ incidence of ADHD, learning disorders, mood disorders, substance abuse, and criminal behavior in adulthood.

TREATMENT

Multimodal:

- Structured environment, firm rules, consistent enforcement.
- Psychotherapy: Behavior modification, problem-solving skills.
- Adjunctive pharmacotherapy may help: Antipsychotics, lithium, selective serotonin reuptake inhibitors (SSRIs).

Conduct disorder is one of the most difficult mental health problems during adolescence.

Conduct disorder is the most common diagnosis in outpatient psychiatry clinics.

ATTENTION DEFICIT/HYPERACTIVITY DISORDER (ADHD)

A 9-year-old boy's mother has been called to school because her son has not done his homework. He claims that he did not know about the assignments. He interrupts other kids and is always getting up during class. His parents report that he cannot sit still at the dinner table. *Think: ADHD.*

ADHD is a common psychiatric disorder present in up to 10% of school-age children. Onset of symptoms occurs before age 7 yr. Inattention and distractibility is the hallmark. Classic triad: impaired attention, impulsivity, and excessive motor activity. Symptoms must be present in two or more situations, such as school and home. The diagnosis of ADHD is clinical.

DEFINITION

Three types predominantly:

- Inattentive.
- Hyperactive-impulsive
- Combined: Most children have the combined type.

DIAGNOSIS

- Six or more of the following for 6 months:
  - Inattention: Problems listening, concentrating, paying attention to details, organizing tasks, easily distracted, forgetful.

The diagnosis of ADHD is clinical.

Onset of ADHD occurs no later than age 7 yr.

The three cardinal signs of ADHD:

- Inattention
- Hyperactivity
- Impulsivity

Symptoms **must** be present in two or more situations for a diagnosis of ADHD.

Up to 15–20% continue to have ADHD in adulthood.

Stimulants used appropriately for ADHD do not cause addiction.

ADHD is the most common significant behavioral syndrome in childhood.

- Hyperactivity-impulsivity: Unable to inhibit impulses in social behavior, → blurting out, interrupting, fidgeting, leaving seat, talking excessively.
- Combined subtype: Six or more symptoms of inattention and hyperactivity-impulsivity.
- Onset before age 7 yr.
- Behavior inconsistent with age and development.
- Impairment in two or more social settings.
- Evidence of impairment in functioning.
- The above may →:
  - Difficulty getting along with peers and family.
  - School underachievement secondary to poor organizational skills.
  - Poor sequential memory, deficits in fine motor skills.
- Medical conditions and sleep conditions must be ruled out before a diagnosis of ADHD is made.
- Important to rule out other situations that can trigger ADHD-type behaviors, such as death in the family, divorce, inner ear infection that causes temporary hearing problems, anxiety or depression, learning disability, child abuse.

ETIOLOGY

- Genetic predisposition.
- Environmental factors.
- Perinatal complications, maternal nutrition and substance abuse, obstetric complications, viral infections.
- Neurochemical/neurophysiologic factors.
- Psychosocial factors, including emotional deprivation and parental anxiety and inexperience.
- Family dysfunction.

PATHOPHYSIOLOGY

- Catecholamine hypothesis, a ↓ in norepinephrine metabolites.
- Hypodopaminergic function, low levels of homovanillic acid.

EPIDEMIOLOGY

- Prevalence: 3–10% among young and school-age children.
- Male-to-female ratio: 3:1.
- ↑ incidence of mood disorders, personality disorders, conduct disorder, and ODD.
- Most cases improve in adolescence; 20% have symptoms into adulthood.

TREATMENT

- Pharmacotherapy:
  - Psychostimulants (first-line drugs): Methylphenidate (Ritalin), dextroamphetamine, pemoline.
  - Atomoxetine (second-line drug).
  - Atypical antipsychotics: On the rise; work by blocking dopamine.
  - Clonidine: Caution when using in combination with methylphenidate.

- Psychotherapy:
  - Behavior modification, cognitive behavioral therapy.
  - Parental counseling: Positive reinforcement, firm nonpunitive limit setting, reduce external stimulation.
  - Group therapy: Social skills, self-esteem.

PERVASIVE DEVELOPMENTAL DISORDERS (PDDs)

DEFINITION

- Group of conditions that involve problems with social skills, language, and behaviors.
- Apparent early in life with developmental delay involving multiple areas of development.
- Include autistic disorder, Asperger syndrome, Rett syndrome, and childhood disintegrative disorder.
- Pervasive developmental disorder not otherwise specified (PDD-NOS; atypical autism): Diagnosed when criteria are not met for any of the above.

TREATMENT

- There is no cure, but goal of treatment is to manage symptoms and improve social skills.
- Remedial education.
- Behavioral therapy.
- Neuroleptics such as haloperidol to control self-injurious and aggressive behavior and mood lability.
- SSRIs to help control stereotyped and repetitive behaviors.

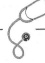
The most efficacious pharmacotherapeutic agents for ADHD are psychostimulants, though behavioral modification and firm limit setting should also be used. Seventy-five percent of patients have significant improvement on Ritalin.

Autistic Disorder

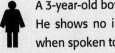
A 3-year-old boy is brought in by his parents because they think he is deaf. He shows no interest in them or anyone around him and speaks only when spoken to directly. He often lines his toys up in a straight line. Hearing tests are normal. *Think: Autism.*

Autism is a spectrum of behaviors that include abnormalities in social interactions, aberrant communication, and restricted repetitive and stereotyped behaviors. The onset is usually before age 3 yr. Speech is typically delayed or may regress. It is often associated with mental retardation.

Seventy percent of children with autistic disorder are mentally retarded, though a few have narrow remarkable abilities (savants). Only 1–2% can function completely independently as adults.

Spectrum of pervasive developmental disorders characterized by various degrees of impaired social interaction and communication and repetitive, stereotyped patterns of behavior.

DIAGNOSIS

- Diagnosis made within the first 3 yr and other causes of the clinical presentation ruled out.
- It is based on behavior, not cause.
- Parents usually notice signs in the first 2 yr of the child's life.

Autism is not caused by thimerosal-containing vaccines.

Standard developmental screening tests have poor sensitivity for autism.

Two areas are particularly affected in autistic disorder:
- Communication
- Social interactions

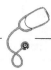

Computed tomography (CT) and magnetic resonance imaging (MRI) in autistic disorder show ventricular enlargement; polymicrogyria; and small, densely packed, immature cells in the limbic system and cerebellum.

Half of children with autistic disorder never speak.

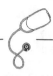

Those with autistic disorder who do speak exhibit echolalia, pronoun reversal, inappropriate cadence or intonation, impaired semantics, and failure to use language for social interaction.

- Characteristic triad: Impairments in social interaction, impairments in communication, and restricted interests and repetitive behaviors.
- At least six of the following (with at least two from qualitative impairment in social interaction, one from qualitative impairments in communication, and one from patterns of behavior):
  - Qualitative impairment in social interaction (at least two):
    - Marked impairment in the use of multiple nonverbal behaviors, including poor eye contact.
    - Failure to develop peer relationships and attachments.
    - Lack of spontaneous seeking to share enjoyment, interests, achievements.
    - Lack of emotional or social reciprocity.
  - Qualitative impairments in communication (at least one):
    - Delay or lack of spoken language (expressive language deficit).
    - Marked impairment in the ability to initiate or sustain a conversation with others.
    - Stereotyped and repetitive use of language or idiosyncratic language.
    - Lack of spontaneous make-believe play or social initiative.
  - Repetitive and stereotyped patterns of behavior and activities (at least one):
    - Inflexible rituals: Unvarying pattern of daily activities.
    - Preoccupations.
    - Highly responsive to intimate environment, stimulus overselectivity, unable to cope with change in routine.

ETIOLOGY

- Genetic predisposition (36% concordance rate in monozygotic twins, 0% in dizygotic twins).
- Prenatal neurologic insult.
- Immunologic and biochemical factors.

PATHOPHYSIOLOGY

- Neuroanatomic structural abnormalities.
- Abnormalities in dopamine and serotonin system: ↑ in serotonin.

EPIDEMIOLOGY

- Prevalence: 10–15:10,000.
- Male-to-female ratio: 4:1.
- Diagnosis first year (25%), second year (50%), after 2 years (25%).
- Significant comorbidity with fragile X syndrome, tuberous sclerosis, mental retardation, and seizures.

PROGNOSIS

- No effective treatment.
- Depends on presence or absence of underlying disorder and speech.

Asperger Syndrome

DIAGNOSIS

- Impaired social interaction (at least two, similar to autistic disorder).
- Restricted or stereotyped behaviors, interests, or activities.
- No substantial delay in language development (unlike autistic disorders).

Rett Syndrome

A 4-year-old girl with prior history of severe mental retardation is brought in for evaluation. She has been developing normally until 18 months of age, when she acquired dementia and her head circumference plateaued. She wrings her hands and has ataxia and marked loss of gross motor skills. *Think: Rett syndrome.*

Rett syndrome is a pervasive developmental disorder. It is a genetic disorder in which developmental arrest typically occurs between 6 and 18 months. Parents may report gross motor development delay, disinterest in play, and loss of eye contact. Hand wringing is a hallmark of this condition. Rapid deterioration may occur. This diagnosis should be considered in a previously healthy child with normal development who develops deceleration of head growth.

> Unlike those with autistic disorder, children with Asperger syndrome have normal language and cognitive development.

DIAGNOSIS

- Normal pre- and perinatal development until between 6 and 18 months of age.
- Normal head circumference at birth, but ↓ rate of growth between the ages of 6 and 18 months.
- Loss of previously learned purposeful hand skills between the ages of 6 and 30 months, followed by the development of stereotyped hand movements.
- Early loss of social interaction, usually followed by subsequent improvement.
- Problems with gait or trunk movements: 50% of females are not ambulatory.
- Severely impaired language and psychomotor development.
- The diagnosis is also supported by a positive mutational analysis of *MECP2*.
- Prone to seizure disorders and gastrointestinal complaints (constipation).

> Generally, autistic disorders more common in boys except Rett syndrome (more common in girls).

EPIDEMIOLOGY

- Classically restricted to females; males are beginning to be recognized due to genetic testing.
- The gene for Rett syndrome is located on the X chromosome.

PROGNOSIS

- Females can live up to 40 years of age.
- Currently, there is no cure.

Childhood Disintegrative Disorder

DIAGNOSIS

- Normal development in the first 2 years of life.
- Loss of previously acquired skills in at least two of the following:
  - Language.
  - Social and self-care skills.
  - Bowel or bladder control.
  - Play skills.
  - Motor skills.
- At least two of the following:
  - Impaired social interaction.
  - Impaired use of language.
  - Restricted, repetitive, and stereotyped behaviors and interests.
- Regression can be very sudden.

EPIDEMIOLOGY

- Onset ages 2–10 yr.
- Four to eight times higher incidence in boys.
- Rare.

TREATMENT

- No permanent cure.
- Behavior therapy: Aims to teach child how to relearn skills that are lost.

TIC DISORDERS

Tics

- Sudden, repetitive, stereotyped movements (motor tics) and utterances (phonic tics).
- Most common motor tics involve the face and head (eg, blinking of eyes).
- Examples of vocal tics include coprolalia (repetitive speaking of obscene words) and echolalia (exact repetition of words).

Tourette Syndrome

 A 13-year-old boy has had uncontrollable blinking since he was 9 years old. Recently, he has noticed that he often involuntarily makes a barking noise that is embarrassing. *Think: Tourette syndrome.*

It is characterized by motor and phonic (or vocal) tics. Tics are defined as involuntary, sudden, intermittent, repetitive movements (motor tics) or sounds (phonic tics). Comorbidities, such as ADHD and obsessive-compulsive disorder, are common. The age of onset is before 18 yr but most children shows readily identifiable symptoms by age 7 yr.

DIAGNOSIS

- Multiple motor and vocal tics occurring multiple times per day, almost daily for > 1 yr (no tic-free period for > 3 months).
- Onset before age 18.
- Distress or impairment in social functioning.

EPIDEMIOLOGY

- Three times more common in boys.
- Onset usually between the ages of 7 and 8 yr.
- High comorbidity with obsessive-compulsive disorder (OCD) and ADHD.

ETIOLOGY

- Genetic: 50% concordance rate in monozygotic twins, 8% in dizygotic.
- Neurochemical: Impaired regulation of dopamine in the caudate nucleus.

TREATMENT

- Most cases are mild and do not require drug therapy.
- Supportive psychobehavioral therapy, education, and reassurance.
- Pharmacotherapy when symptoms interfere with functioning: Haloperidol or pimozide.

> Tics in Tourette syndrome may be consciously repressed for short periods of time.

ELIMINATION DISORDERS

Enuresis

DIAGNOSIS

- Lack of involuntary urinary continence beyond age 4 for diurnal enuresis and age 6 for nocturnal enuresis.
- Occurs at least twice per week for at least 3 consecutive months.
- Types:
  - Primary: Child never established continence.
  - Secondary: Most commonly occurs between ages 5 and 8 yr.
- Rule out the influence of a medical condition (eg, urethritis, diabetes, seizures).

ETIOLOGY

- Genetic predisposition.
- Physical factors: Small bladder, low nocturnal levels of antidiuretic hormone (ADH).
- Delayed or stringent toilet training.
- Psychosocial stressors.

EPIDEMIOLOGY

Prevalence: 7% male and 3% female at age 5 yr; 3% male and 2% female prevalence at age 10 yr.

SIGNS AND SYMPTOMS

- Urination during the day, night, or both on the individual.
- Nocturnal (nighttime only) is the most common subtype.
- Diurnal (daytime only) is more common in females.

TREATMENT

- According to specific causative factors suggested by an adequate psychosocial evaluation.
- Enlist child in cure, offer positive reinforcement, do not punish; older children participate in cleaning up.
- No liquids after dinner; urinate before going to bed.
- Behavior modification therapy (eg, buzzer to wake up child when wetness is detected).
- Pharmacotherapy: Antidiuretics (desmopressin [DDAVP]) or tricyclic antidepressants (imipramine).

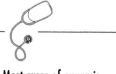

Most cases of enuresis spontaneously remit by age 7.

Encopresis

DIAGNOSIS

- Repeated passage of feces into inappropriate places (eg, clothing or floor) whether involuntary or intentional.
- Behavior must occur once a month for 3 months.
- Individual must be at least 4 years old.
- Rule out the influence of a medication or a general medical condition (eg, hypothyroidism, lower gastrointestinal [GI] problems, dietary factors).

ETIOLOGY

- Anxiety about defecating in a particular place.
- A more generalized anxiety in response to stressful environmental factors.
- Oppositional behavior.
- Physiologic conditions: Lack of sphincter control, constipation with overflow incontinence.

EPIDEMIOLOGY

- Prevalence: 1% in 5-year-old children (less common than enuresis).
- Incidence ↓ with age.
- More common in males than females.
- Associated with other conditions such as conduct disorder and ADHD.

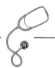

Encopresis in a 7-year-old child likely indicates a more serious disturbance than thumb-sucking in a 4-year-old, which is more serious than a nightmare in a 5-year-old, breath-holding spells in a 2-year-old, and nocturnal enuresis in a 6-year-old.

TREATMENT

- According to the specific causative factors suggested by an adequate psychosocial evaluation.
- Enlist child in cure, positive reinforcement; do not punish.
- Older children participate in cleaning up.
- Choose a specific time every day to attempt bowel movement.
- Stool softeners: Majority of encopresis cases involve constipation.
- Psychotherapy, family therapy, and behavioral therapy.

- Depressive disorders can be classified into three types:
  - Major depressive disorder (MDD).
  - Dysthymic disorder (DD).
  - Depressive disorder not otherwise specified (NOS).
- **Dysthymic disorder:** Symptoms are less intense but last longer than major depressive disorder. Characterized by chronically depressed or irritable mood (at least 1 year) and must have two of the following symptoms: appetite disturbance, sleep disturbance, fatigue, low self-esteem, poor concentration, difficulty making decisions, or feelings of hopelessness.
- **Depressive disorder NOS:** Clinically significant depressive symptoms but does not meet criteria for any specific mood disorder or adjustment disorder with depressed mood.

Fifty to sixty percent of individuals with a single depressive episode can be expected to have a second episode.

Major Depressive Disorder (MDD)

DEFINITION

- Pathologic sadness or despondency not explained as a normal response to stress and causing an impairment in function.
- Recurrent condition that generally continues into adulthood.

ETIOLOGY/PATHOPHYSIOLOGY

- Genetic predisposition.
- Catecholamine hypothesis: Depression is caused by a deficit of norepinephrine at nerve terminals throughout the brain.
- Cortisol hypothesis: Larger quantities of cortisol metabolites in blood and urine, abnormal diurnal variation.

Electroencephalography (EEG) in depression shows ↓ slow-wave (delta) sleep, shortened time before onset of rapid eye movement (REM), and longer duration of REM.

EPIDEMIOLOGY

- Prevalence: 2% of children; 4–8% of adolescents.
- Twenty-eight percent of child psychiatry clinic patients.
- Fifteen to twenty percent incidence in adolescents.
- Two to three times higher in postpubertal girls than boys.
- Other mental disorders frequently co-occur with major depressive episode including anxiety/panic disorders, OCD, eating disorders, substance abuse, borderline personality disorder, ADHD, and ODD.

In suspected cases of depression, be sure to look for other signs or risk factors such as school failure or family history of mental health disorders.

DIAGNOSIS

- Depressed mood with at least five of the following signs lasting more than 2 weeks:
  - Depressed mood.
  - Loss of interest in activities.
  - Plus, four or more of the following for 2 weeks or longer:
    - Sleep disturbance.
    - Weight change or appetite disturbance.
    - ↓ concentration.
    - Suicidal ideation.
    - Psychomotor agitation or retardation.
    - Fatigue or loss of energy.
    - Feelings of worthlessness or inappropriate guilt.

A combination of treatments for depression may be necessary. Childhood depression should be treated with behavior modification before medication.

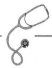

Use of antidepressant medications in adolescents may ↑ risk of suicidal thoughts and behaviors during initial weeks due to disinhabition.

One percent of suicide gestures are lethal.

Seventy-five percent of those who go on to attempt suicide convey their suicidal intentions directly or indirectly.

Girls attempt suicide more but boys are more successful.

Thirty to seventy percent of suicides occur with significant alcohol or drug abuse. Substance abuse disinhibits the individual to complete the act.

■ Always rule out other causes of the clinical presentation (eg, hypothyroidism, nutritional deficiency, chronic infection/systemic disease, substance abuse).

COMPLICATIONS

■ Can persist into adulthood.
■ Up to 15% of patients with depression commit suicide each year.

TREATMENT

■ If suicidal or homicidal, admit to the hospital.
■ Biopsychosocial approach.
■ Cognitive behavior therapy (CBT).
■ Individual and/or group therapy.
■ Family intervention.
■ TCAs, SSRIs. TCAs have risk of lethal overdose—look for convulsions, coma, and cardiac arrythmias in toxicity.
■ Electric shock therapy: Catatonic syndrome or intractable depression.
■ For adolescents, CBT and SSRIs appear to be most effective.

Suicide

DEFINITION

■ Suicide is a complex human behavior with biologic, sociologic, and psychological roots that results in a self-inflicted death that is intentional rather than accidental.
■ Suicide ideation, with or without a plan.
■ Suicide gesture—for attention, without intent for death.
■ Suicide attempt.

ETIOLOGY

■ Genetic predisposition.
■ Psychiatric disorders: Correlations of suicidal behavior and mood or disruptive disorders, substance abuse.
■ Environmental factors: Stressful life events; family disruption due to death or separation, illness, birth, or siblings; peer pressure; physical or sexual abuse.
■ Parental influence: Psychiatric illness, substance abuse, violence, physical or sexual abuse.

EPIDEMIOLOGY

■ Attempted suicides account for 6% of deaths in 10- to 14-year-olds, 11% of deaths in 15- to 19-year-olds.
■ Third leading cause of death for young adults aged 10–19.
■ In the United States, there are about 50–100 attempts for each complete suicide; 8–9% of U.S. adolescents attempt suicide.
■ Boys more frequently complete suicide, but girls attempt more often. (Girls tend to choose less lethal methods like overdose, cutting; boys will choose firearms, hanging).
■ The rate of suicide is higher in Alaskan, Asian-American, and Native American youth.
■ Of the 1–2% of those who attempt suicide, 10% will eventually complete the act.

- **Risk factors:** Look for psychiatric disorders, prior attempts, family clustering of suicides, substance use/abuse, history of sexual abuse, or serotonin abnormalities.

DIAGNOSIS

- Even though risk factors for suicide are known, it is not possible to predict who will commit suicide.
- Assess signs and symptoms, correlate with other clinical variables such as psychiatric and substance abuse history, gender, age, race, prior history of suicide attempts, and recent traumatic life events.
- **Key questions:** Are you having any thoughts about harming yourself or taking your life? Have you developed a plan? What is your plan?

TREATMENT

- Immediate hospitalization; remove all potentially lethal items.
- Psychotherapeutic intervention, trustful atmosphere, coping strategies; remove motivation for suicide; involve parents and relatives, guidance counselor.
- Pharmacotherapy depends on the accompanying diagnosis.

VIOLENT BEHAVIOR

EPIDEMIOLOGY

- Homicide is the second leading cause of death among 15- to 19-year-olds and the leading cause of death in African-American adolescents.
- Rates of homicide are higher in males than in females.
- Death by firearm homicide is highest in the 15- to 24-year-old age group.

RISK FACTORS

- Look for clinical entities associated with violent behavior such as mental retardation, moderate to severe language disorder, learning disorder, ADHD, mood disorders, anxiety disorders, personality disorders, conduct disorders, and ODD.
- Other risk factors: Substance abuse, gang involvement, history/exposure to domestic/child abuse, and access to firearms.

SCREENING

Ask about recent involvement in physical fights, carrying a weapon, firearms in household, concerns that an adolescent has about his/her safety, past episodes of trauma, and social problems in school or neighborhood.

SUBSTANCE ABUSE

EPIDEMIOLOGY

- Alcohol and cigarettes are the most prevalent drugs among school-age young adults.
- Marijuana is the most commonly reported illicit drug used.
- The prevalence of substance abuse varies according to age, gender, geographic region, race, and other demographic factors.

Suicidal ideation, when accompanied by a specific plan, must be taken seriously, and these patients need to be hospitalized for assistance and suicide precautions.

Suicide completers: Male, older, history of depression, alcoholism, schizophrenia, careful planning, high lethality, firearms.

Suicide attempters: Female, younger, history of depression, alcoholism, personality disorder, impulsive, no planning, low lethality, drug overdose.

SIGNS AND SYMPTOMS

See Table 21-1 for signs and symptoms of intoxication and withdrawal due to substances of abuse.

TREATMENT

- Group therapy.
- Narcotics Anonymous.
- Hospitalizations may be necessary for acute withdrawal.
- Alcohol abuse: Rule out medical complications, start benzodiazepine for withdrawal symptoms, and give thiamine before glucose to prevent Wernicke encephalopathy.

TABLE 21-1. Substances of Abuse—Intoxication and Withdrawal

SUBSTANCE	INTOXICATION/OVERDOSE	WITHDRAWAL
Alcohol	↓ fine motor control Impaired judgment and coordination Ataxic gait and poor balance Lethargy, difficulty sitting upright Respiratory depression	Irritability, insomnia, disorientation, tremor, diaphoresis (6–24 hr) Alcoholic hallucinosis (1–2 days) Delirium tremens (2–5 days)—grand mal seizures Rx: Benzodiazepines
Sedative-hypnotics (benzodiazepines, barbiturates)	Drowsiness, slurred speech Incoordination, ataxia Mood lability, impaired judgment Nystagmus Respiratory depression, coma, death Rx: Benzodiazepines—flumazenil (careful, may precipitate seizures); barbiturates—alkalinize urine; both—activated charcoal	Autonomic hyperactivity Insomnia, anxiety, tremor Nausea, vomiting Delirium, hallucinations Seizures—may be life threatening
Stimulants (cocaine, amphetamines)	Euphoria, sweating, chills, nausea Autonomic instability, cardiac arrhythmias Psychomotor agitation, dilated pupils Vasoconstriction—MI, CVA Rx: Benzodiazepines (haloperidol if severe)	Not life threatening Dysphoric "crash," depression, anxiety Hunger, craving Constricted pupils
Opioids (heroin, codeine, morphine, methadone, meperidine)	Drowsiness, slurred speech Nausea, vomiting, constipation Constricted pupils Seizures Respiratory depression Rx: Naloxone/naltrexone, methadone taper	Not life threatening Dysphoria, insomnia Lacrimation, rhinorrhea Yawning, weakness, muscle aches Sweating, piloerection, dilated pupils Nausea, vomiting Rx: Clonidine, methadone taper
Hallucinogens (mushrooms, mescaline, LSD)	Perceptual changes, papillary dilation Tachycardia, palpitations Tremors, incoordination Rx: "Talk down"	May have flashbacks later due to reabsorption of lipid stores

TABLE 21-1. Substances of Abuse—Intoxication and Withdrawal *(continued)*

SUBSTANCE	INTOXICATION/OVERDOSE	WITHDRAWAL
PCP (hallucinogen)	Violence, recklessness, impulsivity Impaired judgment, nystagmus, ataxia Hypertension, tachycardia Muscle rigidity, high pain tolerance Seizures, coma Rx: Benzodiazepines, acidify urine	As with other hallucinogens, flashbacks may occur
Marijuana (THC)	Euphoria, impaired concentration Mild tachycardia Conjunctival injection Dry mouth, ↑ appetite	No withdrawal syndrome, but mild irritability, insomnia, nausea, and ↓ appetite may occur in heavy users
Inhalants	Impaired judgment, belligerence, impulsivity Perceptual disturbances, slurred speech Ataxia, dizziness Nystagmus, tremor, hyporeflexia Lethargy, euphoria, stupor, coma Respiratory depression, cardiac arrhythmias	Does not usually occur, but can Irritability, nausea, vomiting, tachycardia Occasional hallucinations
Caffeine	Anxiety, insomnia, twitching Flushed face, rambling speech GI disturbance, diuresis	Headache, nausea, vomiting, drowsiness Anxiety, depression
Nicotine	Restlessness, insomnia, anxiety ↑ GI motility	Dysphoria, anxiety, irritability, insomnia ↑ appetite, craving

CVA, cerebrovascular accident; GI, gastrointestinal; LSD, lysergic acid diethylamide; MI, myocardial infarction; PCP, phencyclidine; Rx, treatment; THC, tetrahydrocannabinol.

ANXIETY DISORDERS

Separation Anxiety

DEFINITION

- Excessive anxiety beyond that expected for the child's developmental level related to separation or impending separation from the attachment figure.
- Separation anxiety is normal until age 3–4 yr.

EPIDEMIOLOGY

- Prevalence: 4% of school-age children.
- Males and females are affected equally.

ETIOLOGY

Contribution by parental anxiety/excessive concern expressed.

SIGNS AND SYMPTOMS

- May refuse to sleep alone or go to school.
- May complain of physical symptoms in order to avoid anxiety-provoking activities.
- Become extremely distressed when forced to separate, and may worry excessively about losing their parents forever.

TREATMENT

- Family therapy.
- Supportive psychotherapy.
- Low-dose antidepressants.

School Phobia

DEFINITION

- A child who develops emotional upset at the prospect of going to school in the absence of severe antisocial behavior.
- Related to separation anxiety.

ETIOLOGY

- Environmental, hostile, or dependent relationship between a parent and child; stressful events at home or school.
- Concurrent psychiatric disorders, depression, separation anxiety, generalized anxiety, posttraumatic stress, somatoform disorder, avoidant personality disorder.

EPIDEMIOLOGY

- More common in lower socioeconomic classes, younger children in the family, early teenage years, lack of parental interest or education.
- Equal in both males and females.
- Most frequent among younger children.
- Prevalence: 5% of elementary school children, 2% of junior high school children.

SIGNS AND SYMPTOMS

- Avoidance behavior in relation to school; seeks situations that provide comfort and security; once in school, comfortable and productive, fear of school recurs the next day despite positive experience the day before.
- Physical complaints secondary to anxiety: Anorexia, headache, abdominal pain.

DIAGNOSIS

- Marked and persistent fear that is excessive and unreasonable, instigated by the anticipation of the school situation.
- Exposure to school provokes an immediate anxiety response.
- School is avoided.
- School phobia interferes with academic and social functioning.
- Duration of at least 6 months.
- Other mental disorders ruled out.

TREATMENT

- Mainstay of treatment is returning the child to regular school attendance.
- Behavioral therapy, recognize and control anxiety symptoms.
- Anxiolytics or antidepressants for a short period of time when the symptoms are most severe.

Obsessive-Compulsive Disorder (OCD)

DEFINITIONS

- **Obsessions:** Persistent, intrusive thoughts, images, impulses involuntarily intruding into consciousness, causing distress and functional impairment. Common themes are contamination and fear of harm to self or others.
- **Compulsions:** Actions that are responses to a perceived internal obligation to follow certain rituals and rules, which may be motivated directly by obsessions or efforts to ward off certain thoughts or fears.

DIAGNOSIS

Impaired social, academic, or vocational functioning with four or more of the following:

- Preoccupied with details, rules, lists, order, organization, or schedules, resulting in loss of the goal of activity.
- Perfectionism that prohibits task completion.
- Social impairment secondary to preoccupation with work and level of productivity.
- Overconscientious, scrupulous, and inflexible about matters of morality, ethics, or values.
- Unable to discard objects of no worth or sentimental value.
- Preference to work as an individual and not in a group.
- Miserly spending in order to save for future catastrophes.
- Inflexible, rigid, stubborn.
- Characteristics must be ego-dystonic and functionally disruptive versus ego-syntonic and functionally adaptive in OCD.

ETIOLOGY

Genetic predisposition, higher concordance among monozygotic versus dizygotic twins.

EPIDEMIOLOGY

High comorbidity with ADHD and tic disorders.

SIGNS AND SYMPTOMS

- Unproductive because of preoccupation with details, rules, lists, schedules, organization, order.
- Uncompleted tasks secondary to perfectionist tendencies.
- Work habits interfere with social interactions.
- Impossible standards of morals, ethics, or values.
- Inflexible, stubborn, cheap; prefers to work as an individual and not in a group.

TREATMENT

- Long-term therapy is required.
- Maintain a professional distance from the patient.
- Establish ground rules for therapy.
- Behavioral therapy such as self-observation, extinction, operant conditioning, and modeling.
- Pharmacotherapy:
  - First-line agents are SSRIs (ie, fluoxetine, fluvoxamine, paroxetine, sertraline).
  - Clomipramine is a second-line agent.

Habit

DEFINITION

Repetitive patterns of movement used to discharge tension.

ETIOLOGY

- A stressful environment at home or school.
- Concurrent psychiatric disorders including anxiety or depression.

PATHOPHYSIOLOGY

Purposeful movement loses original meaning and becomes repetitive and a means to discharge anxiety or provide comfort.

EPIDEMIOLOGY

- Highest prevalence among 7- to 11-year-olds.
- Males: 1–13%.
- Females: 1–11%.

SIGNS AND SYMPTOMS

- Bruxism (teeth grinding or clenching).
- Tics, repetitive movement, gesture or utterance that mimics some aspect of normal behavior.
- Stuttering, impairment in speech fluency characterized by frequent repetitions or prolongations of sounds or syllables.
- Thumb-sucking, self-nurturing, and comforting behavior.

Individual is often unaware of habitual behavior.

TREATMENT

Behavior therapy: Identify habit, under what circumstances it most often occurs, work on habit reversal.

Habit reversal: Substituting another, more benign behavior for the previous habit.

Selective Mutism

DEFINITION

Not speaking in certain situations (eg, school).

EPIDEMIOLOGY

- Onset usually around age 5 or 6.
- Girls > boys.
- May be preceded by a stressful life event.

TREATMENT

Supportive psychotherapy, behavior therapy, family therapy.

DEFINITION

- **Intense, persistent,** and **pervasive** preoccupation with becoming a member of the opposite sex.
- Patients exhibit a strong and persistent cross-gender identification and a sense of inappropriateness about their assigned sex.

EPIDEMIOLOGY

- Prevalence: 1 in 30,000 males, 1 in 100,000 females.
- Coexisting separation and/or generalized anxiety disorder or depression is common.
- ↑ risk of suicide.
- Onset for boys is usually between ages 2 and 4; less clear for girls because cross-gender behaviors are more often tolerated in girls.

SIGNS AND SYMPTOMS

For genetic men: Overidentification with the mother, overtly feminine behavior, little interest in usual male pursuits, peer relationships primarily with girls.

DIAGNOSIS

- Persistent discomfort with his or her sex.
- Four or more of the following:
    - Stated desire to be or that he or she is the other sex.
    - Wearing clothes appropriate to the opposite sex.
    - Persistent role-playing or fantasies of being the opposite sex.
    - Interest in the habits of the opposite sex.
    - Preference for playmates of the opposite sex.

TREATMENT

Psychotherapy aimed at helping individual to accept his or her anatomic sex, adjustment in social and occupational areas, increasing self-esteem, and building social skills with peers.

Social and occupational adjustment is usually no better after surgery for gender identity disorder.

DEFINITION

Two subtypes:

- Restricting
- Binge eating/purging

Anorexia Nervosa

A 16-year-old girl has a 6-month history of amenorrhea and a 25-lb weight loss. She is thin, with Tanner stage 4 development of breasts and pubic hair. She also reports constipation and feeling of bloating. When you ask her about the weight loss, she states that she is "overweight." She had no menstruation in last 6 months. *Think: Anorexia nervosa.*

Anorexia nervosa is an eating disorder that is characterized by a triad of amenorrhea, weight loss, and psychiatric disturbance. Common presenting symptoms include constipation, intolerance to cold, dry skin, and hair loss. It predominantly affects females. Anorexia nervosa is associated with multiple hormonal abnormalities resulting in amenorrhea. Electrolyte abnormalities such as hyponatremia, hypokalemia, hypophosphatemia, and hypoglycemia may be present.

DIAGNOSIS

- Refusal to maintain body weight at or above 85% of ideal weight for age and height.
- Even though underweight, an intense fear of gaining weight.
- Disturbance in self-perception of body weight and lack of insight into the seriousness of physical condition.
- The absence of at least three consecutive menstrual cycles in women.

ETIOLOGY

- Genetic predisposition (6–10% of female relatives of anorexic patients have the condition, twin studies confirm).
- Psychological need to control, perfectionism.
- Conforming to society's ideal of beauty.
- Stressful life events such as leaving home for college or death in the family.

PATHOPHYSIOLOGY

- A primary hypothalamic disturbance secondary to ↑ corticotropin-releasing factor.
- Central neurotransmitter dysregulation affecting dopamine, serotonin, and norepinephrine.
- Reduced norepinephrine activity and turnover.
- Endocrine abnormalities, ↑ growth hormone levels, loss of cortisol diurnal variation, reduced luteinizing hormone (LH), follicle-stimulating hormone (FSH), impaired response to luteinizing hormone–releasing hormone (LHRH), abnormal glucose tolerance test.

EPIDEMIOLOGY

- Predominance in females (female-to-male ratio 10:1).
- One percent prevalence among women.
- Bimodal onset at 14 and 18 yr.
- More common in industrialized countries.
- Incidence has ↑ over the past two decades.
- More common in activities such as ballet, gymnastics, and modeling.

The most common cause of death in anorexia nervosa is cardiac arrhythmias due to electrolyte disturbances, particularly hypokalemia.

Electrocardiography (ECG) in anorexia nervosa may show low-voltage T-wave inversion and flattening, ST depression, supraventricular or ventricular arrhythmias, and/or prolonged QT intervals.

SIGNS AND SYMPTOMS

- Extreme dieting, special diets such as vegetarianism.
- Refusal to eat meals with family members or in public.
- Rituals surrounding meals.
- Preoccupation with food and its preparation.
- Intense fear of becoming obese, which does not diminish as weight loss progresses.
- Disturbance in the way in which one's body, weight, size, and/or shape is experienced, such as "feeling fat" although one may be emaciated.
- Denial of hunger.
- Obsessive interest in physical exercise.
- Abuse laxatives, diuretics, or stimulants in an effort to enhance weight loss.
- Studiousness and academic success.
- Multiorgan involvement:
  - Amenorrhea.
  - Hypothermia.
  - Constipation.
  - Low blood pressure, bradycardia.
  - Lanugo, hair loss.
  - Petechiae.
  - Pedal edema, dry skin.
  - Osteopenia.
- Electrolyte abnormalities: Alkalosis, hypokalemia.
- Lab abnormalities: Leukopenia, elevated liver function tests (LFTs), elevated triglycerides, carotenemia.

The long-term mortality of anorexia nervosa is 10%.

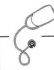

Beware of complications occurring during rehabilitation for anorexia nervosa, including congestive heart failure (CHF), cardiac arrhythmias, and overcorrection of electrolyte abnormalities.

TREATMENT

- Anorexic patients deny health risks associated with their behavior, making them resistant to treatment.
- Individual and family psychotherapy: Target abnormal and destructive thought processes.
- Behavior modification techniques to restore normal eating behavior, set specific weight goals.
- Nutritional rehabilitation: Restore nutritional state and weight.
- Pharmacologic therapy (SSRIs have been used successfully).

Bulimia Nervosa

A 15-year-old girl has bilateral parotid gland swelling and erosion of the posterior aspect of the dental enamel of her upper incisors. She reports frequent vomiting after her meal. *Think: Bulimia nervosa.*

Bulimia nervosa is characterized by recurrent episodes of binge eating defined as the rapid consumption of a large amount of food in a reasonably short period of time. The hallmark of bulimia is a fear of not being able to stop eating when the binge is in progress. Self-induced vomiting and excessive exercise are the compensatory behaviors. Parotid enlargement, dental problems, and abrasions of knuckles are due to biting down on them during self-induced vomiting. The typical age of presentation is during the teenage year.

DIAGNOSIS

- Recurrent episodes of eating within a 2-hr period of larger-than-normal proportions accompanied by a sense of lack of control over actions (binge eating).
- Unlike anorexia, these patients are at or above their expected weight.
- Recurrent compensatory behavior in order to prevent weight gain—self-induced vomiting, laxatives, diuretics, enemas, excessive exercise.
- Episodes occur at least twice a week for 3 months.
- Body shape and weight is the basis of self-evaluation.
- Does not occur exclusively during episodes of anorexia nervosa.

ETIOLOGY

Biopsychosocial.

PATHOPHYSIOLOGY

- A primary hypothalamic disturbance secondary to ↑ corticotropin-releasing factor.
- Central neurotransmitter dysregulation affecting dopamine, serotonin, and norepinephrine.
- Reduced norepinephrine activity and turnover.
- Endocrine abnormalities, low triiodothyronine (T_3), high T_3 receptor uptake (T_3RU), impaired thyrotropin-releasing hormone (TRH) responsiveness, abnormal dexamethasone suppression test.

EPIDEMIOLOGY

- Predominantly found in women (4% prevalence).
- Predominant in whites.
- More common in industrialized countries.
- Culturally dependent.

SIGNS AND SYMPTOMS

- Secretive binge-eating and purging behaviors.
- Abuse laxatives, diuretics, or stimulants in an effort to enhance weight loss.
- Obsessive interest in physical activity.
- Physical manifestations include parotid gland enlargement, dental caries, scars on dorsum of fingers (due to teeth scraping during self-induced vomiting).
- Laboratory abnormalities include dehydration, hypokalemia, hypochloremia, hypomagnesemia, elevated blood urea nitrogen (BUN), and amylase.

TREATMENT

Group therapy is the most effective treatment.

Eating Disorder Not Otherwise Specified (NOS)

DEFINITION

Abnormal eating behaviors or exhibits characteristics of other eating disorders without meeting all criteria. Examples include:

- Meets all criteria for anorexia nervosa except weight falls within normal range or does not have amenorrhea.

- Meets all criteria for bulimia nervosa but binge eating does not meet duration/frequency criteria.
- Binge eating in the absence of purging activities.

Rumination

DIAGNOSIS

- Repeated regurgitation and rechewing of food for a period of at least 1 month following a period of normal functioning.
- Onset is between 3 and 12 months in normal infant; later in the mentally retarded.
- Other medical and psychiatric conditions have been ruled out.

Rumination comes from the Greek root, *ruminare*, meaning "to chew the cud."

ETIOLOGY

- Adverse psychosocial environment.
- Mental retardation.

PATHOPHYSIOLOGY

- Unsatisfactory mother-infant relationship that causes the infant to seek an internal source of gratification.
- Positive reinforcement when attention follows rumination.
- Negative reinforcement when rumination reduces anxiety.

EPIDEMIOLOGY

Highest prevalence in normal infants and mentally retarded adults.

SIGNS AND SYMPTOMS

- Presents with "spitting up" or frequent vomiting.
- Effortless regurgitation, does not involve retching.
- Infants are irritable and hungry between episodes of regurgitation.
- Malnutrition, weight loss, failure to thrive.
- Up to 25% mortality rate.

TREATMENT

- Counseling to improve parent-child dynamics.
- Behavioral intervention.
- Aversive techniques, noxious stimulus is paired with rumination.
- Nonaversive techniques, differential reinforcement or other incompatible responses.
- In infants, the disorder frequently remits spontaneously.

Pica

DIAGNOSIS

- Persistent eating of nonnutritive substances for a period of at least 1 month (eg, clay, dirt, etc.).
- The eating of nonnutritive substances is inappropriate to the level of development.
- Behavior is not culturally sanctioned.
- Rule out other psychiatric disorders.

ETIOLOGY

- Mental retardation.
- Vitamin or mineral deficiencies (eg, iron deficiency anemia, particularly in pregnancy).
- Poverty, neglect, lack of parental supervision, developmental delays.
- Cultural belief.

Pica is found commonly in PDD and schizophrenia.

EPIDEMIOLOGY

- In children aged 18 months to 2 yr, the ingestion and mouthing of nonnutritive substances is normal behavior.
- Most common during the second and third years.
- The prevalence ↑ with the severity of mental retardation.

SIGNS AND SYMPTOMS

- Presenting complaint—"puts everything in his or her mouth."
- Direct observation of pica.
- Complications:
    - Ingestion of paint chips can → lead poisoning.
    - Hair or large objects can cause bowel obstruction.
    - Sharp objects such as pins or nails can cause intestinal perforation.
    - Ingestion of feces or dirt can result in parasitic infections.

TREATMENT

- Often remits spontaneously.
- Treat underlying vitamin deficiency, if present.
- Psychotherapy—assess why pica is occurring.
- Behavior modification.
- Direct observation and removal of potential pica.

SOMATOFORM DISORDERS

See Table 21-2 comparing somatoform disorders, factitious disorders, and malingering.

DEFINITION

- Symptoms without physical cause.
- Symptoms must cause clinically significant distress or impairment in social, occupational, or other areas of functioning.
- Includes somatization disorder, undifferentiated somatoform disorder, conversion disorder, pain disorder, hypochondriasis, body dysmorphic disorder, and somatoform disorder NOS.

TABLE 21-2. **Somatoform Disorders versus Factitious Disorders versus Malingering**

DISORDER	DEVELOPMENT OF SYMPTOMS	REASON FOR SYMPTOMS
Somatoform disorders	Unconscious	Unconscious
Factitious disorder	Conscious	Unconscious (primary gain)
Malingering	Conscious	Conscious (secondary gain)

- Psychodynamic therapy: Gain insight into unconscious conflicts and understand how psychological factors have influenced maintenance of the symptoms.
- Identify and eliminate sources of secondary gain in order to avoid reinforcing the symptoms.
- Improve self-esteem, promoting assertiveness, and teach nonsomatic ways to express distress.
- Group therapy: Learn better coping strategies and improved social skills.

Somatization Disorder

History of many physical complaints, including at least:

- Pain symptoms at more than four sites that are not intentionally produced.
- Two nonpain GI symptoms.
- One sexual or reproductive complaint.
- One pseudoneurologic complaint.
- Age of onset < 30 years old.

Conversion Disorder

DIAGNOSIS

- Sensory symptoms, motor deficits, or pseudoseizures that are not intentionally produced.
- Cannot be explained by an organic etiology.
- Initiation of the symptom or deficit preceded by a psychological stressor.
- Unintentional and involuntary.
- Appropriate investigation leaves no medical explanation of symptoms.
- Symptoms cause impairment in social functioning.
- Other etiologies for the clinical presentation are ruled out.

ETIOLOGY

- Psychodynamic theory: Certain developmental predispositions respond to particular types of stress with conversion symptoms.
- Behaviorists: A learned excess or deficit that follows a particular event or psychological state and is reinforced by a particular event or set of conditions.
- Sociocultural: Predisposition of various ethnic and social groups to respond to stress with conversion symptoms.

EPIDEMIOLOGY

- More common in women, rural areas, and lower socioeconomic classes.
- Rare in children < 10 years.
- Incidence ↑ in children who have experienced physical or sexual abuse and in those whose parents are seriously ill or have chronic pain.

Favorable prognosis for conversion disorder is associated with acute onset, definite precipitation by a stressful event, good premorbid health, and the absence of previous psychiatric illness.

Conversion disorder may be associated in some cases with history of a traumatic brain injury.

A proportion of patients diagnosed with conversion disorder go on to develop demonstrable organic pathology (eg, multiple sclerosis or seizure nidus).

HIGH-YIELD FACTS

PSYCHIATRIC DISEASE

SIGNS AND SYMPTOMS

- Paralysis, abnormal movements, inability to speak, see, hear; pseudoseizures.
- Usually occurs within the context of a primary illness such as major depression, schizophrenia, or somatization disorder.
- *La belle indifference*, the lack of interest in potentially life-altering symptoms, is common in adults, but rarely occurs in children.

Hypochondriasis

A 17-year-old girl becomes very concerned that a small lump in her left breast is "malignant cancer." Her histopathology report showed it to be entirely benign. Despite reassurance by her physician she remains excessively worried. What is the cause of her excessive fear and what is the best possible treatment?

She has hypochondriasis, which is defined as a preoccupation with fears of having, or the belief that one has, a serious disease based on misinterpretation of bodily symptoms. The key feature in this condition is an abnormal concern that one is developing or has a serious illness. Psychotherapy that includes exploration of current life problems often result in symptom resolution.

DIAGNOSIS

- Preoccupation over > 6 months with fear of having a disease based on the individual's misinterpretation of normal bodily sensations.
- Persistent preoccupation despite adequate medical evaluation and assurance.
- Causes impairment in social functioning.
- Other psychiatric diseases ruled out.

ETIOLOGY

- Associated with anxiety, depression, and narcissistic traits.
- Past experience with serious illness as a child or of a family member.

EPIDEMIOLOGY

- There is a 1–9% prevalence in young adults.
- Affects males and females equally.
- The most common age of onset is early adulthood.

Hypochondriasis can → strained social relationships because of preoccupation with perceived condition and the patient's expectation of receiving special treatment.

SIGNS AND SYMPTOMS

- Complaints involving most organ systems.
- Multiple visits to different doctors and deterioration of doctor-patient relationships.
- Individuals often believe that they are not receiving proper care so they pursue more opinions.
- Receive many evaluations and unnecessary surgeries.
- May become addicted to drugs as a result of their chronic ongoing physical complaints.

- The primary aim of therapy is to help the patient identify and manage the fear of serious illness.
- In addition to techniques helpful for somatoform disorders:
  - Behavior modification techniques: Earn points to participate in daily routine despite feeling sick.
  - Educate about physiologic mechanisms.

Body Dysmorphic Disorder

- Preoccupation with imagined defect in appearance or excessive concern about a slight physical anomaly (eg, large nose, small muscles).
- Multiple visits to plastic surgeons or dermatologists are common.

Pain Disorder

DIAGNOSIS

- Pain in one or more anatomic sites of sufficient severity to warrant medical attention but with no physical findings to account for the pain or its intensity.
- Pain causes impairment in social functioning.
- Psychological factors are directly related to the onset, severity, exacerbation, or maintenance of the pain.
- Pain is not intentionally produced or feigned.
- Rule out other causes of the clinical presentation.

ETIOLOGY

Psychiatric—common in conditions such as schizophrenia, somatization disorder, anxiety, dissociation, conversion, and depression.

PATHOPHYSIOLOGY

- A defect in ego function underlying the experience and expression of feelings.
- Psychologically stressful events are converted into somatic symptoms rather than the development and appropriate expression of emotions.

Alexithymia is the inability to express emotion.

EPIDEMIOLOGY

Affects males and females equally.

FACTITIOUS DISORDERS

Munchausen Syndrome

DEFINITION

Intentional production or feigning of symptoms (eg, thermometer manipulation, self-injury, ingestion, injection) for primary gain (eg, relief of anxiety, assuming the sick role).

HIGH-YIELD FACTS

PSYCHIATRIC DISEASE

ETIOLOGY

- Children who make themselves sick may have been victims of Munchausen by proxy.
- Experience of misuse of illness to get attention and reinforcement of these actions.

TREATMENT

- Younger children are more likely than older children/adolescents to admit to deception if approached in a direct and concerned (not accusatory) way.
- Family therapy: Recognize how family communicates through illness and identify more effective ways of communication and getting what they need from family members.
- Involvement of primary care doctor/pediatrician in confrontation.

Munchausen Syndrome by Proxy (MBP)

DEFINITION

- Intentional fabrication or actual production of symptoms in a child by a caregiver (usually the mother) in order to gain attention for themselves.
- A form of child abuse.

EPIDEMIOLOGY

- Adults who commit MBP may have a history of factitious disorders themselves.
- Ninety-eight percent of perpetrators are women.
- Mortality rate is 9%.
- Up to 75% of the morbidity involved relates to physicians trying to treat the unknown conditions.

SIGNS AND SYMPTOMS

- Conditions that do not respond to treatment or whose courses are puzzling and persistent, often:
  - Vomiting/diarrhea (ingestion, syrup of ipecac).
  - Rashes (due to scrubbing with solvents).
  - Failure to thrive.
  - Seizures.
  - Infections.
  - Adding blood or other substances to urine specimens.
- Physical or laboratory findings that are unusual, discrepant, or clinically impossible or do not occur in the absence of the parent.
- Medically knowledgeable/fascinated mother who appears to enjoy the hospital setting, who is reluctant to leave child, and herself is dramatic and desires attention.
- Family history of similar problems or unexplained death in sibling.
- Signs or history of factitious disorder in mother.

TREATMENT

- Appropriate physician suspicion, good medical records, and reporting of abuse (often multiple doctors have been visited, with little continuity).
- Caregiver requires psychiatric therapy, such as for other factitious disorders.

Malingering

DEFINITION

Intentional creation of symptoms for secondary gain (eg, getting out of going to school or doing chores).

PSYCHOLOGICAL IMPACT OF ADOPTION AND FOSTER CARE

DEFINITION

- **Adoption:** Acquiring legal guardianship of an individual.
- **Foster care:** Temporary placement of an individual who has been removed from an unsafe environment.
- **Kinship:** Placement with relatives.

ETIOLOGY

- Questions of who the other parents are and why they left him or her and the subsequent impact of the perceived abandonment.
- Parental assumptions of the behavior and personalities of the people whose union produced the child causes them to be hypervigilant.

PATHOPHYSIOLOGY

- A narcissistic injury resulting in the assumption that they were unlovable, dirty, bad, or unrewarding to the biological parents.
- Some blame the biological parents, assuming they were bad, alcoholic, or mentally ill.
- Assume abandonment could happen again.
- Unconscious rage at having been abandoned.

EPIDEMIOLOGY

- Adoption is common among individuals who are unable to have children and want a family.
- Two percent of population is adopted.
- Foster care is common among children who have been abandoned by their parents or were removed from a dysfunctional environment.

SIGNS AND SYMPTOMS

- Adolescent curious about his or her origins and early life creates conflict within the individual.
- Continually search strangers' faces for resemblances.
- Expression of feelings of abandonment and the desire to find biological parents.
- Foster child relationships may have been disrupted several times before, so the child is ambivalent toward the parents.
- Rage, stemming from initial abandonment, causes aggressive and antagonist behavior.

Child could be coached to say, "I am adopted—so what! So was President Ford!"

TREATMENT

- Individual and family therapy.
- Address disruptive behavior and the etiology.
- Address issues of abandonment.
- Enhance communication between child and parents.

- When to tell the child he or she is adopted?
    - Controversial.
    - Sooner is better (age 3–4 or earlier).
- How to tell the child he or she is adopted? According to development level.

Patterns of behavior that deviate from cultural standards, can begin in adolescence or early adulthood.
- **Cluster A: "Weird"**
    - Paranoid: Distrustful and suspicious.
    - Schizoid: Isolated, a "loner" type with limited emotional expression.
- **Cluster B: "Wild"**
    - Borderline: Unstable mood, impulsive.
    - Histrionic: Sexually provocative, attention seeking.
    - Narcissistic: Needs to be admired, has sense of entitlement.
    - Antisocial: Lacks remorse, violates laws of society, breaks the law.
- **Cluster C: "Worried"**
    - Obsessive-compulsive: See above.
    - Avoidant: Socially inhibited, intense fear of ridicule and being disliked.
    - Dependent: Submissive, needs to be taken care of, cannot be on their own.

Pediatric Life Support

- The great majority of pediatric cardiopulmonary arrests outside the hospital setting occur with parents or their surrogates (ie, teachers, coaches, day care workers, babysitters) nearby. BLS courses should be particularly targeted toward these individuals.
- Most cardiac arrests in children are caused by **progressive respiratory failure** and **circulatory collapse.**

EPIDEMIOLOGY

- Primary cardiac arrest is rather uncommon in children. It is most often **asphyxial,** resulting from respiratory failure or shock, or both.
- Outcomes are generally poor: Out-of-hospital setting 5–12% survival; in-hospital setting about 27% survival.
- The incidence of pediatric arrests is highest during infancy (age < 1) and approaches that observed in adults, but is lower among children and adolescents.
- Survival to discharge is more common among children and adolescents than infants or adults.
- During **infancy,** the leading causes of arrest are **injuries** (intentional and unintentional), **respiratory diseases, airway obstruction** (eg, foreign body aspiration), **sepsis, drowning,** and **sudden infant death syndrome (SIDS).**
- During **childhood** and **adolescence,** the leading cause of arrest is **injury** (intentional and unintentional).
- **Injuries** should be viewed as **preventable** (not accidents), and education about injury prevention is an important aspect of pediatric BLS.

Injury is the leading cause of pediatric arrest in children over age 1 yr.

FATAL PEDIATRIC INJURIES

Most common causes of fatal pediatric injuries:

1. **Motor vehicle injuries:**
   - Nearly 50% of all pediatric injuries or deaths.
   - Risk factors include misuse of child seat restraints, seat belts, and airbags; adolescent drivers; and intoxicated drivers.
2. **Pedestrian injuries:** Leading cause of injury in ages 5–9.
3. **Bicycle injuries:** Helmets reduce morbidity of head and brain injuries by 85–90%.
4. **Drownings:**
   - Twenty percent of drowning victims who survive suffer permanent brain injury secondary to prolonged hypoxia.
   - Children younger than age 4 are at especially high risk.
   - Alcohol is often associated with adolescent drownings.
5. **Burns:**
   - Eighty percent of all fatalities occur from house fires (mostly from smoke inhalation).
   - Smoke detectors can reduce morbidity and mortality of house fires by 90%.
   - Contact burns, electrical burns, and scaldings most often affect children below the age of 4.

Remember, injury in children is not always an accident.

6. **Firearms:**
   - Second leading cause of death in all adolescent males and the leading cause of death in African-American adolescents.
   - Two-thirds of American households have firearms; one-third have a handgun.

Motor vehicles are the leading cause of pediatric injuries.

BURNS

- Upper extremities most frequent, followed by face and neck.
- Pediatric considerations:
  - Larger body surface area-to-body mass ratio.
  - ↑ fluid loss → greater fluid resuscitation requirement.
  - ↑ risk for hypothermia.

PATHOPHYSIOLOGY

Disruption of three functions of skin:

- Regulation of heat loss.
- Preservation of body fluids.
- Barrier to infection.

EPIDEMIOLOGY

Occur commonly in toddlers, due to their curious nature and lack of understanding of danger.

CLASSIFICATION

Four criteria:
- **Depth:**
  - **First degree** (eg, sunburn): Superficial. Only epidermis involved. Erythema, pain, and **absence of blisters.**
  - **Second degree:** Partial thickness. Epidermis and dermis involved, but dermal appendages spared. Red or mottled appearance with associated **blisters.** Painful.
  - **Third degree:** Full thickness. Destroys epidermis and all of the dermis. **Painless, dry, and does not blanch.**
- **Percentage of body surface area:** Rule of nines—does not apply!
  - Head: 9% front, 9% back.
  - Chest, abdomen, and pelvis: 18% (genitals 1%).
  - Gluteals: 2.5% each.
  - Arms: 9% each (4.5% front and 4.5% back).
  - Legs: 14% each (7% front and 7% back).
- **Location:**
  - Assess risk for disability.
  - Worse on face, eyes, ears, feet, perineum, or hands.
- **Association with other injuries.**

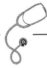

Burns indicating abuse generally do not have a splash pattern, but more linear (eg, placing a child in a hot bath).

TREATMENT

- Airway, breathing, and circulation (**ABCs**) first!
  - **Airway:** Facial or neck burns, singed nose hair, **hoarseness,** or soot around mouth or nares may indicate inhalational injury. Assess for airway patency.

- **Breathing:** Check arterial blood gases (ABGs) and check CO levels.
  - **Circulation:** IV fluid resuscitation.
- Infants: > 10% of body surface area (BSA).
- Children: > 15% BSA.
- IV/IO access and the Parkland Formula:

Parkland formula = [wt kg × % burn × 4 mL/kg] +
maintenance fluid requirements

Administer one-half over first 8 hr and remainder over next 16 hr.

- Superficial and partial thickness:
  - Rapid and effective analgesia.
  - Cold compresses.
  - Antiseptic cleansing.
  - Debride open blisters.
  - Topical antibiotic (silver sulfadiazine).
  - Protect with bulky dressing.
  - Reexamine in 24 hr and serially after for healing and infection.
- Full thickness or extensive partial thickness:
  - ABCs of trauma, especially airway.
  - Fluid and electrolyte replacement (as above).
  - Sedation and analgesia is usually necessary.
  - Clean and manage as above.

CRITERIA FOR ADMISSION/TRANSFER

- Admit:
  - Two to five percent of full-thickness burn.
  - Five to ten percent of body surface.
- Other considerations for admission:
  - Burns involving the face, hands, genitalia, perineum, or major joints.
  - Circumferential extremity burns.
  - High-voltage electrical burns.
  - Significant chemical burns.
  - Inhalation injury.
  - Suspicion of abuse or unsafe home environment.
- Burn unit:
- > 5% of full-thickness burn.
- > 10% BSA.

BLS ALGORITHM

1. Determine unresponsiveness: Stimulate and check for responsiveness.
2. If unresponsive, shout for help (send someone to phone 911) and get automatic external defibrillator (AED). If lone provider: for **sudden collapse**, phone 911 and get AED. First, the airway is assessed, then breathing, and finally circulation. If there is an abnormality at any step of this ABC assessment, intervention must be initiated to stabilize the patient.
3. Airway (open and assess): Head tilt–chin lift maneuver or jaw thrust maneuver (if cervical spine injury is suspected).
4. Breathing: Look, listen, and feel.
   - Look for a rise and fall of the chest.
   - Listen for exhaled air.
   - Feel for exhaled air.

- Provide two rescue breaths if no spontaneous breathing is present.
  - **Infants** (< 1 year old): Place mouth over infant's mouth and nose, creating a seal.
  - **Children** (> 1 year old): Pinch nose and create mouth-to-mouth seal.
- If the chest does not rise, or the breath does not go in easily, reposition the head and try again.
- **If no response, check pulse** (brachial artery or femoral): Definite pulse within 10 sec check, give one breath every 6–8 sec and **check pulse every 2 min.** If no pulse, proceed to Circulation.

BLS: Determine unresponsiveness, call for help, and remember your **ABCs:**
Airway
Breathing
Circulation

Infant Compressions

For < 1 year of age:

- **Single provider:**
  - Place one hand on the head to maintain open airway for ventilation.
  - Place the two middle fingers of the other hand on the sternum one fingerbreadth below the nipple line to be used for chest compressions.
  - Chest compressions of 0.5–1 inch in depth at a rate of *at least* 100 per minute.
  - Coordinate compressions with pauses for ventilation at a ratio of 30:2.
- **Two providers:**
  - Use hands encircling chest method with thumbs on sternum for chest compression.
  - Compression to ventilation ratio is 15:2.
- One minute of BLS is provided to children before activating the Emergency Medical Services (EMS) system, because most cardiopulmonary arrest in children is caused by the development of hypoxemia, and 1 min of ventilatory and circulatory support may delay or prevent the development of cardiac arrest.

Child Compressions

Chest compressions should be initiated if heart rate is < 60 beats/min. For child age 1 to puberty:

- Place one hand on the head to maintain open airway for ventilation.
- Place the heel of the other hand on the lower half of the sternum (take care to avoid the xiphoid).
- Chest compressions of 1–1.5 inches in depth at a rate of 100 per minute.
- Coordinate compressions with pauses for ventilation at a ratio of 30:2 for single provider and 15:2 for two providers.
- High-quality cardiopulmonary resuscitation (CPR):
  - Push hard and fast (100/min).
  - Release completely (allow for full chest recoil).
  - Minimize interruptions during compressions (< 10 sec).

Improper opening of the airway is the most common cause of ineffective rescue breaths.

Foreign Body Airway Obstruction

A 2-year-old boy is found unresponsive on the floor of his bedroom. He was last seen by his mother playing with building blocks. She states she only left the child alone for a few minutes while she went to use the bathroom. When EMS arrives, they find a cyanotic infant, unresponsive, not breathing. Pulses are palpable with a heart rate of 137. What are the initial and critical actions that must be taken?

In this case, foreign body aspiration is highly suspicious. This patient is unconscious, so a Heimlich maneuver should not be attempted. The victim should be placed supine, then the airway is opened with head-tilt chin-lift; *if you see the object,* attempt a finger sweep to remove it. Attempt rescue breathing. If unsuccessful, reposition head and attempt rescue breathing. If still unsuccessful, straddle the victim, placing the heel of one hand on the child's abdomen in the midline just above the umbilicus (avoiding the xiphoid). Place the other hand on top of the first and deliver five quick inward and upward thrusts. Repeat this maneuver until ventilation is successful.

- Foreign body airway obstruction should be considered in any child who suddenly demonstrates signs of respiratory distress, gagging, coughing, wheezing, or stridor.
- These symptoms of airway obstruction can also be caused by infection. Infectious etiologies of airway obstruction are pediatric emergencies and should be suspected if fever, congestion, hoarseness, drooling, lethargy, or atony are present.
- If an infectious cause of airway obstruction is being entertained, the child must be transported immediately to the nearest hospital capable of emergent pediatric intubation.
- **Infant compressions:** Hands encircling chest 0.5–1 inch depth, rate > 100/min, 15:2 ratio (two providers).
- **Child compressions:** Heel of palm 1–1.5 inch depth, rate 100/min, 15:2 ratio (two providers).

Infant Airway Obstruction (< 1 Year of Age)

Back blows and chest thrusts:

1. Activate EMS.
2. Hold the choking infant in one arm, with the infant face down, firmly holding the jaw and allowing the body to rest on your forearm.
3. Deliver five **back blows** using the heel of your free hand directly between the infant's shoulder blades.
4. If no improvement, turn the infant over to the face-up position, maintaining support of the head and neck.
5. Deliver five quick **chest thrusts** using the same technique as for infant chest compressions.
6. Repeat above steps, alternating back blows and chest thrusts, until object is removed or the child loses consciousness.

Ninety percent of foreign body deaths are children under age 5; two-thirds of these are infants.

Child Airway Obstruction (> 1 Year of Age)

- Heimlich maneuver—if **conscious**:
  1. Ask patient if she is choking and if she can speak.
  2. If not, tell patient you are going to help her and activate EMS.
  3. Stand behind the conscious victim, and wrap your arms around the abdomen.
  4. Place the thumb of one fist in the midline of the abdomen just above the umbilicus (well below the xiphoid).
  5. Grasp the fist with the other hand and deliver quick thrusts inward and upward.
  6. Continue until object is expelled or victim becomes unconscious.
- If the victim becomes **unconscious** (witnessed):
  1. Place victim supine.
  2. Open the airway with head-tilt chin-lift; *if you see the object*, attempt a finger sweep to remove it.
  3. Attempt rescue breathing.
  4. If unsuccessful, reposition head and attempt rescue breathing.
  5. If still unsuccessful, straddle the victim, placing the heel of one hand on the child's abdomen in the midline just above the umbilicus (avoiding the xiphoid).
  6. Place the other hand on top of the first and deliver five quick inward and upward thrusts.
  7. Repeat steps 2–6 until ventilation is successful or EMS arrives and takes over.

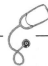

Airway obstruction caused by infection requires immediate transport to the hospital.

Infant airway obstruction = back blows + chest thrusts.

Child (> 1 year of age) airway obstruction = Heimlich maneuver

PEDIATRIC ADVANCED LIFE SUPPORT (PALS)

- Goals: To provide rapid assessment and definitive management of the pediatric arrest situation using advanced airway management techniques, cardiac monitoring equipment, and pharmacologic therapy.
- Respiratory problems are rather common among children, and respiratory arrest is the major cause of cardiac arrest in the pediatric population.
- If respiratory arrest is treated before it progresses to cardiac arrest, survival is markedly improved.
- If respiratory arrest progresses to pulseless cardiac arrest, the chances of survival are poor.
- Early recognition of respiratory failure and effective management of respiratory problems are key elements taught in PALS.

Anatomic Differences in the Pediatric Airway

- Infants are obligate nasal breathers.
- Smaller airway.
- Tongue occupies a greater percentage of the oropharynx.
- Vocal cords are more superior and anterior.
- The tonsils and adenoids are more prominent.
- The epiglottis is larger and more floppy.
- The tracheal rings are less rigid.
- The narrowest part of the airway is just below the vocal cords at the nondistensible cricoid cartilage; endotracheal tube (ETT) size is thus determined by the size of this opening.

Poiseuille's equation:
Resistance (airway) $\times 1/r^4$

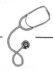

Straight laryngoscope blades are more effective to visualize the pediatric airway. Used to "pick up" epiglottis.

■ Smaller amounts of vocal cord edema can drastically reduce the diameter of the airway (resistance is inversely proportional to the fourth power of the radius).
■ The angle between the base of the tongue and the glottis is more acute.

Pediatric Respiratory Distress

■ The *earlier* you detect respiratory distress or respiratory failure and start the appropriate therapy, the better chance the child has for a *good* outcome.
■ Respiratory distress → hypoxemia (inadequate oxygenation) and/or hypercarbia.

$$\text{Arterial oxygen content} = (1.36 \times \text{Hgb concentration} \times \text{SaO}_2) + (0.003 \times \text{PaO}_2)$$

■ Hypoxemia is readily detected noninvasively with pulse oximetry monitoring.
■ Hypercarbia results from inadequate alveolar ventilation (ie, ↑ CO_2 tension ($PaCO_2$) in the blood.
■ Provide oxygen in the highest concentration available to any child experiencing respiratory difficulty (face tent, blow-by stream, mask, partial nonrebreather).
■ Suction secretions as needed (don't forget the nose in infants).
■ Continually reassess for signs of decompensation; if a trend of worsening respiratory status is noted, assisted ventilation is required to prevent respiratory failure.
■ Upper airway obstruction: Predominantly during **inspiration:**
  ■ Tachypnea.
  ■ Retractions.
  ■ **Stridor:** Classic sign of upper airway obstruction.
■ Lower airway obstruction: Signs of obstruction:
  ■ Tachypnea.
  ■ **Wheezing:** Most common, generally expiratory.

Management of Respiratory Failure and Pediatric Intubation

Timing is everything! If respiratory function is restored promptly, neurologically intact survival is likely:

■ Airway: Open the airway.
■ Breathing: Support breathing using bag-valve-mask ventilation until definitive airway is established (ie, endotracheal intubation). Monitor oxygenation and end tidal CO_2 (after intubation).
■ Circulation: Assess circulation, establish intravenous (IV) access, chest compressions if necessary.

Endotracheal Intubation

■ Endotracheal tube size: For children 1–10 yr:
  ■ Uncuffed endotracheal tube size (mm ID) = (age in years/4) + 4.
  ■ Cuffed endotracheal tube size (mm ID) = (age in years/4) + 3.
■ Cuffed tubes are generally safe for use in the hospital.
■ Keep cuff inflation pressure < 20 cm H_2O.

- Select and prepare all equipment prior to attempting intubation (make sure all are functioning well).
- Laryngoscope blade (Figure 22-1): Size:
  - Infant: Miller (straight) 0.
  - Age < 1: Miller (straight) 1.
  - Age 1–5: Miller (straight) 2.
  - Age > 5: Mac (curved) 2 or Miller 2–3.
- ETT size: Based on above formulas.
- Confirm placement with end-tidal CO_2 indicator.
- Listen in both lung fields for equal breath sounds and confirm absent gastric insufflation.
- If the intubated patient's condition deteriorates, consider the following possibilities (**DOPE**):
  - **D**isplacement of the tube from the trachea.
  - **O**bstruction of the tube.
  - **P**neumothorax.
  - **E**quipment failure.

FIGURE 22-1. Two common types of laryngoscope blades: Macintosh and Miller blades.

(Reproduced, with permissionm, from Lalwani AK. *Current Diagnosis & Treatment in Otolaryngology – Head & Neck Surgery.* New York: McGraw-Hill, 2004: 1700).

Vascular Access

CANNULATION OF PERIPHERAL VEINS

- **Upper extremity:**
  - Median cubital vein.
  - Cephalic vein (and tributaries in the dorsum of the hand).
  - Basilic vein.
- **Lower extremity:**
  - Saphenous veins (especially great saphenous at the ankle).
  - Veins of the dorsal arch.
  - Median marginal veins.

INTRAOSSEOUS CANNULATION

- Rapid and reliable method to deliver fluids and drugs during resuscitation.
- Preferred over ET route for the administration of drugs.
- Temporary route (limit 24 hr).
- Contraindications:
  - Open fracture at proposed insertion site.
  - Signs of skin infection at the insertion site.
  - Previous attempts at site.
- During cardiopulmonary resuscitation (CPR), should be employed after three failed attempts to cannulate peripheral veins (or 90 sec).
- Preferred site of insertion:
  - Proximal tibia: Two fingerbreadths below the tibial tuberosity.
  - Remember to insert needle at an angle pointing **away** from the growth plates.
- Can safely administer fluids, blood products, and drugs. (Anything that can be given via central line can be given by intraosseous route).

COMPLICATIONS

- Rare (< 1%).
- Extravasation → compartment syndrome.
- Infections → cellulitis and osteomyelitis.
- Fractures.
- Injury to the epiphyseal growth plate.

Unpredictable drug absorption when drug administration via the ETT.

LEAN: Lidocaine, epinephrine, atropine, and naloxone (can be administered via ET route if vascular access is not available).

CANNULATION OF CENTRAL VEINS

- Complications (bleeding, infection, pneumothorax, etc.) are more common in the pediatric age group.
- Central catheters should be used only when the benefit outweighs the risks (ie, when central venous pressures need to be monitored).
- Catheters are inserted using the Seldinger (guidewire) technique.
- Common sites include:
  - Femoral vein
  - Internal jugular vein
  - Subclavian vein

The worldwide leading cause of shock is hypovolemia.

Shock and Fluid Resuscitation

- Shock is defined as inadequate oxygen delivery to the tissues and organs.
- Shock can result from:
  - Inadequate blood volume or oxygen-carrying capacity (eg, hypovolemic/hemorrhagic shock).
  - Inappropriately distributed blood volume (distributive shock).
  - Impairment of heart contractility (cardiogenic shock).
  - Obstructive blood flow (obstructive shock).
- All forms of shock require consideration of fluid administration during initial therapy.
- **Hypovolemia** is the worldwide leading cause of shock (inadequate fluid intake plus diarrhea and vomiting can → hypovolemic shock).
- **Septic shock, neurogenic shock,** and **anaphylactic shock** are all characterized by vasodilation, ↑ capillary permeability, and third-space fluid loss that results in an intravascular hypovolemia. These are subcategories of distributive shock.
- **Cardiogenic shock** may even require initial fluid administration before the initiation of inotropic and chronotropic agents ("you must fill the tank before starting the engine"). Judicious use of fluids mandatory to avoid causing pulmonary edema.
- The treatment goal for shock is to prevent end-organ injury and halt the progression to cardiopulmonary failure and cardiac arrest.
- Initial fluid resuscitation:
  - Normal saline or lactated.
  - Ringer's (isotonic).

ADMINISTRATION OF FLUID BOLUS

- Initial bolus should be a rapid infusion of isotonic crystalloid of 20 mL/kg over 20 min.
- Reassess after initial bolus by looking at response in heart rate, capillary refill, level of consciousness, and most importantly *urinary output*. Aim for a urinary output of 0.5–1 cc/kg/hr.
- Remember that only about 25% of crystalloid will remain in the intravascular space; thus, you may need to administer three times the estimated fluid loss (3:1 rule).
- **Blood** is the preferred fluid replacement for trauma victims demonstrating persistent hypovolemic shock *after* two to three boluses of crystalloid (ie, 40–60 mL/kg).
- Maintenance fluids are given by the 4,2,1 formula: 4 mL/kg/hr for the first 10 kg + 2 mL/kg/hr for the second 10 kg + 1 mL/kg/hr for every 1 kg above 20.

3:1 Rule

May need to administer three times estimated fluid loss.

Classification of Shock (Hemorrhagic/Hypovolemic Shock)

Class I
- 0–15% volume loss.
- Normal pulse.
- Normal blood pressure.
- Normal capillary refill.
- Normal respiratory rate.
- Urine output 1–2 mL/kg/hr.

Class II
- 15–30% volume loss.
- Mild tachycardia.
- Mildly ↓ blood pressure.
- Mildly prolonged capillary refill.
- Mild tachypnea.
- Urine output 0.5–1.0 mL/kg/hr.

Class III
- 30–40% volume loss.
- Tachycardia.
- ↓ blood pressure.
- Prolonged capillary refill.
- Tachypnea.
- Urine output 0.25–0.5 mL/kg/hr.

Class IV
- > 40% volume loss.
- Severely tachycardic, bradycardic, or absent pulse.
- Very low blood pressure.
- Greatly prolonged capillary refill.
- Severe tachypnea.
- Urine output 0 mL/kg/hr.

Pressor Support in Pediatric Shock

- First, attempt multiple fluid boluses.
- Try to identify and treat the underlying cause.
- Choose pressor agent according to the type of shock present.

Pharmacologic Agents Used in the Treatment of Shock

- Inotropes:
  - Dopamine
  - Epinephrine
  - Dobutamine
- Phosphodiesterase inhibitors:
  - Milrinone
  - Inamrinone
- Vasodilators:
  - Nitroglycerine
  - Nitroprusside
- Vasopressors:
  - Epinephrine
  - Norepinephrine
  - Dopamine
  - Vasopressin

Hypovolemic Shock

Multiple crystalloid boluses will be necessary (20 mL/kg bolus over 20 min, repeat PRN).

Septic Shock

Multiple crystalloid boluses will be necessary (20 mL/kg bolus over 5–20 min, repeat PRN).

- Consider dopamine 5–20 µg/kg/min if patient is **normotensive**.
- Consider epinephrine 0.1–1.0 µg/kg/min if patient is **hypotensive**.

Cardiogenic Shock

- Initial fluid bolus is usually necessary.
- Consider dobutamine 5–20 µg/kg/min if patient is **normotensive**. (*Note:* Dobutamine may not be effective in infants and young children due to lack of stroke volume response.)
- Consider epinephrine 0.1–1.0 µg/kg/min if the patient is **hypotensive**.

Cardiac Arrhythmias

- Tachycardias.
- Bradycardias.
- No pulse: Asystole, pulseless electrical activity (PEA), ventricular fibrillation (VF), or pulseless ventricular tachycardia (VT).

Tachyarrhythmias

Sinus Tachycardia
- Defined as a rate of sinus node discharge faster than normal for age.
- Age-specific heart rates:
    - 0–3 months (85–205 beats/min): Mean 140 tachycardia > 205.
    - 3 months–2 yr (100–190 beats/min): Mean 130, tachycardia > 190.
    - 2–10 yr (60–140 beats/min): Mean 80, tachycardia > 140.
    - > 10 yr (60–100 beats/min): Mean 75, tachycardia > 100.
- Typically, a response to a **need for ↑ cardiac output** (compensatory tachycardia).
- Common causes include fever, pain, anxiety, blood loss, sepsis, and shock.
- Always assess and **reassess ABCs.**
- Therapy entails treating the underlying cause.

Supraventricular Tachycardia (SVT)
- SVT is **rapid, very regular**, often **paroxysmal.**
- Often exceeds 220 bpm in infants, exceeds 180 bpm in children.
- P waves are absent or indistinguishable.
- QRS complex is typically narrow (< 0.08 sec).
- SVT is most commonly caused by reentry mechanism.
- **SVT algorithm:**
    - Assess ABCs, support as needed.
    - Administer 100% oxygen, ventilate as needed.
    - Document electrocardiogram (ECG)/rhythm tracing: Evaluate QRS—narrow ≤ 0.08 sec.

- Establish IV or IO access:
  - Adenosine 0.1 mg/kg rapid intravenous push, immediately followed by 5 mL of saline flush (maximum dose: 6 mg in children and 12 mg in adolescents).
  - Synchronized cardioversion: 0.5 to 1 J/kg; if not effective ↑ to 2 J/kg (sedate if possible, but do not delay cardioversion).
- If still in SVT: Obtain cardiology consult and consider administration of:
  - Amiodarone 5 mg/kg IV over 20–60 min *or*
  - Procainamide 15 mg/kg IV over 30–60 min. If patient becomes unstable at any time, proceed directly with synchronized cardioversion.
- Management of SVT:
  - Stable: Vagal maneuvers and/or adenosine.
  - Unstable: Synchronized cardioversion.

Ventricular Tachycardia (VT) (with pulse)

- Wide QRS complex (> 0.08 sec).
- P waves not present.
- Very uncommon in children.
- Risk factors include prolonged QT syndrome, cardiac anomalies, drug ingestions, electrolyte abnormalities, underlying cardiac disease.
- **VT algorithm:**
  1. Assess ABCs, support as needed.
  2. Administer 100% oxygen, ventilate as needed.
  3. Document electrocardiogram (ECG)/rhythm tracing (*wide* QRS ≥ 0.08 sec).
  4. Establish IV or IO access or
  5. Synchronized cardioversion: 0.5–1 J/kg; if not effective, ↑ to 2 J/kg (sedate if possible, but do not delay cardioversion).
  6. If still in VT: Call cardiology consult for administration of:
     - Amiodarone 5 mg/kg IV over 20–60 min *or*
     - Procainamide 15 mg/kg IV over 30–60 min.
  7. Obtain cardiology consult as needed.
  8. Identify and treat possible causes:
     - **4Hs:** Hypovolemia, Hypoxemia, Hypothermia, Hyper/hypokalemia.
     - **4Ts:** Tamponade, Tension pneumothorax, Toxins, Thromboembolism.

Ventricular tachycardia:
- QRS wide
- No P waves
- Rare in children

BRADYARRHYTHMIAS

- Age-specific heart rates:
  - 0–3 months (85–205 beats/min); bradycardia < 85.
  - 3 months–2 yr (100–190 beats/min); bradycardia < 100.
  - 2–10 yr (60–140 beats/min); bradycardia < 60.
  - > 10 yr (60–100 beats/min); bradycardia < 60

Bradycardia Algorithm

1. Assess ABCs, support.
2. Administer 100% oxygen, ventilate, prepare to intubate.
3. Establish IV/IO access.
4. Cardiac monitor, pulse oximetry, blood pressure cuff.
5. Reassess ABCs.
   - If stable, continue to support ABCs, admit for observation.
   - If unstable (poor perfusion, hypotension, heart rate < 60, continued hypoxia despite 100% oxygen administration):

1. Begin chest compressions if still persistent bradycardia.
2. Give epinephrine 0.01 mg/kg (1:10,000, 0.1 mL/kg) IV/IO, or via ETT 0.1 mg/kg (1:1,000, 0.1 mL/kg). Repeat every 3–5 min.
3. If ↑ vagal tone or primary AV block, give atropine 0.02 mg/kg IVP. Min dose: 0.1 mg. Max dose: 0.02 mg/kg to maximum of 1.0 mg via ETT dose: Two to three times dose in 5 mL normal saline.
4. Consider external pacing.

PULSELESS ARRHYTHMIAS

A 6-year-old girl with a past medical history of asthma is brought to your ED by EMS in respiratory distress. Her vital signs are heart rate 120, BP 90/50, RR 26, O$_2$ 93% on facemask. Per EMS, the child had been wheezing all morning, and the mother had tried several nebulizer treatments without relief. The mother called 911 when her child seemed to become in more distress. While performing your primary survey the patient becomes unresponsive, the monitor shows v-fib. What are the initial and critical actions that must be taken?

Here the patient is going into cardiac failure/arrest secondary to respiratory distress. The first step is to palpate for a pulse. This patient has ventricular fibrillation, which is a shockable rhythm.

Ventricular Fibrillation (VF)/Pulseless VT
1. Assess ABCs.
2. Continue CPR for 2 min.
3. Confirm rhythm in more than one lead. Is rhythm shockable?
4. Intubate and hyperventilate with 100% oxygen.
5. IV/IO access (do not delay defibrillation for access).
6. If shockable rhythm, defibrillate × 1 with 2 J/kg).
7. Restart CPR for 2 min.
8. Give another shock, 4 J/kg; give epinephrine 0.01 mg/kg (0.1 mL/kg of 1:10,000) IV/IO or ETT 0.1 mg/kg (0.1 mL/kg of 1:1000).
9. Restart CPR for 2 min.
10. Give another shock 4 J/kg; consider giving antiarrhythmics: Lidocaine 1 mg/kg IV/IO/ETT or amiodarone 5 mg/kg bolus IV/IO.
11. Consider magnesium 25 to 50 mg/kg IV/IO for Torsades de pointes (max dose: 2 g).
12. Identify and treat possible causes (4Hs and 4Ts).

Pulseless Electrical Activity (PEA)
- PEA in children, while rare, usually occurs as a result of **progressive respiratory and/or circulatory failure.**
- As with adult PEA, the **differential diagnosis** for pediatric PEA is essential to successful resuscitation.
- **PEA algorithm:**
  1. Assess ABCs.
  2. Continue CPR.
  3. Confirm rhythm in more than one lead.
  4. Intubate and hyperventilate with 100% oxygen.
  5. IV/IO access.
  6. Consider possible causes of PEA (and specific treatments):
     - Hypovolemia (volume—normal saline infusion).
     - Hypoxia (oxygen, intubation, ventilation).
     - Hypothermia (warmed normal saline infusion).

- Massive pulmonary embolism (heparin infusion, thrombolysis).
- Acidosis (sodium bicarbonate).
- Tension pneumothorax (needle decompression).
- Cardiac tamponade (pericardiocentesis).
- Hyperkalemia (insulin/glucose, calcium).
- Drug overdose from TCAs, digoxin, β blockers, calcium channel blockers.
7. Epinephrine (every 3–5 min):
- IV/IO 0.01 mg/kg (0.1 mL/kg of 1:10,000).
- ETT 0.1 mg/kg (0.1 mL/kg of 1:1000).

Asystole

- Most common pulseless rhythm in children.
- Airway management and hyperventilation are the most important interventions.
- Always confirm asystole in more than one lead and ensure that leads are properly connected.
- **Asystole algorithm:**
  1. ABCs.
  2. CPR.
  3. **Confirm rhythm in more than one lead.**
  4. Intubate and hyperventilate with 100% oxygen.
  5. IV/IO access.
  6. Epinephrine (every 3–5 min):
     - IV/IO 0.01 mg/kg (0.1 mL/kg of 1:10,000).
     - ETT 0.1 mg/kg (0.1 mL/kg of 1:1000).
  7. Consider external pacing.
  8. Search for reversible causes.
- Note that atropine and bicarbonate are **not** part of the algorithm for asystole.

- Newborn resuscitation ideally should be performed in the delivery room, neonatal intensive care unit (NICU), or other unit with personnel experienced with treating newborns and equipment appropriate for the task.
- Birth asphyxia accounts for about 19% of the approximately 5 million neonatal deaths that occur each year worldwide.
- Approximately 10% of newborns require some assistance to begin breathing at birth; about 1% need extensive resuscitative measures to survive.

Preassessment and Triage

Always ask the following questions when treating a new born baby:

1. Was the baby born at term (ie, how many weeks' gestation)?
   - Premature babies are at higher risk for intubation and resuscitation, especially if their respiratory system is not fully developed and functional.
2. Was the amniotic fluid clear?
   - Meconium in the amniotic fluid is a sign of a stressed birth, and the baby, if not vigorous, will need to be intubated.

Suction newborn airway aggressively.

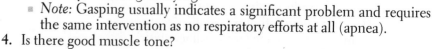

3. Is the baby breathing or crying?
  ● *Note:* Gasping usually indicates a significant problem and requires the same intervention as no respiratory efforts at all (apnea).
4. Is there good muscle tone?
  ● Healthy babies should have flexed extremities and be active.

Newborn Assessment

● **Temperature:** Neonatal hypothermia can be associated with neonatal respiratory depression. Upon delivery, warming and drying with a towel or blanket is often adequate to stimulate breathing in a newborn.
● **Airway:** Position the airway and suction any secretions (neck slightly extended in the "sniffing" position).
● **Breathing:** Observe chest rise and fall, give 100% oxygen if necessary, initiate adequate bag-valve-mask ventilation if necessary (ie, heart rate < 100 beats/min and unresponsiveness; absent or depressed respirations).
● **Circulation:** Assess heart rate and color, provide chest compressions as necessary (if heart rate absent, if heart rate < 60 despite 30 sec of assisted ventilation).

Newborn Resuscitation

Assess every newborn (and give the appropriate support).

1. Delivery outside the delivery room.
2. ABCs—assess and support.
   ● Airway (position and suction).
   ● Breathing (stimulate to cry).
   ● Circulation (heart rate and color).
   ● Temperature (warm and dry).
3. Oxygen (100%).
4. Establish effective ventilation:
   ● Bag-valve-mask.
   ● Laryngeal mask airway (LMA) can be an effective alternative for establishing an airway when bag-valve-mask fails.
   ● Endotracheal intubation (only by trained rescuer competent in neonatal intubations).
5. Chest compressions if pulse < 60 beats/min, despite 30 sec of effective positive-pressure ventilation. Place two hands around infant's chest with thumbs on sternum in the nipple line. Compress to one-third the anterior-posterior diameter.
6. Medications as dictated by the situation.

Start CPR on neonate if pulse < 60.

Newborn ABCs

● Position
● Suction
● Stimulate cry
● Warm and dry

Neonatal Resuscitation

● **Ventilation rate:** 40–60/min (room air or 100% oxygen, with titration to lowest level).
● **Compression rate:** 120 events/min (90 compressions/30 ventilations/min).
● **Compression/ventilation ratio:** 3:1.
● *Note:* The two-finger compression technique is also acceptable.

Meconium Deliveries

1. Deliver head.
2. Aggressively suction hypopharynx while infant is still in birth canal.
3. Complete delivery of infant.
4. Assess temperature and ABCs. If the infant is active and vigorous, continue supportive measures. If any signs of distress (absent or depressed respirations, heart rate < 100, poor muscle tone), proceed with algorithm.
5. Direct tracheal suctioning either following endotracheal intubation or by using ETT as suction catheter.
6. Decision to intubate and perform tracheal suctioning depends on whether the newborn infant is vigorous. Current neonatal resuscitation guidelines define an infant as vigorous if he or she has:
   - Strong respiratory efforts.
   - Good muscle tone.
   - Heart rate more than 100 beats/min.

   In a vigorous and active infant, there is generally no need for tracheal suctioning. In a nonvigorous and depressed infant, drying and stimulation should be delayed. Perform direct laryngoscopy and suction the mouth and hypopharynx, followed by intubation and then applying suction (~100 mmHg) directly to the ETT. A nonvigorous and depressed infant has a low threshold for intubation and direct tracheal suctioning in the presence of thick meconium.

If meconium is present during a delivery, aggressively suction hypopharynx as soon as head is delivered.

APGAR

See Gestation and Birth chapter.

Index

H

H1N1 influenza, 223–225
  vaccine, 80, 225
Habit, 560
Haemophilus ducreyi, 328
Haemophilus influenzae, 270,
    458, 460, 463, 467, 519,
    520
  type B (Hib), 225, 228, 229,
    235, 424, 426
    vaccine, 77–78, 229
Hair loss, 537
Hair pulling (trichotillomania),
    537–538
Hallucinogens, intoxication and
    withdrawal, 556
Hand-foot-mouth disease (cox-
    sackievirus A16), 159, 166,
    539
Hartnup disease, 113, 117
Headaches, 438–442
  cluster, 440
  increased intracranial pressure,
    441–442
  migraine, 438–440
    classic, 440
    common, 439
    complicated, 440
  tension, 440–441
Heart, fetal, 19
Heart defects
  acyanotic, 283–286
    atrial septal defect (ASD),
      284
    patent foramen ovale (PFO),
      285
    subendocardial cushion de-
      fect, 283–284
    ventricular septal defect
      (VSD), 285–286
  cyanotic, 275–283
    hypoplastic left heart syn-
      drome (HLHS), 281–283
    tetralogy of Fallot (TOF),
      275, 277–278
    transposition of the great ves-
      sels, 279–280
    truncus arteriosus, 280–281
Heart murmurs, 253–256
  auscultation maneuvers, 254

innocent, 255–256
normal heart sounds, 253–254
Heavy metal toxicity, 86
Heimlich maneuver, 579
Helicobacter pylori, 187
Hemangioma, 529
Hematocrit screening, 75
Hematuria, causes of, 314
Hemochromatosis, 374
Hemoglobin
  fetal, 21
  normal, by age, 333
Hemolytic disease of the new-
    born, 343
Hemolytic enzymopathies,
    346–347
  glucose-6-phosphate dehy-
    drogenase (G6PD) defi-
    ciency, 346–347
  pyruvate kinase (PK) defi-
    ciency, 347
Hemolytic membrane defects,
    348–349
  hereditary spherocytosis, 348
  paroxysmal nocturnal hemo-
    globinuria, 349
Hemolytic-uremic syndrome
    (HUS), 351
Hemophilia, 355
Henoch-Schönlein purpura,
    271–272, 532–533
Hepatic encephalopathy, 431
Hepatic neoplasms, 219
  amebic abscess, 220
  hepatoblastoma, 219
Hepatitis
  A, 212–213, 437
    vaccine, 81
  autoimmune (chronic), 216
  B, 213–214, 437
    vaccine, 76–77
  C, 214
  D (delta agent), 214–215
  E, 215
  G, 215
  neonatal, 216
Hereditary disease, concepts in,
    126
Hereditary spherocytosis, 348
Hermaphroditism, true, 402–403

Hernias, abdominal, 203–204
  inguinal, 203–204
  umbilical, 203
Heroin
  intoxication and withdrawal,
    556
  maternal use of, 25
Herpes gingivostomatitis (fever
    blisters, cold sores), 523
Herpes simplex, 326, 328, 427,
    515
  perinatal, 32
Herpes zoster (shingles), 164, 427
Herpetic whitlow, 523
Hirschsprung's megacolon, 197
Histoplasma capsulatum, 176
Histoplasmosis, 174, 176–177
HIV. *See* Human immunodefi-
    ciency virus
HIV/AIDS encephalopathy,
    431–432
Hives (urticaria), 131–132
Holoprosencephaly, 100
Homocysteine pathway, 115
Homocystinemia/homocystinu-
    ria, 113, 114–116, 391
Hookworm, 202
Hordeolum (stye), 460
Horner syndrome, 450
Horseshoe kidney, 311
Howell-Jolly bodies, 146
β-Human chorionic gonadotro-
    pin (β-hCG), 23
Human immunodeficiency virus
    (HIV), 33–34, 153–157
  opportunistic infections in,
    155–157
    cryptococcosis, 155–156
    cytomegalovirus (CMV),
      157
    mycobacterial infections,
      atypical, 156–157
    Pneumocystis jiroveci pneu-
      monia, 156
    toxoplasmosis, 155
  perinatal, 33–34
Hunter syndrome, 120
Hurler syndrome, 120
Hyaline membrane disease of the
    newborn, 38–39